Nutrition, Food, and the Environment

Vincent Hegarty, Ph.D.

Michigan State University

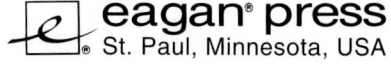 eagan® press
St. Paul, Minnesota, USA

Publisher: Steven C. Nelson

Publication Manager: Miles Wimer

Project Editor: Ann King

Production Editor: Phyllis Albertz

Assistant Editor: Linda Kadlec

Production Manager: Steve Kronmiller

Graphics Coordinator: Patti Ek

Medical Artist: Teri McDermott

Library of Congress Catalog Card Number: 94-61726
International Standard Book Number: 0-9624407-4-4

©1995 by Eagan Press

Printed in the United States of America.

Eagan Press
3340 Pilot Knob Road
St. Paul, MN 55121-2097, USA

The great challenge . . . is to ensure food and nutrition security and sustainable growth in a way that does not place undue pressure on the environment, and leaves the world a place still fit to live in.

World Health Organization, 1992

Think beyond the picture.
What is the nutrition
connection here?

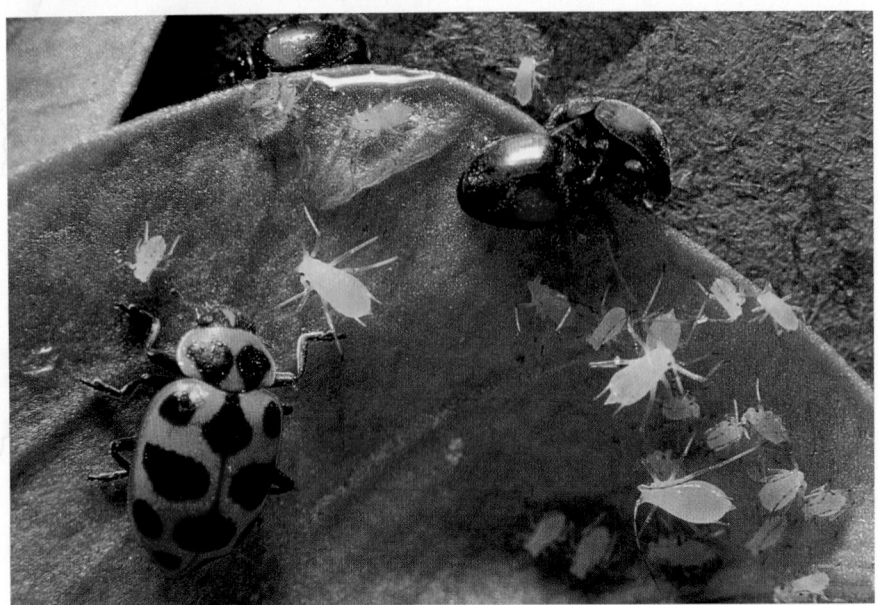

Figure P-1. Aphids (the yellow insects) severely injure plants by feeding on the plant's juices. The ladybugs are natural predators of aphids.

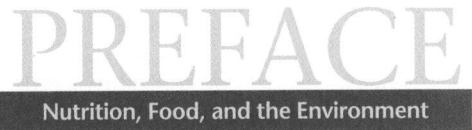

Preface for the Reader

We don't inherit the land from our ancestors, we borrow it from our children.

This proverb has been variously attributed to Native Americans, the Pennsylvania Dutch, and the ancient Hebrews. It is an important message because land and water are the source of our *nutrients*. This book introduces nutrition by linking information on nutrients to an understanding of how food production and processing, and the impact of these on environmental quality, influence each person's *nutritional status*.

Is it the visual impact of television and photographs in magazines and newspapers that first alerts you to *starvation* and suffering in little-known places in the world? To new experiences with food through attractive advertisements? To alteration of the *environment* through chemical pollution or the burning of forests? Probably! Visual impacts encourage us to seek further information on an issue. This book uses the impact of photographs, figures, and tables to draw your attention to major issues in all chapters. You are asked to search each photograph, figure, or table for as much information as you know *now* about nutrition, food, and the environment. Then–"think beyond the picture." A written evaluation of the visual information then follows in the text. Is this too difficult? No. Let's start with the photograph in Figure P-1.

Nutrient: A nourishing substance or ingredient.

Nutritional status: The extent to which the body's need for nutrients is being met.

Starvation: The condition of being without food for a long period of time.

Environment: The conditions under which any person lives. More broadly, the earth's ecosystem.

■ Thinking beyond the picture

Insects on a leaf may seem an unusual first visual message in a book integrating information on nutrition, food, and the environment. But think beyond the photograph and answer the question: What actions on the insects and the plant will have positive or negative effects on our intake of nutrients, the quality of our food, and the well-being of the environment?

You have only a few choices about what to do with the insects. The first choice is to allow them to continue eating the plant. This is good for them but maybe not so good for people. Why? Insects, rodents, bacteria, and other creatures feast on foods that could be eaten by people. They also spread diseases in plants and people. More than 100 million tons of cereals and legumes are lost each year in developing countries. This would meet minimum food energy requirements for about 300 million people–equivalent to more than the total population of the United States.[1] Some experts are worried about the rapid rate of growth of the world population and the ability of agriculture to provide enough food (Chapter 1). About 5.5 billion people exist in the world now, and it is estimated that in 35 years there will be about 9 billion people–whether the food will be sufficient for everybody is a critical question. Even today, there isn't enough food for millions of people in the world. This is due mostly to unequal food distribution.

Pesticides: Any substances intended to control or destroy unwanted animals and plants during production, storage, transportation, distribution, and processing of food, agricultural commodities, or animal feeds.

Your second choice might be to kill the insects. There are too many in the world to stomp on, so let's kill them with *pesticides*. This choice will make more food available for us, but at a price: pesticides may get into our food and water supplies. The significance of pesticides in human health is a matter of some debate (Chapters 2 and 5). There is another problem in killing the insects. We are destroying many insects, plants, animals, and other species to make room for economic development for a rapidly expanding population. However, many ecologists believe that we must preserve as many insects, plants, forests, and animals as possible, thus maintaining biological diversity[2] (Chapter 2). They argue that when biological diversity decreases, we lose genetic material for *biotechnology* (Chapters 1 and 2) and chemicals for medications. Loss of forests may increase global warming, which may have negative effects on the production of some foods.[3,4]

Biotechnology: Application of the techniques of science and engineering to organisms, cells, and parts of cells to produce products and services, including food (bio = life).

A third choice is to prevent increases in the insect population with a process called biological control. How this works in the picture is that the "good insects," the red and black ladybeetles, will eat the aphids who are the "bad insects" in yellow. It is the yellow bugs who eat the plant. By letting other insects do our pest control, we use fewer pesticides and cause less damage to the environment (Chapter 2). This combination of control measures, termed "integrated pest management," uses pesticides only when they are essential.

Your fourth choice is to eat the insects. This may not be very appealing to you, but insects are eaten in many parts of the world–termites in parts of Africa, cheese worms in France, water and wood worms in parts of Brazil. Insects are a rich source of nutrients, especially protein (Chapter 8). All of these choices are legitimate, and different answers will be given by different interest groups–farmers, the pesticide industry, environmentalists, anthropologists, nutritionists, and you, if you are squeamish about bugs in your food.

Can you think of other choices? Each picture, each problem, is viewed by different individuals from slightly different perspectives.

■ What this book is about and how it's organized

Welcome to an introduction to nutrition, to foods important in supplying nutrients, and to environmental issues threatening that relationship. Land, water, and air, the food they produce, and the nutrients we need are indeed related. To understand how we get nutrients, we must know how food is produced, processed, prepared, and distributed. To paraphrase the quotation at the beginning of this preface, we must "borrow" the land and its environment to obtain a nutritious diet and return the land, with its environment unharmed, to supply wholesome food for the next generation. This is an important challenge for all of us.

After reading *Nutrition, Food, and the Environment,* you will understand how nutrients work in the body, why some foods are high or low in individual nutrients, how the body is harmed by deficiencies or excesses of nutrients, and why nutrient requirements change as we get older. Chapter 1 gives an overview of these topics in a definition of nutrition that uses familiar examples from our own experiences. You will be introduced to how food is produced, processed, and distributed in order to furnish these nutrients.

The quality of our diet is influenced by the quality of soil, water, and air; by plants, animals and microorganisms; and by the processing, preservation, preparation, and distribution of food. The food chain is a long one. In exploring it, we visit farms, food factories, supermarkets, and restaurants to understand their influence on the supply of nutrients–some people mistakenly think that nutrition starts in the supermarket or the kitchen refrigerator! We will also see examples of damage to the environment and learn how this may affect nutrient intake and harm our health.

The "Think Beyond" Challenge

Now that we have used the photograph of the insects and the plant to think beyond the photograph, we will use the same approach for many topics in the book. Why are we taking this approach, which is different from that of other books? Education researchers tell us we retain only 20% of what we read, 20% of what we hear, 30% of what we see, but 90% of what we do. When you do a lot of thinking about the visual challenges shown in the photographs, graphs, or tables, the information that follows the visual challenge will be more understandable (you will have done much of the thinking before you read the text). Here is a way you can do this with each "think beyond" challenge in this book:

- Look at the photograph, chart, or table.
- Find as many questions, choices, or solutions as you can think of–we had four choices in our insect-plant example.
- Identify the central question or issue.
- Identify and examine any underlying assumptions. Most of us bring some assumptions and ideas based on our previous experiences.
- Find and evaluate the evidence. Some of that will be provided in the text that follows the visual challenge.
- Consider the implications or consequences of your thoughts.

We can put this process to work by thinking beyond the picture about some specific issues.

Nutrition

Think beyond the picture in Figure P-2 and the graphs in Figure P-3. How can these two extremes in nutritional status be avoided?

The information in the picture and the graphs is familiar in nutrition. Extremes of food intake that may result in starvation and *obesity* are examined in Chapter 13. To think beyond the picture and graph, we will

Obesity: Body weight of 20% or more in excess of ideal body weight. This condition has several negative health effects.

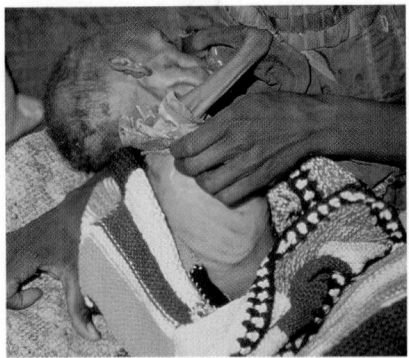

Figure P-2. Starvation occurs because of war, drought, or crop failures. Currently this happens most frequently in developing countries.

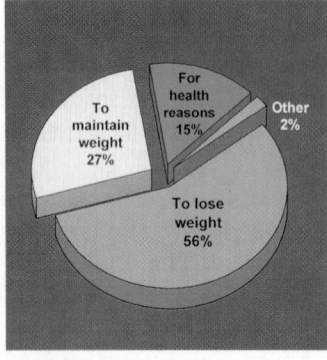

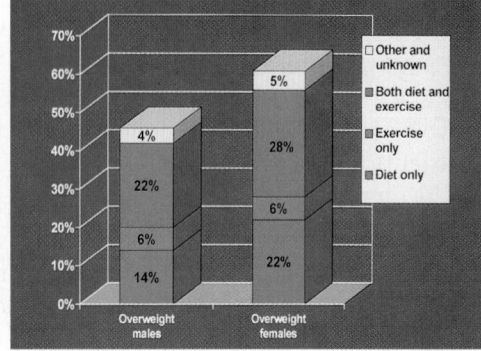

Figure P-3. Reasons why people diet and methods used by the portion of overweight people who try to lose weight. In developed countries weight-loss programs are a big business.

need to get help from the information in Chapter 11 on which foods provide the most energy and how the body uses energy. In Chapter 12, we examine the amount of energy needed for different activities such as sports, jogging, and aerobics. Nutrient needs during pregnancy, lactation, and the early part of life are discussed in Chapter 15 and nutrient needs for adults and the elderly in Chapter 16. Both starvation and obesity frequently involve alterations in how the body uses water, carbohydrates, fats, proteins, vitamins, and minerals (nutrients discussed in Chapters 5–10). Different lifestyles may cause or require different intake of nutrients (Chapter 17). In Chapter 14, we examine some diet-related diseases–coronary heart disease, diabetes, and high blood pressure. A global problem with significant implications in nutrition is *acquired immuno-deficiency syndrome (AIDS)* and the associated human immunovirus (HIV). AIDS produces some symptoms similar to those of extreme starvation.[5] These include "wasting" of the body due to tissue loss, deficiencies of nutrients, decreased resistance to certain diseases, and destructive changes in the digestive tract (Chapter 3). AIDS is also causing another problem in nutrition. "Breast milk may transmit HIV," writes one researcher in the *British Medical Journal*, adding "though the exact risk of transmission is unknown and varies with circumstances."[6] This observation must be confirmed by other studies. It is frightening that the first and best food of life is under such suspicion (Chapter 15).

Acquired immunodeficiency syndrome (AIDS): A disease of the human immune system caused by infection with the human immunodeficiency virus (HIV), usually resulting in death.

Food

Look carefully at the impressive collection of different foods in Figure P-4. Does it surprise you that all the foods in this picture contain soybeans in some form?

Now think beyond the picture.

Food scientists do many things with soybeans. Soybean oil is squeezed out of the seed for use in cooking oils and in the manufacture of margarine and salad dressings. The soybean is a natural source of dietary fiber, and parts are used in breads, cereals, and snacks. Soy flours, soy fiber, bran, and grits are all used in the commercial baking industry.

Now think beyond the food in the picture.

Different types of packages are used with these foods–paper, plastic, glass, and metal. Some are more recyclable or biodegradable than others, causing less of a landfill problem. Some experts predict that many people in the future will consider environmental factors to be as important as nutritional quality when they choose foods. Notice the convenience factor in many of these foods, features that make them easy to store and prepare.

The environment

Think beyond the pictures in Figures P-5 and P-6. Do pesticides harm our food, the environment, or the workers applying pesticides?

The photograph on the left shows how pesticides are often applied to crops in *developed countries* such as those in North America, Europe, and Australia. People working in the sprayed area wear protective clothing, and the amount of pesticides in the food is monitored. Contrast this with the manual application of pesticides that is common in many *developing countries* in Africa, Asia, and Central and South America. The young man

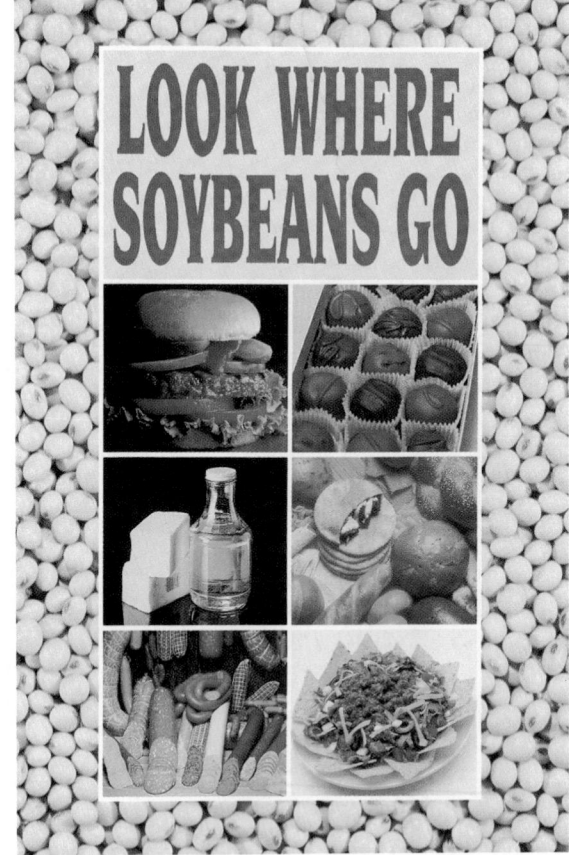

Figure P-4. Foods such as soybeans have multiple uses in many foods. You may not realize how often you eat soybeans unless you read the ingredient lists on foods labels.

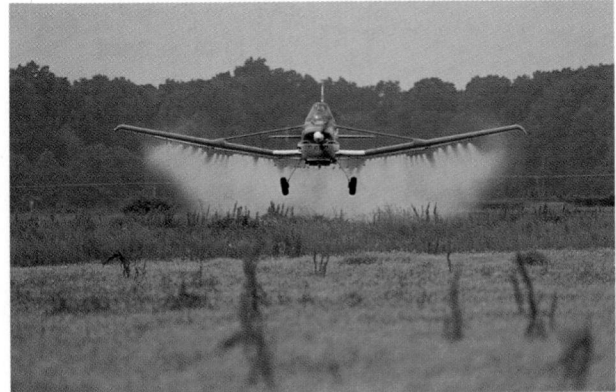
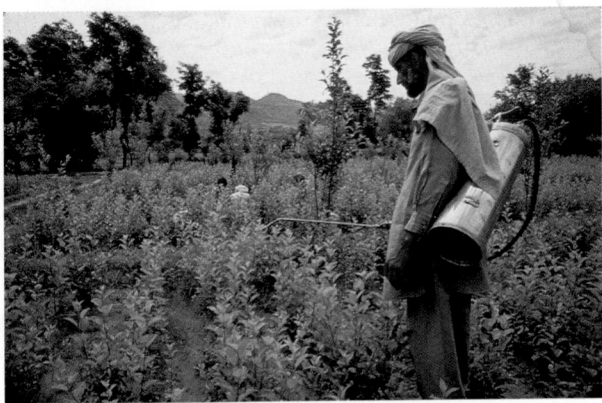

Figures P-5 and P-6. Crop dusting of pesticides from an airplane and hand spraying of pesticides in a rice paddy.

Developed countries: Countries with established industries, agriculture, and services. Includes North America, Australia, New Zealand, Japan, and most of Europe.

Developing countries: Countries in which industries, agriculture, and services are in the developmental stage. Includes most of the countries in Asia, Africa, and Central and South America.

here is spraying pesticides in a rice paddy in Asia (as well as spraying himself, which may be damaging to his health). The worker may have only minimal protection, and often little attention is paid to the pesticides that may be found later in the food supply.

People Are Different

Think beyond these numbers.

It is well known that people in many Asian and African countries consume large amounts of rice. But what about people in the United States?

Consumption of rice in the United States is increasing (Figure P-7). Notice that it is highest along the coasts. People really are different when it comes to food preferences, to food consumption patterns, and, therefore, to the sources of their nutrients. At the end of each chapter is a section called "People Are Different." Each chapter gives the facts about nutrients and food and their interrelationships, along with any environmental concerns. At the end of each chapter, we examine how the information can help us understand the nutritional status of different people.

Test yourself on each of the following topics, which all influence our choice of foods.

See which categories apply to you and whether you differ from family, friends, or people in other parts of the world. You may be surprised by the differences.

- **Age**–Are you eating the same foods you ate 10 years ago?

- **Body weight**–Are you the same body weight you were two years ago? Some people diet to lose weight or to meet weight limits in boxing, fashion modeling, gymnastics, or ballet. Others take nutrient supplements to gain weight, especially to increase muscle mass.

- **Physical condition**–Are you in good physical condition? Some people take supplements in the belief that physical performance will improve. Food intake usually changes when a person is recovering from a severe illness, surgery, or burns.

- **Health**–Do members of your family or your friends consume a special diet for health reasons? Changes in food intake are often recommended for diet-related diseases such as diabetes, coronary heart disease, and high blood pressure.

- **Ethnic origin or race**–Is food an important part of your cultural or ethnic identity?

- **Gender**–Do you eat the same foods as your friends of the opposite gender? Studies show that women and men have different preferences for certain foods.

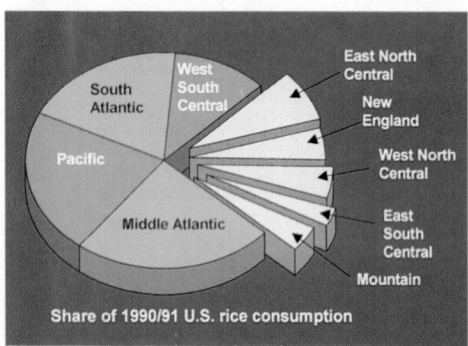

Share of 1990/91 U.S. rice consumption

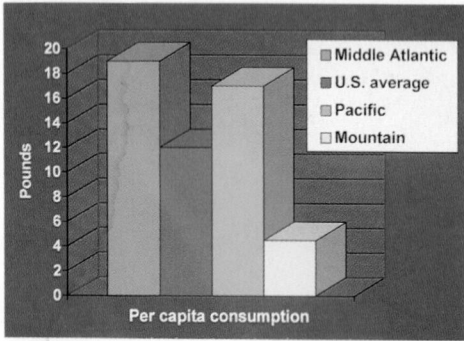

Figure P-7. Consumption of rice in the United States in 1990–1991. Top, shares of the total consumed by different sections of the country. Bottom, per capita direct food use in selected areas.

- **Values**–Are your food choices influenced by certain values–respect for the environment, animal rights, or religious beliefs?

- **Self-concept**–Do you depend on certain foods to improve your status and image?

- **Peer pressure**–Have you felt pressured to eat or not to eat certain foods? This is especially significant during the teen years. Societal and peer pressure to be thin may cause severe problems in self-induced starvation.

- **Parental attitudes**–Do you know if you were breast-fed? Were you influenced to eat certain foods in childhood? Foods that are introduced during the first few years of life may influence food choices later in life.

- **Socioeconomic status**–Are your food choices influenced by what you can spend? The food that is available to people often depends on how much money they have.

- **Television viewing**–Are some of your food choices influenced by advertising? Good commercial reasons exist for advertising certain foods and drinks during sporting events or during television shows for children on Saturday mornings.

- **Nutrition knowledge**–How do you rate your nutrition knowledge? Food choices can be made with either good or poor nutritional knowledge.

- **Food characteristics**–Do you like spicy foods or "squishy" foods?

- **Context**–Is food an important part of your celebrations, holidays, and vacations? These events sometimes involve different or unfamiliar foods.

- **Familiarity**–Do you approach unfamiliar foods with caution? The food industry usually has large budgets to advertise new foods. Relief workers sometimes have difficulty getting starving people to eat unfamiliar foods.

- **Geographic location**–Do you choose the foods you like regardless of where you are? Hamburgers and french fries are now found in most corners of the world. Fruits and vegetables from around the world are available throughout the year in many markets. Is this important to you?

- **Food as an art medium**–Are your taste buds and eyes stimulated by food as an art form?

Nutrition in Your Life

Each chapter opens with brief examples of why the topic is important in our lives. For example, Chapter 6 opens with "Carbohydrate in Our Lives." The list includes the importance of glucose in the body, the recent change from the use of sugar to other sweeteners in many foods and beverages, the importance of fiber in the diet, and other topics of current interest. These opening comments show readers that what they are about to read is relevant to their lives.

Nutrition in Action

At the end of each chapter is a section showing how nutrition information is applied in different circumstances. For example, at the end of Chapter 1 we see how the media use nutrition information. The work of regulatory agencies such as the Food and Drug Administration in maintaining the safety and nutritive value of our food supply is the topic at the end of Chapter 2.

Definitions in the Margins

New or difficult terms are defined in the margin the first time they are used. We have seen some examples above.

Appendixes

The appendixes contain information about the nutrient content of specific foods, including fast foods; reliable sources of nutrition information; readings on the nutrition/environment interface; the Food Exchange System; the Recommended Nutrient Intakes for Canadians; FAO/WHO Recommended Nutrient Reference Values; kilocalories expended in various activities; and a glossary of the terms defined in the margin.

Further Reading

Each chapter ends with a section called "Further Reading." The journal articles and books were chosen carefully to offer useful information if more details are needed. The latest information is listed. Notice also that nutrition information comes from many sources–journals and books specializing in nutrition, food science, biology, agriculture, medicine, and the social sciences, as well as some publications from the popular press. References used in this preface are listed below.

1. World Health Organization Commission on Health and the Environment. *Report of the Panel on Food and Agriculture*, page 25. World Health Organization, Geneva, Switzerland, 1992.
2. May, R. M. How many species inhabit the earth? *Scientific American* 267(4):42, 1992.
3. Cleaver, K., and Schreiber, G. Population, agriculture, and the environment in Africa. *Finance and Development*, page 34, June 1992.
4. Slayter, R. O. Conservation in our changing world. *Environmental Conservation* 18:7, 1992.
5. Singer, P., and others. Nutritional aspects of the acquired immunodeficiency syndrome. *American Journal of Gastroenterology* 87:265, 1992.
6. Cutting, W. A. M. Breast feeding and HIV infection. *British Medical Journal* 305:788, 1992.

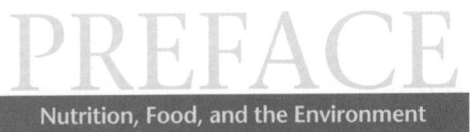

Preface for the Instructor

Food News Blues–The Solution

Well, I read it in the paper
And it made me flip my lid
For it said that oat bran fiber
Didn't work–and never did!
So I stopped my muffin madness
Seeking health another way
Then I read a brand new item
Saying oat bran was OK.
Which is what I've heard for many
Of the foods that kill or cure
Some say, "Eat 'em;" some say "Drop 'em."
Seems that no one's really sure.
Then I found the best solution
Which divorced the guilt from eating.
No, I didn't change my diet.
I quite simply gave up reading!

Perhaps Dr. David Kritchevsky of The Wistar Institute in Philadelphia has poetically defined our challenge and our opportunity.

Our challenge is to cope with the rapid changes in nutrition science and in its applications to the world at large. Integration of the study of nutrition and of food in an environmental context is a new and needed approach to the introduction of nutrition. Our students are challenging us to provide new justifications for some nutrition recommendations. They ask: Is our food safe? Is food produced in a manner friendly to the environment? Why are so many people hungry in our country and throughout the world?

Our opportunity comes from the fact that our students are willing to place nutrition in a larger context. They want to know how is our food produced. For the many students who come from urban backgrounds, the earlier chapters give a brief glimpse of how food moves from our farms to our plates. Acceptance of nutrition recommendations in the future may well depend on the confidence of the next generation in a safe food supply. One way to earn that confidence is to increase their understanding of the long and vital chain linking the food producer, food processor, and food consumer. The information presented in this book on certain food processing techniques–canning, irradiation, fermentation, biotechnology, and others–makes no pretensions to being an in-depth study. It is my hope that it will be the catalyst to further questioning and further study by the student.

Nutrition, Food, and the Environment is an introduction to nutrition. It makes no claims to being a book on the environment. It does lay claim to new approaches in incorporating issues in food processing and on the environment into the very fabric of nutrition. Our professional organizations are taking the lead in acknowledging the importance of environmental issues in relation to nutrition. For example, the American Dietetic Association issued a position paper (1993) endorsing the importance of environmental issues in the training of dietitians. An international nutrition conference held in Australia (1993) was entitled "Nutrition and the Environment." The American Institute of Nutrition scheduled symposia in 1994 on the effect of environmental toxicants and nutrient requirements, on the role of nutrients in modifying toxicants, and on the effects of long-term exposure of toxicants on the nutritional status of the elderly and other vulnerable groups. The role of environmental factors such as unsanitary and toxic environments on the nutritional status of young children is receiving increasing attention. Dr. Noel Solomons and colleagues challenge us to action in a thought-provoking paper entitled: "The Underprivileged, Developing Country Child: Environmental Contamination and Growth Revisited" (*Nutrition Reviews* 51:327, 1993). *Nutrition, Food, and the Environment* introduces the student to the latest information on relationships between nutrition and the other two topics in its title.

This book contains information and illustrations that are consumer-oriented, practical, personalized, and have an international outlook. It is meant to be understandable to readers with limited or no training in science. However, this new approach was not adopted at the expense of the coverage of the nutrition and food safety topics present in other introductory nutrition texts. That coverage is retained here as well.

Our audience will be from many backgrounds and have differing interests in nutrition. You and I are in an important partnership. I provide the challenge in the visual material and discussions that follow many of the photographs, figures, and tables. You bring your teaching style, topics of special interest, student demands, and other requirements. *Nutrition, Food, and the Environment* should be versatile enough to allow you to meet all of your individual requirements. Our students have differing backgrounds in education, culture, interests, occupational goals, recreational interests, health status, and other experiences. Readers of this book also will be from many areas of study–the liberal arts and social sciences, natural sciences, premedical, nursing, agriculture, physical and health education, human ecology, and many others. The book may be used in two- and four-year colleges and universities and in continuing education courses and workshops. Professionals in medical and health areas and in food, agricultural, environmental, recreational, and policy areas will also find it useful.

I look forward to being your companion in stimulating our students to examine and understand the fascinating and important interactions between the nutrients in our diet, the quantity and quality of food our world produces, and our ability to extract the pleasures that food provides us while leaving planet Earth undamaged for the generations that follow us.

Supplementary Materials

Accompanying this text is a complete package of supplementary materials to assist both the student and the instructor.

Free student study guide

A study guide is available on-line or on diskette (IBM PC compatible). It helps the reader by providing an overview of each chapter, study activities, cognitive maps, and self-testing exercises.

Instructor's manual and test bank

Written by the author, this manual includes chapter learning objectives, a summary of each chapter, comments on the "think beyond the picture" challenges, listing of additional readings and resources, and a test bank of multiple choice and short-answer questions grouped by topic categories. The test questions are also available on diskette (IBM PC compatible).

Color transparencies

A set of full-color transparency masters of selected figures and tables for key issues in the text are available to qualified adopters of *Nutrition, Food, and the Environment*.

Diet and fitness analysis software

The Diet Easy for Windows™ software program, a product of First DataBank—The Hearst Corporation (N-Squared Computing), is an easy-to-use nutrition and fitness tool that enables the user to analyze the nutritional content of foods or favorite recipes, to plan menus, and to track personal weight changes. The database contains over 2,400 foods and 80 exercises and activites, and the program is designed to allow the user to edit foods and activites or to add new ones to the database. The software contains a guided tour through a practice session that incorporates many of the Diet Easy for Windows™ functions.

Electronic mail contact with the author

Adopters will have an electronic mail number so that they can communicate directly with the author. They will be alerted to new issues and discoveries in the most current literature on nutrition and nutrition-related subjects.

Acknowledgments

This book breaks new ground by introducing the principles of nutrition within a larger framework that includes the production of food, the availability of nutrients, the environmental consequences of food production, and the nutritional status of individuals. Accomplishing this required thoughtful input from reviewers and consultants and also from people who shared their photographs to make the visual impact of this book different from that of most other introductory nutrition books.

Although many people provided valuable comments and insights during the development and writing of the book, I particularly want to thank Paul Addis, Patricia Berglund, Walter Bushuk, Mary Darling, Swati Elavia, Jack Francis, Joan Gordon, Madge Hanson, Craig Hassel, Robert Hollingworth, Julie Jones, Mindy Kurzer, David Lineback, Lois Lund, Howard Morris, Don Mottram, Rosemary Newman, Patricia Ode, Dennis Savaiano, William Schaefer, David Smith, James Stanton, Elizabeth Van Oss Tymchuk, Zata Vickers, and Joseph Warthesen. While the end result remains my own interpretation, I appreciate the input from a group of scientists for whom I have great respect.

I am also grateful to the people who helped by providing some of the unique photographs and figures: David Anderson, Anita Daniels, Jamie Depolo, Giuditta Dolci-Favi, Mary Garzino, Deborah Kronowitz, Maureen Mackey, Amy Nelson, Stephanie Ockner, Claudia O'Donnell, David Pinkston, Jeanne Sowa, Gertrude Trent, and Jack Watson.

The professionalism and pleasant work environment provided by my colleagues at Michigan State University, especially Mary Carlson, Mary Hempsted, and Carol Shaulis, allowed me to efficiently dispose of my work as chairperson during the day so that I could be effective as a writer after work hours. The superb library and photographic services at Michigan State University eased the load of research for this book.

The Eagan Press "team" were great colleagues at all stages of the book. The skilled editing of Ann King and Elwood Caldwell is much appreciated. Steve Kronmiller and his staff created an intriguing layout. Leslie Gibson and Greg Grahek provided useful advice, and Miles Wimer and Steve Nelson showed faith and confidence in the project at all times.

My sincere thanks go to the special people in my life: my wife Maura for her support, advice, and encouragement; my sons Adrian and Neal, for the "young folks' perspective"; and my parents for the greatest of all gifts, an education.

Vincent Hegarty

About the Author

Vincent Hegarty is professor and chairperson, Department of Food Science and Human Nutrition, at Michigan State University. Previous faculty positions were at the University of Minnesota and University of Houston, the latter accompanied by an adjunct professorship at the University of Texas Health Science Center at Houston. He is visiting professor at the University of Zimbabwe; University College Cork, Ireland; and the United Arab Emirates University.

Dr. Hegarty has taught nutrition courses for over 25 years. While at the University of Minnesota, he won teaching excellence awards from the university and the College of Agriculture. He is the author of the book *Decisions in Nutrition* and over 100 research papers published in nutrition, biomedical, and agricultural journals. He has served on committees at the National Institutes of Health and the U.S. Department of Agriculture.

Dr. Hegarty was Evans Medical Research Fellow while completing his Ph.D. degree in human nutrition at the University of London, England. He has B.Sc. and M.Sc. degrees in biochemistry and a B.A. degree in political economy, philosophy, and history from the National University of Ireland.

CONTENTS

Nutrition, Food, and the Environment

Contents in Brief

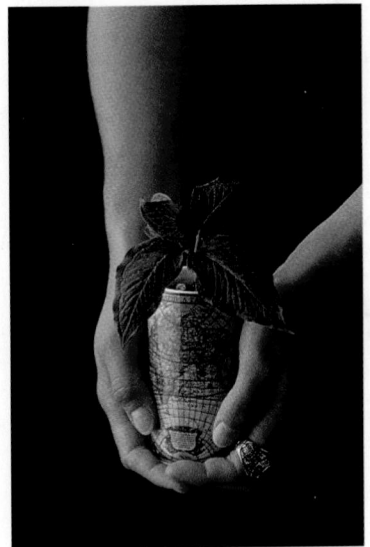

C1. This book will show you the **nutrients**, their food sources, and the effects of deficiencies and toxicities; how you get nutrients from **food** after its safe production, processing, and distribution; and how the **environment** may be affected positively or negatively when food is produced in different parts of the world.

Table of Contents

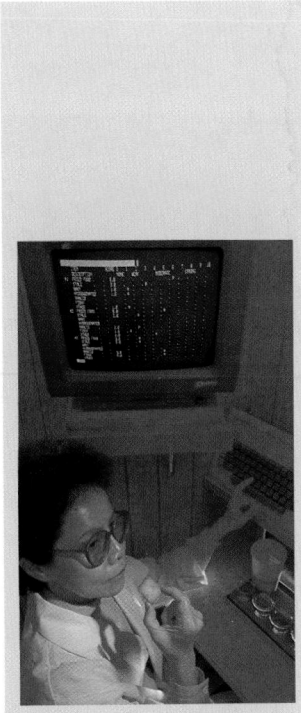

C2. This is one way in
which scientists measure
the sensory qualities of
food and drinks. Your
nutrient intake may be
influenced by the sight,
taste, or odor of food.

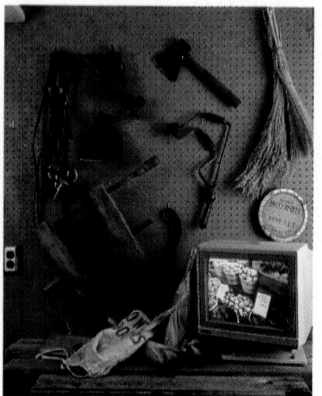

C3. The efficiency of food production has improved greatly in recent years.

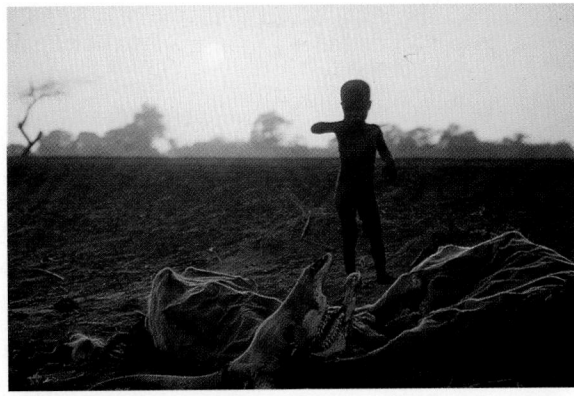

C4. Water is an essential nutrient for people, plants, animals, and microorganisms. Growing things cannot thrive when water is scarce.

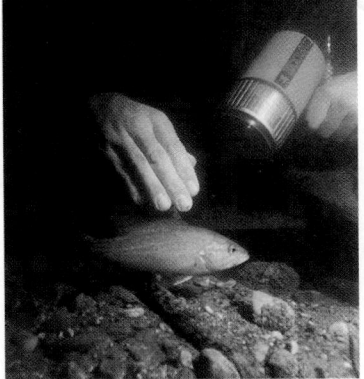

C5. Does your diet contain fish, an important source of protein and other nutrients?

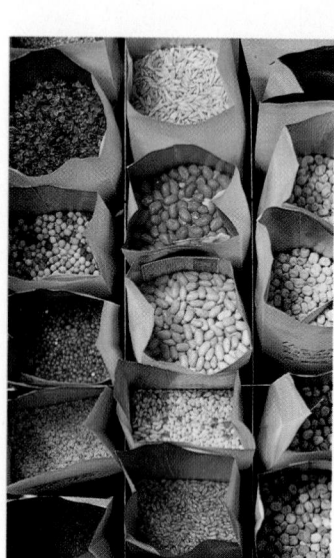

C6. Nuts are an important (and usually inexpensive) source of many nutrients.

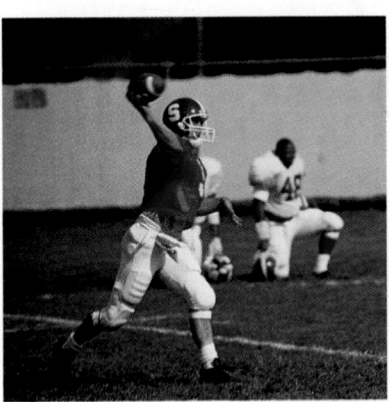

C7. You use energy nutrients for physical activity, for maintaining body temperature and vital processes such as breathing, and for the digestion and metabolism of food.

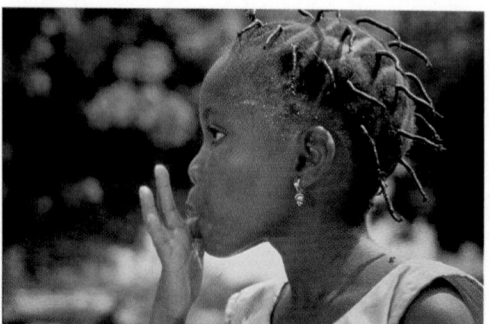

C8. Influences on the food you eat may include age, culture, income, geographic location, and health.

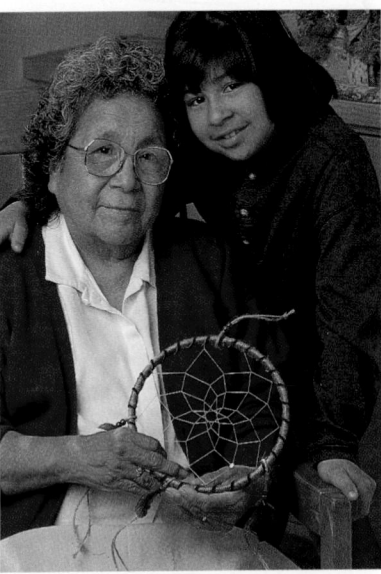

C9. As we grow older, we experience changes in our intake of and need for various nutrients.

Nutrition, Food, and the Environment

**Think beyond the photograph.
Where do we get these chemicals and how do
they influence nutrition?**

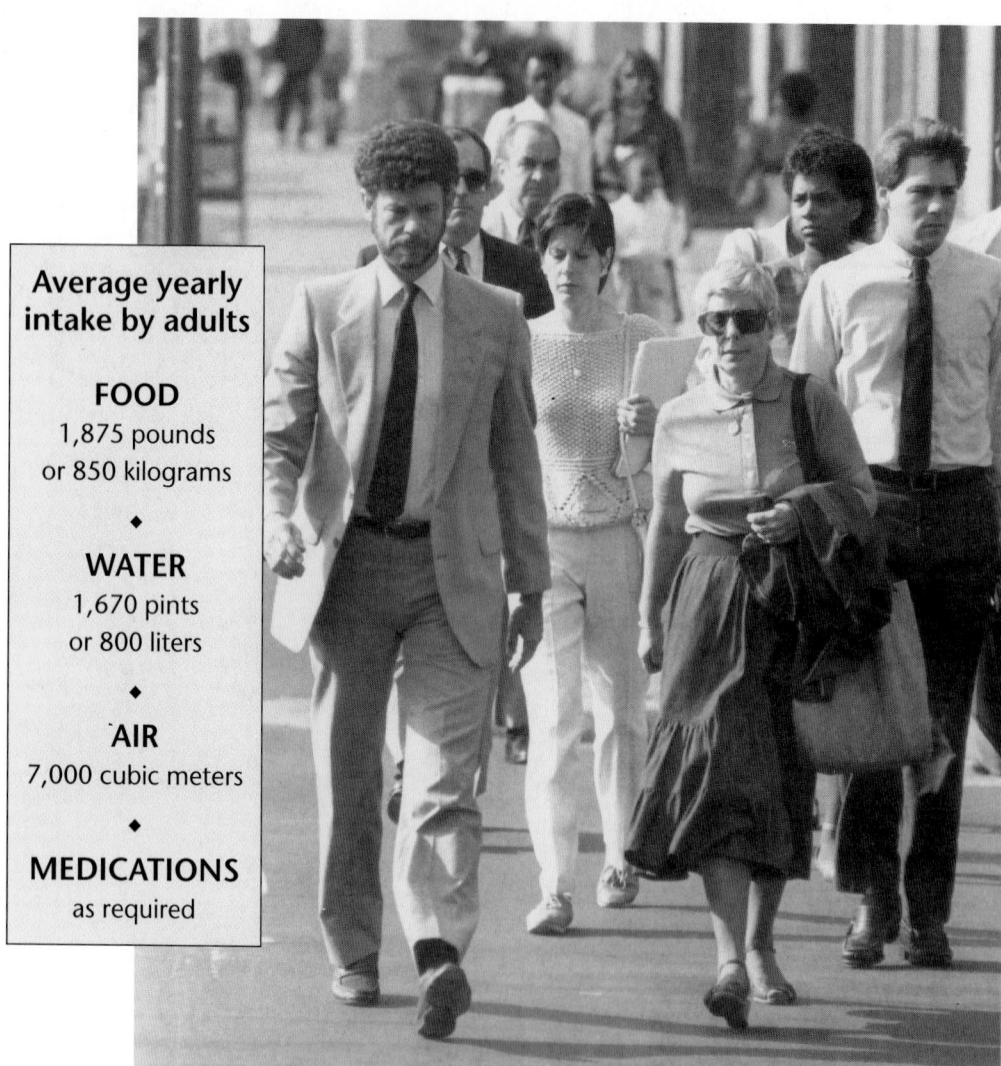

**Average yearly
intake by adults**

FOOD
1,875 pounds
or 850 kilograms

◆

WATER
1,670 pints
or 800 liters

◆

AIR
7,000 cubic meters

◆

MEDICATIONS
as required

Figure 1-1. We are a collection of chemicals, some of which are called nutrients.

## CHAPTER 1

Nutrition, Food, and the Environment– The Interrelationships

■ Some issues about nutrition, food, and the environment in our lives

Our bodies deal with thousands of different chemicals every day. The picture and information on the opening page give an introduction to the most incredible chemical laboratory known–your body.

Food

It may be difficult to understand why hunger exists in the United States when we are told that the amount of *food* consumed by every man, woman, and child averages out to 1,875 pounds per year. This is more than three quarters of a ton of food eaten each year at a cost of $1,910 per person, or $5.23 per day, according to the latest U.S. Department of Agriculture (USDA) data (1988).[1] Clearly, some people spend and eat more than the national average (Table 1-1).

Some of this food is produced on farms close to our homes, some in the far corners of the world. We eat many fresh foods year round because of improved transportation, packaging, and storage of food. At your local supermarket, you can buy grapes out of season from South America, cheeses from Europe, and bananas from Central America. Some hamburger meat may come from cattle raised on land cleared of rain forests in Brazil and Central America. This concerns some experts because loss of rain forests could lead to an increase in global warming. This environmental damage may decrease production of some foods, which we will examine shortly.

Most introductory textbooks in nutrition start with the concerns of people who want to lose weight, are worried about cholesterol intake or the type of fat in different foods, wonder whether they should take vitamin

---

Major Topics in This Chapter

Factors influencing food availability throughout the world

Your body is a remarkable collection of chemicals, which you get from food, water, air, medications, and various contaminants.

■

The nutrients: what they are, how you get them, and what they do for you; a working definition of nutrition

How you get and use information in nutrition

■

People Are Different– Some environmental issues affecting food and nutrition

Nutrition in Action–The media–one of many sources of nutrition information

---

Food: Substances taken into the body that maintain life and growth by supplying energy and building and replacing tissues.

Table 1-1. Annual U.S. Per Capita Consumption

Food	Pounds	Kilograms
Dairy products–milk, cheese, yogurt, ice cream	570	259
Fruits	340	155
Vegetables	226	103
Red meat, poultry, fish, eggs	213	97
Flour and cereal products	183	83
Caloric sweeteners (sugar and other sweeteners)	139	63
Potatoes	127	58
Fats and oils	63	29
Coffee and cocoa	14	6
Total	**1,875**	**853**

supplements, and have a long list of other concerns. These issues are important–and they will be covered. Not all of us need to lose weight or take nutrient supplements, but there is an issue that does affect all of us and future generations as well, so let it be our starting point.

Diet: The usual pattern of food and drink intake by a person or animal.

The world population is about 5.5 billion people, with about 260 million in the United States, and there is more than enough food to feed all of these people if the food were distributed efficiently.[2] Why, then, do we see pictures in magazines and on television of people with signs saying they will work for food or, worse still, of people dying of starvation? Read the following numbers slowly to get a grasp of the dimension of human suffering in the world caused by lack of food and poor diets.

- One in every seven persons (more than 790 million of them) are severely undernourished, according to the latest United Nations statistics.

- About 190 million children under five years of age suffer major nutritional problems because of an inadequate *diet.*

- About 40,000 children under five years of age die *every day,* mostly due to *malnutrition.*

Malnutrition: Poor nutritional status produced by nutrient intakes either below or above the beneficial range of intake.

- More than 2 billion people suffer from deficiencies of vitamin A, iodine, and iron, which can lead to blindness, mental retardation, and even death.

Why does such suffering happen? Poverty is one reason for starvation in some parts of the world and for hunger in some parts of the United States, Canada, and Europe. War, politics, loss of productive farm land due to environmental damage, climate, high birth rates, decreased death rates, and combinations of one or more of these contribute to undernutrition and starvation.

Nutrition problems exist even in the well-fed parts of the world. Death from starvation is rare, but hunger is a growing concern. A 1991 report states that one in eight American children under 12 years of age is hungry and millions more are in danger of hunger. These are alarming statistics, but care is needed in interpreting them because hunger is difficult to measure.

> Hunger, a major social and political concern in the United States, . . . is a measurement problem

caution two nutrition researchers at Cornell University. They continue,

> And this problem is receiving little scientific attention. Even a definition of hunger has not been generally accepted.

Many factors are related to hunger in the United States, including poverty, unemployment, family breakup, inflation, substance abuse, and homelessness. It is ironic that, at the same time, billions of dollars are spent on weight-reducing diets and nutrient supplements such as vitamins and amino acids.

Premature death from diet-related diseases is common in developed countries. These "diseases of affluence" include coronary heart disease, cancer, diabetes, and *hypertension* (high blood pressure). Other food-related problems also are apparent in developed countries. Some people are concerned about the quality and safety of the food supply. Others believe that modern food production methods harm the environment. In response to consumers' concerns about the quality of their diet and the environment, fast-food chains have changed both the nutrient content of their food and the packaging material for food containers. Take a moment to study the implications of the graph in Figure 1-2.

Hypertension: High blood pressure.

Think beyond the graph by asking: if the problems summarized in the long list above are bad now, will they be any better in the year 2032, when we reach an estimated world population of 9 billion people?

Can we solve problems in nutrient deficiencies, food availability, and the quality of the environment when there may be some 3.5 billion *more* people in the world about 35 years from now? These may be uncomfortable questions, but they are challenging opportunities with which to start a study of nutrition.

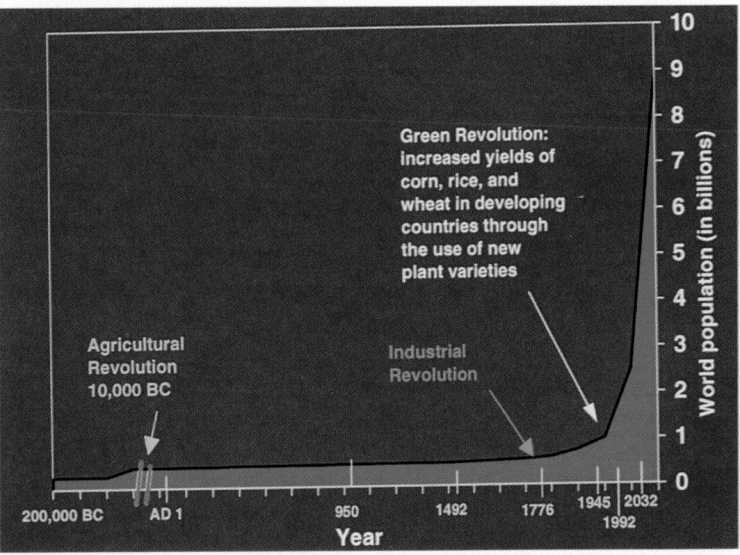

Figure 1-2. The population of the world has increased significantly since 1900.

Consider the many personal, ethical, and religious reasons why some people oppose limitations on population control. Such social and moral issues are beyond the scope of this book, but they are mentioned here to show how factors affecting food intake and nutritional status touch all aspects of our lives.

We have looked at just a small sampling of how nutrition, the supply of food, and the environment have important effects on everybody in the world. Most of us also have individual questions or concerns about some aspect of nutrition. It is not unreasonable to be selfish in personalizing nutrition information. We may have introduced ourselves to nutrition with the question "Is it good for *me*?" The "is it good" part of the question implies an understanding of nutrients and knowledge that production and processing result in foods containing varying amounts of nutrients. Nowadays it can also mean that we wonder whether the food is safe and whether it has any *toxicants* picked up from the environment. The "for me" part allows us to plug in all of the factors we dealt with at the end of the Preface that make each of us a unique individual in our interaction with food. But we saw above that there is more than just "me" to consider. That is why this book takes a global view wherever appropriate–because all of us are involved. Issues of food availability and safety, the quality of the environment, and human suffering from nutrient deficiencies do not respect international borders. With our growing numbers in the world, we all compete for the same food, and we are all responsible for our common heritage in the land, water, and air so vital for our food production.

Toxicants: Chemicals that harm people, animals, or plants.

Water

The average healthy person consumes about 800 liters, or about 1,700 pints, of water every year. Chemistry tells us that water (H_2O) is made up of hydrogen and oxygen. Water can also dissolve many other chemicals, including nutrients in food and in our body, as well as toxic pollutants. It is an essential nutrient. If no fluids are consumed, death occurs, usually after five or six days. Contrast this with the 60–70 days without food before death occurs in healthy adults of normal weight. Close attention will be paid to fluid intake and the quality of the water supply when we get to Chapter 5.

Air

Oxidation: Gain in oxygen, or loss of hydrogen from a chemical compound. An important oxidation process is the use of oxygen from the air to convert carbohydrates, lipids, and proteins in the body into energy, carbon dioxide, and water.

We breathe in about 7,000 cubic meters of air each year (a meter is about 10% longer than a yard). Air is approximately 80% nitrogen and 20% oxygen. Oxygen is vital in nutrition, because it liberates energy from carbohydrates, fats, and proteins in the body by a process called *oxidation*. All cells in the body rely on oxygen to liberate most of the energy needed for life. The brain, in particular, is sensitive to a shortage of oxygen. But oxygen in concentrations higher than in the air we breathe presents problems also. Francis Crick, the famed Nobel Prize winner, has this warning about oxygen:

> Molecular oxygen is a powerful but dangerous compound. It is potentially a highly toxic substance for cells, because cellular processes are liable to produce several lethal derivatives of it . . . . Many cells have special *enzymes* to mop up these life-threatening substances. . . .

Enzyme: A protein that speeds up biochemical reactions in humans, animals, plants, and microorganisms without otherwise becoming part of the reaction.

Nutritionists are interested in the role some nutrients such as iron play in transporting oxygen around the body. But the harmful effects of too much oxygen must be controlled in foods and in the body. That control is done by *antioxidants*, chemical substances frequently mentioned in advertisements and articles in popular magazines. Antioxidants are present naturally in some foods. They prevent fat from becoming rancid during storage. In our bodies, they protect against cell damage that may cause premature aging.

Think for a moment about what was said concerning oxygen–it is vital to life, but too much is dangerous. This is like the many examples we will meet where too little or too much of a nutrient may cause severe health problems. The correct approach is to consume a diet with the proper balance of all nutrients.

Antioxidants: Substances that prevent oxygen from combining with other substances to cause damage to cells, or cause fat in foods to become rancid.

Medications (Drugs)

Drugs are chemical agents used to prevent or treat disease.[3] They have been used throughout history as treatment for diseases and injuries, but it is only recently that we have learned that drugs can be important in nutrition. For instance, they may interfere with appetite or with the digestion, absorption, metabolism, or excretion of nutrients in the body. Here are some other examples of interactions.

> **Too much or too little of any nutrient can damage health.**

- Some drugs can have an effect–negative or positive–on nutritional status. For example, excessive use of aspirin may lead to intestinal bleeding, resulting in deficiencies of iron and a number of vitamins.

- On the other hand, some foods may aid or hinder the action of certain drugs. For example, dietary fat increases the absorption of fat-soluble drugs, while some foods decrease the absorption of certain *antibiotics*, such as penicillin.

- Some foods and drugs cannot be taken together. For example, a drug used for severe depression also inhibits the enzyme monoamine oxidase in the body. This is unfortunate because this enzyme metabolizes potentially toxic chemicals occurring naturally in fermented foods such as cheese, wine, beer, and yogurt. In other words, the drug interferes with the normal body process of detoxifying a naturally occurring toxicant in foods.

Antibiotics: Substances produced by living organisms that inhibit the growth of other organisms. Penicillin is a good example of an antibiotic.

- Drugs can be used in food production, such as the antibiotics given to livestock to prevent infections and promote growth. One concern is that meat and dairy products from treated animals may transfer some of these antibiotics to the humans who consume them. If this happens, the effectiveness of the antibiotic could be reduced in people, thereby lowering their resistance to certain diseases. This happens when the body produces resistant strains of *microbes* due to its constant exposure to antibiotics.

- Nutrients are sometimes given in pharmacologic doses for their drug effect. For example, a synthetic form of vitamin A, retinoic acid, is used for acne, a skin disorder. Although not as toxic as other synthetic forms of vitamin A, it is a prescription drug. Retinoic acid may cause birth

Microbes (bacteria, germs): Tiny one-celled forms of life, producing fermentation, spoilage, decay, and disease.

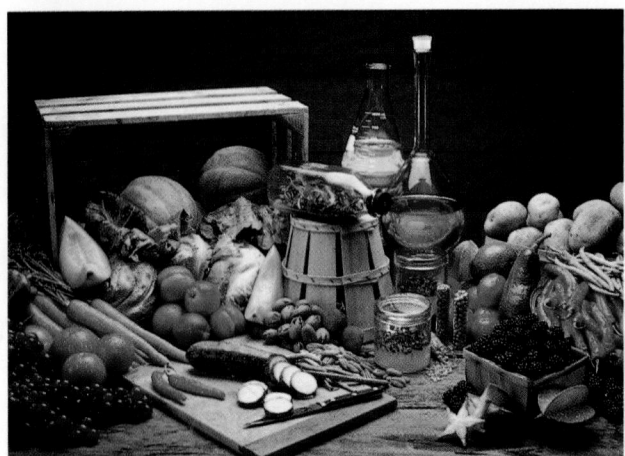

Figure 1-3. A balanced diet comes from eating a variety of foods in moderation. Nutrient supplements are recommended only for medical problems and are not necessary if your diet is balanced.

Balanced diet: A diet providing the recommended intake of all nutrients and containing a wide variety of foods.

defects and interfere with normal body secretions. Too high an intake of nutrients can be damaging to health; some nutrients in high doses can even cause death.

Think beyond the picture in Figure 1-3. Can you get too much of a nutrient from these foods?

It is highly unlikely that you will get toxic doses of a nutrient from food sources–it is virtually impossible if you consume a *balanced diet.* But, considering the availability of nutrient supplements such as vitamin pills and the ease of self-prescribing any dose of any nutrient, it is quite possible to get a toxic dose from supplements. Knowledge of the functions and appropriate intake of all nutrients is important.

In summary, nutritionists are concerned about the quantity and quality of our food, water, and air, as well as the amount of other chemicals that we consume, such as prescription and over-the-counter drugs and nutrient supplements. Illegal drugs also have negative effects on nutritional status. We are now ready to answer an important question.

■ What is nutrition?

The American Medical Association (AMA) defines nutrition as:

> the science of food, the nutrients and other substances therein, their action, interaction, and balance in relation to health and disease, and the processes by which the organism (body) ingests, digests, absorbs, transports, utilizes and excretes food substances.

This is a long definition, but we will break it down into smaller parts and use familiar examples from our experiences. The AMA tells us that nutrition is the "**science of food,** the nutrients and other substances therein . . ."

The Science of Food

Think beyond the message in the advertisement (Figure 1-4).

Think of the many ways nature is copied in much of our processed food. This copying allows the wide variety of foods available today. Increased variety and choices in foods are welcomed by most people. On the other hand, the distinctions between natural and processed foods are not always well defined. Consumers have choices to make, but frequently they may be confused. Should we buy natural food or processed–and is there any difference? But what is "natural" food? Is what nature makes "natural"? This seems logical, but go to the supermarket and you will see some rather unusual foods labeled "natural"–for instance, some candy bars and crackers. The labels and advertisements imply that "natural" foods are somehow more nutritious and healthier than processed food. Most nutritionists agree that such general statements are misleading.

Nature Took Millions Of Years To Perfect The Blend Of Vitamins, Minerals, Fiber, Color And Flavor In This Apple.

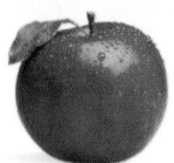

If You Have A *Tighter* Deadline, Call Watson Foods.
1 (800) 388-3481

Figure 1-4. Foods evolved over the centuries by natural selection. Modern scientific methods are now used to modify the nutrient content of foods during their production and processing.

We may be confused further by terms such as "light" or "lite," "low fat," and "high fiber." Help may be on the way! New nutrition-labeling rules took effect in 1994. "The nutrition-labeling revolution is finally coming to a grocery store near you" states *The Wall Street Journal* of December 3, 1992. Note the writer's sense of relief, especially in the use of the word "finally." Formerly undefined terms on labels will in the future have a defined meaning. The Food and Drug Administration (FDA) estimates that labels on 196,000 food products in the United States were changed. This is an important topic. The new nutrition-labeling rules are examined in detail in Chapter 4.

Food science–A brief history

The advertisement we looked at alerts us to the great job nature has done in providing nutrients down through the ages. Our ancient ancestors knew little about nutrients and other chemicals in foods. Nutrition is a relatively new science—the first vitamin was discovered about 80 years ago, and knowledge of how some minerals work in our body was developed within the past 10 to 20 years. But the processing of food and the scientific principles behind various processing techniques go back to ancient times, as seen in Table 1-2.

A 12,000 year time span stretches from the first stone milling of cereal grains to present-day controversies about whether *irradiation* is a safe way to preserve foods. Think a little more about the information in this table. Notice how all of the food processing developments since early times have involved two major impacts on food–making other products from original ingredients, and making food safer and more available by improving storage conditions. For example, other products from stone milling of grain in-

Irradiation: Ultraviolet, ionizing, and microwave irradiation are used to preserve food. Ionizing irradiation from radioactive isotopes destroys microorganisms and insects and inhibits sprouting in plants. It *cannot* make the food radioactive.

Table 1-2. Food Technology Through the Ages

Time		Technology
BC	10,000	Stone milling of cereals
		Baking of flat breads
	4000	Salting, drying, and smoking of fish and meat
	3000	Alcoholic fermentation of barley to beers
		Wine from grapes
AD	200	Yogurt fermentation
	1800s	
	Early	Canning
	Mid	Roller milling for flour
	Late	Cookies; breakfast cereal
		Pasteurization of milk
		Government food regulations
	1990s	
	Early	Quick freezing
		Modified atmosphere packaging for fruit and meat
	Mid	Accelerated freeze drying
	Late	Irradiation

cluded bread from the resulting flour. But then there was a gap of nearly 12,000 years until cookies and breakfast cereals were first made in the 1800s. Food preservation began thousands of years ago with the salting, drying, smoking, and fermentation of certain foods. Then it was discovered that heat and the removal of air preserved food, although the reasons why were not understood at the time. Now we know that microorganisms cause food spoilage and that heat or the lack of oxygen kills most microorganisms. Development of the metal can in the early 1800s was a major breakthrough. Canning is now being replaced by chilling and freezing, and soon possibly by irradiation, as a means of preserving food for reasons of health, economics, environmental preservation, and convenience.

All of the early developments detailed above were made in the Middle East, Egypt, China, or India. For example, yogurt fermentation was perfected in India and the Middle East about 1,800 years ago. Discoveries from the 1600s to present times were made mainly in the United States, United Kingdom, and various European countries. The parting message from this table is that food processing is not a recent creation and is evolving constantly.

Present knowledge in food science and in nutrition allows food processors to alter the nutrient value and chemical content of foods in many ways. Nutrients and chemicals in foods obey the laws of chemistry, physics, and biology to give unique colors, textures, tastes, and odors. All of these are packaged within the billions of cells that make up a plateful of food. Figure 1-5 shows how a tiny portion of a soybean seed cell looks under a powerful microscope.

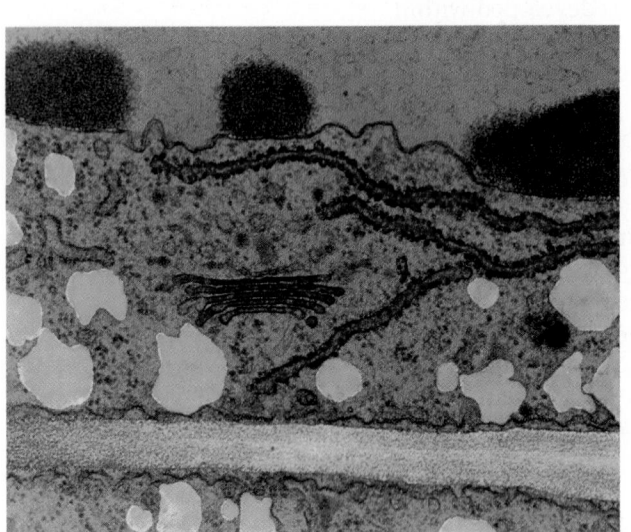

Figure 1-5. A portion of a soybean seed as seen under a microscope, with components colored by computer processing.

Scientists have helped us identify various parts of the cell by computer processing them in colors. They used purple for seed storage protein, yellow for stored oil, and red for cell parts where the synthesis of the stored protein and oil occurs. Food technologists extract the oil and protein from cells for use in a variety of foods. Let's take a quick look at the different kinds of scientists who work on food to make it more nutritious, attractive, plentiful, safer, less expensive, and more adaptable to our busy lifestyles. Improvements by food scientists and farmers are the main reasons why the food supply is more plentiful and safer than at any other time in history.

Scientists and food

Food chemists and sensory specialists work on making food more appealing by changing the taste, texture, and odor of food. Microbiologists use bacteria to make foods such as cheese, yogurt, and bread. They also have an important job in monitoring bacteria and molds that cause food poisoning or spoilage. Food processing experts look for better ways to take food from farms and to process and package it for use in homes and restaurants. Food technologists, food engineers, and biotechnologists make new forms of food. Some of these new foods are called "engineered" or "fabricated" foods. This is done by taking "bits and pieces" of other foods to make a new food that people will enjoy. A good example is surimi, which is inexpensive fish processed into a copy of expensive foods such as lobster, crab, or shrimp. You will find surimi in most supermarkets.

The use of biotechnology gives some people difficulty because of seemingly implied serious dangers to our food supply. Let's put this argument into historical perspective. Take another look at the information in the table about the history of food technology and note that people applied the principles of biotechnology when they first fermented foods over 5,000 years ago. So why are some people concerned today? Recent improvements in techniques to change genes in plants, animals, and bacteria make it possible to speed up the old methods of plant and animal breeding. Where the most difficulty arises for some people is that we now have the ability to transfer genes from one species to another. Stories about mouse genes in tomatoes frighten some people. However, a report from an international panel of experts confirms that there are no known safety problems with food processed by biotechnological techniques.[4] The report does stress that evaluation of all new foods should cover both safety and nutritional value, and it acknowledges that biotechnology raises a number of important nonscientific issues in ethics, consumer perceptions, and food labeling. We will return to this issue in Chapter 2.

"Designer foods" are created from ingredients to meet consumer demands, especially for health-giving properties such as protection from cancer. Another good example is eggs with low or no cholesterol that still look and taste like normal eggs. Various fat replacers made from protein or carbohydrate material have fewer *calories* but the texture and mouthfeel of fat. Consumers want this type of food, and manufacturers are busy providing it, as seen in Table 1-3.

Notice how environmental and health concerns result in foods described as organic, all natural, and having no *additives* or *preservatives*, whereas health concerns alone result in foods low in cholesterol, sugar, fat, salt, and/or calories. These are a few examples of the creativity of food scientists and technologists in extending the variety and versatility of foods.

Food scientists are dependent on farmers to produce the food for processing. The amount and type of food

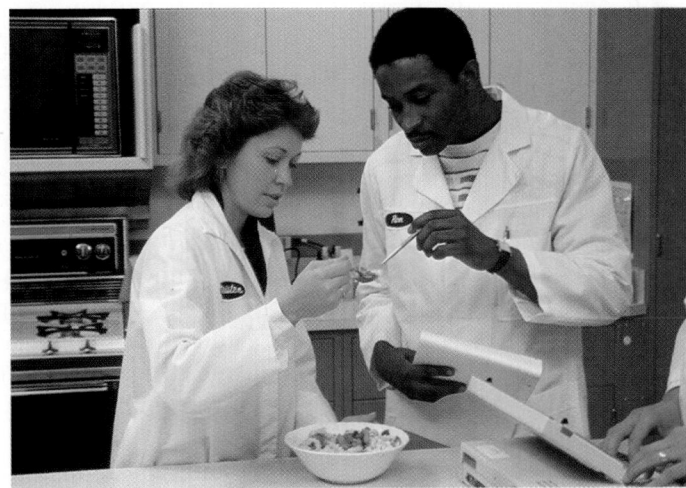

Figure 1-6. Scientists working on new products in a research and development laboratory. Food industries employ nutritionists, food scientists, food engineers, and other professionals. They may work in laboratories, test kitchens, or processing facilities.

Calorie: The term "calorie" is the popular usage for the term "kilocalorie" (kcalorie, kcal) or "Calorie," which is a measure of energy. One kilocalorie equals the amount of heat required to raise the temperature of 1 kilogram of water by 1°C. This book uses "calorie" to represent "kilocalorie."

Table 1-3. Percent Increase in New Foods with Health-Related or Environmentally Friendly Characteristics

New Food Category	Percent Increase in One Year
Organic food	131[a]
All natural	125
No additives or preservatives	99
Low/no cholesterol	78
Reduced/low sugar	76
Reduced/low fat	64
Reduced salt	37
Reduced/low calories	21

[a] The total number of organic foods on the market is less than the numbers in the other categories. Thus, this higher percentage must be interpreted as being derived from a smaller base.

Food additives: All material deliberately added to food to assist in its manufacture and preservation and to improve palatability and appearance.

Preservatives: Additives that protect food from deterioration caused by microorganisms, enzymes, and oxidation.

on people's plates depends on where in the world they live. Climate, availability of water, species of plants and animals, soil quality, use of fertilizer, absence or presence of pests such as insects and rodents, losses of food because of poor refrigeration, storage, transportation, methods of preservation and preparation of food, and the economic and political climate in a country all combine to determine the quantity and quality of food on people's plates. In poor parts of the world, people worry about the very availability of food. Facilities for the processing and storage of food may not exist, so some food will spoil if not eaten immediately or dried in the sun. Contrast this with the large food processing industries, extensive refrigeration, and other storage facilities in stores and private houses in developed countries. Does that mean that we in industrialized countries have nothing to worry about? Some people worry that our food may contain food additives and pesticides; others check the amount of cholesterol, salt, sugar, and type of fat in foods because of their proposed relationship to diseases such as obesity, cancer, coronary heart disease, and high blood pressure. Perhaps the following quotation best summarizes the attitude we should have toward food.

> . . . U.S. consumers should worry less and enjoy more, should be cognizant of real risks but separate them from irrational ones. Food is one of the great pleasures that humankind has, so in addition to being wary, we should make wise choices and then enjoy them.

To implement this good advice from Dr. Julie Jones of the College of St. Catherine, St. Paul, Minnesota,[5] we need a thorough understanding of all aspects of our food supply and of the nutrients it contains.

Nutrients

Nutrition is the "science of food, **the nutrients** and other substances therein . . . ." Nutrients are chemicals in food that nourish the body by providing energy, allowing growth and repair of tissues, and regulating necessary chemical processes in the body. All of the nutrients listed in Table 1-4 are needed from the time we were conceived until the day we die.

Future chapters deal with each of the nutrients in the order listed in this table. It is a long list, but don't be alarmed. It gives you a good first look at all of the nutrients. Look on it as a road map through the nutrients. **Keep returning to this table for an overall summary as we proceed through the book.** However, we can make some general comments on the nutrients at this point.

The body's normal need for nutrients increases during periods of rapid growth (childhood, pregnancy, and lactation) and during recovery from starvation, long illness, or extensive weight loss on a severe diet.

Notice the importance of cereals, fruits and vegetables, meat, and dairy products in supplying various nutrients. Different foods contribute varying levels of nutrients to our diet. It is thus more appropriate to speak of the nutritive quality of *diets* rather than of individual foods. Nutritionists are quick to point out that there are no totally "good" or "bad" foods, only good or bad diets. Different nutrients perform different functions in our

Table 1-4. The Nutrients, Their Functions, and Food Sources

Nutrient	Body Functions	Major Food Sources
Water	Body fluids–blood, saliva, digestive juices, urine	Water, beverages, foods
Energy nutrients		
Carbohydrates (Essential carbohydrate: glucose)	Provides energy; spares body protein	Cereals, fruits, vegetables, milk
Lipid (fat) (Essential lipid: linoleic acid)	Provides essential fatty acids; provides energy; absorbs and transports fat-soluble vitamins (A, D, E, and K); protects vital body tissues; insulates body	Fats and oils, meats, fish, nuts, some seeds, dairy products
Protein (Essential amino acids: histidine, isoleucine, leucine, lysine, methionine, phenylalanine, threonine, tryptophan, valine)	Aids growth and repair of tissues; affects fluid and acid-base balances; is what all enzymes, antibodies, and some hormones (insulin) are made of; provides energy	Meats, fish, dairy products, eggs, nuts, legumes, cereals
Vitamins		
Fat-soluble		
A	Affects vision; health of skin; growth of hair, nails, bones, and glands; prevents infections	Dairy products, liver, carotene in deep green and orange fruits and vegetables
D	Helps absorption of dietary calcium and phosphorus; affects health of bones and teeth	Dairy products, egg yolks
E	Antioxidant–prevents cell damage	Vegetable oils, nuts, seeds
K	Clots blood	Green vegetables, eggs
Water-soluble		
C	Antioxidant–prevents cell damage; causes collagen formation; affects health of teeth and gums	Citrus fruits, green peppers, broccoli, cantaloupe, kiwi fruit, cabbage
B-complex		
Thiamin (B-1)	Affects nerve function; is coenzyme in energy metabolism	Whole grains and enriched cereals, pork, legumes, peanuts
Riboflavin (B-2)	Coenzyme for energy metabolism; protects skin and eyes	Whole grains and enriched cereals, dairy products, eggs, meats, green leafy vegetables
Niacin	Coenzyme for energy metabolism	Meats, fish, nuts, whole grains, eggs
B-6	Aids in metabolism of amino acids and protein	Most high-protein foods
Folic acid (folacin)	Aids metabolism of DNA and RNA (genetic material); prevents a type of anemia	Green leafy vegetables; nuts; legumes; grain products
B-12	Aids metabolism of DNA and RNA; is part of the nerves	Foods of animal origin; microorganisms in fermented foods
Pantothenic acid	Coenzyme for energy metabolism	Most foods of plant and animal origin
Biotin	Coenzyme for energy metabolism	Most foods of plant and animal origin

(Continued on next page)

Table 1-4 (continued) The Nutrients, Their Functions, and Food Sources

Nutrient	Body Functions	Major Food Sources
Minerals		
Macrominerals		
Calcium	Forms bones and teeth; affects blood clotting and nerve function	Dairy products, legumes, dark green vegetables
Phosphorus	Forms bones and teeth; affects body fluid balance; is part of some coenzymes	Dairy products, meats, cereals
Magnesium	Affects nerve and muscle function; is part of some coenzymes	Green vegetables, whole grain cereals
Sulfur	Part of proteins in hair, cartilage, tendons	Sulfur amino acids in dietary proteins
Sodium	Affects nerve and muscle function and body fluid balance	Salt (sodium chloride), soy sauce, salted foods (meats, pickles, some crackers), cheese, butter
Potassium	Affects nerve and muscle function and body fluid balance	Meats, dairy products, fruits and vegetables (especially bananas), whole grains
Chloride	Affects nerve and muscle function and body fluid balance; forms hydrochloric acid in the stomach	Salt, soy sauce, salted foods, cheese, butter
Microminerals (trace minerals)		
Iron	Transports oxygen (in hemoglobin in blood)	Meats, legumes, cereals, eggs
Zinc	Synthesizes proteins; is a coenzyme; heals wounds; affects taste	Meats, fish, whole grains
Iodine	Part of thyroid hormones	Seafood, iodized salt, dairy products, some breads
Selenium	Coenzyme; acts with vitamin E	Seafood, whole grains, meats
Fluoride	Affects tooth and bone structure	Fluoridated drinking water, seafood, tea
Copper	Coenzyme	Seafood, meats, nuts, legumes
Cobalt	Part of vitamin B-12	Foods of animal origin
Chromium	Involved in glucose and energy metabolism	Brewer's yeast, seafood, meat, liver, some vegetables
Manganese	Coenzyme	Whole grains, fruits, nuts, vegetables
Molybdenum	Coenzyme	Cereals, legumes, some vegetables

body. For example, the energy nutrients–carbohydrates, lipids, and proteins–provide the energy for sports, jogging, or just sitting around and the energy needed to maintain body functions such as breathing and pumping blood around the body. There is no mention here of the energy that advertisements tell us that we are supposed to get from vitamin supplements. There is a good reason why they are not listed–vitamins by themselves provide no energy. Vitamins, minerals, and water facilitate the liberation of energy from carbohydrates, lipids, and proteins, but they are not the source of that energy.

Notice also in this table that some nutrients affect specific tissues–vitamin A has its principal effects on eyes, vitamin D on bones and teeth, iron on blood. Understanding nutrition is made easier when the functions of nutrients in the body are first understood. Then you can deduce what goes wrong when the dietary intake of a nutrient is low. For example, calcium is needed for bones and teeth. If children have a low intake of calcium, their bones and teeth will grow at a slower rate. In the case of extreme deficiency of calcium, bones are malformed.

Think about the pictures in Figures 1-7 and 1-8.

The nutrient content of your meal can be calculated by weighing the individual components of the meal and then electronically scanning a database for the nutrient content of each food. An alternative way to determine the nutritive value of your meal is to use the Table of Food Composition in Appendix A.

Remember, in a meal with a wide variety of foods, a single mouthful might contain a little of most of the nutrients on the list above. We cannot deal with a "mouthful" of information on all of the nutrients all at once. That is why the nutrients are presented in separate chapters. This is easier for us to learn, but it is not reality. We will see below that the interactions and balance of nutrients are very important both in the diet and in the body.

> There are no totally good or bad foods, only good or bad diets.

Other Substances

Nutrition is the "science of food, the nutrients and **other substances therein** . . . ."

This category includes some forms of carbohydrates, lipids, and proteins that are nonessential. These should be contrasted with the "essential" nutrients listed in Table 1-4, which are the forms of carbohydrates, lipids, and proteins that must be in a balanced diet. The nonessential forms of carbohydrates, lipids, and proteins are manufactured by our bodies. The body does these fantastic chemical tricks, most times without our knowledge. How the body does this will become clear when we learn more about the energy nutrients.

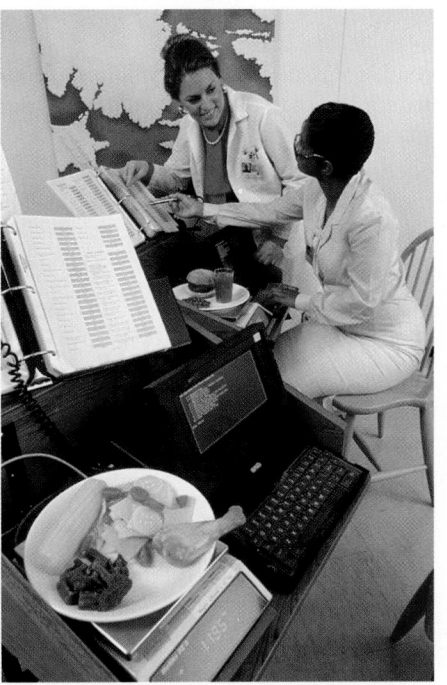

Figures 1-7 and 1-8. Your nutrient intake can be measured by recording the type and amount of food you eat. The nutrient quality of your diet can be quickly analyzed by computer.

Included also under "other substances" are the chemicals that give foods their sensory characteristics of color, texture, flavor, and aroma. Also in this category are naturally occurring toxicants, food additives, bacteria and molds, and environmental contaminants.

Naturally occurring toxicants

Some foods may contain naturally occurring toxicants; usually these are foods of plant origin. Many different plants produce toxic chemicals for one simple reason–protection from animals and microbes. Nature is smart. Plants cannot protect themselves the way animals can; they have no claws to scratch, teeth to bite, feet to escape, or roar to frighten. The alternative is to make toxicants. For example, broccoli and bananas each have five or more defensive chemicals; apples and potatoes have at least two each. Does this mean that we must eliminate these and other foods containing natural toxicants from our diets? Certainly not. The small amount of toxicants in foods in a typical diet presents no known health hazard.

Carcinogens: Substances that cause cancer.

Some foods have naturally occurring *carcinogens*. An expert in toxicology at the FDA estimates that almost all of our foodborne cancer risk is due to naturally occurring carcinogens in ordinary food.[6] Some familiar foods with known naturally occurring carcinogens are listed in the next table.

Table 1-5. Food Sources of Known or Suspected Carcinogens

Carcinogen	Food Source
Naturally occurring carcinogens	Mushrooms, parsnips, celery, spinach, beets, lettuce, radishes, fish, shellfish, garlic, chilies, oranges, spices, flavorings
Carcinogens formed during food processing	Foods that are cured, fried, fermented; broiled meat; smoked, grilled and charred fish or meat, salted and pickled foods
Contaminants	
Dioxins and furans, PCBs	Fatty foods, fish, milk
Chloroform	Drinking water
Methylene chloride	Fatty foods
Benzene	Eggs, cooked meats, fruits and vegetables
Polynuclear aromatics	Grains, vegetables, vegetable oils
Formaldehyde	Fruits
Arsenic	Natural water
Urethane	Alcoholic beverages, bread, olives, soy sauce, yogurt
Nickel	Legumes
Carcinogenic mycotoxins	Corn, peanuts, soybeans, barley, safflower seeds, yellow rice

Think beyond the information in the table by asking yourself how often you consume these foods.

Should you be aware of the problems caused by naturally occurring carcinogens? Of course. Should you be scared? Probably not. Why? The FDA expert stresses that

> our studies show that the real cancer risks in the food supply are low—and almost entirely in the traditional foods themselves.[6]

Let's think about that statement by taking the orange as an example of a traditional food. Oranges contain very small amounts of naturally occurring carcinogens (see Table 1-5 at left). Suppose we decide not to eat oranges because of the risk of cancer. We may now have another problem. A look at the list of nutrients in Table 1-4 shows that citrus fruits, which include oranges, are important sources of vitamin C. Thus, we would be eliminating an excellent source of vitamin C and other nutrients in order to eliminate a negligible risk of cancer.

This topic raises important points. First, many nutrition issues are not black and white, and choices must be made. But we must have reliable information in the proper context to make the correct choice. Second, different people will make different choices for different reasons on this and other issues in nutrition. Third, the examples above deal with numbers.

See how the potentially frightening aspect of naturally occurring carcinogens in some common foods is put into perspective when we learn that only tiny amounts are present. This brings us back to the question asked above: "Is it good for me?". The answer is: "It depends on how much you take." True, this frustrates people, but it is the correct response. Finally, the best and most often used nutrition advice is to eat a wide variety of foods. This will dilute any toxicants in your diet while ensuring that you get an adequate intake of nutrients.

Pollutants and toxins

Environmental and industrial pollutants and toxins can get into the food supply. Concerns include lead, mercury, and other toxic metals in fish; pollutants such as *polychlorinated biphenyls (PCBs)*, found mainly in fish; contaminants from packaging; and pesticide residues, antibiotics, and growth promoters in meat animals. As our knowledge of toxicants in the environment increases, it is important to include this category of "other substances" in a definition of nutrition. These contaminants are undesirable, although it is often difficult to assess the health risks from them. We should work toward reducing their content in food.

Bacteria and molds in our food may be helpful or harmful. Helpful microorganisms make cheese, yogurt, sour cream, bread, wine, antibiotics such as penicillin, and some nutrients—vitamin K, vitamin B-12, biotin, and riboflavin. Harmful microorganisms can spoil food and cause food poisoning, leading to vomiting, diarrhea, fever, and even death. A much feared foodborne disease is *botulism*. We have known about this disease for over 1,000 years. Until recently it was the cause of a number of deaths annually, usually when people ate improperly home-canned foods. Better education on the importance of proper conditions for home canning reduced the occurrence of botulism.

Some molds and fungi may be poisonous. One type of mold produces *aflatoxin*, a powerful carcinogen. However, we are well protected from aflatoxin by strict government regulation and testing of the foods likely to be contaminated—peanuts, grains, and some vegetables.

Action, Interaction, and Balance

Returning to the definition of nutrition—"the science of food, the nutrients and other substances therein, **their action, interaction and balance . . . .**"

Action

Spend some time examining the list of nutrients in Table 1-4 to see their specific actions. For example, carbohydrates, lipids, and proteins provide energy; lipids protect vital body organs such as the kidneys; vitamin K clots blood when you get a scratch; and so on down the list.

Interaction

Many nutrients work together in the body to make important parts of tissues–calcium, phosphorus, and vitamin D are involved in bone forma-

Polychlorinated biphenyls (PCBs): A group of at least 50 widely used compounds containing chlorine. Can accumulate in food chains and may cause a variety of harmful effects including damage to the reproductive cycle of animals and plants.

Botulism: Paralytic disease caused by ingesting a toxin produced by the bacteria *Clostridium botulinum*. Foods most affected are improperly home-canned foods, sausages, and bacon.

Aflatoxin: Toxic substance produced by a mold; a strong carcinogen.

Hemoglobin: The oxygen-carrying, iron-containing protein in red blood cells. (*Hemo* = blood, *globin* = globular protein)

tion; iron and protein form the *hemoglobin* in blood that carries oxygen from the air to all tissues in the body. Hemoglobin is not made at normal rates if dietary iron intake is low. This means there is less hemoglobin to take oxygen to all tissues, where it helps in the liberation of energy from the energy nutrients. We feel this effect by being sluggish and unable to perform intense physical activity. Nutrients interact in many positive ways. For example, marathon runners running 26-plus miles get a lot of energy by utilizing the interactions between the energy nutrients. Carbohydrate, fat, and protein "fuel" stored in the body is broken down in varying proportions depending on the stage of the race. We look at the details of how this is done in Chapter 12.

Balance

"Eat a balanced diet"–surely this advice has been given for many generations. Balance means a wide variety of foods that give the body adequate amounts of all the nutrients listed in the nutrient table. To many people, eating an unbalanced diet usually means eating too little food or not enough nutrients. That is only partly correct. It is equally important to think of unbalanced as meaning too much. We have already discussed how a nutrient can be harmful to our health and may even be deadly. Let's return to vitamin A again as an example–too low an intake causes blindness, and extreme deficiency causes death, but excesses of vitamin A can also be fatal. This can be avoided by not abusing the recommended intake of vitamin A supplements and by avoiding very high intakes of liver, which is very high in vitamin A.

Understanding the concept of balance in nutrient intake gives a better appreciation of the problems caused by too high or too low nutrient intakes and a better appreciation of the benefits of learning to read and understand food labels. We also learn to be cautious of unproven promises of improved health and well-being when some supplements and foods are taken in large amounts.

In Relation to Health and Disease

Nutrition is "the science of food . . . **in relation to health and disease** . . . ." In the first half of this century people in North America, Europe, and Japan were concerned with deficiencies of nutrients in their diets. Vitamin D deficiency was common in children, resulting in rickets (poor formation of bones in the legs). Deficiencies of protein, iron, calcium, iodine, and other nutrients were not uncommon in the general population. Today, these nutritional deficiencies are seen much less frequently in the developed world and are generally associated with poverty. For people with adequate access to food, the concerns are with the possible relationship of high dietary intakes to certain diseases–dietary fat and coronary heart disease to some cancers; sodium (much of it from salt) to hypertension (high blood pressure); and dietary cholesterol to coronary heart disease. Notice the term "possible relationship." Experts differ in their assessments of the significance of dietary components in these complex diseases. Many dietary and nondietary factors may be involved.

Processes by Which Your Body Deals with Ingested Food

The AMA definition of nutrition ends with **"the processes by which the organism (body) ingests, digests, absorbs, transports, utilizes and excretes food substances."**

Now we are near the end of this definition of nutrition, but the nutrients we have been examining still have a fascinating journey to make before they arrive at the tissues where they perform their specific duties as nutrients. Much of this journey is through the *gastrointestinal (GI) tract*, a 30-foot hollow tube from mouth to anus as seen in Figure 1-9.

Now think beyond the figure on the following page by considering the following practical question: What happens if part of the GI tract is removed because of disease?

Digestion and absorption is most active in the upper portion of the small intestine. To lose this part of the GI tract would present considerable difficulty. Knowing how the GI tract works helps in understanding the nutritional implications of diarrhea, constipation, food allergy, and food poisoning. Let's take a brief look at the journey of food and nutrients through the GI tract. The details of digestion will be dealt with in Chapter 3.

Ingestion and digestion

Ingestion is eating and swallowing food and liquid. Which foods and liquids are ingested is determined by the list of factors influencing an individual's food choices (see the People Are Different section of the Preface).

It is a common mistake to think that after swallowing food it is "in you." Yes, it is physically inside you, but the nutrients are not inside the body's cells–yet. That happens only when nutrients are broken free from the non-nutrient parts of foods during digestion in the GI tract, as seen in Figure 1-9.

Digestion is the breakdown of food into its individual nutrients. This is done by the help of various digestive juices. Most dietary carbohydrates, lipids, and proteins are large molecules. During digestion they are broken into their basic components. These are listed in Table 1-4–glucose and other *monosaccharides* for carbohydrates, fatty acids and *glycerol* for lipids, and *amino acids* for proteins. These (and molecules of water, vitamins, and minerals) are small enough to be absorbed from the digestive tract into the blood.

Absorption

The stomach is a reservoir for the food and fluid you consume. Partially digested food passes gradually into the duodenum (the upper part of the small intestine), where further food digestion occurs.[7] Most of the nutrients are absorbed here and move on to the blood for transport to every cell in the body.

If food moves too fast through the digestive tract, as in the case of diarrhea caused by laxative abuse or food poisoning, a lower amount of nutrients is absorbed. Nutrients must be in contact with the cell walls of the GI tract for a reasonable time in order to be absorbed through those cells and

Gastrointestinal (GI) tract: The entire digestive tract from the mouth to the anus.

Monosaccharides: A group name for the simplest carbohydrates, including glucose, fructose, and galactose. Glucose is the most important monosaccharide. (Mono = one, saccharide = sugar)

Glycerol: An organic alcohol that, when combined with fatty acids, forms a fat.

Amino acid: An organic acid containing both an amino (-NH$_2$) and an acidic (-COOH) group. The approximately 20 different amino acids can be linked in varying combinations to form proteins in humans, animals, plants, and microorganisms.

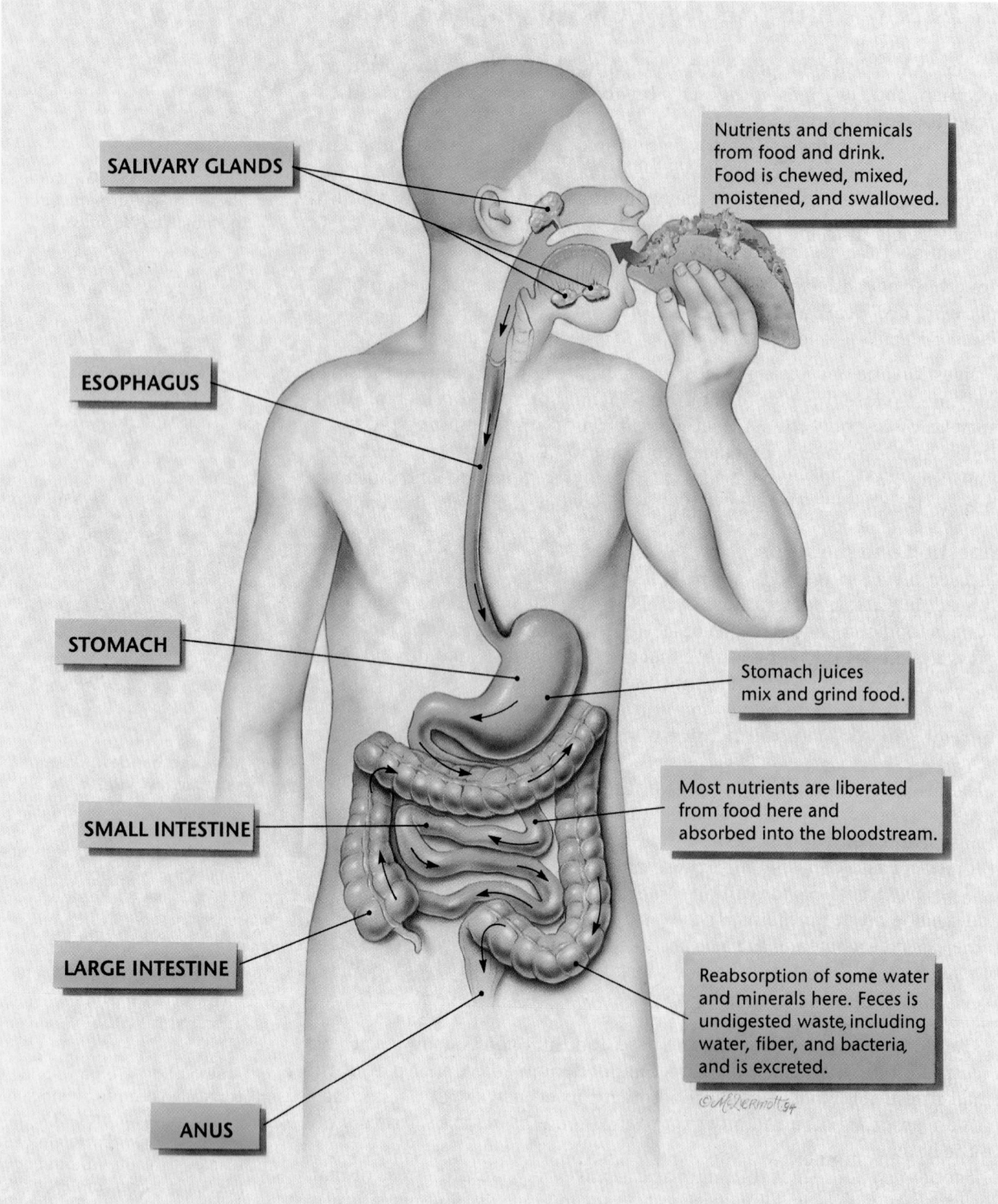

SALIVARY GLANDS

Nutrients and chemicals from food and drink. Food is chewed, mixed, moistened, and swallowed.

ESOPHAGUS

STOMACH

Stomach juices mix and grind food.

SMALL INTESTINE

Most nutrients are liberated from food here and absorbed into the bloodstream.

LARGE INTESTINE

Reabsorption of some water and minerals here. Feces is undigested waste, including water, fiber, and bacteria, and is excreted.

ANUS

Figure 1-9. Digestive activities in the gastrointestinal tract include the chewing and mixing of food, the release of nutrients from food, the absorption of nutrients into the cells, and the excretion of wastes in the feces.

sent onward to the blood. Any nutrients and chemicals in food that are unabsorbed move along the digestive tract to be excreted in the *feces* and are lost to the body.

Feces: Also called stools. Body waste including undigested food, bacteria, and dead cells from the GI tract.

Transportation

Absorbed nutrients are transported in the blood to the liver. The liver is like a processing center–it processes nutrients for dispatch to the cells of tissues around the body for use, and it stores some nutrients. It is a detoxi-fication center for drugs, poisons, and alcohol. Blood is the transportation system to get nutrients to cells and to excrete waste from cells.

Utilization of nutrients

Nutrients have now arrived in cells and are ready to perform their specific functions. Let's turn the words about the function of nutrients from the table into visual reality.

Think about the wonderful coordination of nutrients from food to produce the cells shown in Figure 1-10.

A work of art? Yes, and you own it. Some cells in your body look like this. This magnif-icent structure was made entirely from nutri-ents in your diet. This is the end of the long journey for the nutrients that originated on farms, in seas or lakes, or in your garden. Only one final thing must be done; the waste from digestion of food must be excreted.

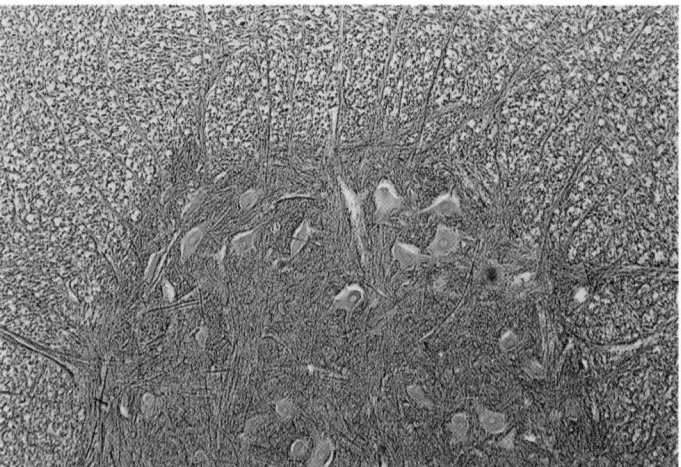

Figure 1-10. Your spinal cord has nerve cells like these. Like all of the other billions of cells in your body, they are made from the nutrients in the foods you eat.

Excretion

Various chemicals are excreted from the body in the form of feces, urine, and sweat. Carbon dioxide and water vapor are excreted through the lungs. Feces contain unabsorbed nutrients, water, and some of the diges-tive juices. Urine is the main means of excretion of water-soluble nutrients and other chemicals after they are absorbed from the digestive tract into the body. If you take an excess amount of water-soluble vitamins, the amount not used by tissues is filtered from the blood by the kidneys and excreted in the urine. Urine analysis is used in many nutritional studies as an indicator of nutrient intake and of nutrient utilization by the body. Perspiration allows loss of water and some salt through the skin. Breast milk may contain some antibiotics and toxicants taken in the diet. Some experts thus consider breast milk to be a means of excretion.

Fat is not water-soluble and cannot be excreted through the urine or sweat. That may appear obvious, but many people are fooled by various weight-reduction programs promising that unwanted fat will "melt away." Think for a moment–once fat has "melted," how will we excrete it? Thousands of people never asked that question when a diet based on grapefruit was popular a few years ago. Supposedly the acidic juices from the grapefruit would "melt" the excess body fat. But we do not urinate away fat or squeeze it out through the pores in the skin. This diet is now among the multitude of unused and forgotten weight-reducing diets.

This is the end of a long journey through a definition of nutrition. You are encouraged to return to it often to insert your own examples into the various parts of the definition. A complete understanding of what nutrition means will help you considerably in your food choices and in understanding nutrition information. Now we need to answer another important question:

■ How is nutritional information obtained and used?

Nutrition is an exciting and ever-changing subject. Researchers obtain new information from many sources. Some of these are outlined in the paragraphs that follow.

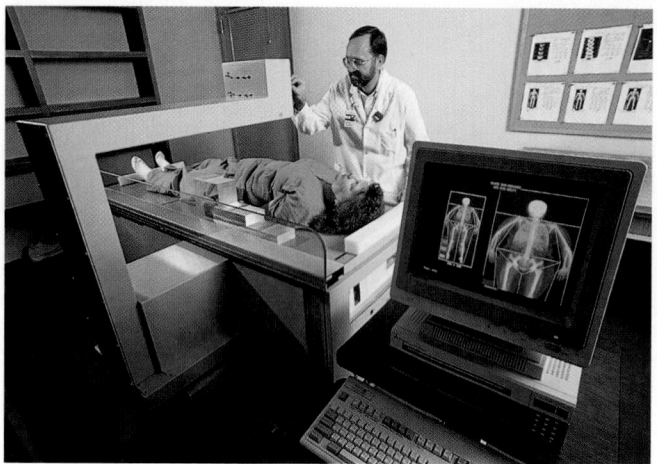

Figure 1-11. Nutritionists can use elaborate scanning instruments to learn how nutrients such as calcium and fluoride affect the growth and maintenance of bones and muscles.

Chemical analysis of foods

Sophisticated instruments can measure large or small quantities of nutrients in food. Values obtained are used on nutrition labels and in tables of food composition (see Appendix A). As many as 1,500 or more new foods are introduced in the United States every year–each of these must be analyzed for nutrient content.

Human experiments and trials

Some experiments may last a few hours–for example, measuring the absorption of nutrients from the digestive tract into the blood supply. Other studies may last up to several years. Such studies include the effect of diet and other factors on heart disease, cancer, and high blood pressure. The experiments are done under strict regulation so that people are not used as "human guinea pigs." Many nutrition trials that could be important cannot be done because they are too dangerous to volunteers.

People with no known nutrition problems can be used to study nutrient requirements of the human body. College students and athletes often volunteer for such studies. One nutrition researcher at Harvard collected toe nail clippings from over 70,000 people. Frivolous research? Not necessarily–these toe nail clippings were analyzed to give further information on the mineral selenium. Check back to Table 1-4 to see why it is important to improve knowledge of selenium. Note that it acts with vitamin E, which prevents cell damage.

The human volunteer in Figure 1-11 is being examined to see if changes in the dietary intake of some minerals such as calcium and fluoride will affect the amount of bone in her body. The television monitor shows an outline of her bones, from which measurements can be made. Return to Table

1-4 for a moment to see that dietary calcium and fluoride are involved in bone and tooth structure.

Clinical records

These give important information on the role of nutrition in certain diseases (such as heart disease, high blood pressure, and cancer) and in recovery from disease. Such studies are done usually in hospitals and may involve chemical analysis of blood, urine, or other body fluids.

In Figure 1-12, the student is measuring blood cholesterol. High cholesterol level is one indication of increased risk of coronary heart disease.

Animal experiments

Nutrition experiments on people are limited by ethical considerations, so nutritionists turn to experimental animals; rats, mice, rabbits, guinea pigs, and monkeys are used most often. Animal experimentation allows nutrition studies that could not be done on humans. For example, healthy animals can be made severely deficient in one or more nutrients. Much of the information on the action of vitamins and minerals in people was obtained from animal studies. Surgical alterations in animals have improved our understanding of both obesity and digestion. Genetic differences within a species of experimental animal are used to determine why people respond differently to diet in diseases such as obesity, high blood pressure, and cancer in which diet may have a role. Research on experimental animals led to the discovery of some vitamins, hormones, and antibiotics, to the development of vaccines, and to organ transplantation.

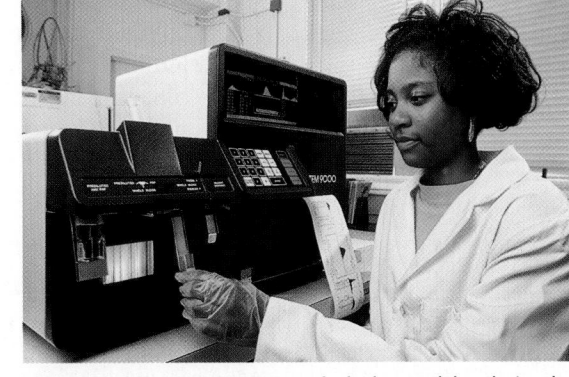

Figure 1-12. Measurement of cholesterol levels in the blood.

Some problems may arise in the use of experimental animals. A few researchers have treated animals without concern for their well-being. This is irresponsible and unscientific. At the other extreme are the irresponsible activities of some animal rights activists. Experiments have been ruined and animal facilities destroyed on some campuses and at research institutes. The appropriate middle ground is to conduct only necessary experiments with no unnecessary pain or suffering inflicted on the animal.[8,9]

Epidemiological studies

Epidemiology tries to answer questions such as why the incidence of heart disease is higher in the United States than in Japan, or why Japanese people have a higher incidence of stroke than Americans. Could differences in the diet be related to these differences in disease patterns? Epidemiologists examine relationships between the type of diet and the pattern of disease in peoples in different parts of the world. Such studies are largely responsible for the great public interest in fiber. Most people are now aware that a high fiber intake may lessen the chances of colon cancer. Epidemiological studies in Africa first suggested that a high fiber intake was associated with a low incidence of colon cancer. The fiber intake for North Americans is lower and the incidence of colon cancer is higher than for most Africans.

Epidemiology: The study of disease patterns, including diet-related disease, in different populations.

Epidemiological work is useful, but it has limitations. Differences in lifestyles, genetic background, and environmental factors, as well as medical services and other factors, must be considered before conclusions on nutritional significance can be drawn.

Comparative and evolutionary studies

Anthropologists provide useful information on the dietary intakes of people in remote parts of the world who still hunt for most of their food. This information on diet and disease patterns is compared to similar information for other people living in industrialized societies.

Wars, natural disasters, and travelers' tales

Nutrition information is obtained from people recovering from starvation after wars or who were trapped for several days without food or fluids after earthquakes and floods. Explorers in the past were useful observers of the effects of spending long periods on poor diets. The British Navy discovered hundred of years ago that if sailors on long voyages ate limes, lemons, and oranges they did not get *scurvy*, a disease that caused sore, bleeding gums. Today we know that such citrus fruits provide enough vitamin C to prevent scurvy (and British people are known as "limeys" in many parts of the world). We are now in the space age, and the effect of space travel on nutrient requirements is receiving much attention.[10]

Scurvy: Deficiency disease of vitamin C; causes soft, spongy, bleeding gums.

■ People are different–Some environmental issues affecting food and nutrition

Think about environmental issues and nutrition.

How will the foods in Figure 1-13 provide a healthy diet and a healthy environment? Are environmental issues important to you? The manufacturers of the foods in the photograph consider environmental issues to be important–note the use of the word "rainforest." This is one example of the increasing influence of environmental issues on food and nutrition. "Environmentally friendly," or as Europeans say, "green," is a term that students of nutrition and food science should treat seriously. Why? Look at what is happening. Large conferences on the environment, including its impact on food production, attract experts from all over the world. Surveys show that some people are willing to pay more for products believed to be environmentally safe, so supermarkets, food processors, and makers of packaging material are working hard to meet the demand. "Greentaxes" and "green funds" are proposed in some countries.[11] Some universities are busy preparing graduates to be "environmentally literate and responsible citizens."[12] We have "ecotourism," and the food garden becomes "edible landscaping."[13] Nutritional and environmental objectives can be integrated,

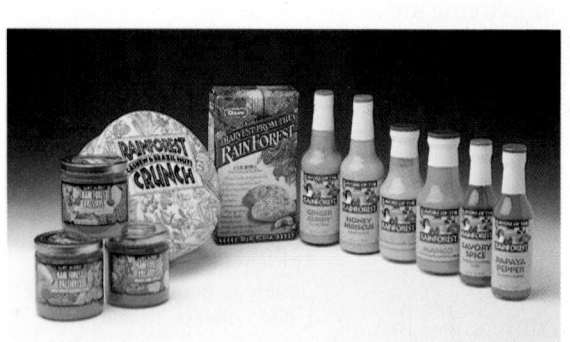

Figure 1-13. The importance of environmental protection is emphasized by the name chosen for these products.

suggests Dr. Kristin McNutt, adding a message for nutritionists that

> consumers might pay more attention to what we think is important about diet and health if we were more responsive to their interests in preserving the health of the planet earth.[14]

In any area with rapidly expanding knowledge, there are bound to be differences of opinion between experts, which create some confusion among some consumers. A major British supermarket chain provides guidelines to a "green" product.[15] As you work through this list, notice that some foods and packages will not meet all qualifications. To be called "green," a product must:

- be energy efficient,
- be nonpolluting,
- make minimum use of packaging,
- not contain harmful substances,
- where possible, be made from renewable resources,
- be recyclable,
- be capable of safe disposal,
- not harm human health,
- be made from locally obtained materials, to minimize transportation costs,
- satisfy a genuine human need.

Here is a suggestion: run through this list again using the banana as the food, to determine whether or not it is "green." The banana will meet most of these criteria. It comes in its own attractive package, which changes color to tell you when it is ready to eat. Now *that* is environmentally responsive packaging!

■ Nutrition in action–The media

There are some excellent science reporters and writers whose stories appear in the popular press as well as in more technical publications. Some of them are quoted throughout this book. However, the media likes controversy, and sometimes the issues it chooses to follow are not those that nutritionists would say were the most important.

Let's say you are a news reporter assigned to write an article about food safety and its impact on nutrition. You are given the information in Figure 1-14 on which to base your choice of topic. It shows actions and objects that entail risk and concern foods.

Which of these groups of foods will you write about? Which will get the

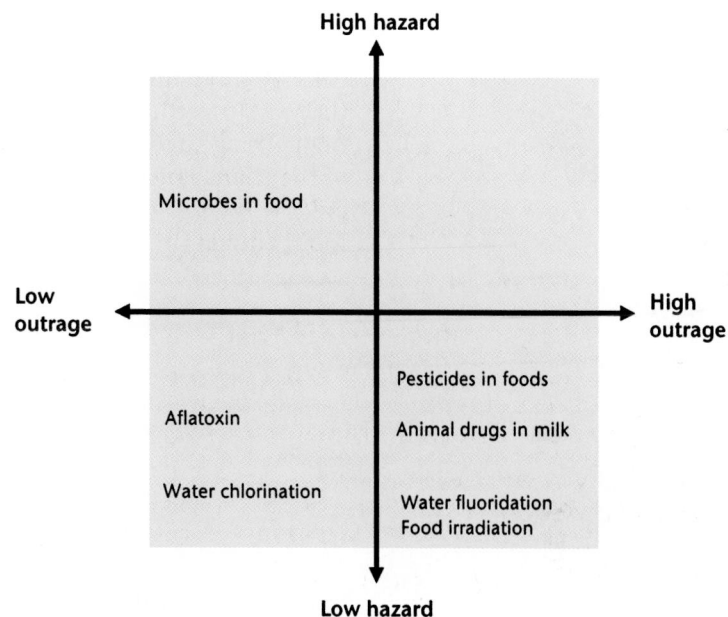

Figure 1-14. Food-related risks are rated according to consumer perceptions of their hazard and the amount of outrage the topic generates.

Hazard: Danger to health and life; involves risk. Measured by the frequency of contact multiplied by the amount of exposure.

most attention and sell the most papers? General knowledge will help with a few answers–the risks on the top half kill far more people than those in the bottom half.[16] More worry and anger is created by risks on the right than by those on the left. Now look at the food items, and you are well on the way to getting your story. Reader attention is captured when there is high outrage, so you will probably take your story from the right-hand side of the chart. The lower right-hand section has a number of food items that are low *hazards* but create high outrage in people. These are pesticides in food, animal drugs in milk, water fluoridation, and food irradiation. The top left-hand section lists microbes in foods, which are a high hazard but do not outrage people, even though food poisoning caused by bacteria results in about 9,000 deaths each year in the United States. In general, what stories are most covered by the media? The ones in the bottom right-hand corner–those with high outrage despite the low hazard involved.

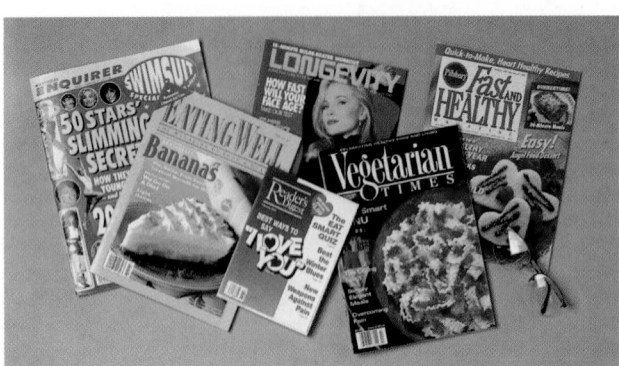

Figure 1-15. Many different magazines and newspapers are sources of nutrition information. As with other current topics, a consumer who reads widely is best able to judge the accuracy and relevance of the information they contain.

Writers for the media have knowledge about nutrition and food to varying degrees. But articles and television programs are only two of the many ways we get nutrition information. We are influenced by food advertisements, although some may have doubtful nutritional information value. Government agencies such as the U.S. Department of Health and Human Services (USDHHS) and the U.S. Department of Agriculture (USDA) distribute messages on food and nutrition. Professional health-related voluntary organizations deal with cancer, diabetes, heart disease, and other nutrition-related diseases. Finally, special-interest consumer groups represent a variety of interests in food and nutrition.[17] The popular media form just one of many groups of information sources available on food and nutrition.

■ Now you know

- The average American spends nearly $2,000 to eat nearly 2,000 pounds of food each year.

- One in every seven persons in the world is severely undernourished, with many nutrient deficiencies.

- Continued rapid growth in the world population could cause increased food shortage and nutrition problems in the future.

- Drugs and over-the-counter medications may have positive or negative effects on nutritional status.

- Nutrition is the study of the science of food and how the human body uses nutrients contained in food and drink.

- Nutritionists are also interested in non-nutrient chemicals in foods–those that give flavor, aroma, color, and texture–and in naturally occurring toxicants.

- Measurement of the excretion of waste and unabsorbed nutrients from the body indicates whether the body is absorbing nutrients efficiently.

- Information in nutrition comes from chemical analysis of food, from studies on people in good health and in illness, from comparing diet-related diseases in peoples in different parts of the world, and from animal studies.

- Environmental issues in food production are important, often very complicated, and sometimes open to misrepresentation.

- The media sometimes look for nutrition and food topics with high outrage but in which the hazards to the public may be minimal.

Further Reading

1. Anonymous. Food supply and use: Per capita consumption of major food commodities. *Agricultural Outlook*, page 64, October 1992.
2. World Health Organization. Commission on Health and the Environment. *Report of the Panel on Food and Agriculture*. WHO, Geneva, Switzerland, 1992.
3. *The Surgeon General's Report on Nutrition and Health*. Chapter 18: Drug-nutrient interactions. Prima Publishing and Communications, Rocklin, California, 1988.
4. Report of a Joint FAO/WHO Consultation. *Strategies for Assessing the Safety of Foods Produced by Biotechnology*. World Health Organization, Geneva, Switzerland, 1991.
5. Jones, J. M. *Food Safety*. Eagan Press, St. Paul, Minnesota, 1992.
6. Scheuplein, R. J. The real cancer risks in our food. In: *Global Food Progress 1991*. D. T. Avery, ed. Hudson Institute, Indianapolis, Indiana, page 155, 1991.
7. Low, A. G. Nutritional regulation of gastric secretion, digestion and emptying. *Nutrition Research Review* 3:229, 1990.
8. Lachmann, P. The use of animals in research–Medical progress depends on it. *British Medical Journal* 305:1, 1992.
9. Porter, D. G. Ethical scores for animal experiments. *Nature* (London) 356:101, 1992.
10. Lane, H. A. Nutrition in space: Evidence from the U.S. and the U.S.S.R. *Nutrition Reviews* 50:3, 1992.
11. Wittwer, S. H. The "greening effect." Implications for consumer food choices. *Food and Nutrition News* 64(3):1, 1992.
12. Cortese, A. D. Education for an environmentally sustainable future. *Environmental Science and Technology* 26:1108, 1992.
13. Barrett, T. M. The rebirth of the food garden. *American Horticulturist* 71(5):1, 1992.
14. McNutt, K. Integrating nutrition and environmental objectives. *Nutrition Today* 25(6):40, 1990.
15. Jones, B. Green consumerism and the supermarkets. *British Food Journal* 93:8, 1991.
16. Groth, E., III. Communicating with consumers about food safety and risk issues. *Food Technology* 45(5):248, 1991.
17. Goldberg, J. P. Nutrition and health communication: The message and the media over half a century. *Nutrition Reviews* 50:71, 1992.

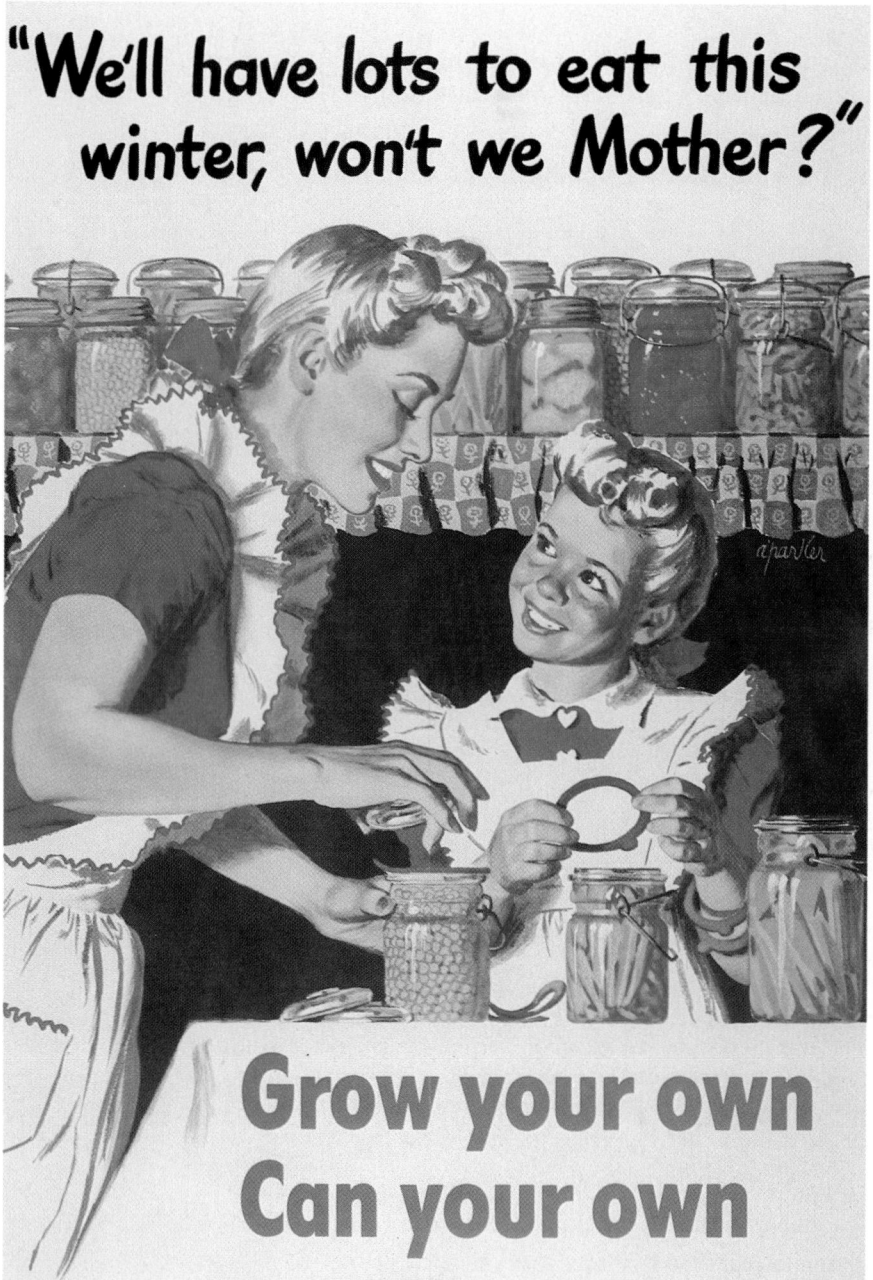

Figure 2-1. Food was in short supply in the United States, Canada, Europe, and elsewhere during World War II (1939–1945). This poster encouraged people to grow and preserve their own food.

Food: From the Field to the Plate

■ Food production and processing affect our lives in many ways

About 50 years ago, people in many parts of the world were concerned about their food supply because of the destruction caused by World War II. Even in the United States, certain foods were scarce, production systems were disrupted, and people were encouraged to contribute to the war effort by growing and preserving their own food.

Have you ever worried that the food supply might not be sufficient to keep you well fed and nourished in the future? Probably not. In the United States and other developed countries, the systems for food production and distribution usually work smoothly, and many people are not even aware of them. Today, some people eat food without any knowledge of how food is produced and processed. Others don't understand the opportunities for increasing food production through biotechnology, or the problems that biotechnology presents. Some may fail to realize that the future provision of food, and thus nutrients, on our plates depends on how many people in the world compete for the same food. Others are beginning to understand the important effect of environmental factors on food production and the availability of nutrients. The students in the Bachelor of Environmental Studies Program at York University in Toronto certainly understood the relationships among nutrition, food, and the environment when, in a letter written in December 1991 to the Prime Minister of Canada, they said,

> to emphasize the importance of a clean, healthy environment, we feel that the Constitution should guarantee that all Canadian citizens have a fundamental right to clean air, clean water, and fertile soil.

Do we realize that traditional foods eaten by people in remote parts of the world, such as the Inuit in the Arctic region of Canada, are contaminated by chemical residues from industrial and other activities around the world?[1] Probably only a few of us do. Concerns about food and the environment often arise from personal experience. Some people debate the benefits and problems of specific food additives. Others question whether food in general is safe to eat and who regulates that safety.

Are we aware that there are competing industrial uses for food produced on the farm? *New Crops, New Uses, New Markets* is the title of a book from the U.S Department of Agriculture (USDA).[2]

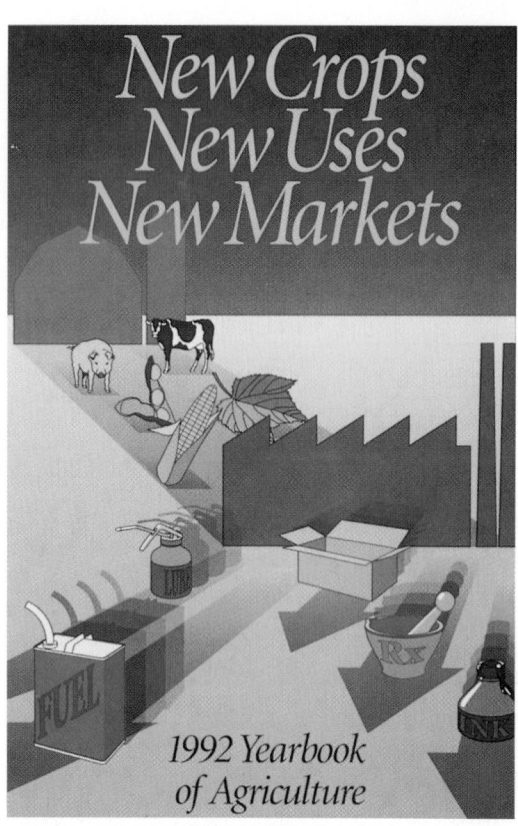

Take a moment to think of the implications of the picture on the front of that book (Figure 2-2).

It tells us that we compete with many nonfood industries for foods and nutrients. For example, oils from plant seeds may end up in food on our plates or may lubricate machines; soybeans may be used for the wide range of foods seen in the illustration in the Preface or may be converted into soy ink. Some medications come from plants and animals. For example, insulin for diabetic people comes from the pancreas of slaughtered meat animals, while plants in the rain forests are the source of many medications such as quinine, which is used to treat malaria.

Figure 2-2. Industrial uses for crops such as soybeans and corn compete with their use as food for people.

■ Food and agricultural factors affect nutrition and health

A "map" of topics that will answer some of these questions is given in Table 2-1. It will guide us as we explore the relationships among nutrition, food, and the environment. Many of these problems and opportunities in nutrition and in food science are global in scope.

Think of how each of the factors in Table 2-1 influences food availability and the intake of nutrients for you and for everybody else in the world.

■ Increased demand for food

Several trends help to increase the demand for food.

Population growth

Large increases in population growth projected for 30 years ahead were seen in Chapter 1 (Figure 1-2). Our inability to correct the poor production and distribution of food and the severe nutritional deficiencies that exist today provides little cause for optimism about improvements for the 3.5 billion more people who may be in the world by the year 2032. Such a large world population will bring about increased nutrition problems due to more poverty, less food, increased spread of disease, depletion of nonrenewable resources such as water and petroleum, loss of soil and water quality, and increased emission of the gases that cause global warming and have negative effects on the *ozone layer*.[3] Science and technology must pro-

Ozone layer: A layer in the upper atmosphere consisting of ozone, a highly reactive gas. Protects life on earth by filtering out harmful ultraviolet radiation from the sun.

Table 2-1. Some Relationships Among Nutrition, Food, and the Environment

I. Food and agricultural factors affecting nutrition and health

A. Increased demand for food influenced by

Population growth

Urbanization

Food losses, wastage, and spoilage

Demand for high animal-protein diets

B. Increased food production influenced by

Productive land

Deforestation

Desertification

Increased productivity

Agricultural chemicals

Aquaculture

Biotechnology

Animal health

Animal wastes

Irrigation

Fuel

Increased exploitation of the seas

Decreased food losses

C. Environmental changes that may have negative effects on food production

Climate changes

Ozone layer depletion

Pest resistance to pesticides

Pathogens resistance to antibiotics and chemicals

Loss of genetic resources

Soil erosion and salinization of soil and water

Over-exploitation of land and water

Inappropriate agricultural systems and/or technology

II. Environmental impact on nutrition and health

A. Potential health consequences of chemical contamination of food

B. Food- and waterborne disease from biological contamination and from irrigation

C. Noncommunicable diseases associated with diet

Malnutrition (under- and overnutrition)

Deficiency diseases

Coronary heart disease, diabetes, some cancers

vide answers for these problems, which will occur during the lifetime of today's young adults.

Death rates of infants and children in developing countries decrease when improvements in nutrition, sanitation, and water supplies and a secure livelihood, better health and education of mothers, and family planning are introduced. These are positive changes, but do they produce such an increase in population that more problems with hunger then arise? Not necessarily. Experience has shown that, in some countries, population growth rates slowed when the economic status improved.

Think of reasons why environments such as the one in Figure 2-3 cause problems in food sanitation and in malnutrition.

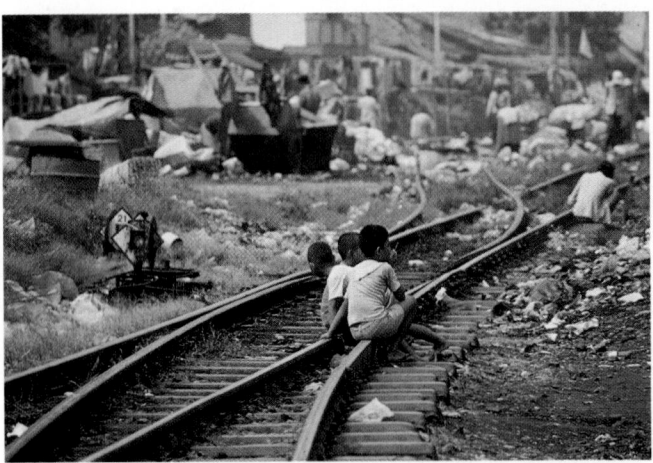

Figure 2-3. Extreme poverty usually leads to poor diets and to overcrowded living conditions, which may include unsanitary conditions for food storage and preparation.

Millet: A cereal with high fiber content grown in parts of Africa, South America, and in India. Used as a gruel or made into a flour and cooked as flat cakes. Usually considered not as attractive in taste as rice or wheat.

Sorghum: Cereal grown in semiarid regions of Africa, India, and China. Used for animal feed in the United States and Australia.

Urbanization

The growth of cities creates problems in food distribution and malnutrition.[3] The following problems become acute when people crowd into cities, especially in developing countries. The people usually change their choice of foods from root crops, maize/corn, *millet*, and *sorghum* to wheat, rice, and other foods requiring less preparation time and to foods from animals. These foods are more expensive and some must be imported, which may cause financial problems for individuals and balance of payment problems for countries. Adding to the nutrition-related problems of urbanization are poor food storage facilities, poor water supply and sanitation, and increased possibilities for the spread of disease.

Food losses, wastage, and spoilage

These are major problems in all countries. Consider the following statement:

> They lie rotting in the California desert, piled 15 feet high over areas the size of football fields. Every year something like 2 billion juicy oranges and millions of lemons have been banned by federal decree from American shops

states a writer in *The Economist* (December 19, 1992). Why?

> . . . to protect the hapless consumer from the havoc that such quantities of fruit would wreak upon prices.

This is a cynical account of how the prices of oranges and lemons are kept high by decreasing their supply. It is an example of an area where government regulations and the principles of supply and demand in economics collide with nutrition and with wastage in the food supply system. We saw in Table 1-4 that citrus fruits are excellent sources of vitamin C and other nutrients.

Wastage is a major problem throughout the world. Wasting less food can be achieved through improvements in biotechnology and in the processing, storage, transportation, and distribution of food. Biotechnology provides better ways to control the ripening and storage of fruits and vegetables. Better use of preservatives, packaging, and transportation systems will get more food to us before it spoils. In addition, education about which foods spoil most easily is needed–the largest percent waste occurs with meat and dairy products, followed by vegetables, cereal products, and fruits.[3] Education about the global responsibility to prevent food wastage is also needed. Some of this wastage is probably through ignorance.

Demand for diets high in animal protein

People in developed countries and high-income people in developing countries want foods high in animal protein, including meats, fish, dairy products, and eggs, rather than foods such as nuts, legumes, and cereals, which also contain protein (see Table 1-4). Some experts are concerned about this use of resources because meats, dairy products, and eggs are usually produced from grains fed to animals. This is inefficient utilization of cereals. Also, less grain is then available. By the year 2000, about a quarter of all cereals may be fed to animals.

■ Increased food production

The high demand for food leads, of course, to more food being produced all over the world in many different ways. The amount of food produced is influenced by many factors–and the production processes have a number of consequences.

Productive Land

This is essential to the growth of crops. But the amount of productive land in the world is decreasing because of losses to urbanization, *deforestation*, and *desertification*.

Deforestation: The permanent clearing of forest land and its conversion to nonforest uses.

Desertification: A process by which the biological productivity of land is reduced, thus causing the spread of desertlike conditions.

Look at the consequences of some of the losses in Figure 2-4.

Tropical forests equivalent in area to the state of Washington are cleared each year.[3] Why should nutritionists be concerned about the loss of forests? Why would a leading medical journal entitle an article "What are the forests worth?"[4] At first glance, these questions are puzzling because deforestation *increases* the area of land for cultivation to feed an increasing population. Forest clearances in North America and Europe centuries ago helped create farms and cities. But when trees are cut now, only short-term gains in usable land are obtained, and ecological harm is done that affects everybody. Trees absorb water and "anchor" soil to prevent it from being blown or washed away. Their leaves decay into

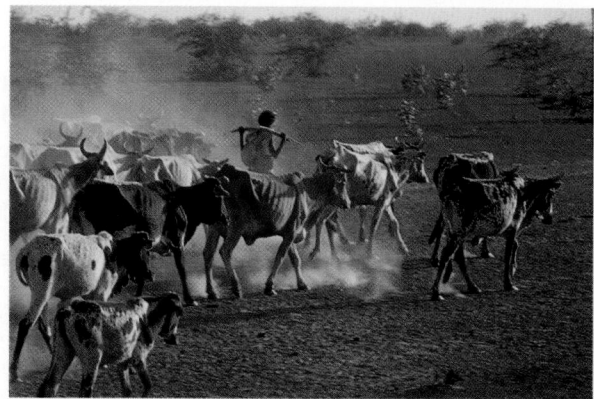

Figure 2-4. Unproductive land cannot ensure adequate food for an increasing world population.

the soil and help to bind it. During flooding, this can help lessen soil loss and the loss of crops and human lives.[3] Removal of trees causes loss of soil because the land is often overgrazed by animals and overused by people. In addition, as people move into the area, the leaves and dead tree parts that would normally decay into the soil are collected for firewood.

Deforestation also removes sources of firewood for future generations. Even today, people in rural Africa travel miles for firewood for cooking (Figure 2-5).

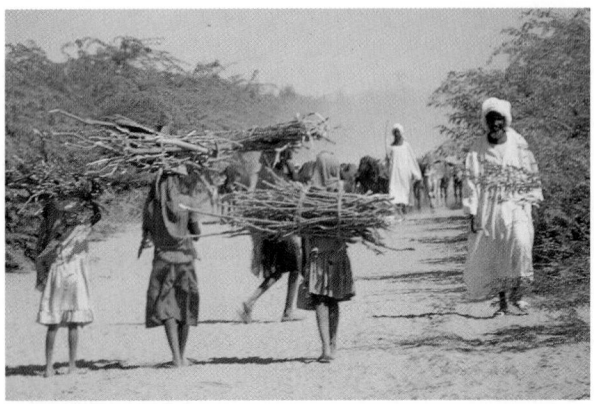

Figure 2-5. Millions of people in the world have no choice but to spend hours each day collecting and hauling firewood for cooking.

Think of the time and energy expended by some people just to get the fuel to cook food.

Without the heat energy from trees and shrubs to cook their staple foods, rural people may be malnourished because they must live off roots and berries. These are of poorer nutritional value than grains or beans and become scarcer as the demand for them grows.[5]

Excessive urbanization has produced large concentrations of people who compete for heat-producing fuels such as trees, shrubs, and brush. Cutting down trees and shrubs turns good land into desert in some areas, resulting in people having to use dried cattle manure and crop residues as fuel. This is a serious problem in parts of Africa and in India. Desertification is produced by human activities–cutting forests, inappropriate agricultural practices, and overgrazing by goats and cattle.

Increased Productivity

If there is no new land to move onto, people must use the land they have in better ways. As science and technology have increased our knowledge, ways have been found to increase the productivity of the land that is available.

Agricultural chemicals–Pros and cons

Chemicals produce mixed benefits in food production. Fertilizers and pesticides increase crop yield and quality when applied appropriately, but if used indiscriminately, they may contaminate the water we drink and the plants and animals we eat.

Think through the list in the margin and decide what factors may affect the quality of the water supply where you live.

Ways must be found to reduce the amount of fertilizers and pesticides used or to prevent them and environmental toxins from contaminating the lakes, rivers, and underground aquifers that supply our drinking water. If not, regulations may be needed that will change the variety, quantity, and quality of farm products and production systems. This could reduce the availability of food, with resulting higher food prices for consumers.[5] Is it unrealistic to think this may happen? Unfortunately, it happens already. People are advised not to eat certain fish from the Great Lakes and some polluted rivers in the United States because of their content of certain environmental toxins.

Think beyond Figure 2-6 to the implications for all of us.

Factors Affecting Water Quality

Application of chemicals to parks and lawns

Crop dusting

Excessive fertilizer application

Livestock waste

Irrigation

Deforestation

Soil erosion

Storm-water runoff

Road-salt runoff

Marine waste

Municipal sewage disposal

Septic system

Hazardous waste disposal

Industrial emission

Strip mining

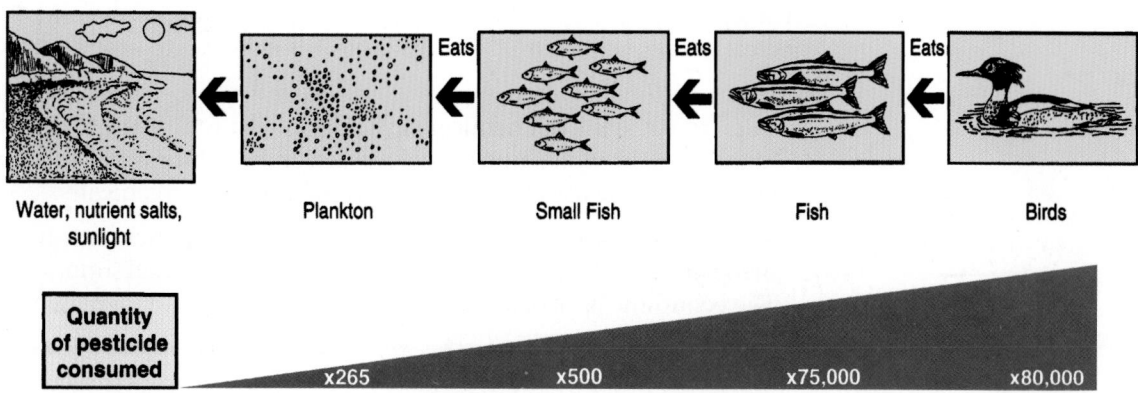

Figure 2-6. Bioconcentration occurs when tiny quantities of chemicals in the environment are concentrated into larger quantities as they pass through the food chain to fish and birds.

Look at how environmental toxins may be concentrated very rapidly in the food chain. Plankton, small animal and vegetable organisms floating in oceans, are eaten by small fish. Then larger fish eat smaller ones, and some birds live entirely on fish. The resulting accumulation of environmental toxins is called *bioconcentration*. This process varies with different toxins and different species; some pesticides nowadays are biodegradable and do not bioconcentrate. But, most pesticides and environmental toxins are soluble in fat. As a result, fish with high fat content, such as lake trout, brown trout, and large salmon, may have the highest bioconcentration of toxins. If these high-fat fish have been caught in polluted waters, they should be eaten in small amounts with as much fat as possible removed.

Bioconcentration: Increasing concentrations of a chemical (toxin, pesticide, pollutant) in organisms further up the food chain. The food chain goes from simple forms of life and small species to larger animals, fish, birds, and ultimately to people.

Think for a moment about how pesticides influence the production and consumption of food.

People have always struggled to find ways to control insects, rodents, weeds, and other pests. They have used magic, prayers, processions, fires, urine, soap suds, tobacco, lime, and in extreme cases, arsenic. (Arsenic, the favored poison of writers of murder novels, is very poisonous.) Pesticides now replace all of these.

Some of the greatest achievements and disappointments in the use of fertilizers and pesticides marked the so-called "Green Revolution," which began in the 1960s, especially in India and other Asian countries. Consider the following thoughts by U.S. Vice-President Al Gore in his book *Earth in the Balance* (1992):

> Although the Green Revolution produced great increases in food production in Third World countries, it often relied on environmentally destructive techniques: heavily subsidized fertilizers and pesticides, the extravagant use of water in poorly designed irrigation schemes, the exploitation of the short-term productivity of soil (which sometimes led to massive soil erosion) . . . .

This, of course, is one opinion. Although some experts on the Green Revolution agree with such an assessment, others disagree.

Do we need pesticides? Yes, according to a recent report from the British Medical Association (BMA),[6] because they do several important things.

- **Improve food quality.** People want the unblemished produce that results from the use of chemical pesticides, and it is difficult to detect any differences in taste, nutritional value, or healthiness between foods grown with the use of chemicals and those grown organically.

- **Reduce food prices.** Pesticides and fertilizers, together with improvements in plant and animal breeding, create an increased supply of food. The economic laws of supply and demand say that an increased supply leads to a reduction in price.

- **Maintain public health.** Pesticides kill disease-bearing insects and rodents, which are a danger to health. This is especially important in developing countries.

- **Promote animal welfare.** Pesticides kill flies that cause irritation and maggots that literally eat sheep alive, and they prevent blindness and gangrene in cattle.

- **Banish hard, exhausting work.** Pulling weeds by hand is backbreaking and exhausting. Herbicides that kill weeds remove the need for this work. However, this success has caused unemployment for some farm workers. The economic impact of unemployment can lower nutrient intakes.

- **Help habitat management.** Herbicides are used in wildlife habitat management, in parks, and by water authorities to control the growth of weeds without harming fish.

- **Are simple and convenient to use.** Herbicides are generally effective and can solve several pest problems at once.

With so many good things to say about pesticides, are there any concerns? Yes, there are two concerns. One is for the health of the environment; the other is for the health of people. We saw above that inappropriate use of pesticides and fertilizers can contaminate the water supply and soil. Public awareness of the dangers to the environment of indiscriminate use of pesticides was widely publicized in 1962 with the publication of the book *Silent Spring* by Rachel Carson. This book still commands public attention, but some of its major conclusions have been challenged. Harvard University nutritionist Dr. Fred Stare observes that people's unfounded fear of chemicals is greater today than when Rachel Carson wrote her book.[7]

To look at human health concerns, we need to make a distinction between two types of exposure to toxic substances. One is *acute exposure*, in which a high single dose results in poisoning. This can occur because of accidental or occupational poisoning, mainly due to inadequate protection of workers. The other is *chronic exposure*–long-term intakes of lower or intermittent doses of pesticides. The health significance of this exposure is more difficult to assess.

Studies among adults indicate that they have the following long-term health concerns about pesticide intake:[6]

Acute exposure to a toxin: A high dose of a toxin, resulting in poisoning.

Chronic exposure to a toxin: Long-term low or intermittent doses of a toxin, resulting in poisoning.

- Carcinogenicity (capacity to cause cancer)
- Mutagenicity (capacity to damage genetic material)
- Teratogenicity (capacity to damage the fetus)
- Allergic and other effects on the immune system
- Effects on the nervous system.

The chronic exposure of children to pesticides is of particular concern to some people.[6] Why? There are several reasons.

- Studies on experimental animals show that some (but by no means all) chemicals, including pesticides, affect the young more than adults.

- The newborn of many species retain more of certain toxins than adults because of their stage of growth and development. They absorb more from the gastrointestinal tract and excrete less.

- There is some evidence of greater cancer risks when exposure to carcinogens is in early life rather than during adulthood.

- Neurotoxins, including neurotoxic pesticides, have possible subtle effects on the developing nervous system of young people. Much of this effect could be the result of the higher consumption of certain foods by children than by adults when consumption is expressed on a per pound or per kilogram of body weight basis.

Even extremely low intakes of pesticides by the mother may result in her breast milk containing pesticides, especially the fat-soluble ones. This can be a problem in some countries for two reasons. First, pesticides may not be controlled, resulting in higher levels in the mother's diet. Second, mothers are advised to breast-feed, exposing a large number of infants to pesticides at an early age. A World Health Organization report on chemical contaminants in food concludes:

> The reported levels of pesticides and other contaminants in human milk at certain times result in estimated intakes by the breast-fed infant that exceed toxicologically acceptable intake levels. Whether such intakes are detrimental to a child's progress in terms of physical or possibly mental development is not known.

Most of the pesticides referred to here are the organochlorines, which are now used mainly in developing countries. In the United States, a report by the National Academy of Sciences on pesticides in the diets of infants and children was published in 1993. Much of the report deals with differences, if any, in the health effects of pesticides among infants, children, and adults. It also deals with the need to make special efforts to assess the risk to infants and children and on ways to provide extra protection for these most vulnerable sections of the population.

Risk assessment—A tool for evaluating chemicals

Think for a moment about risks.

The risk associated with an agent is defined as the exposure (concentration plus frequency of contact) multiplied by the *toxicity*. The key to lowering risk is to lower exposure.

Toxicity: The extent, quality, or degree of being poisonous.

You can implement a number of positive actions to reduce hazard or risk if you remember that nothing in life is risk-free. Unfortunately, common perceptions of risks differ from those of experts–take a look at how experts and college students rank various risks.

How would you rank the risks in Table 2-2?

Notice that college students and experts both rank food preservatives and food coloring low on the risk list. Pesticides are considered a fairly high risk by students. According to a 1991 survey by the Food Marketing Institute, consumers consider pesticides to be the most serious hazard, followed by antibiotics and hormones in poultry and meat, irradiated foods, and artificial colors. However, you can see from the table that experts consider the risk from exposure to pesticides to be much less than the risk from several common activities.

If life has many risks and exposure to pesticides is just one of them, what can we do to minimize this risk? We can take precautions with our own food, and we can encourage food growers and processors to take steps to ensure food safety.

Table 2-2. Ranking of Activities and Technologies in Order of Risk[a]

Risk	Ranking by	
	Experts	College Students[b]
Automobiles	1	5
Smoking	2	3
Alcoholic drinks	3	7
Handguns	4	2
Surgery	5	11
Motorcycles	6	6
X-rays	7	17
Pesticides	**8**	**4**
Food preservatives	14	12
Food coloring	21	20

[a] 1 = highest risk.
[b] Students ranked nuclear power as the greatest risk.

While the jury is still out on studies of effects on children, we can, if we are using commercial baby foods, question manufacturers about their monitoring of pesticides where fruits and vegetables are grown and processed. Most processors are very careful to minimize pesticide residues in their products. For people who prepare their own baby food, here are some tips from the Food and Drug Administration (FDA). As you read through the list, note that these tips can be used in food preparation irrespective of a person's age.

- Wash fresh fruits and vegetables with water and scrub with a brush when appropriate.
- Throw away the outer leaves of leafy vegetables such as lettuce and cabbage.
- Peel and cook produce when appropriate, even though some nutrients and fiber are lost when produce is peeled.

Food processors realize that the health of the public and the reputation of their products must be protected, so they set standards for their products and monitor the production process at various stages.

Look at the many checks proposed for monitoring the amount of pesticides in food (Figure 2-7).[8]

This approach to pesticide control in processed food uses principles of *hazard analysis and critical control points (HACCP)*. This is a management technique that monitors food safety (levels of pesticides, microorganisms,

Hazard analysis and critical control points (HACCP): A method of monitoring food safety by anticipation and prevention of problems. (Other monitoring methods use inspection of finished products.)

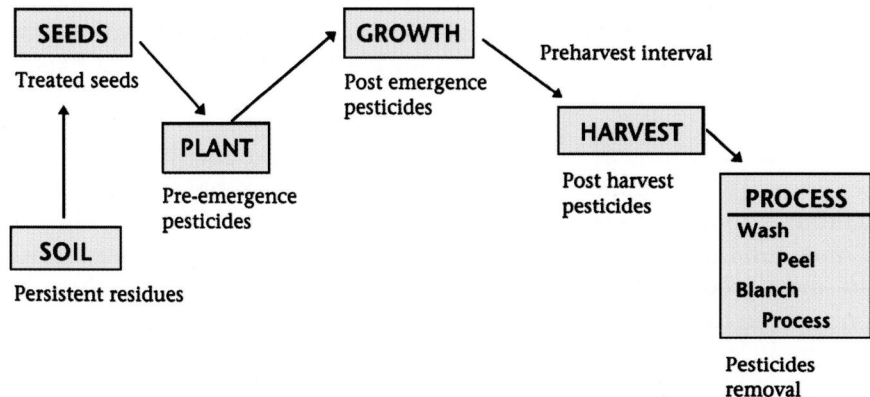

Figure 2-7. An example of hazard analysis and critical control points (HACCP) in the growing and processing of food.

and pollutants) by anticipation and prevention, in contrast to inspection of the result. The HACCP approach is approved by the FDA and USDA as the best way to monitor food safety.

The ideal sought by most people is for pesticides to be used with full knowledge of their safe use and in minimal amounts only as needed. The risk of the consequences above must be balanced against the benefits of pesticides. Experts conclude that pesticides will continue to play a dominant role in animal and plant disease control in the future.[9]

Meanwhile, there are encouraging developments in integrated pest management (IPM), which is used to minimize pesticide use.[10] We had a brief introduction to IPM in the Preface in the four options for what to do with the insects. The third option discussed a biological approach–the insect eating the plant is eaten by an insect that will not harm the plant. Other methods to replace or reduce pesticide use that may be included in IPM programs include proper tillage practices, crop rotation (planting different crops from season to season in the same area), and proper water management.

Before we leave pesticides, here is a parting thought.

Think beyond the numbers in Figure 2-8.

The estimated risk to human health is 50 times *greater* from one mushroom than from the amount of the contaminant PCB in your food. Should you stop eating mushrooms? No. Should you eat a lot of mushrooms often? Probably not. What should you do? You can do something useful immediately that agrees with all experts on the safety of pesticides–eat a balanced diet! This means food from a wide variety of sources, which will dilute the amount of pesticides, naturally occurring toxicants, and other toxic chemicals in your diet. Be alert to the latest reliable information because the debate goes on: "Scientists term food-pesticide cancer risk overrated" is a headline from *The Wall Street Journal* (October 9, 1992). Balance this against the fact that at least 27 pesticides approved for use in the United States are listed as possible carcinogens in humans by the U.S. Environmental Protection Agency (EPA). It is no accident that the word

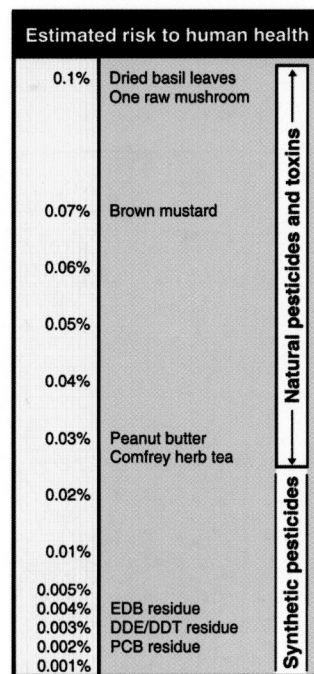

Figure 2-8. The estimated risk to human health is lower from some synthetic pesticides than from natural pesticides and some food toxins.

"balance" is used twice in this paragraph–balance in diet and balance in sources of information. Following this advice will make you better equipped to make the correct choices in your diet.

Aquaculture

Aquaculture: Fish farming.

Aquaculture is another method of increasing the productivity of existing resources. Fish are important sources of protein (see Table 1-4), and aquaculture is found all over the world.[11] In many Asian countries, such as China, rural communities use fish ponds to recycle some food waste. Fish are mass produced in many countries under seminatural conditions in ponds or in floating cages in rivers, lakes, or the sea. Aquaculture is important in increasing food production in many countries. But some environmental and food safety prices must be paid. These systems may be exposed to chemical pollution and oil spills. Many chemicals are used to prevent health problems in the fish–disinfectants to kill bacteria, herbicides to control plant growth in ponds, vaccines to fight certain diseases, and drugs to treat diseases and parasites[12]–and some of them may be used illegally. Drugs and medications are important because diseases spread rapidly in such dense fish populations. Some of these chemicals may remain as residues in the fish flesh. FDA inspectors monitor fish farming, and products passing inspection can carry the seal "Packed Under Federal Inspection" on the label or carton.

Biotechnology

"Biotechnology" is a word that has been around since 1919 to describe interactions between biology and technology. Now it usually means ge-

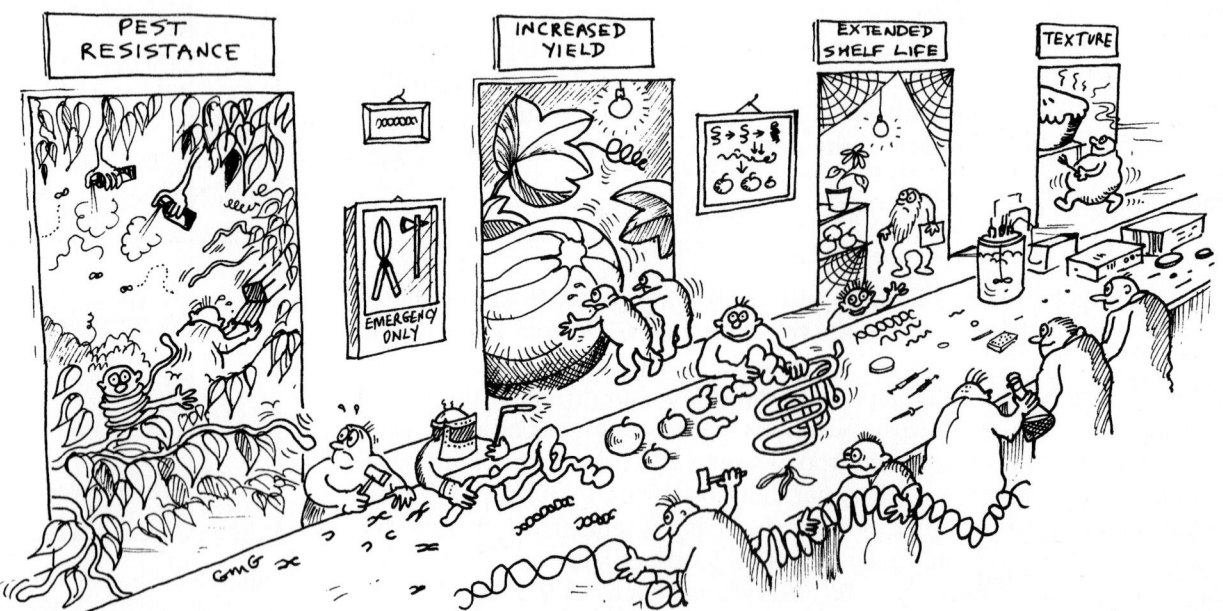

Figure 2-9. A cartoonist's depiction of biotechnology. Notice some of the things biotechnology has created that make food more available.

netic engineering, but the term is constantly evolving. Difficulties in defining and understanding biotechnology cause some of the general public to see biotechnology as pictured in the cartoon in Figure 2-9.

Biotechnology is *not* a bunch of mad scientists playing around unknowingly with our food. As the cartoon demonstrates, biotechnology has improved pest resistance and increased the yield of crops, has extended the *shelf life* of some foods, and has improved food texture. You have "tasted the fruits" of biotechnology. Have you eaten some of the following foods within the past week?

Shelf life: The period during which foods can be stored without spoiling.

Alfalfa	Corn	Rye
Apple	Cotton	Soybean
Asparagus	Cucumber	Sugar beet
Bean	Lettuce	Sunflower
Cabbage	Pea	Sunflower
Cabbage	Pea	Tomato
Carrot	Potato	Wheat
Celery	Rice	

You probably have. Are you disturbed when told that these foods may have been subjected to techniques in biotechnology? These genetic modifications are often made to help the plant resist or tolerate herbicides, insects, and viruses. Now look at the door labeled "Extended Shelf Life" in the Figure 2-9. Shelf life can be extended by various methods. In the case of tomatoes, these are delaying ripening, controlling softening, preventing rotting by fungi, and storing by freezing. This is one example of how biotechnology makes more food last longer at less expense. Other examples are included in Tables 2-3 and 2-4.

Table 2-3. Biotechnology Products for the Food Industry

Product	Use
Enzymes	For cheese making; meat tenderizer; to make "Lite" beer; to make high-fructose corn syrup (sweetener)
Vitamins	Nutritional supplements
Low-calorie products	Non-nutritive sweeteners; food additives
Flavors and pigments	Flavor and coloring agents
Amino acids	Nutritional supplement; production of aspartame (intense sweetener marketed under the brand name NutraSweet)
Single-cell protein	Animal and human food supplement
Organic acids	Food preservatives; acidulants (used in curing and pickling, flavor enhancers, flavoring agents, antioxidants)

Table 2-4. Uses of Biotechnology in Farming

Crop or Livestock	Improvement from Biotechnology
Grains	Pest and drought resistance, higher yields, more and higher-quality protein
Fruits and vegetables	Pest resistance, more flavor, higher nutrition
Poultry	Disease resistance, faster growth, more eggs
Beef cattle, sheep, hogs	Disease resistance, faster growth, leaner meat
Dairy cattle	More milk, improved nutritive value
Fish	Faster growth, larger size, disease resistance

Should nutritionists be interested in biotechnology? Certainly. Consider the following list taken from chapter titles in a recent book on biotechnology and nutrition:[13]

low-calorie diets . . . bioengineering of meat . . . biological conversion of inedible biomass to food . . . changes in carbohydrates, proteins, edible oils . . . nutritional enhancement of vitamins and minerals.

Let's tie all of the above information together with the picture in Figure 2-10.

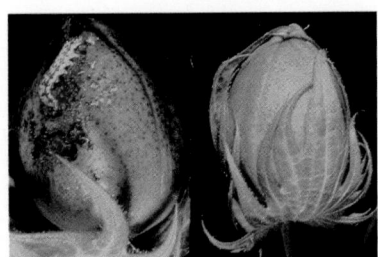

Figure 2-10. Techniques in biotechnology increased the ability of the cotton boll on the right to resist damage from insects. An untreated boll (left) shows typical insect damage.

The cotton plant shown on the right was genetically improved to resist the cotton bollworm, while the conventionally grown cotton plant on the left is heavily damaged by the worms. Maybe your first reaction is: Why is cotton discussed in a book on nutrition, food, and the environment? But look at this–genetic engineering improves cotton, producing positive effects on:

- **Oil quality:** Oil extracted from cotton seeds is used in margarine, cooking oil, and other foods and in the cosmetic industry.

- **Seed protein:** Cottonseed is used for animal feed and in the food industry.

- **Insect and herbicide resistance:** This increases plant yield and improves the ecosystem.

- **Environmental stress resistance** (to heat, drought, and cold stress): This increases plant yield and quality.

- **Fiber modification:** This affects the quality of textiles, carpets, personal care products, and biomedical applications.

At the beginning of this chapter we saw that many of our foods have industrial and other uses. The next time you spread margarine on bread or cook with cottonseed oil, you may be aware of the close scientific relationship between these foods and the cotton clothes you wear.

All of the above looks great, but are there any problems with biotechnology as it applies to our food and nutrient supply? No, says the Institute of Food Technologists.[14] The safety of foods produced by biotechnology will be assured through the same laws and standards that are applied to traditional foods. No, say officials at FDA, but

substances that raise safety concerns would be subjected to closer inquiry. This approach is both scientifically and legally sound and should be adequate to fully protect public health while not inhibiting innovation.[15]

No, says the American Medical Association (AMA).[16] The Council on Scientific Affairs of the AMA recommends that the AMA

endorse or implement programs that will convince the public and government officials that genetic manipulation is not inherently hazardous and that the health and economic benefits of recombinant DNA technology greatly exceed any risk posed to society.

However, the approval of biotechnology by an organization representing food scientists and technologists, a government agency responsible for food regulations, and representatives of the medical profession fails to answer the question of why some people are concerned about biotechnology. Dr. Christine Bruhn of the University of California, Davis, provides three reasons for the concerns.[17] First, the public does not understand biotechnology or its potential uses; people can be influenced by emotions. Second, environmental risks may be associated with the release of engineered organisms into the environment. Third, the social, economic, and ethical implications of biotechnology have the potential to arouse strong public reaction. Her answer to all of these issues is more and better education of the benefits and risks of biotechnology.

Let's look briefly at one technique in biotechnology that has both proponents and critics—the production and use of *bovine somatotropin (BST)*, also called bovine growth hormone. BST is a natural protein produced in all cattle—it is not a steroid. Proponents of BST include some farmers because it increases milk production by 15–20%. If this higher milk production is all consumed, people may have greater intakes of the protein, calcium, phosphorus, riboflavin, and other nutrients that are in milk (see Table 1-4) and at a lower cost. Pharmaceutical companies are happy because projections suggest BST sales of $1 billion per year. Some medical researchers have found that only a very small amount of BST finds its way into milk and that what does is biologically inactive in humans.[18]

Are there any criticisms of BST? Yes. Consumer lobbyists are concerned that BST might be toxic to people when it is eaten and that it causes unnecessary pain to cows, destroys the environment, and might put small farmers out of business. Let's look at these concerns. We saw above that the first argument—might be toxic to people when eaten—is not true based on present evidence. The second, causing unnecessary pain to cows, is an objection with merit. Increased milk yield leads to mastitis (inflammation of the udder) in some cattle. Mastitis is treated with antibiotics that can carry through to the milk and meat we consume if not properly administered, although tests for this are widely available and used. If this happens, people can develop an increased tolerance for antibiotics. Third, destruction of the environment is argued because of the fact that more grass is eaten and, therefore, more waste is created. This argument does not carry much weight, as the numbers are small. Finally, whether or not small farmers go out of business is determined by many factors other than BST, including the law of supply and demand. Increased supply will come from the promised 15–20% increase in milk yield. If there is no increase in demand for milk, the price of milk will decrease. FDA approved BST in the spring of 1994, after its ultimate fate had been wrestled with by lobbyists, scientists, farmers, the pharmaceutical industry, environmentalists, economists, and government regulators.

Let's look at how BST is made. The flow diagram on the left in Figure 2-11 shows the major components in BST manufacture. On the right is the typical pattern of public opinion and government regulation that arises from controversial issues such as biotechnology. The science in this diagram is not intimidating if you remember that genetically manipulated

Bovine somatotropin (BST): A natural hormone produced by cattle that can be produced also by biotechnology. It is injected into cattle, resulting in higher milk yields.

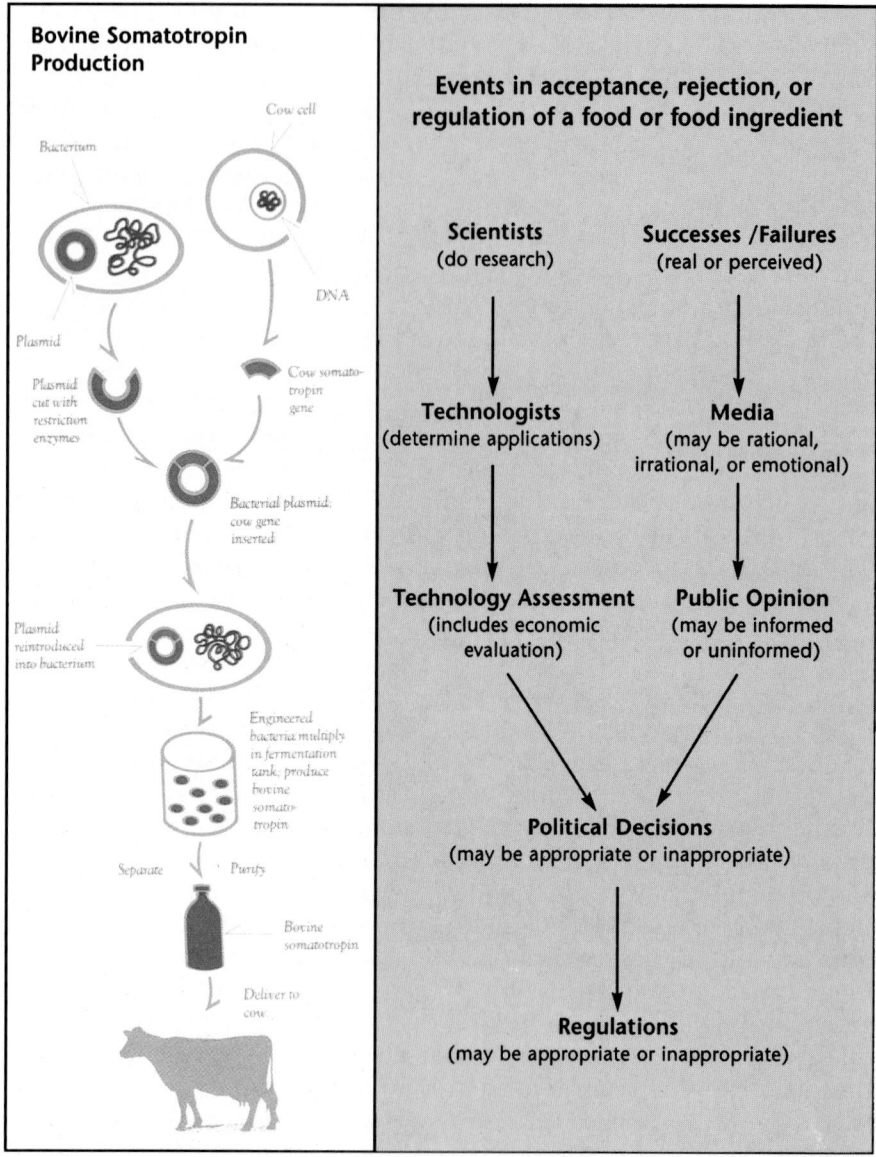

Figure 2-11. Left, process for making bovine somatotropin (BST), or bovine growth hormone. Right, genetically engineered compounds such as BST frequently pass through this sequence of events leading to acceptance, rejection, or regulation.

Plasmid: A small circular form of DNA that carries certain genes and can reproduce independently in a host cell.

DNA (deoxyribonucleic acid): A nucleic acid that contains hereditary information in humans, animals, plants, and microbes. Directs protein synthesis.

bacteria are used as a kind of "factory" to produce large quantities of BST. The two important starting points are the *plasmid* from the bacterium and DNA taken from a cow cell. *DNA (deoxyribonucleic acid)* is the molecule containing hereditary information in humans, animals, plants, and microorganisms. The plasmid is a small circular form of DNA that carries certain genes and is capable of reproducing independently in a host cell. This makes it ideal for combination with the gene from the cow that is coded to make BST. The plasmid is put back into the bacteria, which multiply at a rapid rate. The BST produced by the bacteria is separated and purified and can then be injected into the cow.

Although BST has been available for marketing since 1981, it became available commercially only in early 1994. Yet, in 1990, a 70-foot-high pile of documents on the drug's effectiveness and safety that cost $500 million to collect was submitted to regulatory agencies, reported *The Economist* (August 11, 1990). The parting message is that the introduction of new drugs, additives, and other chemicals into the food supply is a long, uncertain, and costly business.

Animal health

Another factor that affects the amount of food that is produced is animal health. It is a major concern because of its role in nutrition and its interaction with the environment. Animal diseases decrease food production by reducing the amount of meat, dairy products, and eggs available. A look back to Table 1-4 confirms that these foods contribute protein and many vitamins and minerals to our diet. Animal feeds are made from fish meal, bone, and blood and from plant sources such as the cereal grains and soybeans. Much of the animal feed used in many countries is contaminated with *pathogens*, especially *Salmonella*.[11] Many animals become subclinically infected carriers but appear healthy and so the pathogen cannot be detected, although pathogens such as *Salmonella* and *Campylobacter* are passed in their feces. This contaminates the environment–surface water and soil–and also wet surfaces during slaughter, meat processing, and distribution. This infection can cause foodborne diseases in people. To date no effective vaccine is available.

Pathogen: A microorganism or substance capable of producing a disease.

Animal waste

Another factor, animal waste, is a growing concern in both developing and developed countries, as it can be a major cause of water and air pollution.[11] We may have less food from animal sources in the future because of problems with disposal of animal waste. North America and Europe have intensive agricultural systems. A narrow range of crops is intensively grown alongside large feedlots for large numbers of animals. Since chemical fertilizers have replaced animal manure for the fertilization of crops, the manure piles up. We then have not only the possibility of water pollution from the chemical fertilizers, but also problems with the manure, which include nutrients from manure leaching into surface water or groundwater, bad smells near urban communities, and the release of gases to the atmosphere. One of the major gases is methane, which increases global warming (the greenhouse effect). Let's spend a moment examining both sides of the argument on the contribution of meat-producing animals to the production of methane. In 1992, consumer activist Jeremy Rifkin published *Beyond Beef: The Rise and Fall of the Cattle Culture,* a critical examination of the beef cattle industry. Rifkin has this to say on the first page of the book:

> Cattle are also a major cause of global warming. They emit methane, a potent global warming gas, blocking heat from escaping the earth's atmosphere.

Contrast this with what F. M. Byers of Texas A&M University has to say:

The contribution of the U.S. beef cattle industry to annual global methane production (0.1% of all global warming) is not outstanding.

Both writers do agree that much more methane is produced by rice paddies, wetlands, biomass burning, and landfills. The bottom line is that nobody denies that beef cattle do produce methane, but the relevance of its impact on global warming is debatable.

Much plant and animal waste in developing countries is used for fuel for cooking and heating. This creates further possibilities for soil loss, as these materials are not returned to the soil.

Irrigation

Providing water to crops is a long-standing method of making land more productive; it was practiced by Native Americans in what is now the southwestern United States nearly 2,000 years ago. Over the past 150 years, extensive irrigation has been developed in the United States, especially in California and the Southwest.

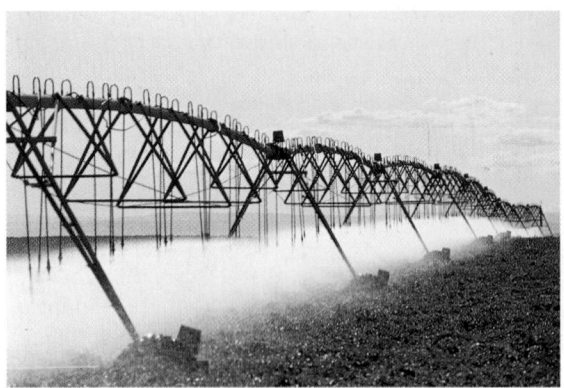

Irrigation (Figure 2-12) helps provide a wide variety of food that would otherwise be less available. In developing countries, many irrigation projects have improved income, food supply, and health. But four problems confront the future of irrigation. One, we may run out of available water in the future–agriculture is in competition with water demands for industry and home use. Two, salt increases in the soil as a result of evaporation, and salinity is harmful to many plants. Three, the cost of fuel to pump water is high. Four, more than 30 diseases are linked to irrigation projects and dams in tropical countries.[3]

Figure 2-12. Irrigation is necessary for crops in many parts of the world. In the future, a shortage of water may restrict the use of irrigation.

Fuel

Fuel is important in modern agriculture for farm equipment and fertilizer production. Higher fuel prices cause problems for many farmers and fishermen, especially in developing countries.

Increased Exploitation of the Seas

A third way in which food production can be increased (besides finding productive land and making it more productive) is to increase our use of the sea. The nutritional and health benefits of eating fish are great. Fish are the major source of protein in some countries, and in others, such as the United States, consumption of fish has increased in recent years as people became more health-conscious. However, the problem of overfishing causes concern. In 1992, Canada implemented a ban on cod fishing off Newfoundland, which was once one of the richest fishing areas in the world. Some modern methods of fishing scoop up all young and old fish and thus lower future stocks of fish.

Decreased Food Losses

We are now at the last of the factors influencing the supply of food in the world–decreased food losses. We can increase our supply of food by taking better care of the food we have. Foods spoil because of microbiological, chemical, physical, or enzyme-induced decay. Decreasing food losses in warehouses, supermarkets, restaurants, and homes is achieved mainly by food preservation and food additives.

Food preservation is simple in some parts of the world, complex in other parts (Figures 2-13 and 2-14).

Since the earliest times, people have struggled to keep food from spoiling. Today we have a wide choice of preservation methods, most involving the addition or removal of heat from food to retard or inactivate spoilage-causing mechanisms. The methods are of several types:

- Physical: Drying, heating, cooling, irradiation

- Chemical: Adding sugar, salt, or chemical preservatives; smoking; and blanching

- Biological: Fermentation

Drying, heating, adding sugar or salt, fermentation, and smoking have been used for thousands of years to preserve food. Canning, refrigeration, freezing, pasteurization, and sterilization are of more recent vintage. Irradiation is the latest method and one that concerns some experts and the general public. But then, pasteurization and canning were not greeted with enthusiasm when they were first introduced.

The preservation technique can affect the nutrient content of the diet. As we look at the methods in more detail, notice which ones increase or decrease nutrients.

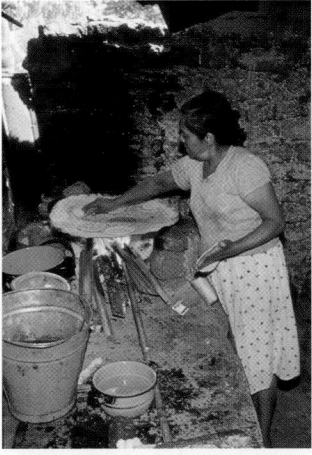

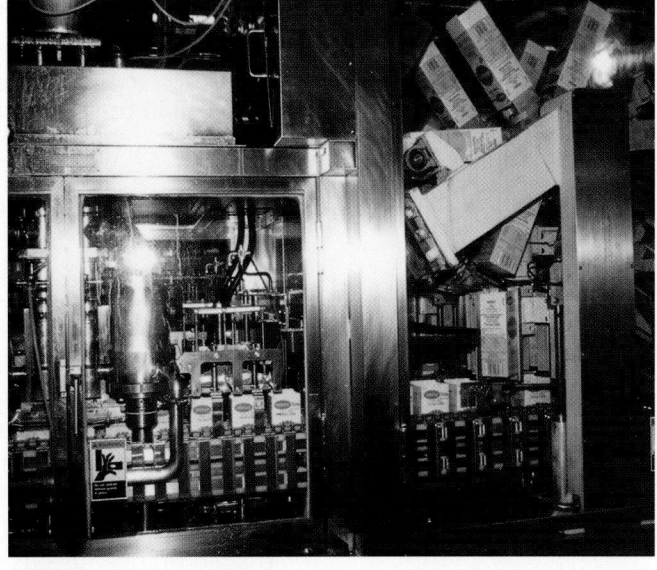

Figures 2-13 and 2-14. Many people in the world must preserve and prepare food under simple time-consuming conditions (left), whereas people with sufficient income can buy convenience as well as greater assurance of food safety (below).

Drying

Drying preserves food because microorganisms cannot survive when water is removed. Even thousands of years ago, people realized that when food was dried it kept longer. Drying was done by sun and wind in ancient times and still is in certain parts of the world. In industrial countries, drying food is expensive because of the high cost of fuel. The food industry uses oven drying, spray drying (mainly for milk products), and freeze-drying. A problem with drying by heating is that it causes loss of heat-sensitive nutrients such as vitamin C, riboflavin, and niacin (see Table 1-4).

Canning

Canning, either commercially or in the home, kills harmful or spoilage-causing microbes and their spores. Heat must be controlled carefully so as to kill all harmful microorganisms but keep nutrient loss at a minimum. Further losses of water-soluble nutrients, such as certain vitamins, occur when the food is canned in water, especially since people usually discard this water before eating the food. Home canning of food must be done with care. Canning temperatures that are too low and improper seals on the canning jars permit botulism poisoning caused by *Clostridium botulinum*. A number of deaths occur each year because of improper home canning; this is very rare with commercially canned foods.

Refrigeration and freezing

These are the two best methods for maintaining the sensory qualities and nutritive value of foods. However, even these techniques are not without problems. When meat is thawed, some vitamins and minerals may be lost in the drippings. The potentially fatal microbe *Listeria* has the ability to grow at certain refrigeration temperatures. Even the home refrigerator has been in the news lately because its cooling system contains chlorofluorocarbons (CFCs), which eventually leak into the atmosphere and degrade the ozone layer above the earth that protects us from the damaging effects of shortwave ultraviolet rays from the sun. A breakthrough may be at hand in the form of a hydrofluorocarbon, which could replace the damaging CFCs.[19]

Pasteurization

Heating foods to a specified high temperature for a short time kills most disease-causing microbes and their spores. Pasteurized food is not sterile, so refrigeration or other preservation techniques must be used also. When milk and fruit juices are pasteurized, considerable amounts of vitamin C are lost. What are the nutrition implications of this? Not much; milk is low in vitamin C. The amount of vitamin C remaining in one cup of heat-treated orange juice is 86 milligrams–an amount greater than the recommended intake for vitamin C.

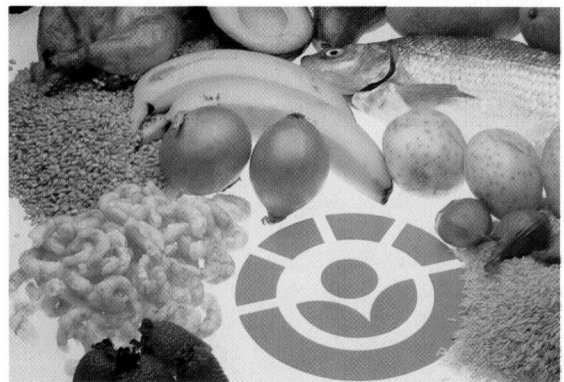

Figure 2-15. Irradiated foods look the same as nonirradiated foods; thus, they must carry the symbol of food irradiation (foreground).

Irradiation

This controversial method of preserving food has been studied for over 40 years. Irradiation reduces microbial contamination of food, kills insects and parasites, and prevents sprouting in seeds. Yet it is a means of food preservation that concerns many people, possibly because of misinformation.

Think about the foods in Figure 2-15 and at the international symbol of irradiation. Do these foods look different from other foods?

Some people think that the international symbol of irradiation looks too clean and harmless. They fear that irradiated food is "nuked" and loaded with radiation. But we live in a world full of radiation. There is radioactivity in our bodies and in soil, sand, and stones no matter where we live. Over 80% of the total radiation received by each American comes from natural background sources, according to a former chairperson of the Atomic Energy Commission. The remaining 18% that is created comes from medical X-rays, nuclear medicine, and consumer products such as smoke detectors, tobacco, and ceramics.

The foods in Table 2-5 have approval to be irradiated in the United States.

In spite of the approval, food manufacturers are not willing to use irradiation to any great extent–consumers may not purchase the food because of doubts about its safety. There are no tell-tale signs of radiation on the food above. We must accept other people's assurance that it was irradiated and that it is safe. To improve consumer information, much effort is going into developing rapid and simple tests to detect irradiated food.[20] Relatively low doses of irradiation eliminate food poisoning bacteria (*Salmonella, Listeria*, and *Campylobacter*) and common food spoilage organisms (*Pseudomonas*) in poultry and fish. Irradiation will not eliminate some spores of the deadly *Clostridium botulinum*. This is a problem, and therefore irradiation to control microbial growth is usually combined with other preservation methods, especially *modified atmosphere packaging*.

Table 2-5. Foods Approved for Irradiation in the United States

Food	Purpose
Wheat and wheat flour	To kill insects
White potatoes	To inhibit sprout development
Dry and dehydrated vegetables, including herbs, seeds, spices, vegetable seasonings, and blends of any of these, and turmeric and paprika when used as color additives	To kill insects, to disinfect
Pork	To control *Trichina* parasites
Fresh fruits and vegetables	To delay ripening and spoilage
Poultry	To kill *Salmonella* bacteria

Laws on food irradiation differ among countries. Germany has a total ban on irradiated food and Japan a partial ban, but many irradiated foods are permitted in The Netherlands. The foods allowed to be irradiated in the United States are those in Table 2-5. Which country is correct? We don't know. The long-term effects of irradiated foods on people are unknown, but most food scientists in the United States believe them to be non-existent.

Is irradiation necessary? The discussion above emphasizes the question of safety, but some people wonder whether we *need* irradiation to begin with. Some foods spoil *faster* after irradiation–pears, apples, citrus fruits, and pineapples among others. Radioactive waste material from irradiation facilities must be disposed of safely. Simpler remedies may be possible. For instance, unsanitary poultry processing plants were much criticized in the media in the early 1990s. Although most have now been restored to satisfactorily safe operation, high levels of harmful bacteria could still reach the supermarkets. Critics of irradiation of poultry contend that poultry processors should pay more attention to improper sanitation in their plants instead of trying to mask it by irradiating the poultry.

Although food scientists and government agencies endorse food irradiation, consumers apparently consider that the scientific/medical/consumer jury is still evaluating its safety. Much progress is anticipated in the next few years as better information on some of the above issues is obtained.

Modified atmosphere packaging: Changing the atmosphere within a package by extracting air and/or using various gases (such as nitrogen) to extend the shelf life of a food.

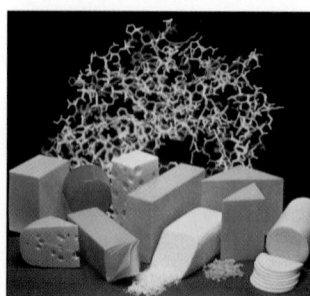

Figure 2-16. This is how a chemist "sees" chymosin, the key enzyme used in cheese manufacture.

Additives

Adding sugar, salt, and chemical preservatives influences both the shelf life and the sensory properties of food. Sugar caters to a "sweet tooth," and both sugar and salt add taste, flavor, consistency, and improved appearance to food. Both act as preservatives by lowering the *water activity* of foods. Several common chemicals prevent the growth of food-spoiling microbes. These include vinegar (acetic acid), as well as citric acid, which is used in salad dressings, relishes, and jams. Mold growth in bread is prevented by calcium propionate. Bacon has nitrite added to kill microbes that cause botulism. Nonmicrobial spoilage of food is also prevented by chemicals. For example, *BHT* and *BHA* prevent the fat in food from becoming rancid. Slightly rancid food has some of its vitamin A destroyed by the chemical process that causes rancidity. Very rancid food is not eaten by most people because of its poor taste and aroma.

Smoking

Smoke treatment kills bacteria in food and protects fat in meat. As with other methods discussed above that involve heating food, a proportion of the heat-sensitive nutrients are destroyed. Liquid smoke extract is used commercially now because it contains a lower amount of cancer-causing chemicals.

Blanching

This method (typically done by dipping vegetables in boiling water before freezing, canning, or dehydration) was first used more than 100 years ago. The heat inactivates enzymes that cause undesirable flavors and colors during storage. The least damage to heat-sensitive nutrients during blanching is done by microwaving, followed by steaming. The most damage is done by the use of boiling water.

Fermentation

Fermentation is becoming more popular because of increased demand for yogurt, soy products (tofu and miso), bread, and aged cheese. Also produced by fermentation are pickles, sauerkraut, wine, and beer. Fermented dairy products have as long a history as wine and beer–the ancient Greeks offered cheese to the gods. It is only recently that we have understood the chemistry behind such ancient practices. Figure 2-16 shows the chemical structure of one of the enzymes required to manufacture these cheeses.

Increased sales of fermented foods will probably continue because of several factors:

- Public interest in more natural products of plant origin and in more healthy foods
- The increased shelf life and convenience of many fermented foods
- Cultural and religious reasons
- Consumption of more plant foods because of population increase
- The recent scientific interest in fermented foods
- The decreased possibility of food poisoning from fermented foods

Various microbes are used in fermentation, depending on which food is produced. Some fermented foods have a high sodium content. High sodium intakes are associated with hypertension in people sensitive to sodium.

In general, processing techniques that preserve food are beneficial. Among the advantages of food preservation are:

- Food is available year around.
- Fresh foods alone cannot feed the growing world population.
- Heat applied during preservation may make foods such as beans and legumes more digestible.

■ Environmental and food production changes may have negative effects on the food supply

Climate changes and ozone layer depletion continue to appear in headlines in the news media. Whether an increase in global warming is actually occurring is a topic of debate among the experts. The implications for food production and nutrient supply are not really known. But, information on ozone depletion is now available while you eat your hamburger. A major fast-food company recently changed its containers for hamburgers from polystyrene foam shells to more environmentally friendly packaging. The polystyrene foam shells were made of materials that may damage the ozone layer. The change is a positive one, even though the paperboard alternatives also can have some adverse effect on the environment.

Emphasis on saving the planet may have significant effects on nutrition.

> Consumers may get to the point where they choose "earth-healthy" over "individual-healthy" products,

speculates nutritionist Kristin McNutt. Dr. McNutt's statement is interesting. It suggests that a study of nutrition must take environmental changes into account because our global food supply may be in danger.

Is there evidence that such dangers exist? Unfortunately, the information is incomplete. The best available evidence suggests that acid rain may not be a problem for many plants. Scientists at the USDA claim that many crops, from lettuce to winter wheat, can tolerate it. Results of the greenhouse effect are not as well understood. A British writer claims that grain yields will tumble if global warming from the greenhouse effect continues.[21] Not so, say scientists at the USDA; yields in wheat, rice, and corn will benefit from extra carbon dioxide (CO_2), a gas plants need for photosynthesis. Carbon dioxide is the gas most responsible for the greenhouse effect, and most CO_2 comes from emissions from cars, factories, planes, and homes. Other scientists do not seem to be especially worried about global warming.[22]

Pest resistance to pesticides can be triggered by a rapid evolutionary selection of existing rare resistant forms, which allows the pest to survive.[6] Put simply, those pests with advantageous differences in biology or behavior avoid death from pesticides and are then free to breed. Subsequent generations are increasingly able to continue their mischief.

Pathogen resistance to antibiotics and chemicals is the same type of process. Microbial populations can acquire resistance to the effect of antibiotics. This is a major problem in disease control in both people and animals and is the reason why many people are concerned about antibiotic residues in meat and dairy products.

Loss of variety in genetic resources (also called biological diversity or biodiversity) will be costly for the food supply of the future.[23] More than 90% of the world's land-dwelling plants and animals live in forests, particularly in tropical countries. Loss of forests and the plants in them decreases biodiversity, with negative effects on plant breeding and on resistance to disease. If plant breeders do not have access to new genetic material, all the plants in a large area may have the same genetic makeup, with the same weaknesses and susceptibility to the same microorganisms. This may have disastrous effects on the food supply and thus on the nutritional status of people, especially in developing countries. An example is the loss of over $1 billion to U.S. farmers in 1970 when a disease swept through uniformly susceptible corn varieties. Similarly, the Irish potato famine in 1846, the Russian and Ukrainian wheat crop losses in 1972, and the citrus canker outbreak in Florida in 1984, which ruined many orange trees, all arose from reductions in genetic diversity.[6] These examples have significant implications in nutrition. We should ponder well the words of Harvard biologist E. O. Wilson, who called the loss of biodiversity "the folly our descendants are least likely to forgive us."

Soil erosion, over-exploitation of land and water, and inappropriate agricultural systems and/or technology remove productive land and water from food production. This is troubling in light of the expected increases in the number of people to be fed in the future.

The issues dealing with the impact of environment on nutrition and health will be a recurring theme throughout the rest of the chapters.

■ Food additives

Think beyond the contents of the pie in Figure 2-19.

Consider the positives in this collection of food additives. Calorie reducers are much appreciated by people on weight-loss diets. Flavors add interest and variety to our food. Process and formulation aids allow a wide variety of foods to be processed and "put together." (Think about

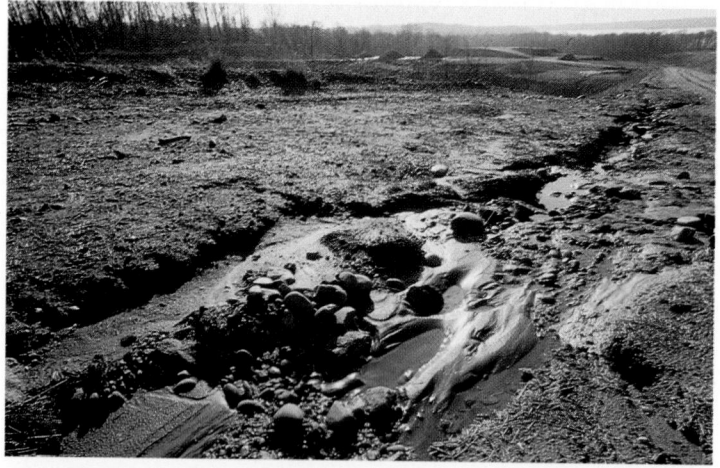
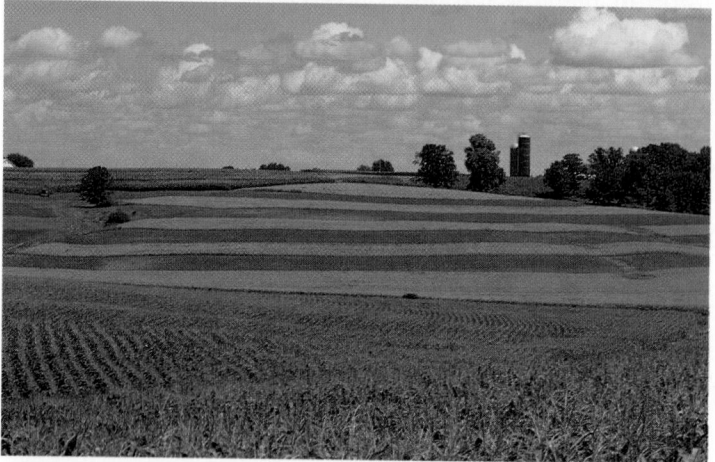

Figures 2-17 and 2-18. Good nutrition starts with the soil. If the soil is exploited and allowed to erode, as in the picture on the top, people cannot get nutritious food, no matter how knowledgeable they are about nutrition. The picture on the bottom shows an Iowa farm that uses strip-cropping and contour farming, two techniques to preserve the soil.

it–we don't grow pizza, mayonnaise, or cookies.) Preservatives extend the shelf life of many foods. Acidulants control the food's acidity. For example, in the production of cottage cheese, lactic acid is added as an ingredient or is produced by bacteria that ferment lactose (milk sugar). The lactic acid makes the cottage cheese more acidic, which slows the growth of spoilage organisms.

Colorants make food attractive. Nature does a superb job of providing a great collection of colors in foods. Many colorants now used in food occur naturally. Some consumers are concerned for health reasons about the addition of synthetic or artificial colors to foods. However, the Food Additives Amendment to the U.S. Food, Drug, and Cosmetic Act, passed in 1958, requires advance testing procedures to assure consumers that food additives are safe. There is also a "GRAS list." *GRAS* stands for "Generally Recognized as Safe." These were the key words in a phrase used in the Food Additives Amendment that described commonly used substances with a long history of safe use (such as phosphates or vegetable oils). The amendment defined them as not being food additives subject to its regulation and thus not requiring additional testing and justification. A list of over 700 such substances has resulted and is monitored by the FDA. However, if their safety to human health is questioned, substances are removed from the list and tested as food additives.

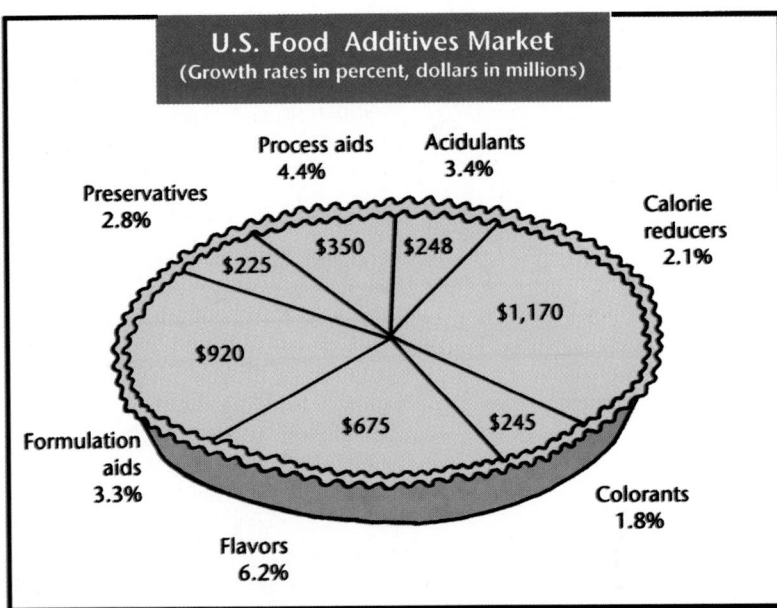

Figure 2-19. The food additive market in the United States (1991 data), with growth rates in percent and dollars in millions.

GRAS (Generally Recognized As Safe): Term applied to a group of historically common food additives judged by the FDA to be safe in food use.

Think beyond the list of substances added to foods (Table 2-6, next page).

Scan the headings on the left in the table to see how food preparation might be more inconvenient and the food itself less interesting, less palatable, and maybe less healthy, as in the case of vitamins and minerals, if we did not have these additives in our food. Look for them on the labels of some foods and understand that each substance is usually used for a good reason.

■ People are different–Organic food

This chapter has taken us from the field and the farm to the food processing plant. Material from plants and animals was subjected to chemicals and processing to increase food yields, to improve and preserve the food, and to make it more attractive and convenient. The way these things were done and the reasons for doing them are not understood by some people. Others have reservations about the effects of such actions on our health

Table 2-6. Common Uses of Additives

Additive Function	Examples[a]	Likely Food Use
Impart or maintain desired consistency	Alginates, lecithin, mono- and diglycerides, methyl cellulose, carrageenan, glycerin, pectin, guar gum, sodium aluminosilicate	Baked goods, cake mixes, salad dressings, ice cream, processed cheese, coconut, table salt, chocolate
Improve or maintain nutritive value	Vitamins A and D, thiamin, niacin, riboflavin, pyridoxine, folic acid, ascorbic acid, calcium carbonate, zinc oxide, iron	Flour, bread, biscuits, breakfast cereals, pasta, margarine, milk, iodized salt, gelatin desserts
Maintain palatability and wholesomeness	Propionic acid and its salts, ascorbic acid, butylated hydroxyanisole (BHA), butylated hydroxytoluene (BHT), benzoates, sodium nitrite, citric acid	Bread, cheese, crackers, frozen and dried fruit, margarine, lard, potato chips, cake mixes, meat
Produce light texture; control acidity and alkalinity	Yeast, sodium bicarbonate, citric acid, fumaric acid, phosphoric acid, lactic acid, tartrates	Cakes, cookies, quick breads, crackers, butter, soft drinks
Enhance flavor or impart desired color	Spices, fructose, aspartame, saccharin, FD&C Red No. 40, monosodium glutamate, caramel, annatto, limonene, turmeric	Spice cake, gingerbread, soft drinks, yogurt, soup, confections, baked goods, cheeses, jams, gum

[a] Includes GRAS and prior-sanctioned substances as well as food additives

Organic foods: No single definition. Description of foods as "organic" implies the use of organic rather than synthetic or artificial fertilizers and no use of pesticides. "Organically processed" foods implies that they have received no treatment with antibiotics, hormones, synthetic additives, preservatives, colorants, or waxes.

and may choose to address these reservations by buying *organic foods*. "Organic" food products can include meats, vegetables, fruits, raw milk, and also processed foods–flour, honey, potato chips, and baby food. This is what the American Dietetic Association advises about organic foods:

- An organic food that is grown and processed properly is not necessarily free from pesticides. There is cross-contamination from wind drifts, soil shifts, or groundwater.

- Eat a variety of foods to ensure a balanced nutritional intake and to lessen contamination from any one source. Be aware that restricting your food choices to a limited number of foods may mean that you are not meeting your nutrition needs.

- In spite of the use of fertilizers and pesticides, populations that eat a large amount of fruits and vegetables have a lower rate of cancer. The benefits of eating this produce may outweigh the risks.

- Be willing to pay more for organically grown foods, but do not expect greater nutritional value or better flavor. Don't expect organic produce to look as "pretty" and unblemished as fruits and vegetables grown with modern farming methods.

- Shop at stores with ethical selling practices, where the foods sold are really what they are advertised to be. Shop on days that produce is delivered in order to buy the food of highest quality.

- Always wash fruits and vegetables thoroughly. Some fruits can be scrubbed with a brush under running water. Wash produce in water containing two drops of dishwashing liquid and then rinse it thoroughly. Discard outer leaves.

- Keep bread without preservatives in the refrigerator to retard mold growth.

Figure 2-20 shows what you may pay for organic foods compared to the price of the same foods conventionally grown. The choice is yours.

■ Nutrition in action–The nation's food protectors

Food that is safe, clean, and wholesome is important for good nutrition. The food we eat at home, at work, in restaurants and fast-food outlets, hospitals, and elsewhere is inspected for safety by the following groups.[24]

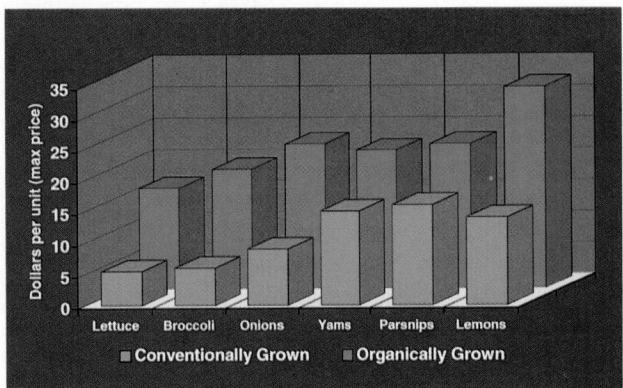

Figure 2-20. Organic foods usually cost more than conventionally grown foods.

U.S. Department of Agriculture

The Food Safety and Inspection Service (FSIS) inspects meat and poultry, including imported meats. This is a mandatory program that assures the public that products are safe, wholesome, and accurately labeled. Unsafe or suspect foods can be recalled. About 7,000 slaughtering and processing plants in the United States are regularly inspected–meat and poultry products are the most intensively inspected foods. FSIS also has a consumer education program on proper care and handling of food, including a toll-free meat and poultry hot line.

The Agricultural Marketing Service (AMS) inspects egg products for both domestic and foreign sales. AMS inspectors keep restricted or "problem" eggs from wholesale markets. Food processors who use eggs–for mayonnaise, egg noodles, ice cream, and other foods–and institutions like nursing homes and hospitals are assured that eggs are safe. Presently, the biggest problem is *Salmonella* bacteria inside some unbroken shell eggs, which could cause food poisoning.

U.S. Department of Health and Human Services

The Food and Drug Administration (FDA) ensures safety and wholesomeness of all foods sold in interstate commerce except meat, poultry, and some egg products. Table 2-7, which lists how much of several defects is allowable in food, may surprise you.

Many parts of this book stress that we compete with two-, four-, and multilegged creatures for food. Some of the defects on the not-very-pleasant list of defect action levels (DAL) will sometimes end up in our food.

Table 2-7. Examples of FDA Food Defect Action Levels[a]

Product	Defect	Action Level
Cocoa beans	Mold	More than 4% by count are moldy
	Insect filth	More than 4% by count are insect-infested, including insect-damaged
	Mold and insect filth	Total of moldy plus insect-infested beans exceeds 6%
	Mammalian excreta	10 milligrams per pound or more
Peanut butter	Insect filth	Average of 30 or more insect fragments per 100 grams
	Rodent filth	Average of 1 or more rodent hairs per 100 grams
	Grit	Gritty taste and water-insoluble inorganic residue of more than 25 milligrams per 100 grams
Tomato puree	Drosophila fly	Average of 20 or more fly eggs per 100 grams; or 10 or more fly eggs and 1 or more maggots per 100 grams; or 2 or more maggots per 100 grams

[a] Defect action levels represent the limit at or above which FDA will take legal action against the product to remove it from the market. They are not average levels at which defects occur; averages are actually much lower. The defect action levels on this list are periodically reviewed and lowered as technology improves.

Why are these materials permitted in our food at all? Why not prohibit them in so many words in the food regulations–zero molds, zero insect fragments, zero rodent hairs, etc.? The answer is that it is not possible to produce food at any price that would meet these requirements. Food comes from fields, barns, orchards, and forests that are inhabited by rodents, insects, and microorganisms. Then why not write limits directly into regulations, instead of using DAL? To do so would appear to endorse the levels stated, which would be misleading. Also, the less formal DAL, while having all the force of law, can more easily reflect the changing situations with which FDA is continually confronted. Change can be for the better, and usually is. But public opinion and other changes can also require the easing of DALs to maintain our food supply. Thus, they should not be enshrined in Congressional law or official regulations.

Inspectors make unannounced visits and take food samples for testing. FDA also monitors pesticide levels in food and checks the safety of food additives. It inspects about 60,000 food processing plants. This number is given to impress on you the size of the U.S. food industry. Given this size, the inspection process is impressive in assuring safe food. FDA also regulates imported food, drugs, and medical devices.

Environmental Protection Agency (EPA)

EPA regulates the manufacture, labeling, and use of all pesticides. It approves or "registers" pesticides to ensure their proper use. EPA sets tolerance levels, or maximum legal limits, for pesticide residues in foods. It also sets national drinking water standards for all public drinking water supplies. The FDA standards for bottled water sold nationwide are modeled closely on these standards.

National Marine Fisheries Service

This agency runs a fee-for-service inspection program for safety, sanitation, and label information for fish products.

State and Local Governments

Cooperative federal and state inspection programs exist for fish, dairy, and other foods. About half the states have their own meat and poultry inspection programs. Local governments inspect restaurants and fast-food outlets and have the power to close establishments for sanitation violations. They also regulate the pesticide level in food.

■ Now you know

- We compete with many industrial uses for available food resources.

- Increased demand for food is due to population growth, urbanization, food losses, and desires for high-protein diets.

- Deforestation and desertification have negative effects on food production.

- Agricultural chemicals (pesticides and fertilizers) increase food production but should be used sparingly so that the environment and human health are protected.

- Biotechnology and aquaculture increase food availability, but environmental concerns must be investigated further.

- Food preservation includes the use of drying, heating, cooling, irradiation, chemicals, and fermentation. Most experts consider irradiation to be safe and appropriate, although some consumers are still reluctant to buy irradiated foods.

- Climate changes, ozone loss, and decreased biodiversity may reduce food production in the future.

- Additives perform many useful functions in food. Like all chemicals, they must be continuously monitored for safety.

- Organic foods are an alternative to foods produced using pesticides, chemical fertilizers, and other chemicals.

- Many federal agencies–USDA's FSIS and AMS and USDHHS's FDA, as well as EPA and National Marine Fisheries Service–and state and local governments regulate the quality of our food supply.

Further Reading

1. Kinlock, D., Kuhnlein, H., and Muir, D. Inuit foods and diet: A preliminary assessment of benefits and risks. *The Science of the Total Environment* 122:247, 1992.
2. 1992 Yearbook of Agriculture. *New Crops, New Uses, New Markets.* U.S. Department of Agriculture, Washington, DC, 1992.
3. Report of the WHO Commission on Health and Environment. *Our Planet, Our Health.* World Health Organization, Geneva, Switzerland, 1992.
4. Fellows, L. What are the forests worth? *Lancet* 339:1330, 1992.
5. Crutchfield, S. Agriculture and water quality conflicts. *Food Review* 14(2):12, 1991.
6. British Medical Association. *The BMA Guide to Pesticides, Chemicals, and Health.* Edward Arnold, London, 1992.
7. Stare, F. J. Some more comments on *Silent Spring. Nutrition Reviews* 50:61, 1992.
8. Dunaif, G. E., and Krysinski, E. P. Managing the pesticide challenge: A food processor's model. *Food Technology* 46(3):72, 1992.
9. WHO Technical Report Series, No 813. *Safe Use of Pesticides.* World Health Organization, Geneva, Switzerland, 1991.
10. Zalom, F. G., and Fry, W. E., eds. *Food, Crop Pests, and the Environment.* The American Phytopathological Society, St. Paul, Minnesota, 1992.
11. WHO Commission on Health and Environment. *Report of the Panel on Food and Agriculture.* World Health Organization, Geneva, Switzerland, 1992.
12. Corey, B. Life on a fish farm: Food safety a priority. *FDA Consumer* 26(6):18, 1992.
13. Bills, D. D., and Kung, S.-D., eds. *Biotechnology and Nutrition.* Butterworth-Heinemann, Boston, 1992.
14. Office of Scientific Public Affairs, Institute of Food Technologists. Biotechnology applied to foods. *Food Technology* 46(9):30, 1992.
15. Kessler, D. A., and others. The safety of foods developed by biotechnology. *Science* 256:1747, 1992.
16. Council on Scientific Affairs, American Medical Association. Biotechnology and the American agricultural industry. *Journal of the American Medical Association* 265:1429, 1991.
17. Bruhn, C. M. Consumer concerns and educational strategies: Focus on biotechnology. *Food Technology* 46(3):80, 1992.
18. Mepham, T. B. Bovine somatotrophin and public health. *British Medical Journal* 302:483, 1991.
19. Stone, R. Warm reception for substitute coolant. *Science* 256:22, 1992.
20. Griffith, G. Irradiated foods: New technology, old debate. *Trends in Food Science and Technology* 3:251, 1992.
21. Pearce, F. Grain yields tumble in greenhouse world. *New Scientist* 134(1817):4, 1992.
22. Moffat, A. S. Does global change threaten the world food supply? *Science* 256:1140, 1992.
23. Reid, W. V. Conserving life's diversity. Can the extinction crisis be stopped? *Environmental Science and Technology* 26:1090, 1992.
24. Gantz, H. The nation's food protectors–Who are they? What do they do? *Food News* 6(4):4, 1990.

Think beyond these pictures. What factors affect your choice of food?

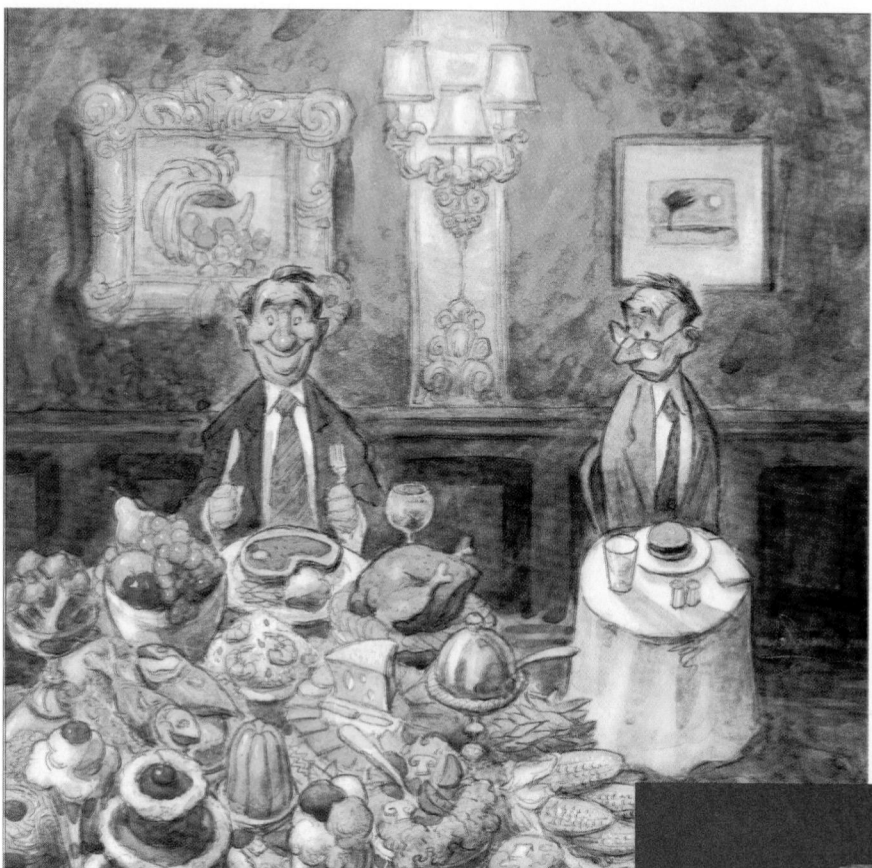

Figure 3-1. Some people have the luxury of eating all the food they wish or of denying themselves food even though it is available.

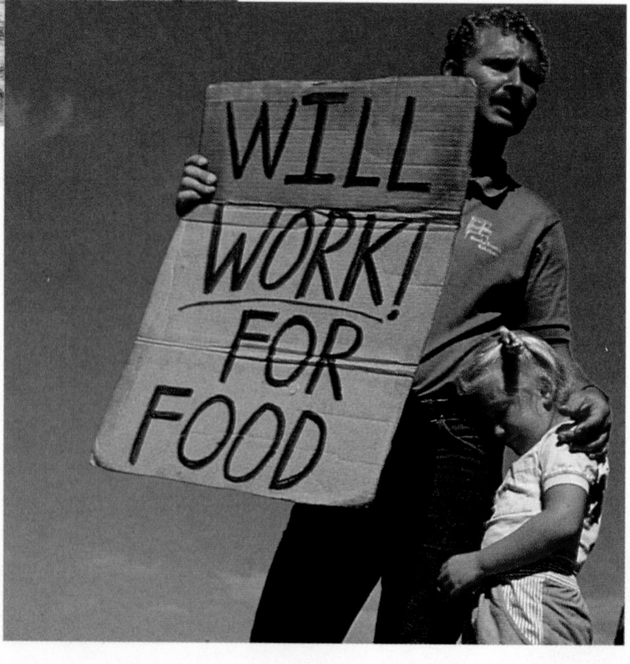

Figure 3-2. For reasons that may be social, economic, or personal, many people in the world do not have enough food.

## CHAPTER 3

Nutrients: From the Plate to You

■ Nutrition and food in your life–
Food on your plate, nutrients in your cells

In Figure 3-1, the person on the left evidently can afford to eat–and does eat–whatever he wishes. This is often seen in developed, industrialized countries. Diseases of affluence (obesity, coronary heart disease, some cancers, and hypertension) may be related to this type of eating. There may be several reasons why the individual on the right has so much less food on his plate. He may have chosen his food carefully to idealize the two Q's of eating–quantity and quality. In other words, he might have selected the correct amount of food containing the nutrients listed in Table 1-4 in the correct proportions. In Chapter 4 we will see how this is done. Or the reason for having less food may be that he is on a weight-loss diet, a concern of many people in developed countries. A condition in which people deliberately eat either very small or very large amounts of food or a limited type of food is called an *eating disorder*. In the United States, this is most typical in teenage girls from middle- and upper-income families. Eating disorders are examined in Chapter 13.

In contrast, the man and girl in Figure 3-2 represent a growing phenomenon in many countries. High unemployment and/or a lack of job opportunities because of poor educational skills mean that many people are hungry. In both the developing and the developed countries, many people do not have wide food choices because of a lack of money.

Although there are many reasons why plates are empty or full of food, differences in most adults' requirements for nutrients are minor. And all healthy people have similar means of delivering the nutrients to every *cell* in the body, from the first bite or mouthful to the last.

Major Topics in This Chapter

Food on your plate; nutrients in your cells

Role of social, psychological, and economic influences on your food choices

■

Sensory evaluation of food

How safe is the food you eat? Bacteria and chemicals

Digestion, absorption, and utilization of nutrients

■

People Are Different–Allergies

Nutrition in Action–Diarrhea: Its nutritional consequences

Eating disorder: Unusual pattern of food intake. Anorexia nervosa is self-induced denial of food, and bulimia is binge eating followed by vomiting.

Cell: Unit of structure of all animals and plants; the physical basis of all life processes.

■ Social, psychological, and economic, as well as nutritional, reasons determine what we put on our plates

Think beyond the information in the Table 3-1. Ask yourself when you last used food for other than nutritional reasons.

Table 3-1. Some Social and Psychological Functions of Food

Function	Example
Aesthetic and creative satisfaction	Special dishes and treats; dinner parties; banquets
Maternal satisfaction; caring	Cooking for the family
Fulfilling social and kinship obligations; friendliness; demonstrating mood and individuality; love	Family meals; "teatime," coffee breaks, eating out; romantic dining; gifts of food
Interpersonal acceptance; friendliness; in-group identity	Slimming clubs; teenage food habits; diet fashions and fads
Prestige; status–political power	Display of foods and wines; cocktail parties; large dinner parties; banquets
Economic purposes and use of food as currency; influencing behavior of others	Business dinners; gifts in return for services; bartering; rewards; punishment
Recreation; adventure; humor	Pleasure of eating with friends; consuming unusual foods; picnics; barbecues; midnight feasts
Relieving tension; security	Social drinking; breast milk to a baby
Religious significance and satisfaction	Jewish, Muslim, and Catholic observances
Symbolism; mythology; superstition; magic	Fish as brain food; oysters and sexual potency; salt over the shoulder; hot cross buns; Halloween
Ceremonial	Christmas dinner; Thanksgiving dinner; wedding receptions; christenings; wakes
Medicinal, health-producing	Slimming foods; herbal products; whole foods; tonics

Are you surprised by the number of social and psychological functions of food that apply to you? Now reread the list to see how members of your family and friends relate to these functions. Notice how food is used for relief, as a distraction, for celebrations, as a means of doing business, and for many other reasons. Both the food service and the food processing industries pay close attention to this–think of all the food created especially for the functions listed. We are better able to use information on the safety and nutritive value of food when we understand these social and psychological functions of food.

Other factors also influence our decisions about which foods to put on our plates. Pleasure, health, and convenience are important considerations. Do you consider hot dogs and hamburgers to be healthy, conve-

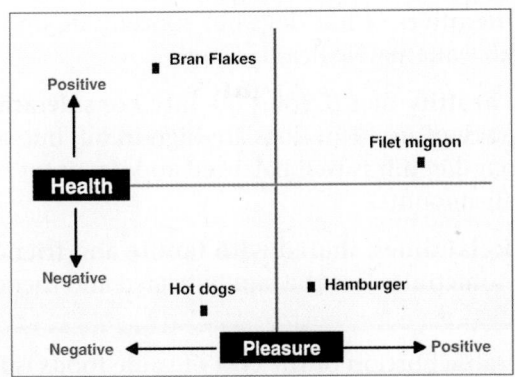
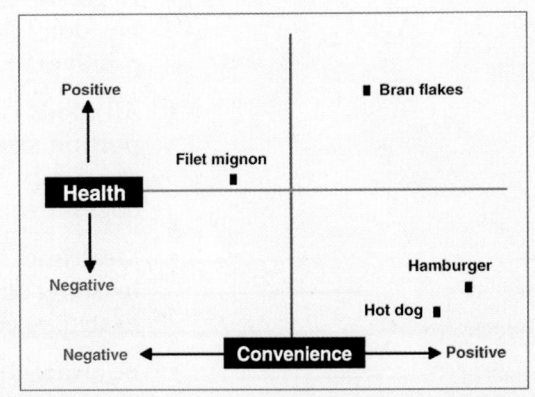

Figure 3-3. Foods ranked on a grid of health and pleasure (left) and on a grid of health and convenience (right). Information like this tells food policy makers and the food industry how consumers make decisions on certain foods.

nient, and pleasurable to eat? Let's see what people in a study at Kansas State University thought about hot dogs, hamburgers, and other foods (Figure 3-3).

Let's pick two foods, hot dogs and hamburgers. Look at the left figure first, where hot dogs are in the bottom left quadrant. People in this study saw hot dogs on the negative side of both pleasure and health. Now move to the right figure and see that hot dogs are in the bottom right quadrant. People still rated them negative on health, but they considered them positive for convenience. Combine the information from both figures, and you can conclude that hot dogs were thought of as not very healthy and not a great source of pleasure, but very convenient. Now do the same for hamburgers. These remain in the lower right-hand quadrant for both the pleasure-health and the convenience-health comparisons. Hamburgers were thus considered pleasurable and convenient but not very healthy. Where do *you* rank these foods or other foods? Such information is used by nutritionists and educators and also by marketing and advertising people working for food companies.

Getting Health and Pleasure from Food the Correct Way

Julia Child is a name familiar to many through her cookbooks and programs on television. She is concerned about the growing "fear of food" in the United States.[1] With help from some nutritionists, she has developed a new way of looking at the way we eat that balances taste and health. They advise this: in matters of taste, consider nutrition, and in matters of nutrition, consider taste. Here are some examples of how to do that.

- **Instead of balancing food choices food by food, or meal by meal, balance them over several days.**

- **The keys to blending taste and health are moderation, variety, and balance.** You can dilute the undesirable aspects of some foods by eating other, healthier foods as well.

> In matters of taste, consider nutrition, and in matters of nutrition, consider taste.

- **Negative, restrictive approaches to nutrition do not work.** For example, don't linger on the negatives of hot dogs but concentrate on the positives of some acceptable alternative healthy food.

- **All foods can fit into a healthy diet if you take into consideration portion size and frequency of use.** Hot dogs are high in fat, but you can still have them in your diet if it is well balanced and if you eat hot dogs infrequently in small amounts.

- **Mealtimes should be special times, shared with family and friends.** In eating on the run, we sometimes lose the family-related and friends-related aspects of food.

- **Be aware that a considerable portion of the cost of some foods is for the convenience component.** We all have busy lifestyles. Some people think that valuable time is "lost" in shopping for, preparing, cooking, and eating food. Convenience increases food costs because other people have cleaned, cooked, packaged, and delivered the food to you. They will also add the costs of advertising and testing, as well as their profit. There is nothing wrong with this–food is a commodity like cars, clothes, and houses.

  However, food is also different because it is so essential for life. *Food as a Human Right* is the title of a book published in the mid-1980s by the United Nations. Do you think that the right to food is comparable to the right to free speech? Think about it–it is a difficult issue involving economics, politics, ethics, and health, among other considerations.

- **Exercise should be part of a healthy lifestyle;** it controls body weight and appetite.

- **Education is critical for healthy eating.** Children should have projects in both culinary and nutrition skills. The next generation must have better nutrition information to make correct food choices.

- **Home preparation and cooking of food should be encouraged.** This allows us to keep control over the foods we eat and helps children learn healthful food choices and preparation techniques.

Sensory Properties of Food and Drink Are Major Reasons for Their Acceptance or Rejection

Chemical senses: The senses of taste and smell, which work by the effect of chemicals in food and drink on the nervous system.

We are now at an important crossroads in following food in its long journey to become the nutrients within us. Food has moved from the field through processing and preparation and is now on our plate to be eaten or rejected. We will make that decision based on important input from our taste buds, eyes, nose, and even our ears (we want our cereal to crunch, not be soggy), all under the master control of the brain. Psychologists tell us that the *chemical senses* are the most primitive of specialized sensory systems, with an evolutionary history of about 500 million years.[2] Yet our chemical senses served us well over the millions of years in picking diets that maintained health and the reproduction of the species. Nowadays, *sensory analysis* is an important part of the training of the next generation of food scientists. Food companies spend large amounts of money determining which sensory aspects of food will appeal most to us.

Sensory analysis: Measurement of the taste, odor, appearance, texture, and sound of food and drink.

Think beyond the photographs in Figures 3-4 and 3-5. This is how sensory evaluation of food is done in a large company. Did you realize that the sensory characteristics of your food are measured so carefully?

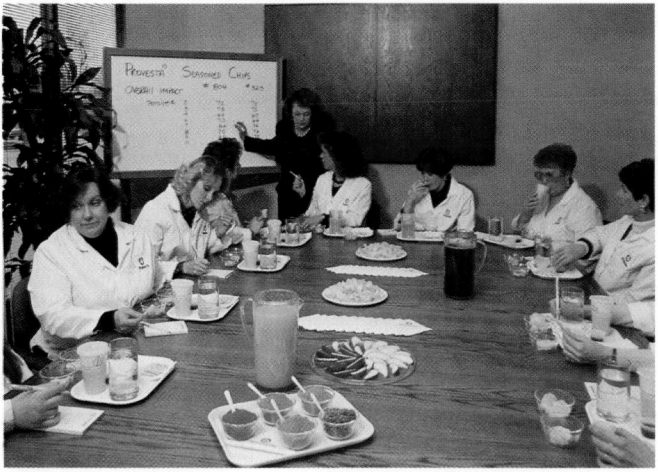
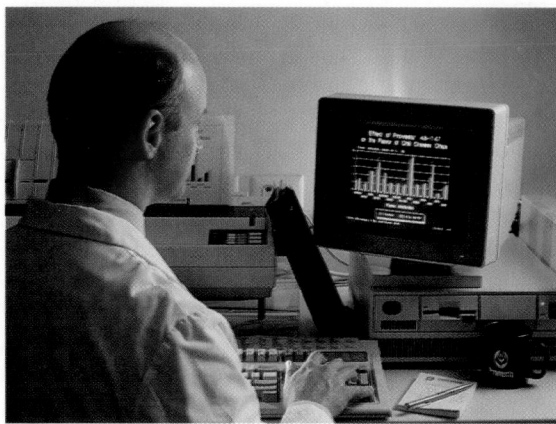

Figures 3-4 and 3-5. Sensory evaluation of foods, either by taste panels or computer programs, is important to the food industry in determining consumer preferences and to the dietetic and medical professions in monitoring sensory changes caused by disease.

Unlike most scenes in a food science laboratory, Figure 3-4 shows no elaborate instrumentation–just people whose senses will help determine whether a food or drink will be liked by the general public. A variety of measurements can be made. Descriptive analysis describes the taste, aroma, or texture of the food in a way that results in a sensory profile. Intensity analysis ranks the intensity of sweetness or other specific characteristics of the food. A *hedonic* measurement determines how much each panelist likes or dislikes a particular characteristic of the food or indicates the overall level of acceptance. Because panelists respond differently, results from many panelists are entered into a computer (Figure 3-5) for statistical analysis that can determine the significance of the response at the range of values likely to be encountered.

Hedonic: Describing the extent of liking or disliking for a food.

Sensory analysis is used also to measure changes in food during storage and distribution and differences in the sensory perception of food by elderly people, children, pregnant women, and people who are sick. Cancer and other illnesses can cause negative changes in the sensory perception of food, resulting in the patient losing interest in food. A recent study of women in the second trimester of pregnancy found that they consumed significantly more sweet food, but not salty food, as compared with women at any other point in pregnancy.[3] The reason for this change, or its physiological significance, if any, is not known.

This is but a brief overview of how the sensory properties of food influ-

Factors Influencing Acceptability of Food

People factors
  Experience, exposure, taboos
  Expectations
  Sensitivity
  Physiological state
  Personality, security
  Occasion/values
  Cost
  Mood
Product factors
  Breed, cultivar
  Environment
  Maturity
  Processing, packaging
  Storage
  Preparation, cooking
  Contamination
  Availability

ence nutrient intake. Other factors influence our food choices as well. To complete this section, you need to go to work again.

Think of a food and see which of the factors listed in the margin influence your acceptance or rejection of it. For example, choose broccoli, raw fish, goat's cheese, or caviar. Then think about whether the reactions of a friend or family member would be the same as yours.

Health and pleasure from food are important, but you may also be concerned about food safety, so it is appropriate to consider that topic.

■ How safe is the food we eat?

This question was answered in a recent editorial in a leading medical journal.[4]

> For healthy persons, there is reason to continue to assume that foods that we eat are safe.

This conclusion is reassuring, especially since some people have concerns about the safety of food associated with biotechnology and with possibly toxic pesticide, antibiotic, and environmental residues in food. Other people are worried about the safety of food additives and food irradiation and the ability of regulatory agencies to assure the safety of our food (see Chapter 2). Although food safety is a growing concern for many consumers,[5] much of this concern may be misplaced. On the basis of the latest and best information, many people believe that the benefits outweigh the risks associated with biotechnology, irradiation, and the other issues just listed. In the opinion of many experts, consumers are distracted from a more serious and potentially deadly concern–food poisoning from microorganisms (also called microbes). However, before we condemn all microbes as villains, let's see what good and harm they do.

Microbes in Our Food and in Our Bodies–Some Helpful, Some Harmful

The positive and negative effects of microbes in nutrition are given little attention in many nutrition books. When discussed, they are usually grouped as the "bad guys"– causing food spoilage, food poisoning, sickness, even death. This is unfortunate, because

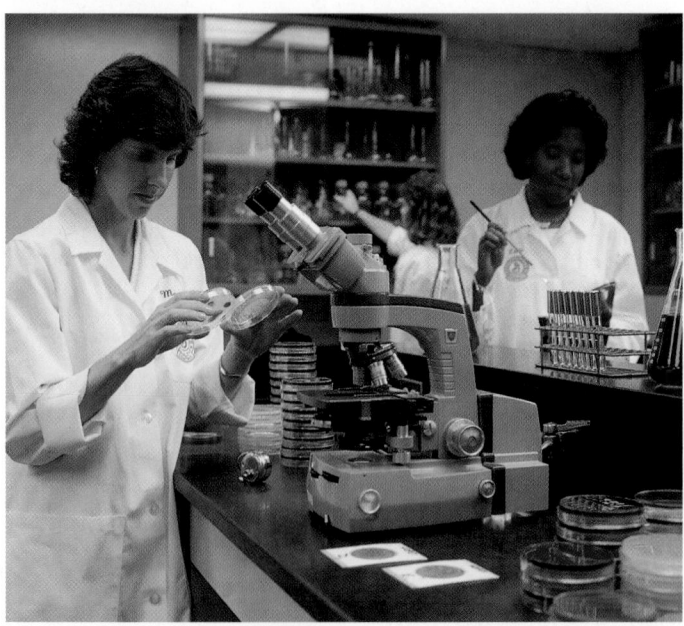

Figure 3-6. These women work in the microbiology laboratory of a national chain of seafood restaurants to ensure consumer safety. They analyze new varieties of seafood and food from new seafood vendors to be sure that safety criteria are met.

microbes are everywhere. In the air, in soil, in water, on our skin and hair, in our mouths and intestines, on and in the food we eat, microbiologist John Postgate tells us in the opening lines to his book *Microbes and Man.*[6] He continues,

> They make the soil fertile; they clean up the environment; they change, often improve, our food; they make vitamins for us inside ourselves; some protect us from less desirable microbes. Yet most people are scarcely aware that they exist–except, sometimes, when they become ill. Microbes as "germs" are regarded as nasty, unpopular because a few can cause disease, a few can spoil food, a few can destroy valuable materials. Only when such misfortunes befall them are most people conscious of microbes at all.

Much of what Postgate says about the influence of microbes on nutrition is positive. Throughout this book we look at the positive influences of microbes in nutrition–the synthesis of vitamin B-12, vitamin K, and other nutrients and the role of microbes in making cheese, yogurt, bread, vinegar, and other foods. So, why are they ignored until they do damage such as causing food poisoning? At least part of the reason is that microbes are out of sight and therefore out of mind. We can see them only with the aid of a microscope (Figure 3-7), and even then not necessarily very well. The inset in Figure 3-7 contains a few microbes "up close and personal."

Food spoilage: Any change in food causing undesirable appearances, flavors, and textures in foods.

Food poisoning: An imprecise term for an illness caused by ingestion of foods containing poisonous substances.

A further reason why microbes are ignored in nutrition is our tendency to get terms mixed up. Let's spend a moment to make an important distinction.

Food spoilage is any change in food that causes the development of an undesirable appearance, flavor, or texture in the food. Microbes take some of the blame here. For example, they are responsible for the souring of milk and the molding of bread, both of which produce changes in appearance, flavor, and texture of the product. But microbes are not to blame for all food spoilage. Vegetable oils become rancid because of chemical changes. Some foods spoil because of physical changes such as crushing and bruising.

Food poisoning is caused by any one of the following: harmful microbes, toxic chemicals, chemical contamination, or allergic reactions to certain proteins.

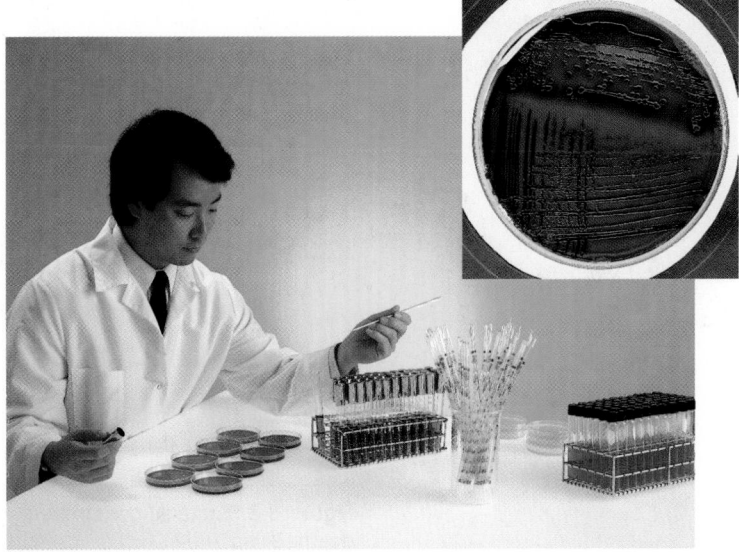

Figure 3-7. Meet a microbiologist at work and see microbes as he sees them through a microscope. The plate contains *Escherichia coli*, which causes many problems in food safety.

Microbes are thus not necessarily to blame for food poisoning. However, this is not to minimize the danger of the food poisoning they do cause.

Food poisoning resulting from foodborne infectious diseases affects about one in every 40 Americans each year, resulting in national economic losses of $1–10 billion annually.[7] This wide range in the estimated cost results from the unknown, but probably high, proportion of foodborne illnesses that go unreported to medical authorities. People often do not report food poisoning. They endure the diarrhea and vomiting for a few days and return to work. The attention of health authorities and the public is captured only when large numbers of people are affected or deaths occur. An example was an extensive outbreak of food poisoning among passengers on a commercial flight from Miami to Minneapolis/St. Paul in 1992.[4] In normal circumstances, it would probably have gone undetected because passengers would have scattered to different destinations and would probably have attributed their illnesses to something other than airline food. What attracted media (and thus public) attention in this case was that a professional football team from Minnesota was on board. The food poisoning was due to an extensive *Shigella* outbreak after contaminated cold sandwiches were served. Contamination occurred in the flight kitchen from workers infected with *Shigella*.

Consider the numbers in Figure 3-8 carefully. They are for the confirmed cases of foodborne illness in the United States between 1983 and 1987.

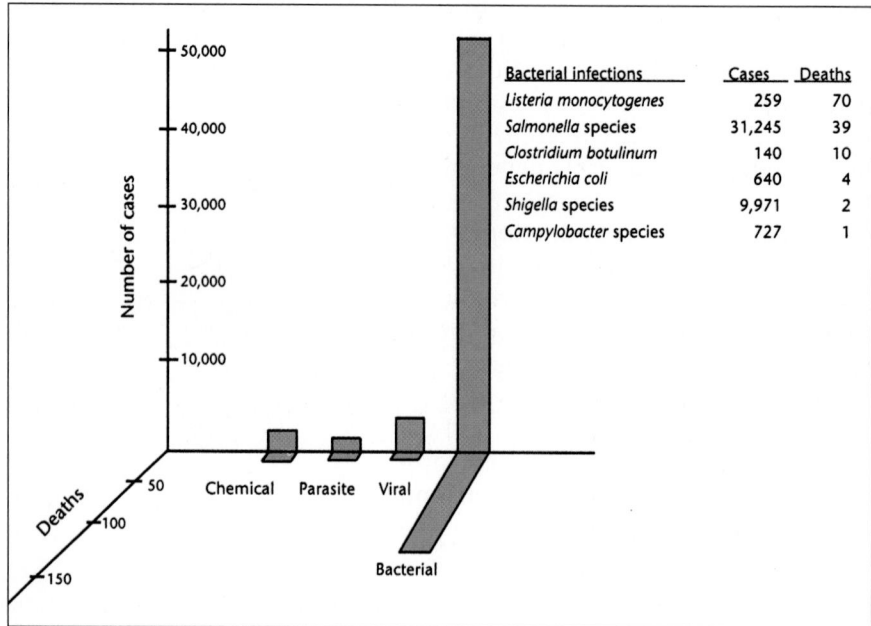

Bacterial infections	Cases	Deaths
Listeria monocytogenes	259	70
Salmonella species	31,245	39
Clostridium botulinum	140	10
Escherichia coli	640	4
Shigella species	9,971	2
Campylobacter species	727	1

Figure 3-8. Bacterial contamination is the most frequent cause of foodborne illness or death.

Foodborne illnesses and deaths are much greater from bacterial toxic agents than from chemical, parasitic, or viral toxins. But people's outrage focuses on chemical toxins because of media attention and public awareness. Note that *Shigella* species, the agent in the food poisoning of football players and other passengers on the Miami-to-Minneapolis flight, caused two deaths during the four-year reporting period. The numbers show clearly that death from bacterial food illness is far more prevalent than that from chemical, parasitic, or viral agents. These disturbing numbers raise another question: What foods are involved most often in food poisoning?

Be careful in studying the numbers in Figure 3-9. First, not all deaths are due to microbes. Look at the figures for mushrooms. Eleven deaths from

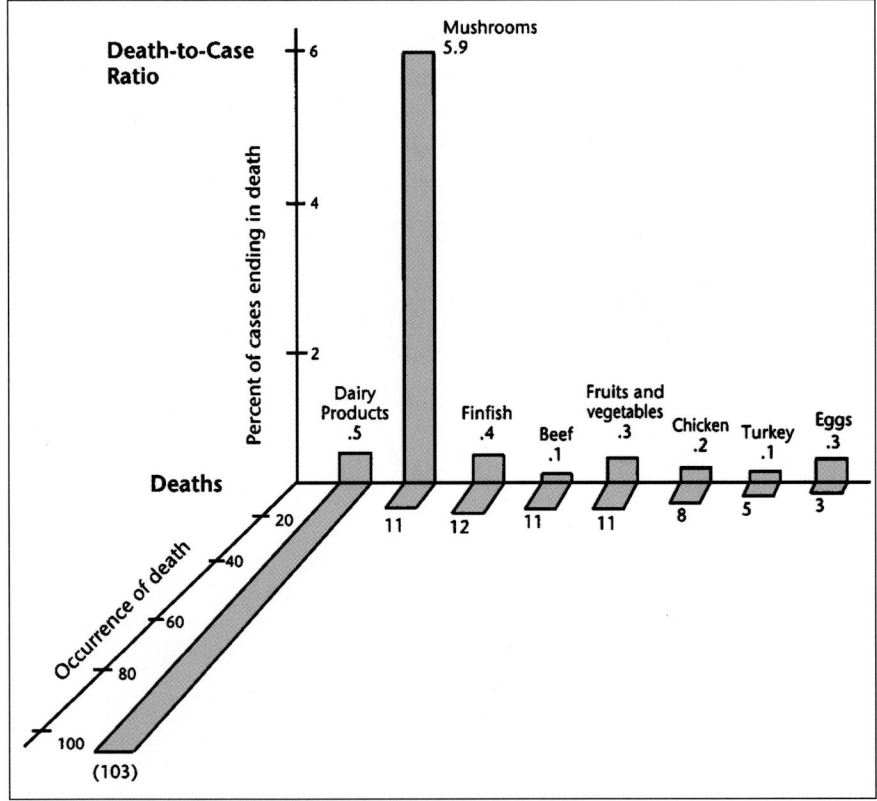

Figure 3-9. Total deaths and deaths per 100 known outcomes of food poisoning for selected foods.

eating mushrooms occurred during the reporting period. These deaths occurred from eating poisonous mushrooms by mistake, since commercial mushrooms are not poisonous. Such mistakes can be costly–mushrooms have the highest death-to-case ratio of all foods listed. A mistake with non-commercial mushrooms may cost a life. The lower figures for other foods mean that many reported cases produce illness but not death.

Why are some foods associated with greater risks than others? There are many reasons, including the fact that some foods must be handled more than others, allowing the possibility of bacterial contamination from handlers. Others are the temperature and time of preparation and holding (improper temperatures could lead to bacterial growth), the acid level of food (many microbes do not like an acid environment), and the presence in the food of sugar or salt, which inhibit bacterial growth. These factors are frequently not as well controlled in fresh foods as in processed foods. Perhaps Dr. Kristin McNutt summed up our modern food supply best with the phrase: Fresh is healthier, but processed is safer.

It is important to emphasize that none of the foods listed in Figure 3-9 need to be eliminated from your diet. But you must know the rules of food safety. They include controlling foodborne pathogens by the use of cooking, *pasteurization, acidulation,* and sanitation (Table 3-2).

The U.S. Center for Disease Control in Atlanta gives guidelines (Table 3-3)

> Remember the 2-40-140 rule: Allow food to stay for no more than 2 hours between 40°F and 140°F (15°C and 53°C). This is the time and temperature danger zone for food safety.

Pasteurization: The killing of food-spoiling bacteria by mild heat treatment. It prolongs shelf life of foods, but usually for a limited period only. Sterilization, which requires higher temperatures, kills all bacteria and spores.

Acidulation: Increasing the acid content of a food.

Table 3-2. How to Control Foodborne Pathogens

Organism	Control
Listeria monocytogenes	Hygiene, sanitation, pasteurization
Salmonella species	Hygiene, cooking, pasteurization
Clostridium botulinum	Appropriate heat treatment, curing, acidulation
Escherichia coli	Sewage control, hygiene
Shigella species	Hygiene, cooking, sewage control
Campylobacter species	Sanitation, cooking, pasteurization

for the approximate incubation periods for the various agents in food poisoning.

We can summarize bacterial food poisoning by placing foods in three categories based on the risk of producing illness.[4]

- **Foods with higher risk:** Unpasteurized milk, uncooked eggs, raw seafood (including uncooked oysters and clams), and moist food maintained and served at room temperatures in hot climates or left unrefrigerated too long in temperate climates.

- **Occasionally unsafe foods:** Cheese, salad bar items, berries and grapes that have not been carefully washed, sandwiches, hamburgers, and foods served on commercial airlines.

Steps to Food Safety

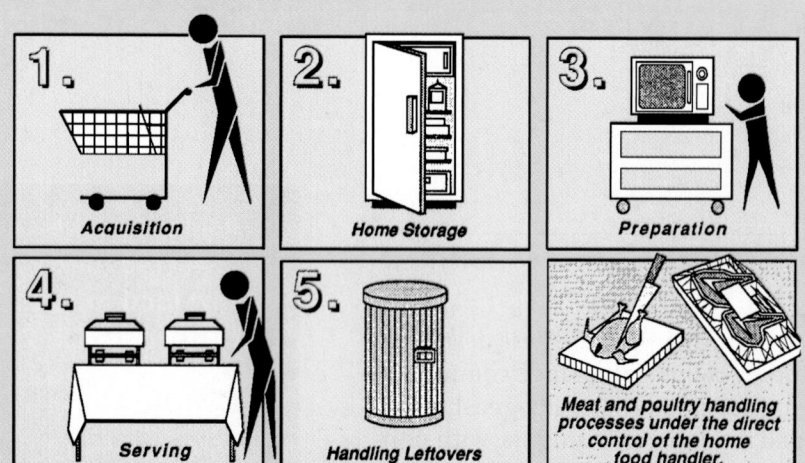

1. Acquisition
2. Home Storage
3. Preparation
4. Serving
5. Handling Leftovers

Meat and poultry handling processes under the direct control of the home food handler.

1. Shopping

- Shop for food last. Take it right home to the refrigerator. Don't leave food in a hot car.
- Don't buy anything you won't use by the use-by date.
- Buy food in good condition. Refrigerated food should be cold. Frozen food should be rock-solid. Do not buy cans with dents, cracks, or bulging lids.

2. Storage

- Run your refrigerator at 40°F and your freezer at 0°F.
- Freeze fresh meat, poultry, or fish immediately if you can't use it within a few days.
- Put packages of raw meat, poultry, or fish on a plate before refrigerating so that they do not drip on other foods. Raw juices can contain bacteria.

3. Preparation

- Wash your hands in hot soapy water *before* preparing food and *after* using the bathroom, changing diapers, and handling pets.
- Bacteria can live in kitchen towels, sponges, and cloths. Wash them often. Replace sponges every few weeks.
- Keep raw meat, poultry, and fish and their juices away from other food. For instance, wash your hands, cutting board, and knife in hot soapy water after cutting up chicken and before dicing salad ingredients.
- Use a plastic cutting board rather than a wooden one. Bacteria can hide in grooves.
- Thaw food in the microwave or refrigerator, *not* on the kitchen counter. Bacteria can grow in the outer layers while the inner layers are thawing.
- Cook red meat to 160°F. Cook poultry to 180°F. Check with a meat thermometer.
- Cook eggs until the yolk and white are firm. Scramble them to a firm texture. Don't use recipes in which eggs remain raw or only partially cooked. Salmonella bacteria can grow inside eggs, even fresh unbroken ones.
- Refrigerate large amounts of food in small, shallow containers to ensure rapid cooling.
- Microwave ovens sometimes leave cold spots in food where bacteria can grow. Cover food with a lid or plastic wrap so the steam can help cook. Vent the wrap. Stir and rotate the food for even cooking. Allow standing time after the microwave is off so food can finish cooking.

- **Rarely unsafe foods:** Peeled fruits; syrups, jellies, and other foods with high sugar content; and items served steaming hot or kept refrigerated.

Regulatory Agencies Protect Our Food, But the Final Decisions Affecting Food Safety Are Up to Us

Food regulation by federal, state, and local agencies is one major reason why we have a safe food supply. Safety of meat is monitored by USDA inspectors (Figure 3-10), who take samples for microbial inspection. Raw meat contaminated by pathogenic bacteria as seen under the microscope is shown in Figure 3-11. The food industry also plays an important part in producing safe food because loss of food due to spoilage or poisoning results in a costly immedi-

Table 3-3. Symptoms of Toxins

If Symptoms Appear in	Toxin is
<1 hour	Probably chemical poisoning
1–7 hours	Probably *Staphylococcus* food poisoning
8–14 hours	Probably *Clostridium perfringens* food poisoning
>14 hours	Other infectious or toxic agents, such as *Salmonella*

- Check the temperature of the food with a meat thermometer. Insert it at several places.

4. Serving

- Serve food on clean dishes, not ones that held raw or partially cooked food.
- *Never leave cooked or perishable food out of the refrigerator for more than 2 hours.*
- Use a cold pack in lunches and picnic baskets. Do not leave food in the sun.
- For a party, make several small platters and keep them in the refrigerator until they are needed. Divide hot foods into small serving platters and keep the platters refrigerated until time to warm them up for serving.

5. Handling leftovers
- Put leftovers in small, shallow containers for quick cooling in the refrigerator.
- Remove stuffing from poultry or other stuffed meats. Refrigerate it separately.
- To reheat, bring sauces, soups, and gravies to a boil. Heat other leftovers thoroughly to 165°F.
- Microwave leftovers using a lid or vented plastic wrap.

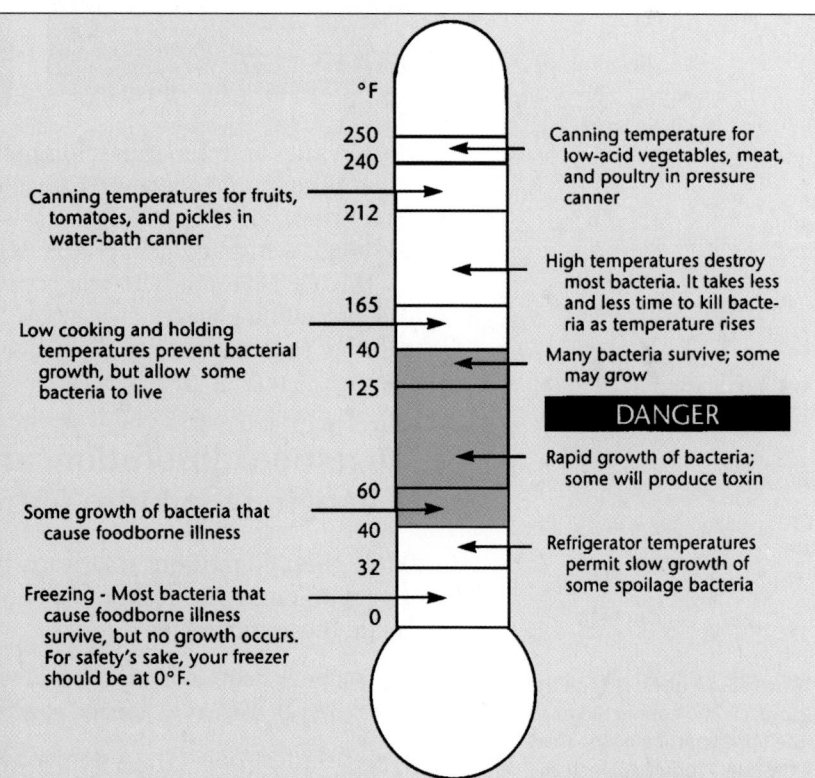

- Discard food after its expiration date.
- Do not taste food that looks or smells strange. If in doubt, throw it out.
- If you cut out mold in hard cheeses and salamis and firm fruits and vegetables, remove a large area because molds can't always be seen. Most moldy food should be discarded.

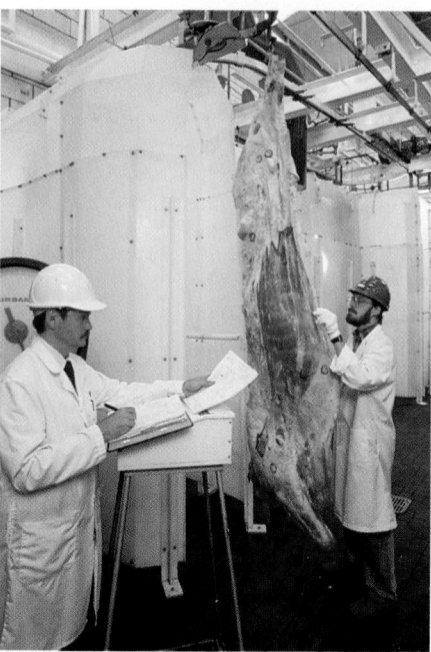 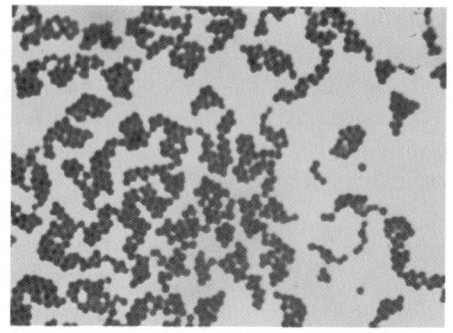

Figures 3-10 and 3-11. Inspection of meat ensures a safe meat supply for the consumer (left); spoilage bacteria on meat (right).

ate loss in sales and sometimes long-term market losses. Most people in the food processing and food service industry realize that training programs are important.[8] In Chapter 2, we saw that the food industry uses hazard analysis and critical control points (HACCP) to monitor food safety. A personal HACCP that will help you control your own food safety was shown on the preceding pages.

It is now time to see how food is converted into nutrients to be used in the body.

■ Digestion, absorption, and utilization– Changing food into nutrients

"More than 80 million Americans live with and suffer from chronic digestive problems," the author of a book on gastrointestinal health tells us.[9] Who are these people?

> . . . sufferers may be of any age and background–for gastrointestinal problems cross all barriers of age and economics.

The gastrointestinal (GI) system obviously is a source of problems for many people. It is also misunderstood, as evidenced by the misuse of antacids and other digestive aids. The introductory information on the GI tract in Chapter 1 is supplemented in this chapter with information on how the brain, liver, *pancreas*, and *gallbladder* influence digestion and metabolism. These tissues act and interact in remarkable ways in getting nutrients out of food and into you. Let's see how they do this important job as we work through the information in Figure 3-12.

Pancreas: A gland behind the stomach and connected to the upper portion of the small intestine. Produces pancreatic juice (important in digestion) and hormones–insulin and glucagon.

Gallbladder: Pear-shaped sac near the liver holding bile from the liver until it is discharged into the GI tract.

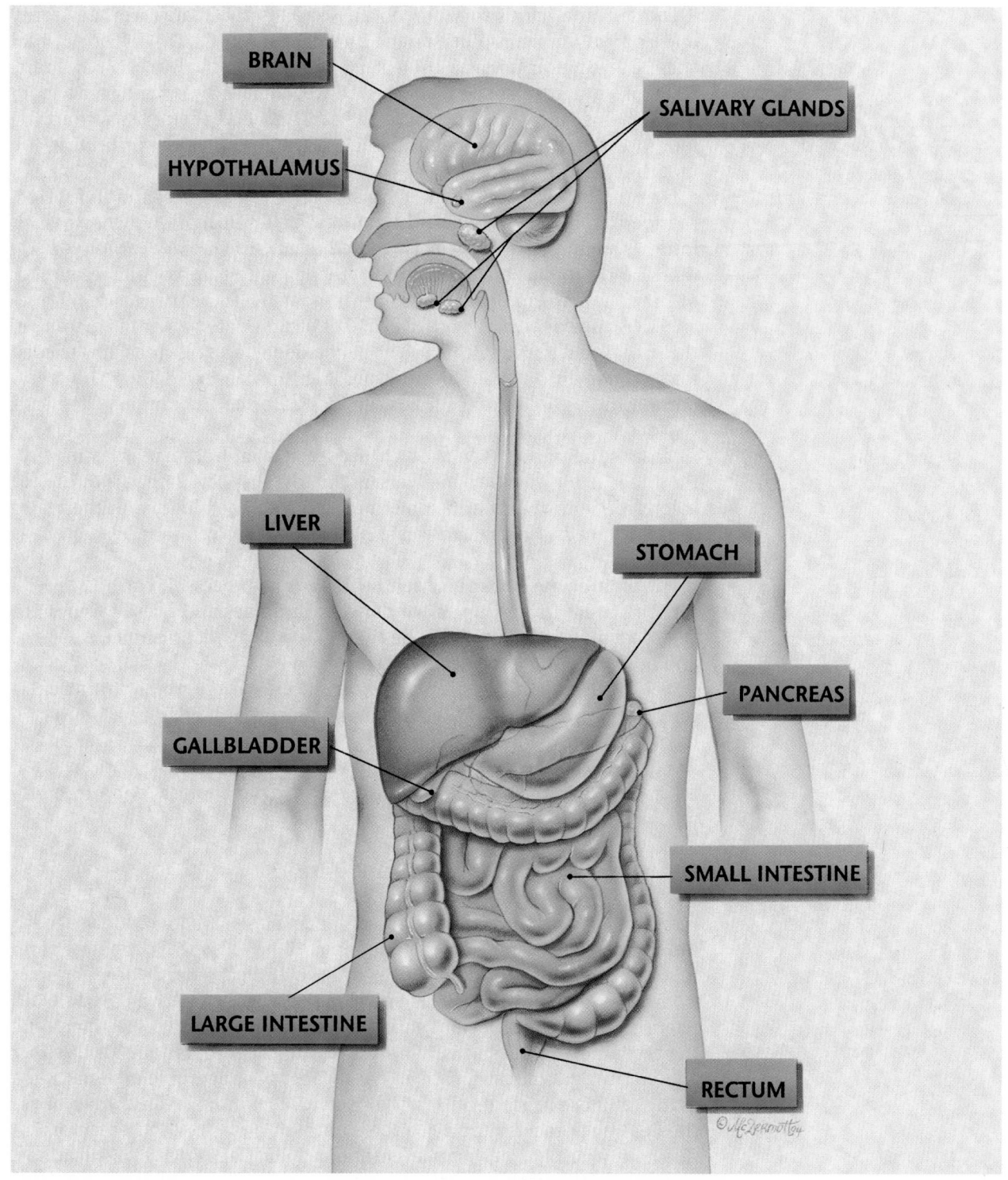

Figure 3-12. The digestive system takes nutrients from food and transfers them to the body.

The salivary glands in your mouth secrete saliva. Saliva contains only one enzyme, which splits starch into smaller units. This is not a vital chemical reaction because the total digestion of starch to glucose units takes place in the small intestine. However, saliva also moistens food, which helps it to be chewed and mixed. The food then passes from the mouth through the esophagus, which is the long "pipe" connecting the mouth to the stomach.

The stomach is a sack containing strong acid, enzymes, and fluid. Here the food is mixed, tossed, and ground. The resulting liquid mass passes into the small intestine. This is where most of the dietary carbohydrates, lipids, and proteins are digested into their smallest units. A large number of enzymes perform this work. Some of them are in the pancreatic juice secreted by the pancreas, which also makes bicarbonate to neutralize some of the strong acid in the stomach. The gallbladder stores bile until it is needed for secretion into the small intestine. Bile is made in the liver and is important in the digestion of lipids. Besides enzymes, it contains chemicals that act as detergents.

Most of the nutrients in food are absorbed from the small intestine into the blood supply, which delivers them to cells. The large intestine, or colon, reabsorbs water and some minerals into the blood, and these also are sent to cells. Undigested waste is passed to the rectum for excretion as feces.

The brain is the control center for this whole process. It controls the digestive system by an impressive network of nerves and chemical messengers. The master control is in the hypothalamus, which regulates appetite and hunger.

We will deal with the specifics of digestion of each group of nutrients–carbohydrates, lipids, proteins, vitamins, and minerals–in Chapters 6 through 10. In the next sections, we concentrate on getting a better understanding of digestion and metabolism through answers to questions often asked by the general public and answered by nutritionists and other biomedical professionals.

How Can We Digest Food So Rapidly?

More than three-quarters of a ton of food per year is a lot of food for each of us to digest. Each meal is digested in about 3–4 hours.[10] The time from ingestion of food to the excretion of feces (called "transit time") ranges from 24 to 72 hours in a healthy person. Why is there a two-day time difference in the range for transit time? Many factors are involved, including the type of diet and especially the amount of fiber it contains. If the fiber content is high, transit time is reduced. Fiber is indigestible material, such as the cellulose in plant cell walls. It is nature's natural laxative that moves the digestive process quickly to the elimination of feces. Other factors influencing transit time include emotions, physical activity, medications, and various illnesses.

Layers of muscles squeeze and push food along the GI tract in a process called *peristalsis*. The activity of these muscles decreases as we grow older.[11] This is one reason why some elderly people have problems with constipation. The muscles are not active enough to move the feces quickly along the large intestine for elimination. Water is absorbed from this slow-moving fecal mass, thus hardening it to a state of constipation.

A number of digestive juices contain chemicals to speed up digestion. For instance, enzymes are important in speeding up the breakdown of complex nutrients. Proteins and starches are digested into their smallest basic parts, amino acids and glucose, respectively.

Think about this puzzling question: Why doesn't the stomach digest itself?

Believe it or not, this question was the cover feature of *Nature*, one of the leading scientific journals in the world. It is *not* a trick question. We put all kinds of food into our mouths, and most of it is digested and the waste excreted. The strong acids and other chemicals in the GI tract do their job well. So, what protects the walls of the GI tract from being digested? A highly viscous substance, the *gastric mucus*, is secreted into the GI tract and lines the walls. It cleverly alters its chemical microenvironment continuously to prevent the strong acid in the stomach from digesting the stomach itself.[12] Speaking of acids brings us to the next question.

When Do You Need an Antacid?

Americans seem to think *antacids* are needed often. Almost $1 billion per year is spent on over-the-counter antacids.[13] They may not always be needed, and if they are overused they cause problems. Frequent and prolonged use can cause heart, kidney, and bone problems. If you must use antacids, moderation is the key. You can make the use of antacids unnecessary and yet prevent heartburn or indigestion by observing a few simple rules:

- **Don't eat big meals.** They need more acid to digest them.
- **Eat more slowly.** Eating quickly produces more acid.
- **Cut down on caffeine.** It makes the stomach produce more acid.
- **Cut back on alcohol and smoking.** They irritate the lining of the stomach.
- **After you eat, don't lie down right away.** Lying down prevents gravity from moving food from the stomach to the intestines. For the same reason, don't eat big meals just before going to sleep.
- **Don't wear tight-fitting garments.** They squeeze your stomach, forcing the stomach's acid back into the esophagus, where it gives a burning sensation.

Peristalsis: Coordinated muscle contractions that move food along the GI tract.

Gastric mucus: "Gastric" means relating to the stomach. Mucus is a viscous fluid.

Antacid: An agent that neutralizes acidity in the GI tract.

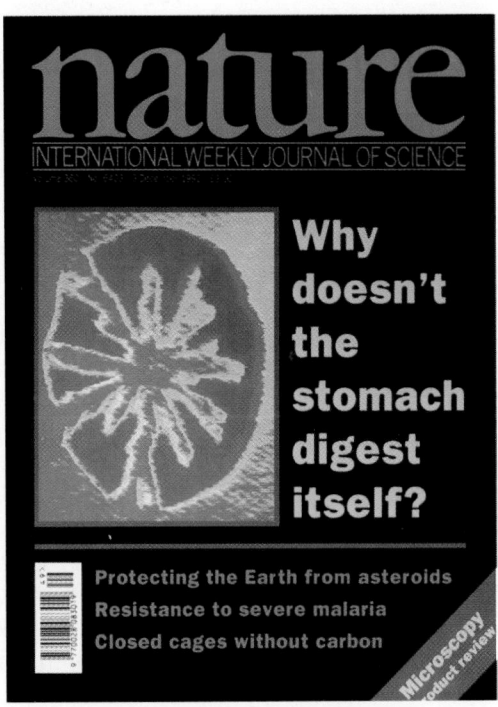

Figure 3-13. The cover of a famous international science journal poses an interesting question.

Why Does Stress Affect the Digestive System?

The brain-gut connection is very real.[9] Nerves from the brain go to the esophagus, stomach, gallbladder, pancreas, small intestine, and colon. When you look at or smell food, these nerves stimulate stomach and intestinal contractions and the secretion of digestive juices. Stress causes excessive nervous activity, which in turn causes GI activity. Stress will make ulcers and other disorders worse.

Do We Have Invited and Uninvited Guests in the Digestive System?

Yes. "A microscopic zoo" is how one writer describes the human body, including the GI tract.[14] The contents of our colons contain about 10 billion microbes per gram–if you don't think metric, that is about 280 billion microbes per ounce. Is this trivial information? Think of it this way: the number of microbial cells in our GI tract exceeds the number of cells in our entire body. It is reasonable to suggest that we get to know the contributions made by our guests in the human digestive system.

They are considered normal residents, and they do some nice and some not-so-nice things for us. Bacteria synthesize vitamin B-12 and vitamin K. Bacteria in the mouth convert sugars to an acid that dissolves tooth enamel, causing dental caries. Resident microbes create intestinal gas, bad breath, and body odor. Scientists now realize that resident microbes may be more important than previously thought.[15] Experimental evidence suggests that bacteria in the gut may convert certain food additives, contaminants, and natural non-nutrient components of food into cancer-causing chemicals. Other bacteria in the GI tract are known to inactivate potential carcinogens. All of this is very speculative at the moment. However, don't be surprised if books on nutrition in the future have much more to tell us about how these bacteria interact with the nutrient and non-nutrient components of our diet.

We also have guests that are not microscopic. Parasites in the GI tract can cause nutrition problems. For example, hookworms drain iron from the intestinal system of infected people in tropical countries. Tapeworms create problems for people in areas such as Mexico, Latin America, and southern Africa. They live in the small intestine of a person, some growing to a length of 30–45 feet when pulled out to full length.[16] These parasites must be fed, and their food comes from predigested food. This loss of food to the parasite is serious for people with low nutrient intake.

Odd objects can accumulate in the GI tract also. It is foolish to follow health fads without understanding the chemistry of what you are eating.[17] For example, "diet pills" containing guar gum are sold as a way to reduce body weight. They are supposed to produce weight loss. The idea is that the guar gum will soak up water and swell in size 10- to 20-fold. This swollen mass gives a full feeling in the GI tract because there is less room available for other food. Guar gums are classified in the fiber group. They pass from the body undigested in the feces, thereby contributing no calories to the body. However, in a few cases where too much guar gum has been ingested, surgery has been needed to remove the mass from the GI tract.

Another mass in the GI tract requiring surgical removal occurred when a previously healthy man took very large amounts of a vegetable-derived oil said to contain lecithin.[18] He bought the oil at a health food store in the belief that lecithin lowers blood cholesterol and improves memory. But in the amounts he took the lecithin just gave him gastric blockage.

These two instances should be convincing evidence that we must know the composition of what we put into our mouths and understand what happens after it is swallowed.

Which Foods Produce Gas?

Most gas, or flatulence, is produced by bacteria in the body, although some comes from swallowed air. It is produced mainly by plant foods. Strong odors come from sulfur-containing plant foods such as beans and other legumes, cabbage, cauliflower, dried apricots, and broccoli, and flatulence can be reduced by eating only small quantities of these foods.

Belching air through the mouth is reduced by giving up carbonated drinks, refraining from chewing gum, and not smoking.

Can Medications Interfere with the Absorption of Nutrients?

We know that eating certain foods is beneficial when we are sick. Folk medicine advises us to feed a cold and starve a fever. Chicken soup is a long-time favorite remedy for illness. What many people do not know is that the chemicals in food sometimes interact with medications to decrease their effectiveness.[19] To avoid this, read the labels of *over-the-counter (OTC) drugs* and, if in doubt, consult your pharmacist. However, some foods can increase the effectiveness of medication. Here is a sampling of how some foods and drinks interact with medications.

Over-the-counter drugs: Medications not requiring a prescription; for example, aspirin, antacids, and cold relief medications.

- Dairy foods, which are high in calcium, affect the action of some antibiotics and of iron supplements containing ferrous sulfate. The calcium can combine with these drugs and supplements, which then cannot be absorbed from the GI tract into the blood. These medications should be taken on an empty stomach.

- High-fiber diets reduce the absorption of some drugs such as Tylenol.

- A high-protein diet can increase the absorption of aspirin.

- Caffeine is in coffee, some tea, and some soft drinks. It is related to the medication theophylline, which is taken for asthma and bronchitis. People taking this drug should avoid caffeine-containing foods and beverages.

- Alcoholic drinks, including beer and wine, do not mix well with some prescription or OTC drugs. Attempts to cure hangovers sometimes involve aspirin, which may cause a bleeding ulcer. Alcohol combined with antihistamines has a depressive effect on the central nervous system, causing drowsiness. Many OTC cold remedies contain antihistamines, so don't mix alcohol and cold medications, especially if you are going to drive, operate machinery, or take a nutrition test!

- Other medications: Oral contraceptives decrease the absorption of folic acid. Antacids, if taken regularly, decrease iron absorption. Some diuretics (medications given to increase urine flow from the body) may cause potassium deficiency. To avoid this, foods high in potassium, such as meats, dairy products, fruits and vegetables (especially bananas), and whole grains, should be eaten by people on diuretics. Some of the steroid drugs inhibit the body's ability to use amino acids and decrease the amount of calcium that gets into bones.

What Are the Differences Between Hunger and Appetite?

Hunger: A physiological response to lack of food. Hunger pains coincide with powerful contractions of stomach muscles.

Appetite: A pleasant sensation based on previous experiences causing a person to seek food for taste and enjoyment.

Hunger and *appetite* are words that are well known to us but difficult to define. Look back to the photographs at the beginning of this chapter. Appetite may be huge for the man on the left and small for the man on the right in Figure 3-1. They may or may not be hungry. The people in Figure 3-2 are probably hungry. Some factors controlling hunger and appetite are under our voluntary control; others are not.

Take a moment to review the information in Figure 3-14 and insert your own experiences where appropriate.

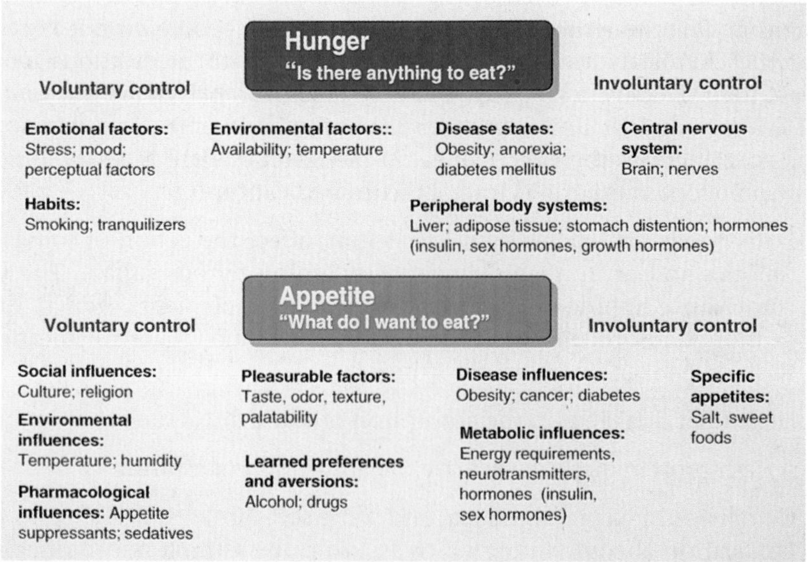

Figure 3-14. Voluntary and involuntary regulation of hunger (top) and appetite (bottom).

Why do some people have difficulty in controlling excess body weight? One answer can be seen in the above information. Notice that in the regulation of appetite and hunger, only a few factors are under our voluntary control. An understanding of this distinction will assist us later when we study obesity, weight-reducing diets, and eating disorders.

When *satiety* (the feeling of fullness) occurs, eating usually stops. The relevance of a number of controls on satiety is now being debated.[10] The latest research suggests that distension (stretching) of the stomach and small intestine is one of the most significant influences on eating. The search is on for a chemical involved in switching on and off the urge to eat. Just think of the vast income to be generated for the group that discovers a safe chemical to effectively regulate food intake. There are a few clues as to which chemical may be the "magic bullet." The brain is thought to have two regulatory centers, one for hunger and one for satiety. Some scientists believe that fat, amino acids, hormones, or neurotransmitters brought to the brain by the blood have the greatest influence on satiety. Other scientists suggest that the liver is the primary regulator of food intake. The liver is the reception site for nutrients after digestion and absorption. It makes physiological sense that this organ would play at least some part in food intake regulation. This brief introduction to the important area of regulation of eating behavior is a useful example of the complex but fascinating interactions involved in most nutrition issues.

Satiety: The condition of being full to satisfaction.

Is the Liver the Body's Chemical Factory and Detoxification Center?

Yes. The liver is a busy organ, the site of hundreds of different chemical reactions after every meal. The liver is busy even in a starving person as it mobilizes nutrients from around the body in an effort to maintain life. It also stores some absorbed fat and carbohydrate. All nutrients pass through the liver and are then sent to every cell in the body. Sometimes nutrients are packaged by the liver for distribution to the cells. For example, vitamin A is soluble in fat, but the blood must have vitamin A in a water-soluble form to transport it to the cells. The liver obliges by making it water-soluble when it hooks a protein onto vitamin A.

Detoxification is the process by which a harmful material is chemically converted into a harmless one. The liver detoxifies harmful substances in food and drink. Alcohol is the best known toxin detoxified by the liver. However, excess alcohol intake over long periods may cause cirrhosis, or hardening of the liver.

How Do Nutrients Get to Cells?

A cell is the smallest subdivision of a *tissue* that is capable of independent life when kept alive in tissue culture. Nutrients come from cells in foods of plant and animal origin to form cells within our body. Notice the order and relatedness in the sequence shown in Figure 3-15.

Tissue: A group or collection of similar cells that act together to perform a particular function; e.g., muscles and nerves are each classified as tissues.

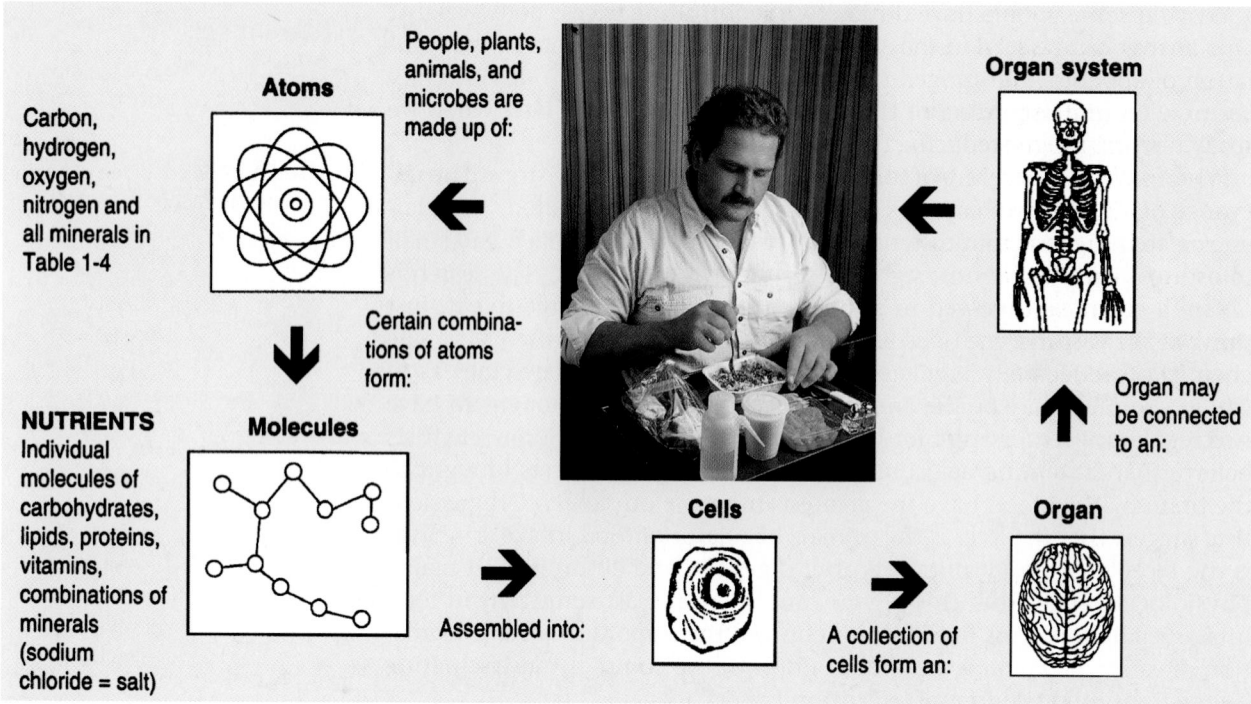

Figure 3-15. "You are what you eat." The body can be viewed on different levels of increasing complexity.

If you look at a cell under a microscope, you will see a brilliant collection of little specialized structures. Those of most significance in nutrition are pictured in Figure 3-16.

Cells are like little independent republics "doing their own thing" and requiring energy to do it. Without energy they die. Glucose is the main source of their energy (see Table 1-4).

Let's see how glucose from your diet gets into cells. Most of the glucose in the body comes from carbohydrates in your diet. Digestion of carbohydrates produces glucose, which is absorbed from the GI tract into the blood and taken to the liver. The liver may store some of the glucose for energy use in emergencies. The remaining glucose is sent through the blood to every cell in the body. However, it needs a helper to cross the *cell membrane*, the wall around a cell.[20] The membrane is an impressive double sheet of lipids that keeps the liquid environments inside and outside the cells apart because they differ in chemical composition. The details of these differences will be important in the discussion of body fluids in Chapter 5. But the problem for glucose and other water-soluble nutrients is that they cannot dissolve into the lipid of the membrane. So glucose hooks onto a special protein, the transporter molecule. This combined glucose-protein structure can squeeze through tiny pores in the membrane to get into the cell. Once inside the cell, glucose is unhooked from the protein and can then be stored or broken down for energy. (Notice that a lot of

Cell membrane: A thin, soft layer of tissue surrounding a cell or lining a tube or cavity.

squeezing, hooking up, and breaking down go on within us so that we can use nutrients.)

The *nucleus* of a cell contains DNA, the genetic material controlling heredity. This is the blueprint for our entire existence–it determines the number and composition of cells in a tissue. The cell also contains other structures. *Mitochondria* supply the energy for all its activities. *Ribosomes* make proteins for all parts of the cell and export them through the *Golgi complex*. *Lysosomes* break down unwanted cell parts and foreign matter that may enter the cell. Most of the subcellular parts described here are affected by nutritional stresses, such as those occurring in starvation, disease, growth during childhood, pregnancy, and recovery from disease.

■ People are different–Allergies

Allergies interfere with the process of getting nutrients from the plate to you. A discussion of allergies requires clear definitions at the beginning. It is appropriate that we discuss food allergies under the heading "People are Different." Public perception of the importance of food allergies far exceeds their actual prevalence. This is a problem for nutritionists because people may avoid some nutritious foods in the mistaken belief that they cause an *allergy*.[21] The following is an important distinction.

Food allergy or food hypersensitivity is an abnormal or exaggerated response of the *immune system* as a result of eating a food. These changes in the immune system can be seen in clinical tests for true food allergies. Some foods have naturally occurring *allergens*, combinations of protein and carbohydrate that cannot be broken down during digestion and that are stable when heated. If minute amounts of intact allergens are absorbed into a susceptible body, they cause an allergic reaction. Food allergies seem to be greatest in the first few years of life, but most infants outgrow the problem.[22]

Food intolerance is a reaction to a food or food additive that does not involve the immune system. The symptoms of a nonallergic reaction to a food may be very similar to those of an allergic reaction. A good example of food intolerance is the nausea, vomiting, and diarrhea experienced by

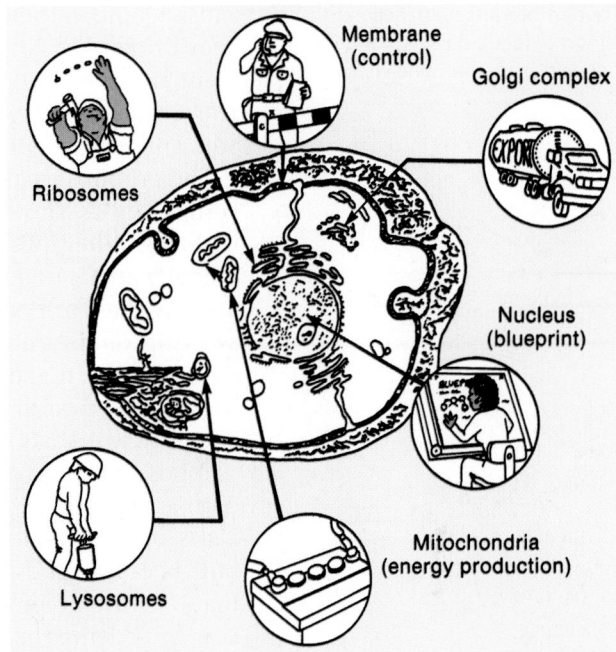

Figure 3-16. One of the billions of cells in your body and the functions of its various parts. The functions can be represented by familiar activities.

Nucleus: The essential part of a cell; involved in growth, metabolism, reproduction, and transmission of characteristics of a cell.

Mitochondria: Tiny rods within a cell; "power houses" of cells because they produce energy. They are involved in protein synthesis and lipid metabolism.

Ribosomes: Tiny structures in cells that synthesize proteins.

Golgi complex: A structure situated near the nucleus in most cells. It concentrates and packages newly formed cell material.

Lysosomes: Tiny particles within cells; contain enzymes to break down proteins and certain carbohydrates within cells.

Allergy: An abnormal tissue reaction to a specific foreign substance (allergen) that, in similar amounts, produces no effect in nonsensitive persons.

Food allergy or food hypersensitivity: Abnormal or exaggerated response of the immune system due to eating certain foods.

Immune system: A system in the body that protects against certain infectious diseases.

Allergen: Any substance that causes allergy. Common allergens include foods, inhalants (dust, pollen, smoke), some drugs, infectious agents (bacteria, viruses, fungi), contactants (chemicals, animals, plants), and physical agents (heat, cold, light).

Food intolerance: A reaction to a food or food additive that does not involve the immune system.

most people in the world (except those of northern European origin) when they drink milk. Milk contains lactose, a sugar, and many people lack sufficient amounts of the enzyme lactase, which is needed to digest lactose in the small intestine. Thus, they cannot tolerate a large intake of milk and some other dairy products.

The proportionately small group of persons with problems in tolerating certain foods should consult an allergist before making major dietary changes. What follows is a brief guideline to causes and treatments of food allergies and is not a substitute for medical advice. Symptoms of allergic reactions due to food include skin reactions involving rashes, hives, and swelling of the mouth, tongue, and throat. Digestive reactions include nausea, vomiting, diarrhea, cramping, gas, and abdominal pain and bloating. The respiratory system may react with sneezing, nasal congestion, coughing, and asthma.[22] Severe allergic reactions may result in death.

Foods that may cause allergic reactions in some people include wheat, corn, soy, nuts and peanuts, eggs, seafood and shellfish, cow's milk, and fruits and vegetables. Understanding information on food labels is important because foods that cause allergic reactions may be included in the manufacture of another food. For example, milk causes food allergy problems for some people.[21] Dairy products are easily recognized; however, the presence of milk or chemicals from milk in other foods may be missed. Casein is a milk protein used in some bakery products, salad dressings, frozen desserts, creamed foods and soups, and processed luncheon meat.[22]

Distinguishing true cases from misdiagnosed cases of food allergy is important. An increasing number of parents, teachers, day care providers, and restaurant personnel are recognizing that they need to learn more about the nutritional and other significances of food allergies.[23]

■ Nutrition in action–Nutritional consequences of diarrhea

Diarrhea is the frequent passage of watery bowel movements. Nutritionists are concerned about prolonged diarrhea because it causes dehydration and ultimately death if not corrected. It also reduces the amount of nutrients absorbed from food. Diarrhea is an inconvenience and a brief irritant for most people in developed countries, but in developing countries it is a major cause of death–about 4 million infants and children with it die each year. The main cause of diarrhea is bacterial contamination of food or water. Clean water is not taken for granted in many countries. Other causes of diarrhea include food allergy and intolerance and some drugs such as antibiotics and ulcer drugs.

Foods high in protein–meat, chicken, fish, and eggs–are more likely than carbohydrate-rich foods to provide the conditions needed by the bacteria that cause food poisoning. Dry foods are less likely than moist foods to support the growth of these bac-

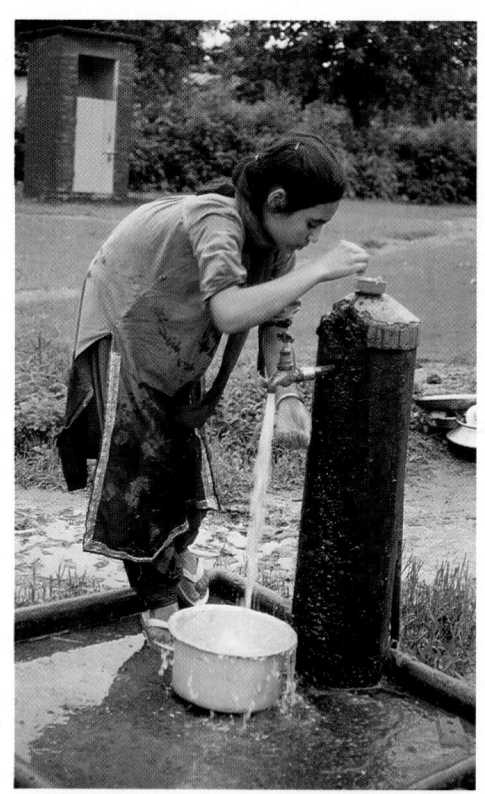

Figure 3-17. Clean water may not be available in some parts of the world. Poor water quality can cause diarrhea and other problems, causing negative effects on people's nutritional status.

teria. Proper refrigeration of perishable food is a key to prevention of diarrhea caused by bacteria.[9]

Travelers' diarrhea happens to people traveling in many parts of the world due to toxins from bacteria in food and water. The traveler may not be immune to some microbes newly met in a foreign country. Prevention includes drinking bottled or boiled water, soft drinks, or fruit juices and avoiding ice cubes, because freezing does not kill bacteria. The foods most involved are uncooked fruits and vegetables. Washing fruit and vegetables in local water is not sufficient. A good rule is: if you can't peel it yourself, don't eat it.

During the 1991 war against Iraq (Desert Shield and Desert Storm), there were numerous outbreaks of diarrhea among the U.S. forces. The microbial villains were *Escherichia coli* and *Shigella*.[24] (*Shigella* was the cause of the food poisoning from a commercial airline meal mentioned previously.) The military made extensive efforts to secure a safe supply of food and water and a high level of sanitation–it seems that throughout history the military has had to fight an extra war against diarrhea.

The effects of diarrhea can be kept under control in extreme cases by giving a glucose-based solution to replace the fluids and nutrients lost. The person drinks a mixture of water, sugar, and essential salts. Rice-syrup solids are also effective. These inexpensive and effective ways of treating diarrhea are being used in many countries.

■ Now you know

- The quantity and quality of food intake varies widely among people as a result of social, psychological, economic, nutritional, pleasure, health, and convenience factors.

- Healthy eating integrates health and pleasure messages about which foods to eat.

- Microbes are important in making some foods (cheese, bread, yogurt) and in the digestion of food. Some bacteria cause food poisoning.

- Food spoilage causes undesirable appearance, flavor, and texture in foods.

- Food safety problems are controlled when rules are observed in purchasing, storing, preparing, cooking, microwaving, serving, and reheating food and handling leftovers.

- The sensory properties of taste, aroma, and texture have important effects on the choice of food.

- Understanding the GI system explains: why so many people have digestive problems; variations in transit time and the reasons for constipation, especially in the elderly; how enzymes and digestive juices work; why antacids are usually not needed; the negative effects of stress on digestion; the role of microbes; which plant foods produce gas (flatulence); and why certain drugs, such as antibiotics, interact with foods and influence the absorption of nutrients.

- Hunger and appetite both influence food intake.

- The liver is important in nutrition–it is a chemical factory for nutrients and a detoxification center for toxins, including alcohol.

- Allergies may not be as prevalent as the public perceives. They are abnormal responses of the immune system to allergens in such foods as milk, wheat, corn, soy, nuts and peanuts, eggs, seafood, shellfish, and fruits and vegetables.

- Diarrhea causes 4 million infant deaths each year. Bacterial contamination of food and water is the main cause. Inexpensive mixtures of sugar and certain salts are effective treatments.

Further Reading

1. Callaway, C. W. The marriage of taste and health: A union whose time has come. *Nutrition Today* 27(3):37, 1992.
2. Scott, T. R. Taste: The neural basis of body wisdom. *World Review of Nutrition and Dietetics* 67:1, 1992.
3. Bowen, D. J. Taste and food preference changes across the course of pregnancy. *Appetite* 19:233, 1992.
4. DuPont, H. L. How safe is the food we eat? *Journal of the American Medical Association* 268:3240, 1992.
5. Senauer, B. Consumer food safety concerns. *Cereal Foods World* 37:298, 1992.
6. Postgate, J. *Microbes and Man, 3rd edition.* Cambridge University Press, Cambridge, 1992.
7. Cody, M. M., and Keith, M. *Food Safety for Professionals: A Reference and Study Guide.* The American Dietetic Association, Chicago, 1991.
8. Cruickshank, J. G. Food handlers and food poisoning. Training programmes are the best. *British Medical Journal* 300:207, 1990.
9. Peikin, S. *Gastrointestinal Health.* Harper Perennial, New York, 1992.
10. Read, N. W. Role of gastrointestinal factors in hunger and satiety in man. *Proceedings of the Nutrition Society* 51:7, 1992.
11. Barrett, J. A. Colorectal disorders in elderly people. *British Medical Journal* 305:764, 1992.
12. Bhaskar, K. R., and others. Viscous fingering of HCl through gastric mucin. *Nature* (London) 360:458, 1992.
13. Cramer, T. A burning question: When do you need an antacid? *FDA Consumer* 26(1):18, 1992.
14. Lewis, R. The bugs within us. *FDA Consumer* 26(7):37, 1992.
15. Coates, M. E., and Walker, R. Interrelationships between the gastrointestinal microflora and non-nutrient components of the diet. *Nutrition Research Reviews* 5:85, 1992.
16. Despommier, D. D. Tapeworm infection–The long and the short of it. *New England Medical Journal* 327:727, 1992.
17. Lewis, J. H. Esophageal and small bowel obstruction from guar gum-containing "diet pills": Analysis of 26 cases reported to the Food and Drug Administration. *American Journal of Gastroenterology* 87:1424, 1992.
18. Hsu, H. H., and others. Gastric bezoar caused by lecithin: An unusual complication of health faddism. *American Journal of Gastroenterology* 87:794, 1992.
19. James, C. T. Food and drugs: Do they mix? *Health Sciences Review*, page 24, Spring 1991.

20. Lienhard, G. E., and others. How cells absorb glucose. *Scientific American* 266(1):86, 1992.
21. Sampson, H. A., and Metcalfe, D. D. Food allergies. *Journal of the American Medical Association* 268:2840, 1992.
22. Dobler, M. L. *Food Allergies.* The American Dietetic Association, Chicago, 1991.
23. Yunginger, J. W. Lethal food allergy in children. *New England Journal of Medicine* 327:421, 1992.
24. Hyams, K. C., and others. Diarrheal disease during Operation Desert Shield. *New England Journal of Medicine* 325:1423, 1991.

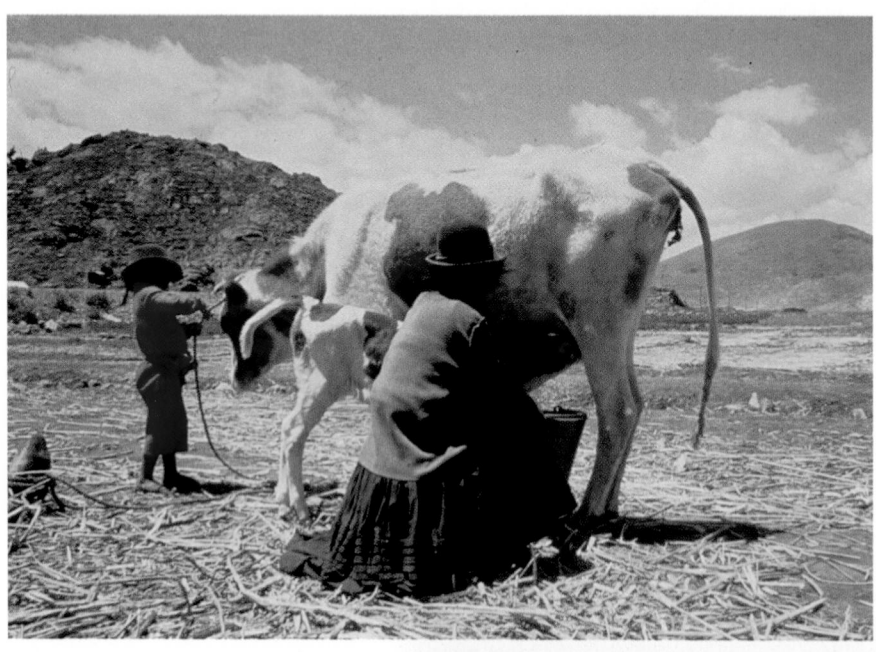

Figures 4-1 and 4-2. A South American woman getting milk direct from the source of supply (left); people choosing among processed foods in a modern supermarket (below).

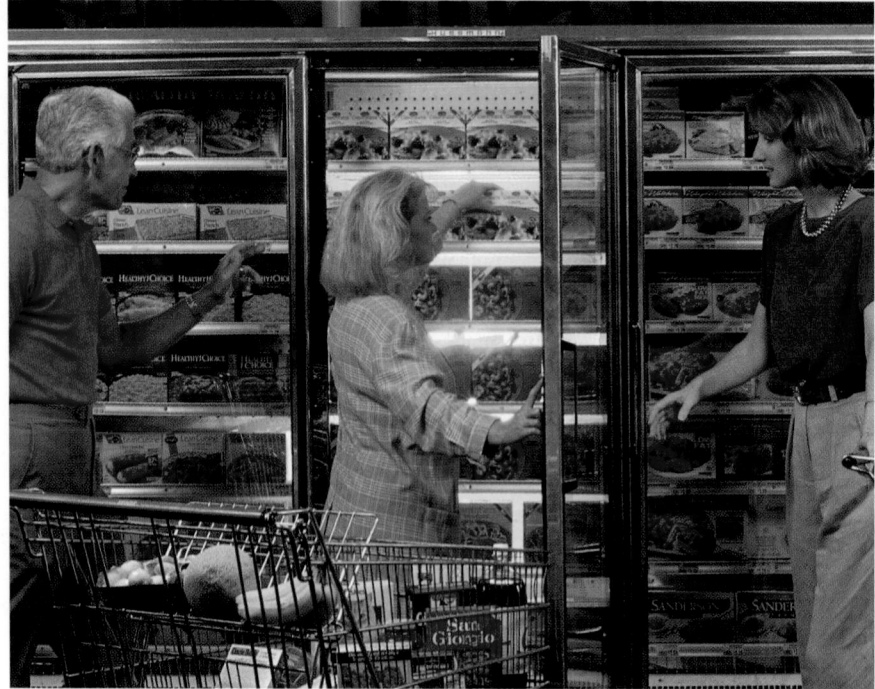

Eating Right–
The Right Balance

■ Nutrition in our lives–The right balance of the right foods

The woman on the left is from a rural area of Peru. She goes directly to the fields to get her supply of milk. Most people in developed countries, and in urban environments in developing countries, go directly to the supermarket or food store. The contrast between these two food delivery systems is great. Yet, in both cases, the important question is: Are the people getting the right balance of foods? Good nutrition is based on the right balance of all nutrients listed in Table 1-4, which come from a wide variety of foods.

People down through the centuries obtained food by cultivating seeds and taming animals. Until quite recently, climate and pests determined how much food reached their tables. Their life expectancy was 35–40 years of age. Regrettably, for millions of people living in developing countries today, the same situation exists.

The ancient Egyptians considered many foods to have medicinal properties, including effects on behavior. Onions were thought to induce sleep, cabbage and almonds to help relieve the effects of excessive alcohol, lemons to protect against the evil eye, and salt to stimulate passion.[1] We aren't much different today, judging by a report published in 1993 that showed nearly $14 billion spent annually in the United States on *unconventional medicine*.[2] Included in this amount is $1.2 billion for commercial diet supplements and $0.8 billion for *megavitamin supplements*. Such supplements are taken mainly for their medicinal value–for example, vitamin E to slow aging. A balanced diet should provide sufficient nutrients to make consumption of supplements unnecessary, or at least of marginal value.

Unconventional medicine: Medical practice not taught widely at U.S. medical schools or generally available at U.S. hospitals.

Megavitamin supplements: Vitamin intake greater than 10 times the RDA, taken in pill, powder, or liquid form.

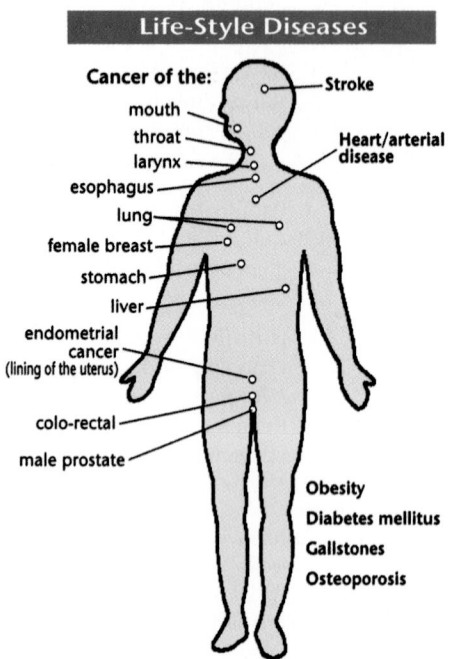

Figure 4-3. Food and nutrition topics frequently make cover stories. This is a Canadian magazine.

Food composition: The amount of nutrients, chemicals, and ingredients in a food.

Think about the topics that made the front page of a Canadian weekly newsmagazine (Figure 4-3).

Phrases such as "Food for Living" and "The Best and the Worst" suggest that the search for health-giving properties in foods is still in progress. The statements that celebrities make about food seem to be taken as dietary guidelines by some people. Some experts suggest that such information and misinformation create the fear of not eating healthfully, even though the fear is not realistic considering the availability and quality of food for most people. The food supply is better than at any time in history and has been a significant contributor to the increase in life expectancy to about 75 years in developed countries.

The ancient Egyptians and people down through the centuries were probably more knowledgeable about where their food came from than we are. They were directly involved in all aspects of food production–the planting, growing, and reaping of crops and the killing of animals for meat. In our modern, urban, industrialized world, many people are unaware of where food comes from, how it is manufactured, its chemical composition, and its effects on health. Most people fear the unknown, and some people are willing to profit from the fear that comes through ignorance. That is why we need labels on food–to tell us about their *composition* and nutritional value. It is why we need dietary guidelines to tell us what proportion of foods to eat for maximum health. And it is why we need to learn from scientists the relationships between certain foods and some diseases.

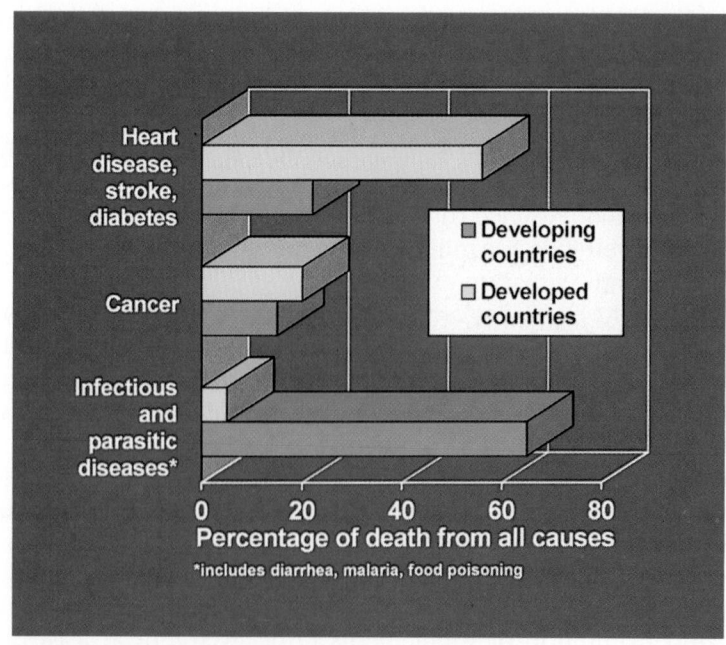

Figure 4-4. Diet-related lifestyle diseases include heart disease, some cancers, stroke, obesity, and diabetes.

Figure 4-5. In developed countries, the greatest causes of death are heart disease, stroke, diabetes, and cancer. In developing countries, most deaths are from infectious and parasitic diseases.

Consider the diet-related life-style diseases, also called "diseases of affluence," shown in Figure 4-4.

The foods and nutrients involved in these diseases will be examined in Chapter 14–an overview is given here. For many years, experts have suggested that a strong linkage exists between coronary heart disease and the amount of fat, the type of fat (saturated), and the amount of cholesterol in the diet. High dietary fat intake may also be associated with some cancers, especially cancers of the colon and prostate. Low fiber intake may be associated with colon cancer. High sodium intake, much of it from salt, may cause stroke in some people. Many of these relationships are still controversial. We do know that death from these diseases is significant in the United States and other developed countries. The greatest killers in developing countries are not the life-style diseases but infections and *parasitic diseases*, as seen in the Figure 4-5.

Parasitic diseases: Diseases caused by parasites, organisms that live within, upon, or at the expense of the host. An example with nutritional implications is the loss of blood (and therefore iron) to hookworms in the GI tract.

Consider the following fact. People in modern affluent societies have higher intake of fat, sugar, and salt than their ancestors did.

Our typical diet in the United States is low in fruits and vegetables–foods that have low fat, sugar, and salt when unprocessed but are high in starch and fiber. However, life expectancy was much less for the hunter-gatherers and peasant farmers than for people in modern affluent societies. Clearly, diet is only one of many factors influencing life expectancy.

Table 4-1. Changing Lifestyles, Changing Dietary Patterns

	Diet (percent of energy)				Diet (grams per day)	
	Fat	Refined Sugar	Starch	Protein	Salt	Fiber
Hunter-gatherers						
(pre-agricultural revolution)	15–20	0	50–70	15–20	1	40
Peasant farmers						
(post-agricultural revolution)	10–15	5	60–75	10–15	5–15	60–120
Modern affluent societies						
(post-industrial revolution)	40+	20	25–30	12	10	20

■ Dietary guidelines for disease prevention

Governments in many countries issue dietary guidelines after receiving advice from nutrition and medical experts.[3] In 1990, the USDA and the US-DHHS issued *Nutrition and Your Health: Dietary Guidelines for Americans*. This publication is an update of two previous editions of guidelines.[4] The guidelines, which are for people aged two years and older, emphasize enjoyable and healthful eating through variety and moderation. Previous editions took a more negative approach by emphasizing dietary restrictions. The Dietary Guidelines make seven recommendations. Let's look at which foods are affected by these recommendations. In later chapters we will see how they influence the intake of specific nutrients.

- **Eat a variety of foods**. This is the best way to get the nutrients needed for health. No single food provides all the nutrients in the amounts you need. Milk comes close to providing all nutrients, but it is low in iron, and some people are intolerant of it. Varying your intake also means

Fortified foods: Foods with added nutrients, usually vitamins and minerals.

not consuming just a few highly *fortified foods* or supplements. Variety is the secret to selecting a nutritious diet.

- **Maintain healthy weight.** This means avoiding being too fat or too thin. Obesity is linked to coronary heart disease, stroke, hypertension, diabetes, certain cancers, and other illnesses. Recommended body weights will be examined in Chapter 11.

- **Choose a diet low in fat, saturated fat, and cholesterol** because of their association with coronary heart disease, obesity, and certain cancers. Eating less fat from foods of animal origin helps to lower cholesterol, total fat, and saturated fat in the diet.

- **Choose a diet with plenty of vegetables, fruits, and grain products.** Vegetables include dry beans and peas, and grain products include breads, cereals, pasta, and rice. Variety in your choices here will provide important vitamins, minerals, fiber, and less fat.

- **Use sugar only in moderation** because sugar supplies only calories and negligible amounts of most nutrients. Reading labels correctly is important because sugar comes in many forms–table sugar (sucrose), brown sugar, honey, syrup, corn sweetener, high-fructose corn sweetener, *molasses*, glucose (dextrose), fructose, maltose, and lactose.

- **Use salt and sodium only in moderation** because high blood pressure is common in populations with high salt intake. Surveys show that some Americans consume too much salt and sodium.

- **If you drink alcoholic beverages, do so in moderation.** This is excellent advice for several reasons. Alcoholic beverages supply calories with little or no nutrients. Alcohol is linked to many health problems, can lead to addiction, and can cause accidents. Taken during pregnancy, it can cause mental disabilities and physical deformities in the baby. Alcohol should not be taken with any medications, including over-the-counter preparations.

Molasses: Residue left after sugar refining.

The Dietary Guidelines define moderate drinking as no more than one drink per day for women, and no more than two drinks per day for men. A drink is classified as 12 ounces of regular beer, or 5 ounces of wine, or 1½ ounces of distilled spirits (80 proof).

The *Nutrition Recommendations for Canadians* were published in 1990.[5] According to them, the Canadian diet should

- Provide energy consistent with the maintenance of body weight within the recommended range
- Include essential nutrients in amounts recommended in the Recommended Nutrient Intakes for Canadians (RNI)
- Include no more than 30% of energy as fat, of which no more than 10% is saturated fat
- Provide 55% of energy as carbohydrate from a variety of sources
- Include no more than 5% of total energy as alcohol, or two drinks daily, whichever is less
- Contain no more caffeine than the equivalent of four regular cups of coffee per day

In addition,

- The sodium content of the Canadian diet should be reduced.
- Community water supplies should have 1 milligram of fluoride per liter of water.

Dietary guidelines were introduced in Japan recently. The traditional Japanese diet is changing to a Western-type diet high in fat, sugar, and salt and low in fiber, so guidelines are needed. The Japanese introduce an interesting guideline not mentioned in the American, Canadian, or British guidelines, an emphasis on the importance of the social aspects of eating. Eating should be enjoyable and shared with family and friends if possible. They believe that this leads to the incorporation of positive recommendations and is as important as the health promotion aspects of eating.

Planning Healthy Diets–Putting Dietary Guidelines into Practice

Planning a healthy diet means choosing nutritious foods to meet your nutrient requirements. Here we look at the foods that will achieve this, while acknowledging that personal, economic, health, and other situations will also intervene in determining what foods you choose to eat. We look at two major diet plans that fulfill the recommendations of the Dietary Guidelines. They are the Food Guide Pyramid and the Exchange Lists of Foods.

Food Guide Pyramid: A research-based food guidance system, developed by the USDA, in which foods necessary in large amounts are at the base of the pyramid and foods to be eaten sparingly are at the top.

The Food Guide Pyramid

The *Food Guide Pyramid* replaced the Basic Four Food Groups in 1992 as the basic graphical depiction of dietary guidelines. The USDA studied many designs before deciding on a pyramid as the most effective way of presenting the information to the public.[6] The audience is the same as for the Dietary Guidelines–healthy Americans over the age of two years.

Think about your diet and compare it with the recommendations in the Pyramid.

The goals for the Food Guide Pyramid are many. It emphasizes overall health and not just the prevention or treatment of any single disease. It is based on up-to-

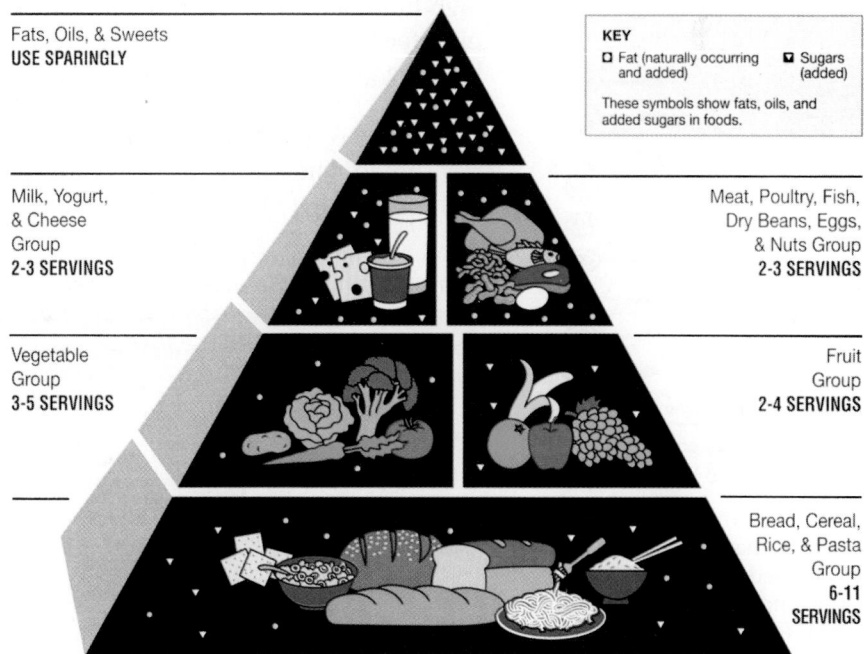

Food Guide Pyramid
A Guide to Daily Food Choices

Fats, Oils, & Sweets
USE SPARINGLY

KEY
▢ Fat (naturally occurring and added) ◪ Sugars (added)
These symbols show fats, oils, and added sugars in foods.

Milk, Yogurt, & Cheese Group
2-3 SERVINGS

Meat, Poultry, Fish, Dry Beans, Eggs, & Nuts Group
2-3 SERVINGS

Vegetable Group
3-5 SERVINGS

Fruit Group
2-4 SERVINGS

Bread, Cereal, Rice, & Pasta Group
6-11 SERVINGS

Figure 4-6. The Food Guide Pyramid.

A

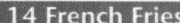

One Baked Potato

Calories: 120
Fat: trace

14 French Fries

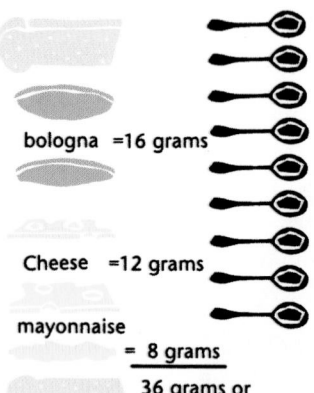

Calories: 225
Fat: 11 grams

B

bologna = 16 grams

Cheese = 12 grams

mayonnaise
= 8 grams

36 grams or
9 teaspoons of fat

Figure 4-7. The amount of fat in a food may depend on how it is cooked and served. A, the same amount of potato in different forms. B, calories can add up quickly when certain foods are combined.

date research. The Pyramid focuses on the total diet and not on individual foods, and it is user-friendly for consumers. No one food group is more important than another–for good health you need them all. Maximum flexibility can be achieved by using food substitutions. For example, instead of emphasizing specific low-fat choices, the Pyramid shows that consumers can balance a high-fat dessert such as a rich ice cream with selections from other groups that have less fat. Let's start our explanation of the Food Guide Pyramid at the top, with the fats, oils, and sweets group.

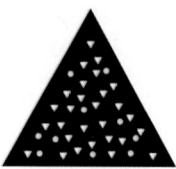

Typical foods here include salad dressing and oils, cream, butter, margarine, sugars, soft drinks, candies, and sweet desserts. These foods provide primarily calories and should be eaten sparingly. Notice that the symbols for fats and sugars are also in the other groups. For example, sugar is added to some foods in the bread, fruit, meat, and milk groups. The fat in these groups may be naturally occurring or may be added.

Let's apply this information to the preparation of some well-known foods. For example, consider the fat content of foods that are usually not consumed in their original form. Boiled potatoes are in the vegetable group and are naturally low in fat. But Figure 4-7A shows what happens to the fat content and the number of calories when potatoes are converted into french fries. Another example is croissants and doughnuts, which are high in fat although the main ingredient, flour, is low in fat. In addition, most foods consumed today are complex, not simple. Notice in Figure 4-7B how the grams of fat add up when a bologna and cheese sandwich is put together.

The Dietary Guidelines recommend that no more than 30% of your calories should come from fat. You can calculate for yourself the number of grams of fat that provide 30% of calories in your daily diet.

Table 4-2. Sample Diets for a Day at Three Calorie Levels

Food	Lower (about 1,600 cal)	Moderate (about 2,200 cal)	Higher (about 2,800 cal)
Bread group, servings	6	9	11
Vegetable group, servings	3	4	5
Fruit group, servings	2	3	4
Milk group, servings	2–3[a]	2–3[a]	2–3[a]
Meat group, ounces[b]	5	6	7
Total fat, grams	53	73	93
Total added sugars, teaspoons	6	12	18

[a] Three servings for women who are pregnant or breast feeding, teenagers, and young adults to age 24.
[b] Total ounces per day.

Multiply your total day's calories by 0.30 to get the allowable calories from fat per day. *Example: 2,200 calories × 0.30 = 660 calories from fat.*

Divide this number by 9 (each gram of fat has 9 calories) to get the allowable grams of fat per day. *Example: 660 calories from fat ÷ 9 = 73 grams of fat.*

The USDA provides a guideline (Table 4-2) to help you choose a balanced diet with no more than 30% of calories coming from fat.

A simple check shows that the number of calories from fat totals about 30% in each of the three sample diets. For example, a person consuming the 1,600-calorie diet should consume no more than 53 grams of fat, which equals 477 calories (because there are 9 calories in each gram of fat). This 477 calories is 30% of the 1,600-calorie diet.

Common sense is needed to meet the target of 30% of calories from fat. The example that follows has correct mathematical calculations but poor nutritional practice. Unfortunately, some people play the numbers this way, but you will quickly realize that this is *not* the healthy way to get the maximum of 30% of total calories from fat. Meet Mr. Baseball at the ballpark as he buys a hot dog. He may not know which foods are high in fat and that 1 gram of fat has 9 calories. Here is an analysis of his fat intake as he eats his hot dog, bun, and relish, all washed down by beer or a cola drink while he watches the game.

Table 4-3. Percent Calories from Fat in Food at the Baseball Game

	Fat (grams)	Calories from Fat	Total Calories	Percent Calories from Fat
1 hot dog	17	153	184	83
1 bun	2	18	115	16
Relish	<0.1	0.9	20	4.5
Total	19.1	172	319	54
Add 1 beer, regular, 12-oz can	0	0	146	0
Total	19.1	172	465	37
Or add 1 cola, regular, 12-oz can	0	0	151	0
Total	19.1	172	470	37

Suppose Mr. Baseball is determined to reach 30% of calories from fat instead of the 37% he now has consumed. All he needs to do is add one extra can of beer or cola to "wash down" the hot dog.

	Fat (grams)	Calories from Fat	Total Calories	Percent Calories from Fat
Former total	19.1	172	470	37
Add one more beer	0	0	146	0
New total	19.1	172	616	28

Bingo! He is now at less than 30% of total calories from fat because of the diluting effect of the beer or cola, which does not contain any calories from fat. All of the numbers are correct, but the method of achieving them is poor nutrition.

Table 4-4. Fat in Fats, Oils, and Sweets Group

Food	Amount	Grams of Fat
Butter or margarine	1 tsp	4
Mayonnaise	1 tbsp	11
Salad dressing	1 tbsp	7
Reduced-calorie salad dressing	1 tbsp	...[a]
Sour cream	2 tbsp	6
Cream cheese	1 oz	10
Sugar, jam, jelly	1 oz	0
Cola	12 fl. oz	0
Fruit drink, ade	12 fl. oz	0
Chocolate bar	1 oz	9
Sherbet	½ cup	2
Fruit sorbet	½ cup	0
Gelatin dessert	½ cup	0

[a] Check product label.

Table 4-5. Sugar Added by Processing

Food	Amount	Added Sugar (teaspoons)[a]
Bread group		
Bread	1 slice	0
Muffin	1 medium	1
Cookies	2 medium	1
Danish pastry	1 medium	1
Doughnut	1 medium	2
Ready-to-eat-cereal, sweetened	1 oz	...[b]
Pound cake, no-fat	1 oz	2
Angel food cake	1/12 of a tube cake	5
Cake, frosted	1/16 of average cake	6
Pie, fruit, two-crust	1/6 of 8-inch pie	6
Fruit group		
Canned in juice	1/2 cup	0
Canned in light syrup	1/2 cup	2
Canned in heavy syrup	1/2 cup	4
Milk group		
Milk, plain	1 cup	0
Chocolate milk, 2%	1 cup	3
Low-fat yogurt, plain	8 oz	0
Low-fat yogurt, flavored	8 oz	5
Low-fat yogurt, fruit	8 oz	7
Ice cream, ice milk, or frozen yogurt	1/2 cup	3
Chocolate shake	10 fl. oz	9
Other		
Sugar, jam, or jelly	1 tsp	1
Syrup or honey	1 tbsp	3
Chocolate bar	1 oz	3
Fruit sorbet	1/2 cup	3
Gelatin dessert	1/2 cup	4
Sherbet	1/2 cup	5
Cola	12 fl. oz	9
Fruit drink, ade	12 fl. oz	12

[a] One teaspoon equals 4 grams of sugar.
[b] Check product label.

Fat is present in high concentrations in some foods in the fats, oils, and sweets group. Even small servings, such as 1 tablespoon of mayonnaise, provide a lot of fat.

Sugar is found in many foods (see Table 4-5). Some of it is natural, as in fruits, and some is added in cooking or processing.

Salt is a combination of sodium and chloride ions. Most foods contain some sodium and chloride naturally. The USDA recommends that we restrict sodium intake to a maximum of 2,400–3,000 milligrams per day. Much of this comes from salt added during cooking or at the table. One teaspoon of salt provides about 2,000 milligrams of sodium. However, as Table 4-6 shows, we get sodium from a wide variety of foods.

Some people are advised to further restrict sodium intake because of the relationship between sodium and hypertension. However, some researchers have found that only about 10% of people are sensitive to salt. If there is a history of hypertension in your family, you should talk to a doctor and dietitian.

Table 4-6. Sodium in Food

Food	Amount	Sodium (milligrams)
Bread, cereal, rice, and pasta group		
Cooked cereal, rice, or pasta, unsalted	1/2 cup	Trace
Ready-to-eat cereal	1 oz	100–360
Bread	1 slice	110–175
Vegetable and fruit groups		
Vegetables, fresh or frozen, cooked without salt	1/2 cup	Less than 70
Vegetables, canned or frozen, with sauce	1/2 cup	140–460
Tomato juice, canned	3/4 cup	660
Vegetable soup, canned	1 cup	820
Fruit, fresh, frozen, or canned	1/2 cup	Trace
Milk, yogurt, and cheese group		
Milk	1 cup	120
Yogurt	8 oz	160
Natural cheeses	1½ oz	110–450
Processed cheeses	2 oz	800
Meat group		
Fresh meat, poultry, fish	3 oz	Less than 90
Tuna, canned, water pack	3 oz	300
Bologna	2 oz	580
Ham, lean, roasted	3 oz	1,020
Other		
Salad dressing	1 tbsp	75–220
Ketchup, mustard, steak sauce	1 tbsp	130–230
Soy sauce	1 tbsp	1,030
Salt	1 tsp	2,000
Dill pickle	1 medium	930
Potato chips, salted	1 oz	130
Corn chips, salted	1 oz	235
Peanuts, roasted in oil, salted	1 oz	120

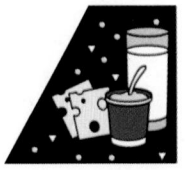

Dairy products are high in protein, vitamins, and minerals except iron. Milk, yogurt, and cheese are the best sources of calcium. Two servings are recommended for most people, with three servings for pregnant and lactating women, teenagers, and young adults to age 24. Notice in Table 4-7 that some foods in this group, such as natural and processed cheese, are high in fat.

Table 4-7. Fat in the Milk, Yogurt, and Cheese Group[a]

Food	Amount	Servings	Grams of Fat
♦ Skim milk	1 cup	1	Trace
♦ Nonfat yogurt, plain	8 oz	1	Trace
Low-fat milk, 2%	1 cup	1	5
Whole milk	1 cup	1	8
Chocolate milk, 2%	1 cup	1	5
Low-fat yogurt, plain	8 oz	1	4
Low-fat yogurt, fruit	8 oz	1	3
Natural cheddar cheese	1½ oz	1	14
Processed cheese	2 oz	1	18
Mozzarella, part skim	1½ oz	1	7
Ricotta, part skim	1/2 cup	1	10
Cottage cheese, 4% fat	1/2 cup	1/4	5
Ice cream	1/2 cup	1/3	7
Ice milk	1/2 cup	1/3	3
Frozen yogurt	1/2 cup	1/2	2

[a] Eat two to three servings a day.
♦ = One of the lowest fat choices in this food group.

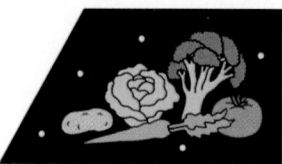

This group provides protein, B-complex vitamins, iron, and zinc. Dry beans, nuts, and eggs are included because they are similar to meat in their content of protein and most vitamins and minerals. The two to three servings recommended per day should total about 5–7 ounces of cooked lean meat, poultry, or fish per day. (Three ounces of meat is about the size of a deck of cards.) High-fat foods in this group include nuts, peanuts, bologna, some other processed meats, and heavily marbled meat that has not been trimmed, such as prime rib.

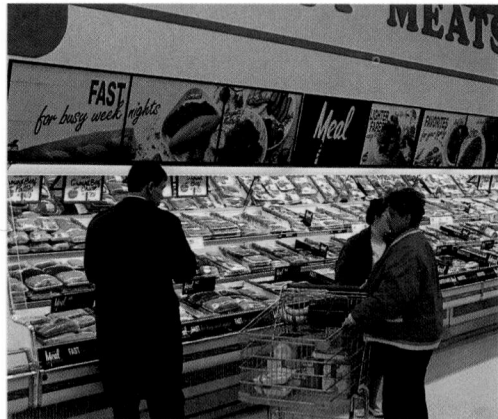

Figure 4-8. Meat is a nutritious food, but it is wise to select low-fat lean cuts.

Table 4-8. Fat in the Meat, Poultry, Fish, Dry Beans, Eggs, and Nuts Group[a]

Food	Amount	Counts as This Much Meat	Grams of Fat
♦ Lean meat, poultry, fish, cooked	3 oz	3 oz	6
Ground beef, lean, cooked	3 oz	3 oz	16
Chicken, with skin, fried	3 oz	3 oz	13
Bologna	2 slices	1 oz	16
Egg	1	1 oz	5
♦ Dry beans and peas, cooked	1/2 cup	1 oz	Trace
Peanut butter	2 tbsp	1 oz	16
Nuts	1/3 cup	1 oz	22

[a] Eat 5–7 oz daily.
♦ = One of the lowest fat choices in this food group

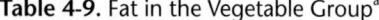

Table 4-9. Fat in the Vegetable Group[a]

Food	Amount	Servings	Grams of Fat
♦ Vegetables, cooked	1/2 cup	1	Trace
♦ Vegetables, leafy, raw	1 cup	1	Trace
♦ Vegetables, nonleafy, raw, chopped	1/2 cup	1	Trace
Potatoes, scalloped	1/2 cup	1	4
Potato salad	1/2 cup	1	8
French fries	10	1	8

[a] Eat three to five servings a day.
♦ = One of the lowest fat choices in this food group

Vegetables are rich sources of vitamins A, C, and folic acid, of fiber, and of the minerals iron and magnesium. They are naturally low in fat. But beware–the fat content is high in some foods because of fat added in preparation. You can see again in Table 4-9 what happens to the fat content of potatoes when they are made into potato salad or french fries.

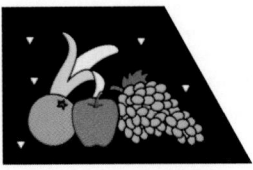

Table 4-10. Fat in the Fruit Group[a]

Food	Amount	Servings	Grams of Fat
◆ Whole fruit: apple, orange, or banana	Medium-sized	1	Trace
◆ Fruit, raw or canned	1/2 cup	1	Trace
◆ Fruit juice, unsweetened	3/4 cup	1	Trace
Avocado	1/4 whole	1	9

[a] Eat two to four servings a day.
◆ = One of the lowest fat choices in this food group.

Fruits and fruit juices are important for their vitamin A and C and potassium content. They are naturally low in sodium and fat. One exception is avocados, which are high in fat.

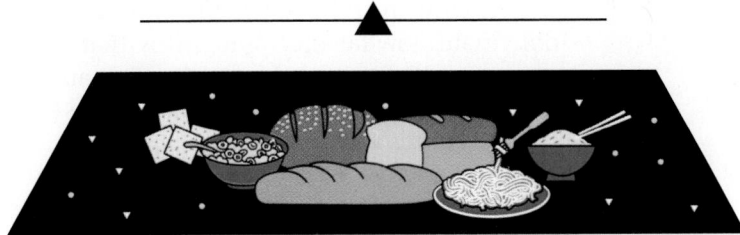

Complex carbohydrates (starches), vitamins, minerals, and fiber are contributed by this group. Starchy foods are no more fattening than other carbohydrate or protein foods and a lot less so than foods containing fatty acids. Of course, their calorie content is increased by the addition of butter or margarine on bread, by cheese or cream sauces on pasta, and by sugar and fat added in cookies, pies, and cakes.

Table 4-11. Fat in the Bread, Cereal, Rice, and Pasta Group[a]

Food	Amount	Servings	Grams of Fat
◆ Bread	1 slice	1	1
◆ Hamburger roll, bagel, English muffin	1	2	2
Tortilla	1	1	3
◆ Rice, pasta, cooked	1/2 cup	1	Trace
Plain crackers, small	3–4	1	3
Breakfast cereal	1 oz	1	...[b]
Pancakes, 4-inch diameter	2	2	3
Croissant	1 large (2 oz)	2	12
Doughnut	1 medium (2 oz)	2	11
Danish	1 medium (2 oz)	2	13
Cake, frosted	1/16 of average-sized cake	1	13
Cookies	2 medium	1	4
Pie, fruit, two-crust	1/6 of 8-inch pie	2	19

[a] Eat six to eleven servings daily.
[b] Check product label.
◆ = One of the lowest fat choices in this food group

Exchange lists: Lists of interchangeable foods with similar caloric contents. Used in diet planning and weight-loss programs.

Exchange Lists of Foods

Exchange lists of foods estimate the energy, carbohydrate, protein, and fat content of a food or meal. Each list has foods with similar distributions of carbohydrate, protein, and fat and therefore a similar number of calories per serving. Any food in the portion size listed can be "exchanged" for any other food on the same list. Attention to portion size is important; otherwise nutrient intake will be different. Some examples of how exchange lists work are shown in Table 4-12.

The concept was developed by the American Diabetes Association and The American Dietetic Association. Exchange lists are used by people with diabetes, and modified versions are used in some weight-reducing programs. They emphasize high-carbohydrate, low-fat diets and stress that meal planning must be flexible to meet the taste and needs of the individual. Photographs of food from the six exchange groups are shown here.

In applying this information to meal planning, any of the foods from the vegetable exchange can be traded because they have similar caloric content. Similar trades can be made within the starch/bread list and the meat list. Since the caloric content of foods listed for the starch/bread and the meat exchange lists are similar (60–65 calories), they can be traded between each other also. The vegetables listed have approximately one-third the calories of the starch/bread and meat items. Because of this, three times the amount of these foods can be traded for one listed amount of starch/bread or meat. Further details on the Exchange List of Foods and examples of foods in the six groups are given in Appendix D.

Table 4-12. Examples of Exchanges in Three Food Groups

Foods	Amount	Calories
Vegetables		
Tomato juice	1/2 cup	22
Cauliflower, raw	1 cup	24
Mushrooms, cooked	1/2 cup	21
Vegetable juice	1/2 cup	22
Starch/bread		
Cornflakes	3/4 cup	66
Bread	1 slice	68
Popcorn, popped	3 cups	69
Beans, cooked	1/3 cup	73
Meats		
Tenderloin, broiled, lean	1 oz	59
Ham, fresh (pork leg), roasted	1 oz	62
Chicken, no skin, dark meat, roasted	1 oz	58
Shrimp, canned	2 oz	66

■ Recommended dietary allowances (RDAs) are guidelines to balanced diets

Recommended Dietary Allowance (RDA): The daily intake of energy and selected nutrients recommended for the U.S. population.

Most countries have a dietary standard for their population. In the United States it is called the *Recommended Dietary Allowance (RDA)*; in Canada it is known as the Recommended Nutrient Intake for Canadians (RNI) and in the United Kingdom as the Reference Nutrient Intake.[7] Dietary standards are set also by the World Health Organization and by the Food and Agricultural Organization of the United Nations. In the United States, the RDAs were first published in 1943 "to provide standards serving as a goal for good nutrition." World War II was in full swing that year, so the new RDAs also acted as a "guide for planning and procuring food supplies for national defense." The latest edition of the RDAs is the 10th. A summary is presented inside the back cover of this book. There are RDAs

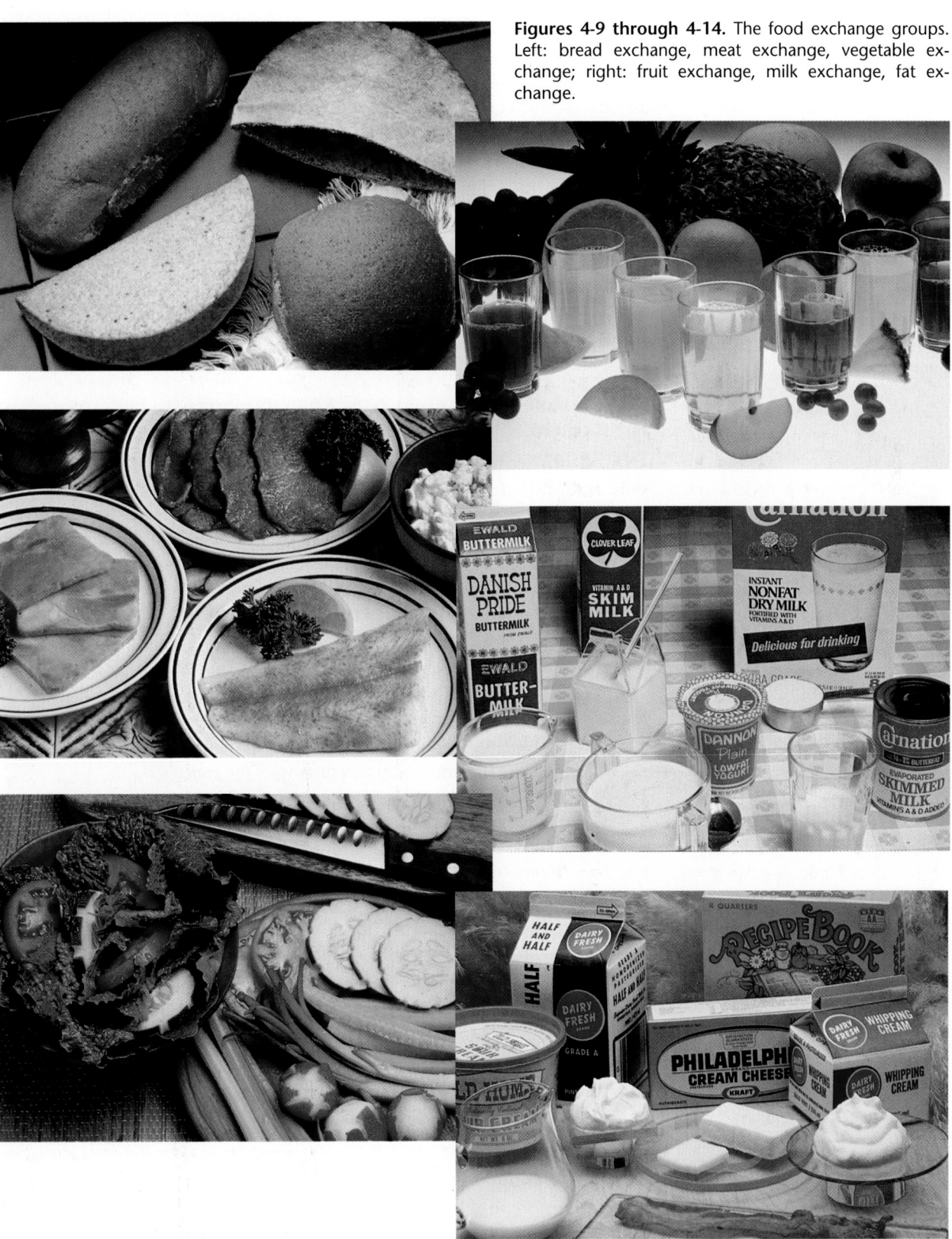

Figures 4-9 through 4-14. The food exchange groups. Left: bread exchange, meat exchange, vegetable exchange; right: fruit exchange, milk exchange, fat exchange.

for eleven vitamins and seven minerals and for protein. The additional tables include two more vitamins and eight more minerals plus RDAs for energy (calories). The Recommended Nutrient Intake for Canadians is given also, in Appendix E. Notice that specific values are given for different ages, for men and women, and for use during pregnancy and lactation. Individuals vary in their need for food because of several factors.

- **Body size**–For a larger body, more nutrients are required.
- **Growth and pregnancy**–Periods of rapid growth and of pregnancy and lactation call for more nutrients than for normal maintenance.
- **Gender differences**–Males and females over 10 years of age have different nutrient requirements because of differences in growth rate, body weight, and body composition. For example, women have higher proportions of body fat; men have more muscle. Women require more iron because of the loss of iron in red blood cells in menstruation.

Compare the nutrients listed in the RDA table inside the back cover with the list of nutrients in Table 1-4.

Not all nutrients appear in the RDA table. Insufficient knowledge about some nutrients is the reason for lack of RDA values now–an indication that nutrition is still a young science. It is important to emphasize that wherever possible the RDAs should be achieved by eating a variety of foods and not by taking supplements or adding nutrients to single foods.

RDAs Are for Groups, Not for Individuals

RDAs are used for the following purposes:

- To interpret food composition records of groups of people
- To set guidelines for the nutrition labeling of food
- To check whether food supplies meet nutritional needs–for example, in planning menus for school lunch, hospitals, prisons, or the armed services
- To establish guides for public assistance programs
- To support the development of new food products by industry
- As a guide in planning and buying food for groups of people
- As a guide in developing nutrition education programs

Metabolic disorders:
Unfavorable alterations in energy changes and in the chemical changes that are associated with growth, maturity, and aging.

Chronic diseases: Disease having a slow onset and lasting a long time–e.g., coronary heart disease, cancer, hypertension.

RDAs are often misinterpreted. It is important to be aware that the RDAs are *not* designed to evaluate individual diets (the RDAs deal only with groups of healthy people) and are *not* for evaluating special nutritional needs arising from *metabolic disorders*, *chronic diseases*, injuries, premature birth, infections, other medical conditions and illnesses, and drug therapies.

People differ in their need for food.

In any group of twenty or more subjects, with similar attributes and activities, food intake can vary as much as twofold

stated a group of well-known British nutritionists as they debated the question: How much food do humans require? The short answer to this question is that we don't know exactly. So, the RDAs cover 97.5% of the population. You are probably covered, but not necessarily so.

Let's use an important nutrient, iron, to show how RDA values are used correctly. RDAs correct for undigested or unabsorbed nutrients. For example, a young girl requires 1.8 milligrams of iron per day. Physiologists tell us that only 10% of dietary iron is absorbed. Therefore, to ensure that the girl gets the required 1.8 milligrams of iron, the RDA must be 18 milligrams.

Vitamin C gives us another insight into RDAs in use. The average daily *requirement* for vitamin C is 10 milligrams. Over time, intake below 10 milligrams per day causes a vitamin C deficiency called scurvy–bleeding gums and teeth that fall out. The RDA for vitamin C for adult men and women is 60 milligrams, and other countries recommend intake ranging from 30 to 100 milligrams per day. Notice that the *RDA value* for vitamin C is higher than the average *requirement*. RDA values are higher than average requirement values for all nutrients with the exception of energy.

Requirement: Minimal amount of a nutrient needed to maintain health and to avoid nutrient deficiency.

How many days can a person go without vitamin C intake before scurvy occurs? Probably 60–120 days–the length of time to deplete vitamin C reserves in the body of a healthy adult. The figure above shows the amounts of different foods needed to meet the 10-milligram vitamin C requirement or the RDA (60 milligrams). It also shows the range of amounts of the vitamin in commercially available vitamin C tablets. Notice that they can contain as much as 1,000 milligrams of vitamin C. Think what unrealistic amounts of food would have to be consumed to give a dietary intake of 1,000 milligrams of the vitamin–probably not many people would eat 25 cups of spinach or 33 potatoes in one day. Also, nutrient supplements like the 1,000-milligram vitamin C tablet give *only* vitamin C and no other nutrients. In contrast, vitamin C *and* many other nutrients are obtained from oranges, grapes, spinach, and other foods. For details on which extra nutrients are provided by these foods, see the Table of Food Composition in Appendix A.

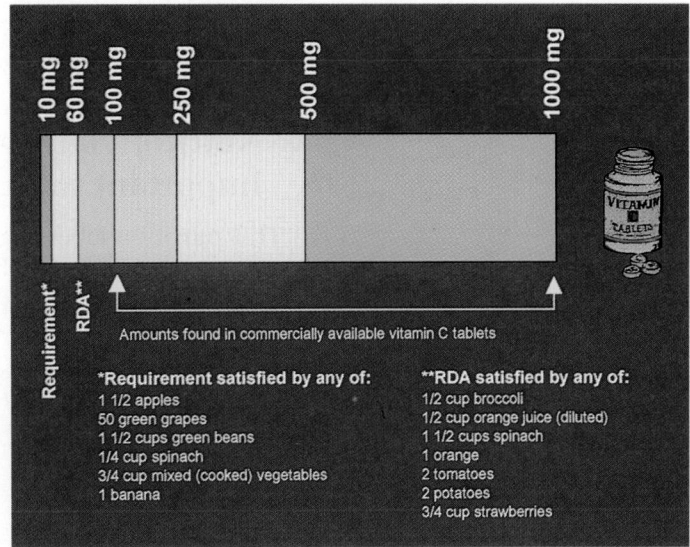

Figure 4-15. The vitamin C content of foods meeting the average requirement and the RDA for vitamin C. Compare these amounts with those provided by commercially available vitamin C supplements.

RDAs for Energy

The example for vitamin C above shows how RDAs for this vitamin and for other nutrients allow for a generous extra amount above the requirement for the nutrient. The exception is the RDA for energy (calories). If the same generous allowances were made for energy intake, it would encourage obesity, as the excess calories would be converted into body fat. RDAs for energy are set at the median of the requirement for each age and gender grouping. Up to 20% additional energy intake is allowed for growth, large body size, and activity, which all require extra calories. Inactive people, the elderly, and those with small body size have lower energy requirements, and, accordingly, recommended energy intake for these groups is 20% below the median values.

Energy is provided by carbohydrates, proteins, lipids, and alcohol. There are no RDA values for carbohydrates and lipids because they are common nutrients in the typical diet. Alcohol is a toxin and is not a nutrient, although it does provide calories.

International travel and seasonal changes may alter your energy requirements because of changes in climate. In hot climates, the requirement for energy decreases, but the recommendation stays the same. The need for vitamins involved in energy metabolism–including thiamin, riboflavin, and niacin–decreases also.

■ Nutrition labels–
Important sources of information

This nutrition label (Figures 4-16 and 4-17) is a common sight on food packages. It was required beginning in 1994.[8] Much of the following information comes from a government publication called the Federal Register (Volume 58, No. 3, January 6, 1993).

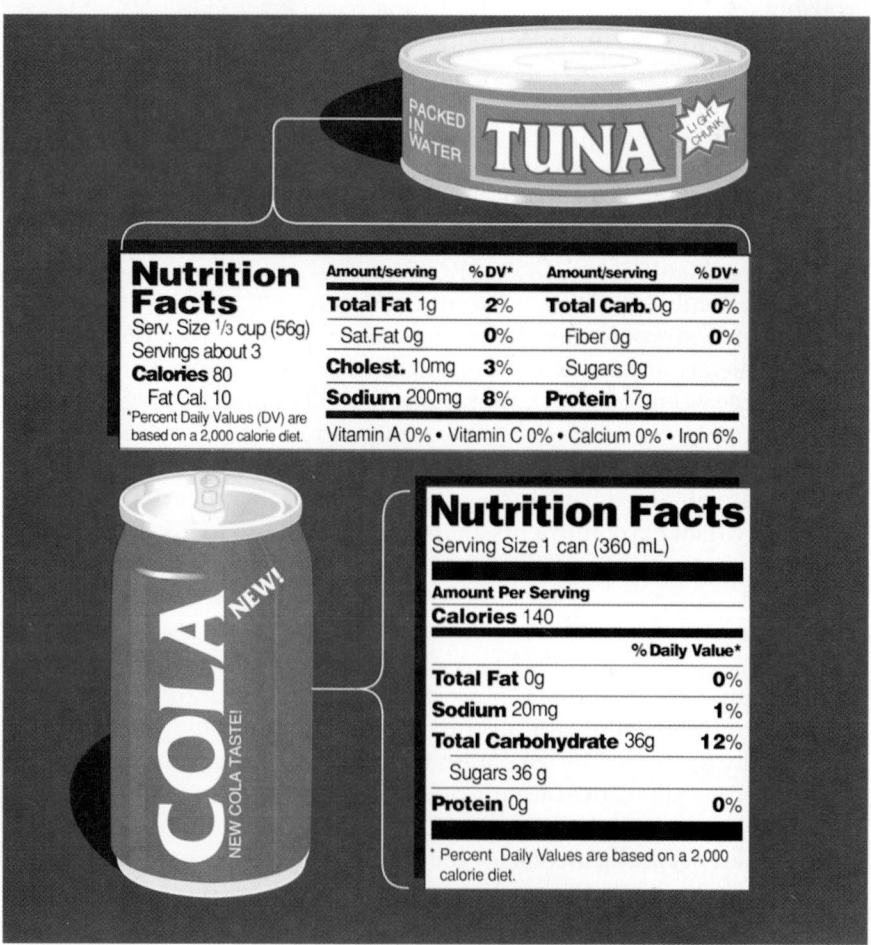

Figures 4-16 and 4-17. The new food labels introduced in 1994.

Look on the food label as a map showing the way through a food supply that has great variety in choices, is complex in its composition, and (for some foods) is increasingly associated with either the cause of or the cure for certain diseases. Clearly, we need help in making the correct food choices, and that help is provided on food labels. But who reads food labels? An interesting assortment of people according to two British researchers.

See if you fit into one or more of these categories of food label readers. They are nutrition- and health-conscious, dieters or weight-watchers, time-savers, quality-oriented, or people who are trying the product for the very first time. Also playing a role in who reads nutrition labels are gender, education, age, and family income.

Some surveys show that only a small proportion of the population reads and understands food labels–those not using food labels include men, people with low incomes, and those with high school educations or less. Some people turn to popular magazines and tabloids rather than to nutrition labels for information on nutrients in their food.

Consumers want food labels to be simple but informative. The U.S. Nutrition Labeling and Education Act (NLEA) of 1990 represents an attempt to meet this requirement. It made FDA responsible for implement-

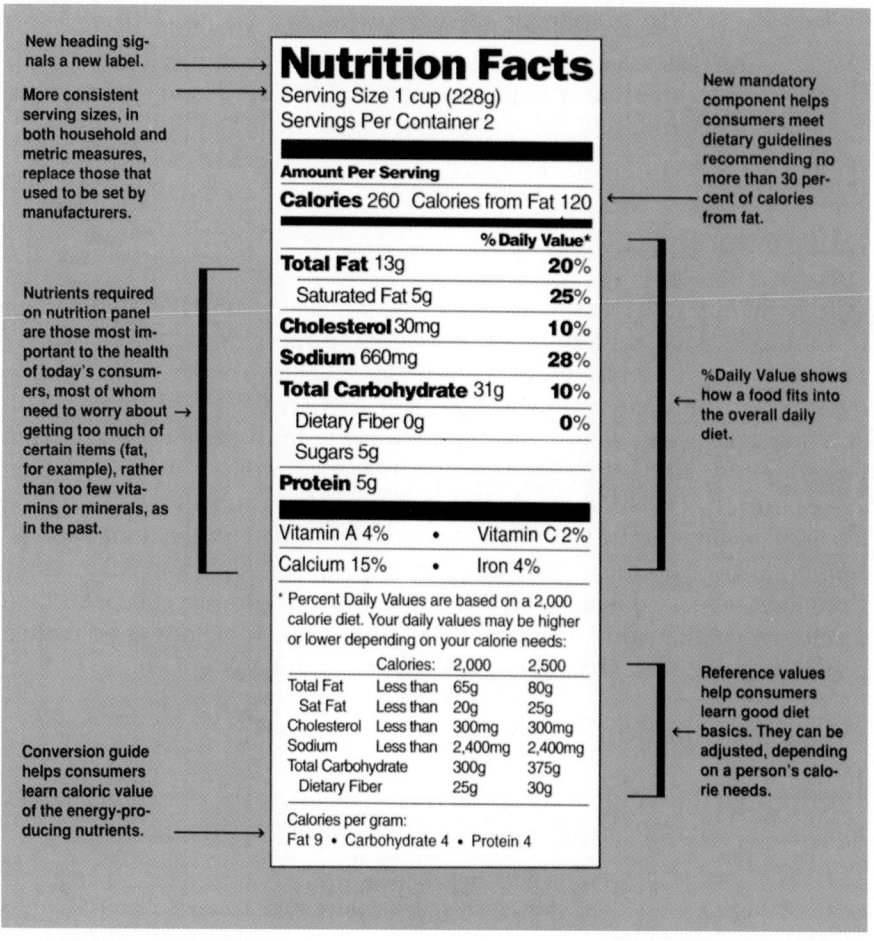

ing new labeling requirements by May of 1994. This law was intended to clear up consumer confusion, encourage product innovation by food manufacturers, and incorporate new knowledge in nutrition learned since labels were last modified in the early 1970s.

Nutrition labeling will be mandatory for most foods. Exceptions not requiring nutritional labels are limited to foods of no nutritional significance, foods sold to restaurant or restaurant-type services, foods prepared on-site in retail establishments and sold from self-service bars or behind deli/bakery counters, raw fruits and vegetables, fresh fish, infant formulas and medical foods (both regulated by different laws), foods shipped in bulk form, foods for institutional food service use, foods processed by small businesses, and food in small packages. For this last category, however, the information must be available by mail or phone, with the address or phone number available at the point of purchase. Be aware that a nutritional label is not required for some foods you eat.

The new label places emphasis on relationships between nutrition and diet-related diseases, rather than simply giving vitamin and mineral information. For example, some experts stress that dietary intake of fat, saturated fat, cholesterol, and sodium are related to some of the life-style diseases mentioned above. People need to know how much of these are in the food they are buying. Therefore, labels must carry a nutrient disclosure statement if specific nutrients and other chemicals are present in the food at or above certain levels. Table 4-13 gives some examples.

Table 4-13. Nutritional Disclosure Requirements for Food Labels

Component	Level at Which Disclosure Statement Is Required
Total fat	11.5 grams
Saturated fat	4.0 grams
Cholesterol	45.0 milligrams
Sodium	360.0 milligrams

Daily Values

Daily Value (DV): Figures on food labels showing how a food fits into the overall daily diet.

In the sample label (Fig. 4-16), the percent of *Daily Value (DV)* is given for the amount of fat, cholesterol, sodium, total carbohydrate, sugars, dietary fiber, protein, vitamins, and minerals. Daily Values are derived from two measures of nutrient concentration called Reference Daily Intake (RDI) and Reference Daily Value (RDV). These new terms were included in regulations published by the FDA in early 1993. For simplicity, they were converted into the Daily Value, which is the term that you will see on all food labels. The American Dietetic Association and other professional groups supported the FDA in making these changes.[9] The RDIs and RDVs came from RDA values pooled for all age and gender groups (except for women during pregnancy and lactation). RDA values, which we discussed earlier, are given in the table inside the back cover of this book.

Other Information on Labels

Apart from the required Nutrition Facts panel (i.e., the nutritional label), food labels will still carry the following mandatory information:

* The common or usual name of the product.
* The name and address of the food manufacturer, packer, or distributor.

- The net contents–weight, measure, or count.
- Ingredients, in decreasing order of concentration by weight.

For example, you will find all of the above information on any carton of breakfast cereal. The amount of any major ingredient in your favorite breakfast cereal can be obtained by checking where it comes in the list of ingredients. If it is listed third, then it is the ingredient in the third highest concentration.

Health claims on labels are controlled also. Only seven direct health/ nutrition claims are allowed on food packages. They are statements that claim a connection between:

- Calcium and *osteoporosis*
- Fat and cancer
- Saturated fat and cholesterol and coronary heart disease.
- Fiber-containing fruits, vegetables, and grain products and cancer.
- Fiber-containing fruits, vegetables, and grain products and risk of coronary heart disease.
- Sodium and hypertension.
- Fruits and vegetables and cancer.

Osteoporosis: Softening of bone during aging; develops mainly in women after menopause.

In the past people were confused and frustrated by the lack of either common or official definitions of words used to describe or imply the nutritional value of food products. Words such as "light," "lite," "reduced," "low," and others were used and abused. The FDA issued the following definitions to help us make the correct food choices.

- **Free (including "without," "no," and "zero")** means that a product contains no amount of, or trivial or "physiologically inconsequential" amounts of, the component. It can apply to fat, saturated fat, cholesterol, sodium, sugars, and/or calories.

- **Low (including "little," "few," and "low source of")**. The term "low" is defined in terms of a reference amount in each case.
  Low fat: 3 grams or less
  Low saturated fat: 1 gram or less
  Low sodium: 140 milligrams or less
  Very low sodium: 35 milligrams or less
  Low cholesterol: less than 20 milligrams
  Low calorie: 40 calories or less

- **High** may be used if the food contains 20% or more of the Daily Value for a particular nutrient.

- **Good source** means that one reference amount of a food contains 10–19% of the DV for a particular nutrient.

- **Reduced** can be used when a nutritionally altered product contains 25% less of a nutrient or of calories than the regular, or reference, product. A "reduced" claim cannot be made for a product if its reference food already meets the requirement for a "low" claim.

- **Less (includes "fewer" and "reduced")** means that a food, whether altered or not, contains 25% less of a nutrient or of calories than the reference food. For example, pretzels that have 25% less fat than potato chips can carry a "less" claim.

- **Light or lite** can mean two things: first, that a nutritionally altered product has one-third fewer calories or half the fat of the reference food; second, that the sodium content of a low-calorie, low-fat food has been reduced by 50%. If a food derives 50% or more of its calories from fat, the fat content must be reduced by at least 50% to qualify for a "light" claim.

   "Light in sodium" can be used on food in which the sodium content has been reduced by at least 50%.

   The term "light" can still be used to describe texture and color, so long as the label explains the intent–"light brown sugar" or "light and fluffy."

- **More** means that a serving of food, whether altered or not, contains more (at least 10% of the DV more) of a nutrient than the reference food does.

- **Percent fat free** means the product must be a low-fat or fat-free product. The claim must accurately reflect the amount of fat present in 100 grams of food–if a food contains 2.5% fat per 50 grams, the claim must be "95% fat free."

- **Lean and extra lean** describe the fat content of meat, poultry, seafood, and game meats. "Lean" is less than 10 grams of fat, less than 4 grams of saturated fat, and less than 95 milligrams of cholesterol per serving and per 100 grams. "Extra lean" is less than 5 grams of fat, less than 2 grams of saturated fat, and less than 95 milligrams of cholesterol per serving and per 100 grams.

- **Fresh** means that a food is raw or unprocessed, not heated or frozen, and contains no preservatives (blanching and irradiation at low levels are allowed). Terms such as "fresh frozen," "frozen fresh," and "freshly frozen" can be used if foods are quickly frozen while still fresh. "Fresh" may be used on a food that is refrigerated, if other requirements are met.

- **Healthy** was a term that could be used, when the regulations were first published, if limits on fat, saturated fat, and sodium were met. However, it was expected that this requirement would be strengthened and made more specific.

- **Serving sizes** are based on the amounts of food customarily consumed per eating occasion.

What is the price that you, I, and the food industry must pay for these changes? FDA did a cost-benefit analysis and came up with some answers to the question: Who will pay for nutrition labeling?

FDA estimates that benefits over the 20 years will be $4–20 billion for deaths prevented. They estimate about $100 billion for healthier lives, improved quality of life, and reduced health care costs. You should read and understand the label–you are paying for it. These changes in nutrition la-

---

Who Will Pay for Nutrition Labeling?[a]

Total cost to food manufacturers and food stores

$315 million the first year

$60 million in subsequent years

Number affected

21,000 food companies

120,000 food stores

77,600 labels

Cost to consumers

On average, $3.15 per household the first year

60 cents per household in subsequent years

[a]Preliminary analysis.

beling did not come easily. Some observers view the present situation with cynicism.[10]

> The politics of food labeling is seldom elegant, occasionally disastrous, and sometimes serviceable. Whichever category applies here, however, it can at least be said that the 1990 Nutrition Labeling and Education Act is what Congress and FDA think the people want.

Strong words indeed.

■ Nutritional status is measured in many ways

Measuring nutritional status should be easy. After all, we know what we eat, and the visual effects of starvation or excessive food intake are obvious. Look again at the pictures of the starving child and the obese person early in the preface–their nutritional problems are obvious. But these are at the extreme ends of a spectrum that includes people with less severe nutrition problems. Such problems are usually not seen easily. Some of the most important measurements in nutrition are the least accurate. We will see why this is so by examining how food intake measurements are made.

Measuring How Much Food We Eat Is Not Easy

Take a moment to recall what you ate yesterday.

Do you know how much of each food you ate? This seems easy until you get down to the details. You are not alone if you find it difficult to estimate your consumption of each food. Patients at the Obesity Research Center in New York City were puzzled about why they were not losing weight. Careful studies showed that their diets had twice the number of calories they thought they were consuming.[11] Nutritionists measure food intake by several methods.[12]

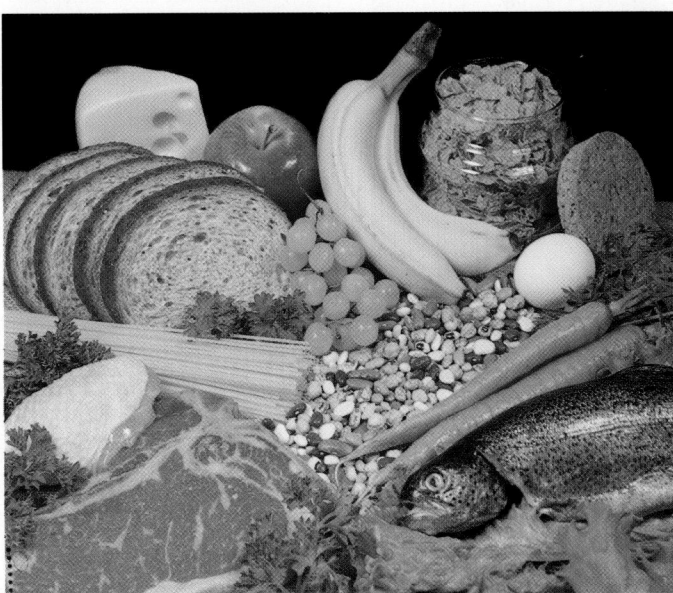

Figure 4-18. Getting all the nutrients is easy when you eat a balanced diet containing many types of foods.

- **Dietary recalls** require people to remember the amounts of food eaten during a given period, usually 24 hours. The method is quick but is open to errors in memory. Reliability of recall may be variable due to the age and health of the person.

- **Food records** are obtained when people record their intake as they eat. People may estimate the amount they eat, or it may be measured. Accuracy of record-keeping may decrease in long studies.

- **Diet histories** are taken by asking questions on usual food intake. Food models may be used to help people estimate usual portion sizes. Additional questions on method of food preparation, recipes, and the influence of time of year can be asked. Nutritionists consider this a good method of determining food intake, but it is time-consuming and may be subject to errors due to memory loss.

- **Food frequency questionnaires** are similar to the diet history method but the person responds to questions regarding the frequency of intake of specific foods from a list of foods. For example, how often do you eat hamburgers or drink milk? Food lists can be made to vary greatly in length and in complexity. Care is needed in constructing these lists because of the dietary diversity in today's multicultural society. A high proportion of the U.S. population does not eat from all the major food groups each day, and only about 3% eat the desired number of servings for each food group. The greatest problems with restricted food choices were found most often among ethnic minorities and those with limited income and formal education.[13]

Ethical Considerations Sometimes Limit Measurements of Nutritional Status

Detective work is needed by the dietitian and physician to determine the nutritional status of a person. "Feeling poorly" may be a complaint that hides a number of nutrition problems. Lack of energy can be due to a poor diet in general, to a deficiency of iron (which helps take oxygen to cells to liberate energy from stored carbohydrate and fat), or to low reserves of thiamin, riboflavin, and niacin (vitamins involved in the liberation of energy). Nutritional assessment is important, but we can deal only with the outlines here.

In addition to considering dietary intake, conclusions on the nutritional status of a person are made from specific measurements.

- **Anthropometry** measures the height, body weight, and the amount of body fat. These measurements are compared against body weight standards.

- **Laboratory tests** may include analysis of blood, urine, and feces, depending on which nutrient deficiency is suspected. Blood samples taken many hours after a meal are more indicative of the body's store of some nutrients. Blood tests may include hemoglobin and protein measurement. Glucose level in the blood is an important measurement for diabetics. About 2 million people in the United States are *insulin-dependent diabetics*. They must prick their fingers several times a day to draw blood, which they then analyze for glucose content using a test kit. A new test is painless and uses a sophisticated instrument called an infrared spectroscope that can measure glucose through the skin.[14]

Urine contains chemicals unused by the body, including chemicals absorbed but not used. For example, if you consume amounts of water-soluble vitamins in excess of the amount needed by the body, the excess is carried by the blood to the kidneys. There it is filtered out of the blood and dumped into the urine. Diabetics excrete the excess glucose

---

The ABCDs of nutrition status or nutrition assessment:

Anthropometry

Biochemical (laboratory tests)

Clinical (including physical examination)

Dietary

Insulin-dependent diabetes: A disorder characterized by inadequate production of insulin, causing alterations in carbohydrate metabolism and resulting in the loss of glucose in the urine.

that cannot be used because of a shortage of insulin. Urine also contains waste products of metabolism, including waste nitrogen from protein metabolism.

- **Physical signs** that may indicate a problem in nutritional status include changes in hair, eyes, lips, gums, tongue, skin, lower extremities, muscular system, nails, and face.

■ People are different–Cultural and ethnic influences on food choices

Our discussions so far have dealt with general principles of a healthy diet. In implementing these principles, we must be aware of the powerful social and psychological functions of food. Take a moment to review the list of these functions in Table 3-1 and note especially that satisfaction and religious significance are factors. Now superimpose the influence of ethnic and geographic origins and you will see why it is important that we consider how and why people are different in the foods they eat.

Take a moment to think why you may differ from other people in food choices. Does your cultural or ethnic identity influence your food choices?

The presence of a wide variety of ethnic foods in the United States is a direct result of the multicultural nature of our society. We will explore a few of the contributions made by specific ethnic groups by examining some traditional foods of Native Americans, African-Americans, Chinese-Americans, and Hispanics. "If taste buds can indicate social change," writes Dr. Elaine Monsen, editor of the *Journal of The American Dietetic Association*, "the United States is undergoing an ethnic explosion."

Native Americans

The approximately 1.5 million Native Americans in about 400 Native American and Alaskan Native nations throughout the United States represent great cultural diversity, including dietary diversity. What follows are generalized statements on the transition from traditional foods to the typical foods eaten today.

The traditional diet included corn (the main cereal), beans, and wild rice, a wide variety of fruits and vegetables, meat from a variety of wild animals, fish, eggs, and no dairy products. The lack of milk products was perhaps associated with the condition of lactose intolerance discussed in Chapters 3 and 6. Native American foods that are now part of the general American diet include corn, squash, beans, cranberries, and maple syrup.

The present-day diet includes many fruits, beef, pork, lamb, and processed meats. Wild game are

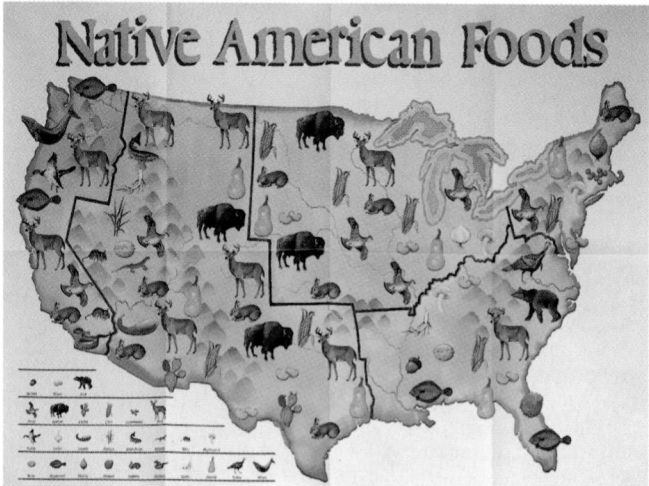

Figure 4-19. Native Americans contributed a wide variety of foods to the North American diet.

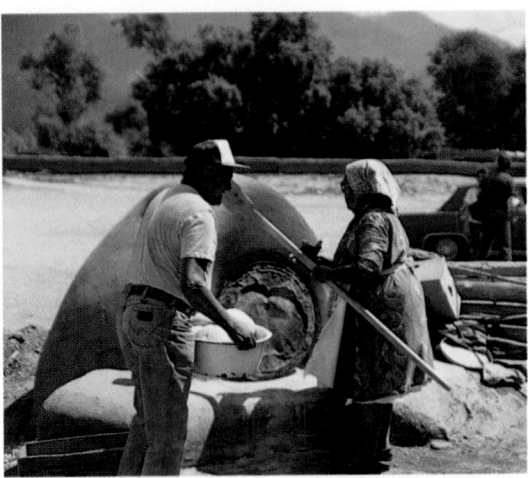

Figure 4-20. Bread is still made in traditional ways in many parts of the world. These are Native Americans in Taos, New Mexico.

less frequently eaten although valued. Vegetable intake is low and variety limited. Powdered and evaporated milk are now included. Bread is still often made in the traditional manner, as in a photograph (Figure 4-20) from Taos, New Mexico.

Sources of fats and oils have changed as the traditional diet adapted to changes in the availability of foods. The role of food in spiritual and physical health is still important to many Native Americans.[15] Corn is especially important in some healing ceremonies.

A recent study of the diet of Alaskan Natives found it to be higher than the national average for energy, protein, fat, carbohydrate, iron, and vitamin A and C but lower in calcium; they consumed six times more fish but fewer fruits and vegetables.[16]

Lack of food and lack of food choices is a problem in some Native American households, mainly as a result of low incomes.

African-Americans

Traditional foods of African-Americans include foods of West Africa in the 17th and 18th centuries and foods of the southern United States. Some of these are: biscuits, corn (corn breads, *hominy*, grits); a variety of green leafy vegetables, okra, potatoes, yams, and collard; a variety of fruits and meats; legumes such as black-eyed peas, peanuts, and different varieties of beans. The traditional diet had many nuts and many seasonings, including salt, garlic, and hot-pepper sauce. Dairy products were never consumed in large amounts, as lactose ("milk sugar") intolerance is estimated to be as high as 60–95% in the African-American community.

Today's diet includes both typical American foods and traditional foods. Some dairy products (ice cream, milk puddings, and some cheese) are consumed. The intake of fruits and vegetables is lower than the national average.

Chinese-Americans

Eating patterns are diverse among Asian Americans, with great differences among Chinese, Thai, Japanese, Korean, Vietnamese, Indonesian, or Filipino diets. We will focus on Chinese-American foods.

A wide variety of fruits and vegetables are popular. Beans, soy, and peas are used in many dishes. Meat (such as beef and pork) is usually served in bite-sized pieces. Although fresh fish is preferred, some fish are preserved by salting and drying, and some shrimp and legumes are made into pastes. Rice remains the primary staple, but noodles, wheat bread, corn, and millet are eaten also.

Seasonings are very popular, especially *monosodium glutamate* (MSG), which increases the sodium content of foods, spices, various fish sauces, and vinegar. Sugar was not widely used in the traditional diet but is increasing in the Chinese-American diet.

Hominy: Corn kernels that have been soaked in a caustic solution, such as lye, to remove the hulls. Grits are ground hominy.

Monosodium glutamate: A flavor enhancer often added to meats, soups, and sauces such as soy sauce. Increases sodium intake.

Most Asian foods are low in fat and cholesterol and high in sodium and carbohydrates. Dairy product consumption is low; thus, the intake of calcium is low. However, this nutrient is also obtained from tofu fortified with calcium and from small bones of fish and poultry.

Hispanics

Hispanics have a wide variety of foods in their traditional dishes, which are unique to Mexico, Puerto Rico, Cuba, and Central and South America. We concentrate here on Mexican food, which is a mixture of Native American and Spanish traditions.

Tortillas: Large, flat pancake made from ground corn or wheat.

Tacos and *tortillas* in other forms are among the most widely consumed Mexican foods. Tortillas are made from corn and from wheat. "California and Texas, which have large Mexican populations, are the two biggest markets for tortillas," states the *New York Times* (September 23, 1992). "Many supermarkets in these states carry up to 20 different brands." Rice is also consumed.

Vegetables are served as part of a dish, not separately. Fruits, beans, chili peppers, and potatoes are popular. Spices and sauces are used in many foods. Various meats, eggs, and dried beans are typical protein sources.

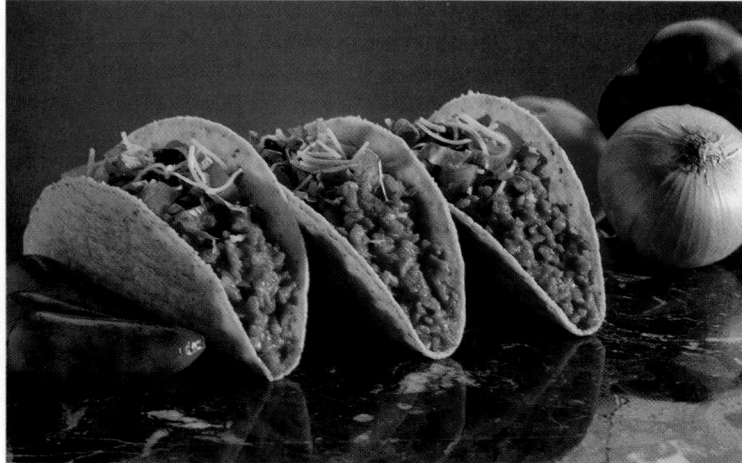

Figure 4-21. Tacos are one of the many creative ways to incorporate cereals into your diet.

Aged cheese, ice cream, and some milk are consumed by Hispanics in the United States. A high incidence of lactose intolerance limits the use of dairy products. However, calcium is supplied by corn tortillas as a result of the lime water used to steep the corn before grinding.

Religious Influences on Food Intake

Religions have always had an influence on food choices.[17] About 60% of people in the world belong to one of five major religions: Christianity, Islam, Hinduism, Buddhism, and Judaism. These religions have specific requirements involving food. Here are some examples.

Food restrictions. Followers of Islam (Muslims) don't consume pork, blood, or alcohol, whereas Hindus don't kill or eat any animal. Jews who follow kosher dietary restrictions may eat only animals with cloven hooves and that chew the cud; cattle, sheep, goats, and deer can be consumed, but not swine. They are also restricted to eating only fish with scales and fins, and they cannot mix meat and dairy products in the same meal.

Days of the year. Until the 1960s, Roman Catholics did not eat meat on Fridays. Devout Jews, Seventh Day Adventists, and Mormons must prepare food before the Sabbath.

Kosher foods: Foods specially selected and prepared to meet traditional Jewish ritual and dietary laws.

Time of day. Fasting between sunrise and sunset is required in some religions. This applies to Muslims during the holy month of Ramadan. Seventh Day Adventists do not eat between meals.

Preparation of food. *Kosher foods* are important in Judaism. Muslims also have ritual slaughter of meat animals. Devout Brahmins clean themselves by ritual bathing and the wearing of clean clothes before eating. "Meals emphasize eating and not linguistic banter or psychological exercises" is how Hindu Brahmin eating rituals are described by one writer.[17]

Fasts. Muslims fast during Ramadan, and Greek Orthodox followers fast every Wednesday and Friday. Devout Jews fast on specific holy days such as the Day of Atonement.

We have just scratched the surface of the interface between food and ethnicity, race, and religion. Irrespective of what eating pattern you may have, The Food Guide Pyramid should be useful to you. The challenge is to incorporate the dietary opportunities and restrictions from various traditions into the dietary recommendations we have been discussing in this chapter.

■ Nutrition in action–Our changing food supply

Agriculturalists and Nutritionists Are Rediscovering Some "Forgotten Crops"

Next time you walk through a supermarket or grocery store, remember that North Americans owe the rest of the world a debt of gratitude for being the centers of origin for many foods. Of all the crops grown in the United States, 98% are based on species originating beyond the U.S. borders.[18]

Look at Figure 4-22 to see how the modern American diet has benefited from grains and oilseed crops from other parts of the world.

About 150 plants are eaten regularly worldwide, but more than 90% of the world's food is provided by only 15 plant species. Three plant foods–rice, corn, and wheat–produce almost two-thirds of this amount.[18] With 5.5 billion people now in the world and an expected world population of about 9 billion people within the next 40 years, agriculturalists are turning to other foods to lessen our dependence on rice, corn, and

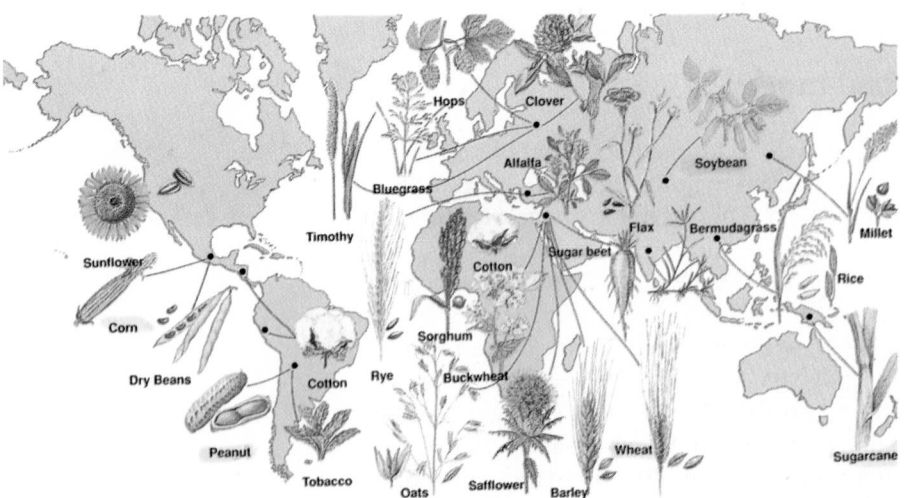

Figure 4-22. Many familiar grains and oilseeds originated in different parts of the world.

wheat. One way to increase the food supply is to grow crops that were plentiful once but are no longer cultivated. The job will not be easy.

"It is even harder for an old crop to make a comeback than for a forgotten film star," is how a writer in *The Economist* (January 27, 1990) describes the task.

> Agricultural scientists who are trying to restore ancient foods to the world's diet are nonetheless determined to do it. They know that it took Americans a century to accept the soybean and Europeans two centuries to accept the potato.

Some of those so-called "forgotten crops" *are* making a comeback. They are grains (including amaranth, quinoa, and millet), and fruits and vegetables such as banana and sweet potato. These crops can be developed for increased production. Let's take a quick look at amaranth and quinoa. Amaranth has been grown all over the world but was particularly important to the Aztecs of ancient Mexico. A staple food crop, it was also used in religious ceremonies. Now it is despised in many countries–it is called "pigweed" in Zimbabwe and in the United States. So why put any faith in what seems to be a loser? Well, it can be grown in hot climates from sea level to 10,000 feet above sea level. It grows in semiarid regions. Both the grain and leaves are eaten–the leaves taste like spinach. The protein and fiber contents of amaranth are higher than those of wheat, rice, and corn. It resists drought, heat, and pests. However, its disappointing yields must be improved by agricultural scientists.

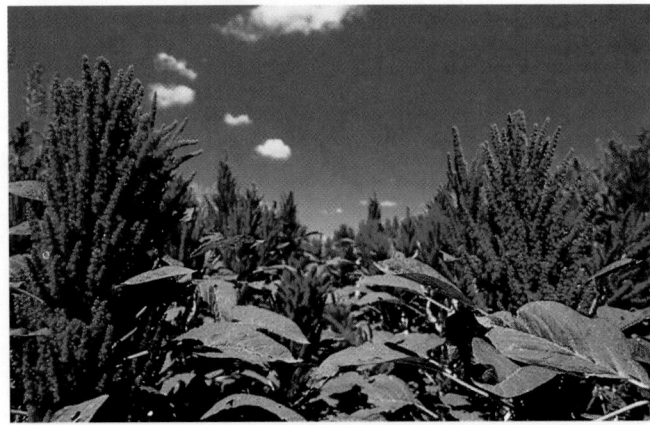

Figure 4-23. Amaranth may be one of the "foods of the future." Both the grains and the leaves can be eaten.

One of the benefits of quinoa is that it grows best in mild climates. Like wild rice, it is sold mainly in health and specialty stores in developed countries. It is regarded as a weed by many farmers in Latin America. But you will hear more about amaranth and quinoa in the future–you may even be eating significant amounts of them.

"Designer" Foods of the Future

Food scientists and the food processing industry are also busy *designing* foods to meet the dietary guidelines for healthy eating. They are aware that the four main influences on why we choose foods are: expense, health, taste, and status. Take a walk down the food aisles in your store and notice that the store owners emphasize their price competitiveness and the food manufacturers emphasize health (with such names as "Healthy Choice," "Slender," and "Right Choice"). Some foods carry Nathan Pritikin's name because he developed an eating pattern with which he guaranteed a long, healthy life. Some brands claim they are light on fat, sugar, and salt/ sodium. Taste is emphasized by impressive photographs of mouth-watering food on the packages–our eyes can almost "taste" the food inside.

Status is captured by a few key words such as "gourmet" or "Le Menu." But the status or prestige value of a food may vary over time. Researchers at Syracuse University studied how the status or prestige of some foods either grew or shrank between the early 1970s and the mid-1980s.[19]

Table 4-14. Some Winners and Losers in the Food Prestige Race

Winners	Losers
Skim milk	Whole milk
Fresh fruit	Pies
Chicken	Hard liquor
Whole wheat bread	Homemade bread
Strawberries	Cantaloupe
Broccoli	Sherbet
Orange juice	Cranberry juice

Think about the list in Table 4-14 and decide which are *your* winners and losers.

Notice how dietary guidelines for healthy eating influence the prestige value of food. For example, increased consumption of low-fat milk, fresh fruit, and broccoli lead to lower fat intakes and to increased fiber intake, which are recommended by dietary guidelines. A look at the top 20 new food product categories in the last 10 years is instructive (Table 4-15).

Table 4-15. New Food Products and Factors Influencing Their Development

Primary Influence	Product Category
Interest in healthy eating	"Light" anything
	High-fiber cereals and breads
	Nondairy spreads
	Fat-free desserts, cheeses, salad dressings
	Poultry-based luncheon meats, sausages
	Fresh frozen yogurts
	Oat bran cereals, breads, and muffins
Interest in convenience	Single-serve entrees, side dishes, desserts
	Dried food snacks
	Microwave breakfast and luncheon entrees
	Dry beer (fermented to reduce residual unfermented sugars in the wort)
	Wine coolers
	Flavored and juice-based waters and seltzers
	Aseptically packaged juices and drinks
Interest in international foods	Mexican sauces, entrees, condiments, flavors
	Surimi-based seafood
	Pasta sauces and pasta varieties
	Ramen soups (soups based on ramen or oriental noodle—made without eggs)
	Rice cakes
	Herb and flavored teas

By understanding the past, we have some chance of predicting the future. This is how trends in food manufacturing, sales, and attitudes during the past 25 years appear to one food expert.[20]

- The number of new food products continues to grow.
- Most "new" foods are variations of existing products.
- New food categories continue to emerge. During the past 25 years, we saw frozen yogurt, granola bars, microwavable mixes, and reduced-calorie frozen entrees grow in sales as new food categories.
- Consumer sophistication leads to foods with more exotic recipes, ingredients, and formulas.
- Ethnic foods expand–Italian, Chinese, Mexican, and others.
- Nutritionally oriented foods expand. Those low in fat, calories, salt/sodium, sugar, and caffeine are among the new products.
- High-fat, high-sugar foods are popular–soft drinks, snacks, cookies, desserts, super-premium ice creams.
- Microwavable products are popular.
- Side dishes move to the center of the plate–rice, pasta, potato, and vegetable main dishes are new on the scene.
- Fresh products are in high demand, as noted by the title of an article in a food trade journal: "Processors attracted to 'temptations of the fresh'."
- Packaging innovations please and disappoint. The pleasing aspects include single-serving packages, microwavable packages, aseptic boxes, and squeeze bottles. Less popular so far include modified- and controlled-atmosphere packages and environmentally friendly packages.
- Fast foods drive new supermarket introductions. Fried chicken, pizza, and Mexican foods are now found in supermarkets as well as in fast-food outlets.
- Activists, the press, and government keep food manufacturers under pressure–attention to food safety and environmental issues has increased greatly in the past 25 years.

Pyramids or triangles seem to be a popular geometric form for nutritionists. We have studied the Food Guide Pyramid. Here is a triangle of foods and ingredients with properties that can possibly prevent cancer. They increase in importance from the base to the apex of the triangle. About 40 such foods have been identified.[21]

Examine the list of foods in Figure 4-24 and see how many you consume on a regular basis.

The next triangle, developed by Canadian nutritionists, helps us to summarize

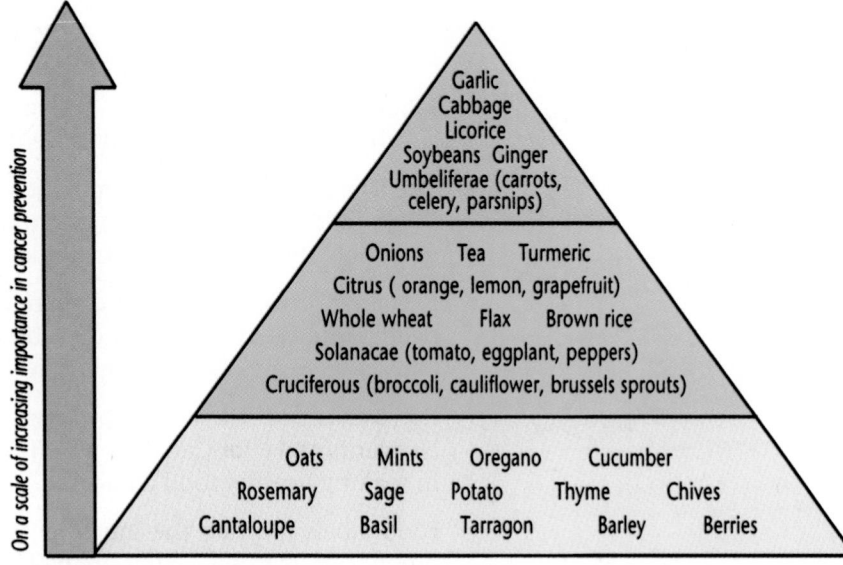

Figure 4-24. The number of foods considered to have anticancer properties is increasing. Foods near the top of the triangle are thought to have the most anticancer properties.

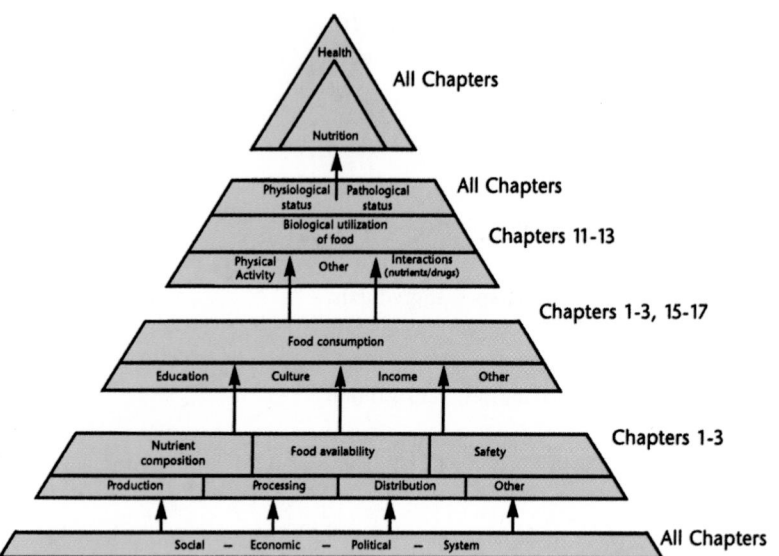

Figure 4-25. Good health, based on proper nutrition, is the goal of all aspects of the food system. Many social, agricultural, medical, and biological forces interact to produce it.

what we have studied in the last four chapters, and sets the scene for the remaining chapters.

We are climbing up this triangle–already we have met examples in which nutrition interfaces with food, with the environment, and with social, economic, and political systems. Food availability was covered in Chapters 1–3. This chapter dealt with food consumption and how it is measured. We are now ready to move on to the study of each individual nutrient, the section called "biological utilization of food." This is what nutrition is all about, and the ultimate objective is at the apex of the triangle– good health.

■ Now you know

- Since ancient times, people have been puzzled about food–its health-giving properties, and its safety.

- Lifestyle diseases, or diseases of affluence, include coronary heart disease, hypertension, diabetes, stroke, certain types of cancer, and gallstones.

- Modern diets are higher in fat, refined sugar, and salt and lower in starch and fiber than diets in ancient times.

- The Dietary Guidelines recommend eating a variety of foods low in fat, sugar, salt; avoiding alcohol; maintaining a healthy body weight; and eating plenty of vegetables, fruits, and grain products.

- Exchange lists are used by diabetics, weight-reducing programs, and people interested in healthy diets because they show how foods can be chosen to create high-carbohydrate, low-fat diets.

- Recommended Dietary Allowances (RDAs) and the Recommended Nutrient Intake for Canadians (RNI) are standards to guide populations in making healthy food choices.

- Food labels indicate the ingredients and the nutritional value of the product. Nutritional claims are better controlled now than in the past.

- Nutritional status is assessed by measuring dietary intake and by anthropometry, laboratory tests, and physical signs.

- Cultural diversity leads to a variety of eating patterns. Religious beliefs also influence food choices.

- Most of the plant foods in North America originated in other parts of the world. Some "forgotten crops," such as amaranth and quinoa, are being redeveloped.

- "Designer" foods of the future must meet criteria for expense, health, taste, and status. Foods are designed now to meet consumers' demands for healthy eating and convenience and to satisfy their interest in tasting new foods from different parts of the world.

Further Reading

1. Kanarek, R. B., and Marks-Kaufman, R. *Nutrition Behavior.* Van Nostrand Reinhold, New York, 1991.
2. Eisenberg, D. M., and others. Unconventional medicine in the United States. Prevalence, costs, and patterns of use. *New England Journal of Medicine* 328:246, 1993.
3. Rosenberg, I. W. Nutritional requirements and dietary guidelines: The globe shrinks. *Nutrition Reviews* 50:88, 1992.
4. Peterkin, B. B. What's new about the 1990 Dietary Guidelines for Americans? *Journal of Nutrition Education* 23:183, 1991.
5. Murray, T. K. Nutrition Recommendations, 1990. *Journal of the Canadian Dietetic Association* 51:391, 1990.
6. Welsh, S., and others. Development of the Food Guide Pyramid. *Nutrition Today,* page 12, November/December, 1992.
7. Salmon, J. Excerpts from Dietary Reference Values for food energy and nutrients for the United Kingdom: Introduction to the guide and summary tables. *Nutrition Reviews* 50:90, 1992.
8. The American Dietetic Association. ADA's timely statement on proposed revision of U.S. RDAs for use on food labels. *Journal of The American Dietetic Association* 92:361, 1992.
9. Scarlett, T. The politics of food labeling. *Food Technology* 46(7):58, 1992.
10. Rhein, R. Food labels in U.S. to make clearer health claims for consumers. *British Medical Journal* 306:83, 1993.
11. Lichtman, S. W., and others. Discrepancy between self-reported and actual caloric intake and exercise in obese subjects. *New England Journal of Medicine* 327:1893, 1992.
12. Freudenheim, J. L. A review of study designs and methods of dietary assessment in nutritional epidemiology of chronic disease. *Journal of Nutrition* 123:401, 1993.
13. Kant, A. K., and others. Dietary diversity in the U.S. population, NHANES II, 1976–1980. *Journal of the American Dietetic Association* 91:1526, 1991.
14. Robinson, M. R., and others. Noninvasive glucose monitoring in diabetic patients, a preliminary evaluation. *Clinical Chemistry* 38:1618, 1992.
15. Nobmann, E. D., and others. The diet of Alaska Native adults: 1987–1988. *American Journal of Clinical Nutrition* 55:1024, 1992.
16. Kittler, P. G., and Sucher, K. *Food and Culture in America. A Nutrition Handbook.* Van Nostrand, New York, 1989.

17. Several papers from a symposium entitled: Religious and philosophical bases of food choices. *Food Technology* 46(10):92, 1992.

18. Paoletti, M. G., and others. Agroecosystem biodiversity: Matching production and conservation biology. *Agriculture, Ecosystems and Environment* 40:3, 1992.

19. Crockett, S. J., and Stuber, D. L. Prestige value of foods: Changes over time. *Ecology of Food and Nutrition* 27:51, 1992.

20. Friedman, M. Twenty-five years and 98,900 new products later. *Prepared Foods New Products Annual*, page 23, 1990.

21. Caragay, A. B. Cancer-preventive foods and ingredients. *Food Technology* 46(4):65, 1992.

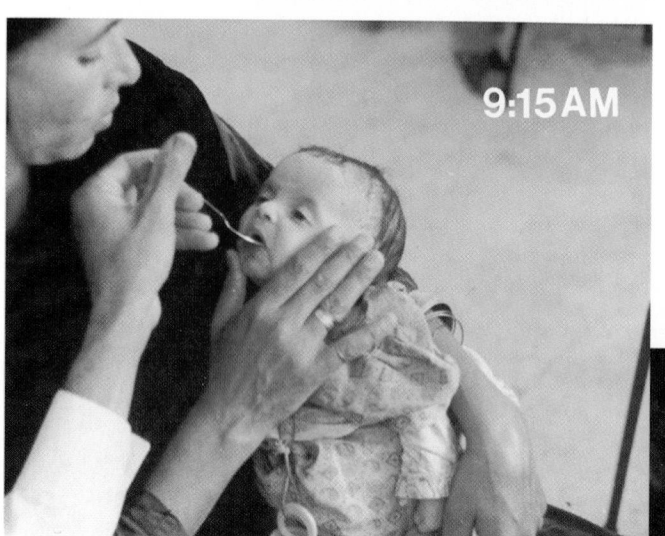

9:15 AM

Figure 5-1. Severe diarrhea causes dehydration, which is fatal if untreated, especially in infants. Lost body fluids are quickly replaced by a simple mixture of glucose and salt dissolved in clean water in a process known as oral rehydration therapy (ORT).

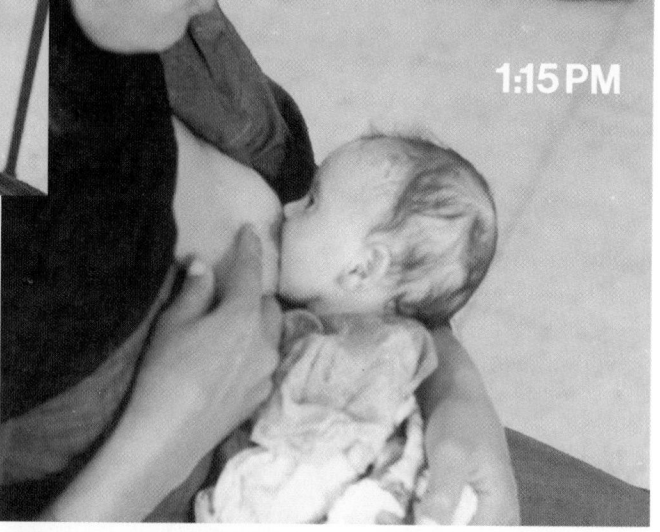

1:15 PM

Figure 5-2. An infant with fetal alcohol syndrome (FAS) and the same child several years later. FAS produces a distinct facial appearance and marginal intellectual capabilities that remain throughout life.

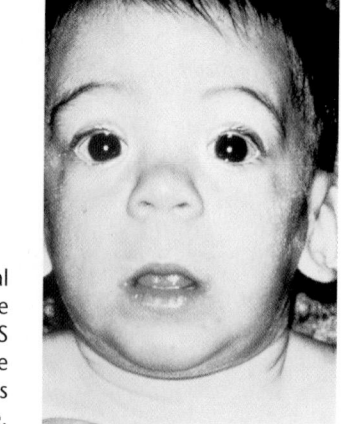
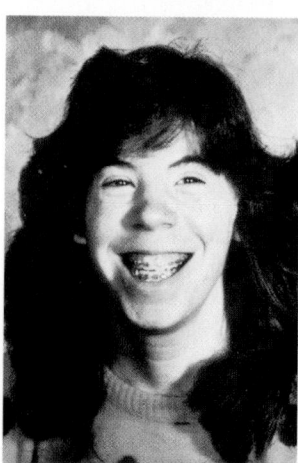

## CHAPTER 5

Water–Beverages and Brewing

■ Nutrition in our lives–Water, alcohol, and other beverages

The top photograph shows a child recovering from a lack of a vitally important nutrient–water. His dehydration has resulted from extreme diarrhea. In contrast, the young person in the bottom pictures suffers from *fetal alcohol syndrome (FAS)*, resulting from her mother's excess intake of a toxic substance–alcohol. FAS occurs when the developing fetus is exposed to alcohol. These nutrition-related problems cause great suffering. However, there is reason to believe that better education will lead to the elimination of these problems in the future.

Dehydration caused by diarrhea is life-threatening and is usually caused by food and water contaminated with diarrhea-causing microorganisms. A major factor contributing to the problem is improper sewage disposal in overcrowded cities. Correction of this environmental problem is the long-term solution in developing countries, where diarrhea kills a worldwide total of up to 5 million children each year. A short-term solution for people dehydrated by diarrhea is fluids that are inexpensive and easy to use and that do save many lives each year. Look closely at the times on the two photographs on the left. At 9 a.m. the child was weak from dehydration and had to be coaxed by his mother, who held him while a clinic worker fed him. For the next 3 hours he was fed a simple mixture mainly of glucose and salt dissolved in clean water. This process is known as *oral rehydration therapy (ORT)*. The salts are available in foil packets, so preparation of the ORT solution is simple. Effects are positive and rapid–body water is quickly returned to its normal level and the child becomes hungry, as seen in the second photograph, after the child has had 3 hours of ORT treatment.

Fetal alcohol syndrome does not have such a satisfactory outcome–the child on the right retains the distinctive facial appearance observed in in-

---

Major Topics in This Chapter

Water is vital for many body processes.

Water is critical for survival.

■

Water quality is a growing concern in many parts of the world.

Water in foods is important for quality and preservation.

There are nutritional implications when you consume caffeine, soft drinks, or alcohol.

■

People Are Different— Effect of alcohol on nutritional status

Food Science in Action— Brewing

Fetal alcohol syndrome (FAS): Lifelong disabilities and malformations, especially to the face, caused by alcohol use by the mother during pregnancy. FAS is the leading known cause of mental retardation in the United States.

Oral rehydration therapy (ORT): Feeding a mixture of sugar, salt, and clean water to dehydrated children, especially those with severe diarrhea.

fancy and has marginal intellectual capabilities. Growth rate is reduced, head size is abnormally small, and IQ is below average, resulting in low academic achievement, especially in math. Children with FAS have poor judgment, are easily distracted, and have difficulties in social interactions. FAS is now recognized as the leading known cause of mental retardation in the United States.[1]

The damaging effects of alcohol were described by William Shakespeare in the play *Othello.*

> I have very poor and unhappy brains for drinking: I could well wish courtesy would invent some other custom of entertainment.

Shakespeare suggested, and scientists now tell us, that alcohol is toxic to the body.

Water, on the other hand, is essential for life. One main message in this chapter is that we should value the importance of water for our health and survival. According to inventor and diplomat Benjamin Franklin, "When the well is dry we know the worth of water." Some people in affluent countries say the well is not dry but polluted. A new growth industry has developed around bottled water–Americans spend more than $2 billion each year on bottled water and water-purifying systems.

■ Water in the human body–Vital in many body processes

Think beyond the photograph in Figure 5-3. Your nutrient requirements began shortly after fertilization when you were just a few cells.

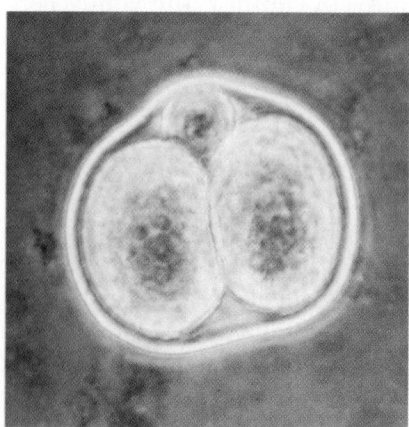

Figure 5-3. Your highest fluid concentration was at the time of your conception and in the period of rapid growth during pregnancy. Water is critical for the division and growth of cells.

Water was critical for maintaining life and allowing the cells to multiply throughout childhood into the billions of cells that form your body. Each of these cells has its own water content that contributes to the 12 gallons of water that walk around with us. No, we are not "all wet" and it does not slosh around within us–water is one of the most closely regulated chemicals in the body. With 12 gallons of body fluids in us, it might seem that we could go without fluids for a long time. Wrong–death occurs usually within about 4 days if there is no fluid intake. A similar fate awaits animals in extreme drought.

Contrast this with the approximately 60 days that can pass without food before death occurs in most healthy adults. Political prisoners know these time differences well–hunger strikes give time to stimulate public opinion and to negotiate a settlement. The first known "thirst strike" was reported recently.[2] A prisoner claimed to have taken no fluid for 13 days, although this could not be confirmed. However, his extreme physical condition suggested to researchers that he had been without fluid for much longer than 4 days. The amount of body weight lost, the degree of kidney failure, the decreased skin quality, and the chapped lips attested to this. The researchers concluded that

> the voluntary refusal of liquid needs exceptional determination since thirst is one of the most powerful behavioral drives. The craving for water can become intense enough to dominate all other thoughts or sensations.

Let's see where and how we use the 12 gallons of water within each of us.

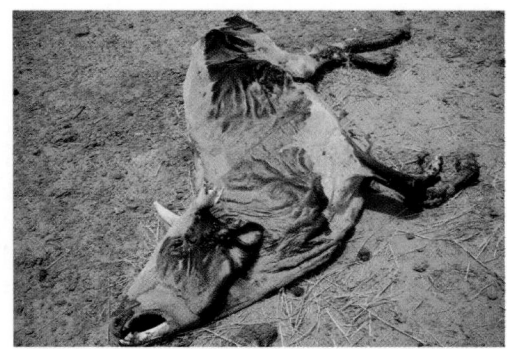

Figure 5-4. A victim of drought. Water is a nutrient that is vital for the survival of humans, animals, plants, and microbes.

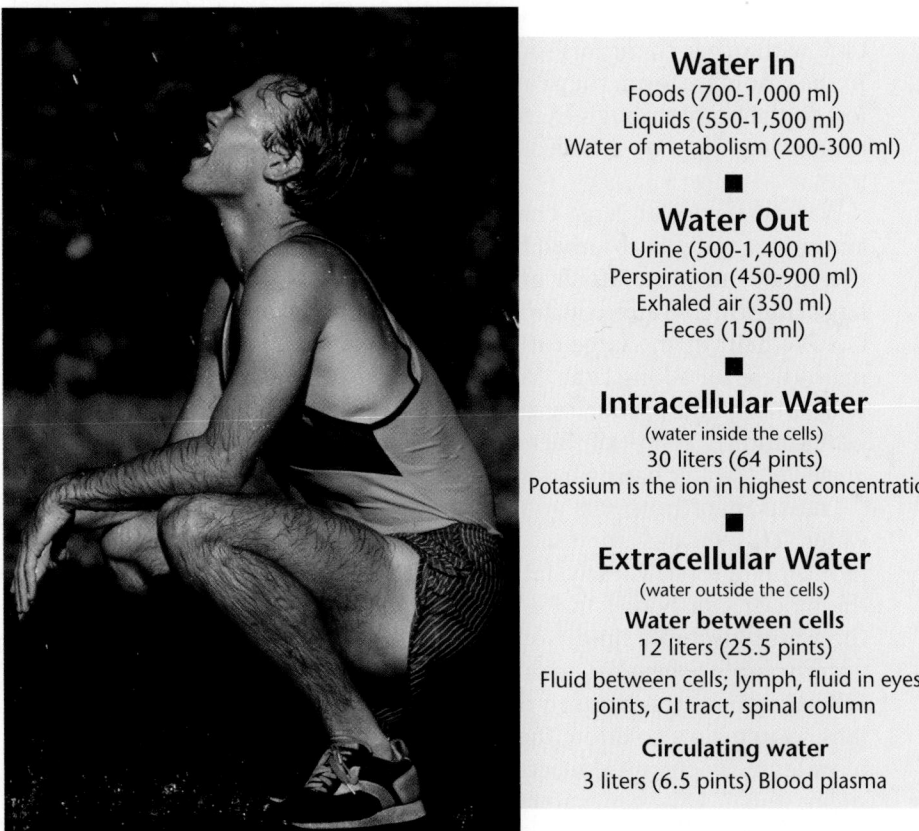

Water In
Foods (700-1,000 ml)
Liquids (550-1,500 ml)
Water of metabolism (200-300 ml)

∎

Water Out
Urine (500-1,400 ml)
Perspiration (450-900 ml)
Exhaled air (350 ml)
Feces (150 ml)

∎

Intracellular Water
(water inside the cells)
30 liters (64 pints)
Potassium is the ion in highest concentration

∎

Extracellular Water
(water outside the cells)
Water between cells
12 liters (25.5 pints)
Fluid between cells; lymph, fluid in eyes, joints, GI tract, spinal column

Circulating water
3 liters (6.5 pints) Blood plasma

Figure 5-5. Water in the body comes from three sources: liquids, water in foods, and water of metabolism (produced when the energy nutrients carbohydrates, lipids, and proteins are metabolized to energy, with the consequent liberation of water and carbon dioxide). Water exists inside and outside every cell in the body. It leaves the body in urine, perspiration, exhaled air, and the feces. Perspiration plays an important role in heat loss.

Water Is Vital for Many Body Processes

Let's follow a mouthful of food washed down by a mouthful of fluid as it moves through the digestive system.

Lubrication in the mouth is done by saliva, which is about 99.5% water. *Hydrolysis* ("breaking with water") liberates nutrients from food. Digestive juices contain enzymes that break down carbohydrates, lipids, and proteins into their simplest components. Bile, about 85% water, is produced by the liver and stored in the gallbladder to assist in the digestion of fat. Other digestive juices are secreted by the stomach, small intestine, and pancreas.

Absorption of nutrients from food needs the fluid medium provided by digestive juices. After enzymes in digestive juices liberate nutrients from food, the nutrients must remain soluble in the watery medium of the GI tract in order to be absorbed into the blood supply. These nutrients include simple sugars, amino acids from digested proteins, some fatty acids and glycerol from lipids, as well as minerals and vitamins. Minerals such as iron, zinc, and calcium can become insoluble in the GI tract if they combine with other chemicals such as phosphorus, oxalic acid, or phytic acid. In the insoluble form, they cannot be absorbed into the blood and are thus lost to the body through excretion in the feces. The *bioavailability* of these nutrients is thereby reduced because they are not absorbed from the GI tract.

Water does not undergo change as it passes through the GI tract. A small amount of water is absorbed from the stomach, but most is absorbed from the small intestine. Much of the remaining water is absorbed from the large intestine. Water continues to be absorbed from the feces as long as feces remain in the large intestine, giving rise to constipation if they remain there for a long time. We saw previously how fiber binds water, providing bulk and producing the desire to defecate. Chemists describe the water-binding ability of fiber as a *hydrophilic* ("water loving") reaction; *hydrophobic* ("water hating") describes the opposite reaction.

Transport of nutrients and waste is done by the blood, which is 85% water. This creates an interesting question–What about the fat in the mouthful of food? Clearly, fat is not soluble in water, so how is it carried in the blood? Our bodies make many clever chemical changes. In this case, the water-insoluble lipid is chemically hooked onto a protein to form a water-soluble *lipoprotein*, which can be transported in the blood.

Biochemical reactions in the body need water as a medium or as a reactant. Water can also dilute the concentration of reactants. New knowledge of water in biochemical reactions is emerging–"water is looking like pretty sticky stuff."[3] How can water be "sticky"? It seems to "stick" to other molecules so as to influence their conformation or shape, thereby allowing them to carry out some vital body function. One good example is the water involved in the delivery of oxygen from the air to every cell in the body. We all know that oxygen is essential for life–a few minutes without it causes permanent brain damage; a little longer causes death. As a result, how oxygen gets to cells (including brain cells) is very important. Oxygen from air inhaled into the lungs hooks onto hemoglobin, the pigment in

Hydrolysis: (Literally, "breaking with water.") A process that occurs when the OH^- and H^+ ions that make up a water molecule (H_2O) split a substance into two parts. For example, table sugar (sucrose, $C_{12}H_{22}O_{11}$) is hydrolyzed by the addition of H_2O into $C_6H_{12}O_6$ (glucose) and $C_6H_{12}O_6$ (fructose).

Bioavailability: Degree to which a substance is able to be digested and utilized by the body in the amount or form in which it is present; usually refers to nutrients in foods.

Hydrophilic: Literally means "water loving." Refers to something that chemically attracts water.

Hydrophobic: Literally means "water hating." Refers to something that chemically repels water.

Lipoprotein: A protein combined with lipids such as cholesterol, phospholipids, and triglycerides; water-soluble for transportation in the blood.

red blood cells. Scientists have learned that when four oxygen molecules hook onto one hemoglobin molecule, 60 water molecules hook on as well. This is a remarkable amount of water, although what it does we do not know yet. Clearly, all this water is not along just for the ride!

Water also assists some enzymes. *Hydration* is involved in the synthesis of large carbohydrate, lipid, and protein molecules in the body. Water is involved also in the breakdown (hydrolysis) of these same large molecules to produce water, carbon dioxide, and energy, plus nitrogen compounds in the case of proteins. The water produced here is called *water of metabolism*, and the excess is excreted through the urine.

Hydration: The addition or absorption of water.

Excretion of body wastes requires water in large quantities. Routes of excretion are urine, feces, perspiration, and exhaled air. More body fluid is lost in the urine than by any other route.

Water of metabolism: Water produced in the body when carbohydrates, lipids, proteins, and alcohol are broken down for energy.

Urine is 93–97% water plus dissolved chemicals such as chlorides (including sodium chloride), sodium, phosphorus, potassium, and ketone bodies. Nitrogen-containing substances such as urea, creatinine, and creatine are also present. Urine from most people has a tiny trace of glucose (2–3 milligrams per 100 milliliters) after a heavy meal. However, diabetic people can lose up to 100 grams of glucose in the urine every 24 hours. Sometimes urine is cloudy, which could have several causes. One is the excretion of excess phosphorus from a meal containing a large amount of meat, which is high in phosphorus. Urine is the main excretion mechanism for all water-soluble substances. For example, excess intakes of water-soluble vitamins (vitamin C and the B-complex vitamins) are excreted in the urine.

Perspiration is not a major means of waste excretion. Sweat does taste salty, but even in a marathon run or a long game, the loss of sodium is not critical. Taking salt or sodium pills is not necessary because food taken after the event quickly replaces the lost sodium. When we study minerals in Chapter 10, we will learn that the typical North American diet is high in sodium.

Heat loss from the body is important, and water and perspiration play a vital role in this. Heat is produced when carbohydrates, lipids, and proteins are burned in the body to produce energy. This influences body temperature, which must remain within the range of 80–108°F (27–42°C). Death occurs outside this range, so the body has protective mechanisms to prevent wide changes in its temperature. When heat is lost from your body, such as during exercise or a fever, additional blood is sent to the skin to increase heat. If you get too hot, you perspire, or sweat. Excess body heat is removed only when perspiration is evaporated from the skin. About 85% of the body's heat loss is through the skin, with the remainder being lost via the breath, urine, and feces. However, the efficient evaporation of sweat is prevented by high humidity. Thus, intense physical activity is dangerous in high humidity because internal body temperatures can rise to harmful levels.

If you get too cold, the reverse of perspiration happens–blood is drawn from the extremities (hands, legs, and feet) to decrease heat loss through the skin. You also shiver by contracting and relaxing muscles and in so doing generate heat from the breakdown of the energy nutrients.

Amniotic fluid: The liquid that protects the developing fetus.

There are some **other functions of water in the body.** One is its role as a cushion for body tissues. For example, *amniotic fluid* surrounds and protects the fetus during pregnancy. In addition, tears act as a lubricant for the eyes, and synovial fluid allows bones to move freely against each other at joints. Water gives cells their shape and rigidity.

Increased Fluid Intake Is Important for Many People

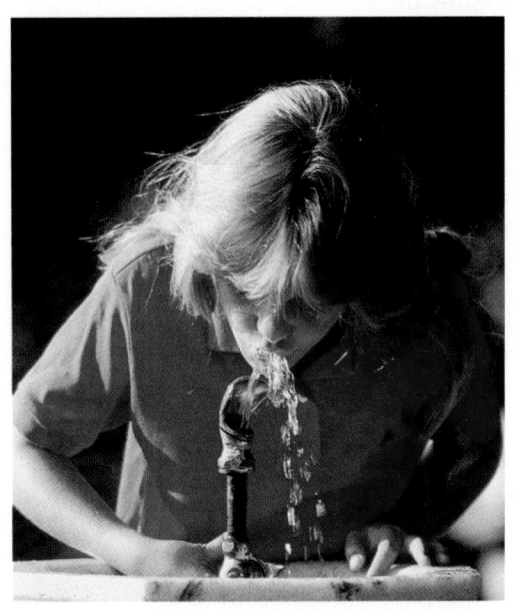

Figure 5-6. Adequate fluid intake is necessary at all times. In some periods of our lives and in certain diseases and environments, we need to increase fluid intake.

Having now established that we have a high water content and that water performs vital functions in the body, we should note that it is especially important for certain members of the population to pay particular attention to their fluid intake.

- **Pregnant and lactating women.** Production of amniotic fluid, the developing fetus, and the synthesis of breast milk all have a high requirement for water.[4] A low fluid intake may stop the production of milk.

- **Infants.** Babies and children have a higher concentration of body water than adults. The concentration of total body water decreases from about 80–85% in the infant to 65–70% in adults. The total amount of water in a person increases during growth due to the rapid increase in the size of tissues with high water content (blood, muscle) as well as tissue with lower water content such as bone and fat.

- **People suffering from diarrhea and vomiting**–especially young children. Diarrhea causes dehydration (up to 1 liter or nearly 2 pints of fluid loss per hour). Vomiting removes stomach secretions.

- **Elderly people** have decreased sensitivity to thirst and decreased ability to conserve body water. Some of this is due to decreased efficiency of the kidneys.

- **People with fever.** The high fluid loss caused by elevated body temperature must be replaced.

Solutes: Substances dissolved in a liquid.

Kidney dialysis: Mechanical purification of blood to remove liquids and chemicals that the kidneys would normally remove if they were not diseased.

- **People with some types of kidney disease** need high fluid intake to dilute the urine. High concentrations of *solutes* put a strain on the kidneys. Low fluid intake in measured amounts is needed by people on *kidney dialysis* or with minimal kidney function.

- **People on high-protein diets** should increase their fluid intake. Some weight-reducing diets and some supplements for athletes are high in protein. When protein is broken down for energy, nitrogen compounds are created as end products. These must be excreted in the urine, and additional fluid intake is required to ensure that their concentrations are kept diluted–kidney damage results if they are not. This information has practical applications; authors of weight-reducing diets requiring high dietary protein intake recommend the drinking of up to 8 glasses of fluid every day.

- **People doing hard physical work**. Fluids lost through perspiration must be replaced.

- **People in hot weather or high environmental temperatures.**

- **Air travelers**. On a 3½ hour flight you can lose up to 2 pounds of water. Cabin air is dry and circulates rapidly.

- **Athletes**. The winning or losing of some sporting events depends on body fluid levels. Marathon runners who don't take enough fluid during a race may not perform well. When boxers and wrestlers take diuretics to lose body water to quickly meet a body weight limit, they may qualify but lose the match. We return to this important topic in Chapter 12.

Water can be consumed in large amounts without harmful effects, but there is an upper limit to the amount of water an individual should consume. People rarely reach this upper limit without a conscious effort to consume large quantities of water so as to achieve water intoxication.

Control of Body Fluids

To understand how we control body fluids, we must discuss some terms much used by physiologists–*ions*, *pH*, and *buffers*.

Ions

Pure water (H_2O) contains hydrogen ions (H^+) and hydroxyl ions (OH^-). An ion consists of an atom or atoms carrying an electric charge. The hydrogen ion in water carries a positive charge and the hydroxyl ion a negative charge. Now add a salt that dissolves in water by dissociating (breaking) into ions. A good example is sodium chloride ($NaCl$), commonly called table salt, which dissociates into two ions, Na^+ and Cl^-. In the human body, about 90% of the ions in the *extracellular fluid* are Na^+ and Cl^-. Physiologists refer to this as the "internal sea" because the composition is similar to that of seawater, suggesting our origins in the distant past. The potassium ion (K^+) is in highest concentration in the *intracellular fluid*. Both Na^+ and K^+ are important in maintaining body fluid balance within and outside cells. Nerves need sodium, potassium, and calcium ions in order to function. Important negatively charged ions in the body include chloride, bicarbonate, and sulfate. "Electrolytes" is the term used by nutritionists and physiologists for sodium, potassium, and chloride in solution. In general scientific terms, *electrolytes* are solutions that conduct electricity.

pH

Hydrogen ions (H^+) are released by some substances when dissolved in water, which makes the solution acidic. Hydrochloric acid (HCl), which is secreted in the stomach and is the strongest acid in the body, dissociates into H^+ and Cl^-. It is the concentration of the hydrogen ion (H^+) that makes HCl such a strong acid. However, if a solution contains more hydroxyl ions (OH^-), the solution is alkaline, or basic. The body has no strong alkaline fluids.

The strength of acids and bases is measured by the pH scale (Figure 5-7).

Ion: An atom or group of atoms with an electrical charge. Ions are created when a salt such as NaCl is put into solution, where it is ionized into sodium (Na^+) and chlorine (Cl^-) ions.

pH: Abbreviation for potential hydrogen. A measure of the concentration of hydrogen ions (H^+) in a substance, which in turn measures its acidity or alkalinity.

Buffers: Substances that resist change in acidity or alkalinity.

Extracellular fluid: The fluid outside cells.

Intracellular fluid: The fluid within cells.

Electrolytes: Compounds that ionize in water, which can then conduct electricity.

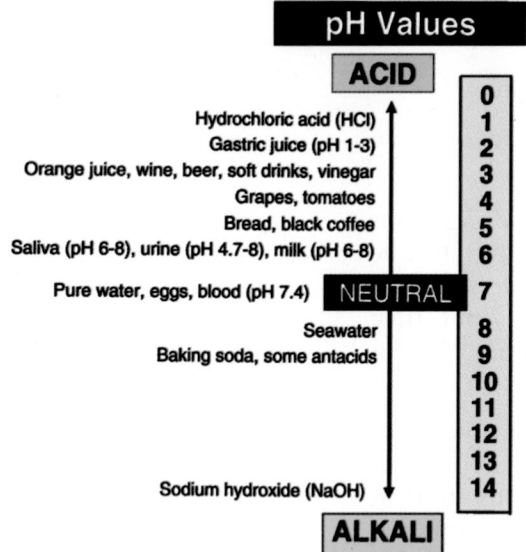

pH Values

ACID

Hydrochloric acid (HCl)	0
Gastric juice (pH 1-3)	1
	2
Orange juice, wine, beer, soft drinks, vinegar	3
Grapes, tomatoes	4
Bread, black coffee	5
Saliva (pH 6-8), urine (pH 4.7-8), milk (pH 6-8)	6
Pure water, eggs, blood (pH 7.4) NEUTRAL	7
Seawater	8
Baking soda, some antacids	9
	10
	11
	12
	13
Sodium hydroxide (NaOH)	14

ALKALI

Figure 5-7. The pH scale measures the degree of acidity or alkalinity of body fluids, tissues, and foods. Neutral pH is 7.0. At a pH level less than 5.0, milk proteins coagulate (which can be seen in yogurt and cheese making or when milk is mixed with fruit juice). Pickling foods in vinegar lowers their pH even farther, and the acid environment prevents the growth of spoilage microorganisms.

One reason that nutritionists and biologists are interested in the pH scale is that enzymes usually work within narrow pH ranges. For example, stomach enzymes involved in digestion are in a very acidic environment of about pH 1.5. As the partially digested food passes into the small intestine, the enzymes there continue the digestive process at a slightly alkaline pH of 8.0. If you could swap the enzymes in the stomach with those in the small intestine, none of them would work. They would have been inactivated because they were not in a pH range in which they could be active.

Buffers

It is critical to maintain pH within close ranges so that enzymes and other body functions can perform their vital activities at a maximum rate. Therefore, the body has buffers such as proteins, carbonates, and bicarbonates, which prevent wide swings in pH values by absorbing excess H^+ or OH^- ions. The acid-base balance of the blood is thus kept under tight control and maintained at about pH 7.4. If blood becomes too acidic (a condition called "acidosis") or too alkaline or basic ("alkalosis"), coma or death results. This is due mainly to the denaturation of blood proteins, which produces a breakdown in the transport of oxygen, other nutrients, and waste by the blood.

Water Balance is Critical for Survival

Water balance is said to exist when the intake and output of water are equal. Fluid intake is a more appropriate term than water intake because fluid intake includes water, juices, milk, broths, soups, tea, coffee, and cocoa. Any of these will help to meet the requirement of a minimum intake of about 2 pints of fluid per day. This amount is needed to balance the loss of a minimum of 2 pints of water each day in the elimination of body wastes. A lower intake can damage kidneys because the nitrogen end products of protein metabolism referred to above are not diluted sufficiently in the urine.

Nutritionists are concerned when levels and distributions of body fluids are altered. *Edema* is an excessive accumulation of tissue fluid, mainly in the extracellular space. Figure 5-8 shows what it looks like.

The extra fluid causing edema comes from the blood and accumulates in the legs, arms, and belly. Many factors contribute to edema, including undernutrition and failure of the kidneys, liver, or heart. The undernutrition results from a diet low in protein, which causes a decreased level of blood proteins. This in turn results in movement of fluid from the blood into the extracellular spaces. Affected areas are spongy to the touch and leave a depression when pressure is applied.

Edema: Excessive accumulation of fluid in tissues.

Diuretics increase urine volume. Extensive use of diuretics causes a loss of potassium in the urine, resulting in a severe depletion of body potassium. Alcohol and chemicals in coffee and tea act as diuretics. Many people come into contact with diuretics through the use of slimming aids. Dieters may be happy that body weight is decreasing after taking various diuretics. However, they should be aware that they are losing body weight because they are losing body water and *not* body fat.

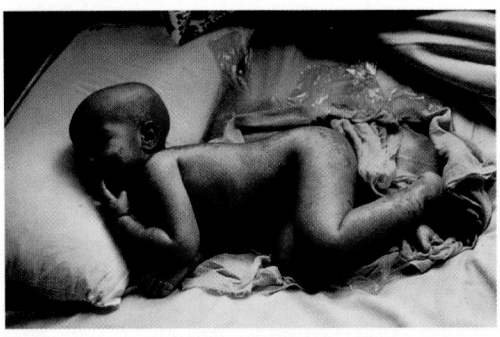

Figure 5-8. Edema is the accumulation of excess fluid outside cells. Nutritionists may see edema in certain types of protein deficiency.

■ Water quality is a growing concern in all parts of the world

Think of the contrasts shown in Figures 5-9 and 5-10, in photographs from different parts of the world.

In the first one, scientists from the U.S. Department of Agriculture and students from Ohio State University are measuring the effects of farm pesticides and nitrogen from fertilizers on groundwater quality. In developed countries we expect water to be clean, odorless, colorless, and *safe*. Water is easily accessible, and therefore, unfortunately, sometimes easily wasted. It is often forgotten that until this century, water purity was of great concern in the cities of North America and Europe. Surface water from rivers, lakes, and reservoirs was frequently contaminated by infectious agents from human and animal waste, and epidemics of cholera, dysentery, and typhoid were common in New York, London, and other cities. Contrast this with the picture of a woman drawing water from the river, which is a common sight in developing countries. Many of last century's concerns about water safety in developed countries are now concerns in developing coun-

Diuretics: Substances that increase the excretion of urine.

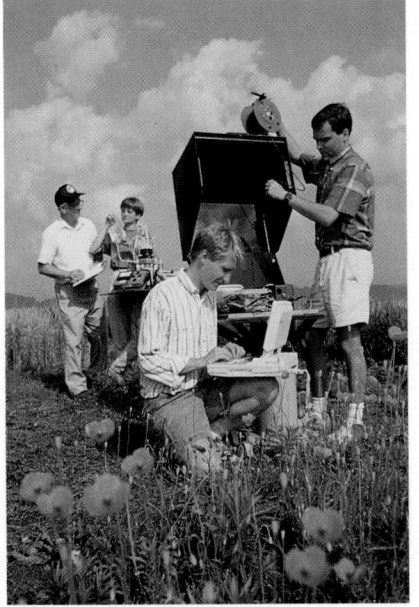

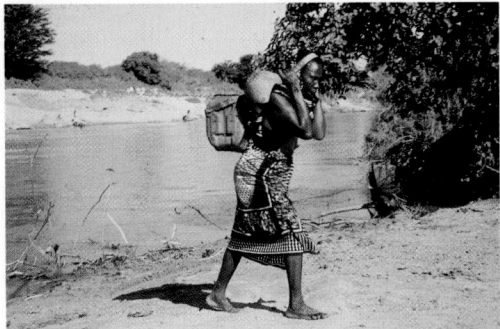

Figures 5-9 and 5-10. A safe and available supply of water is a concern all over the world. Pollutants from industry and agriculture that contaminate groundwater are monitored in many countries. Some citizens in all countries must draw their water directly from rivers and wells.

tries. This contrast leads us to a brief discussion on absolute safety versus relative safety, using water as the example.

What Does "Safety" Mean?

Absolute safety is the assurance that damage or injury from use of a substance is impossible.[5] Absolute safety of food, water, or any other commodity is a scientific impossibility. There will always be a certain risk, usually very slight, from eating food and drinking water. Relative food safety is defined as the practical certainty that injury or damage will not result from a food or ingredient of normal quality used in a reasonable and customary manner. All of this sounds rather legalistic, so let's go back to the two photographs for examples.

Neither the water from the tap nor the water from the river is absolutely safe. Water is one of those chemicals with a great ability to dissolve other chemicals. Instruments are now so sensitive that tiny amounts of chemicals dissolved in water and other liquids can be measured. Newspaper and magazine articles sometimes refer to the amount of a troublesome chemical as being present in amounts of parts per million (ppm) or parts per billion (ppb). The example in the margin indicates how tiny these parts are.

Hold up a glass of tap water to the light. In all probability it looks "clean" and has no color, taste, or smell. But it may contain some useful and some harmful chemicals and other matter. Depending on the source of the water, it may include some or all of the following useful chemicals.

- **Calcium and other minerals** from rocks and soil. These make water a reasonable dietary source of some minerals.
- **Fluoride**, which may be added to increase the intake of fluoride in areas where foods or water are low in this nutrient (see Table 1-4).
- **Chlorine**, which kills harmful microorganisms. (However, some evidence suggests that chlorine may increase the risk of cancer.)

Harmful chemicals that may be present in water include:

- **Nitrate** from commercial fertilizers, livestock manure, and sewage. This is an environmental problem. Drinking-water wells in some rural communities have nitrate levels above the levels recommended for health.[6]
- **Lead** from lead piping, which affects brain development (see Chapter 10).
- **Microorganisms** from human and animal wastes.
- **Organic chemicals** such as pesticides.

Absolutely pure water is not possible for the general community, so absolute safety is out of the question. But in most countries, we can be sure that our water is relatively safe. That is because we have the means of testing the quality of water from springs and wells and elaborate treatment plants to take contaminants from river water. Chemicals such as chlorine are added to kill microorganisms.

Let's examine the risk-benefit of using chlorine in drinking water. Lack of chlorination of water is considered the main reason why about 4,000 peo-

If you dissolved one sugar cube in 730 gallons (2,700 liters) of water (enough to fill a truck), the concentration of sugar would be *1 part per million* (ppm, $1:10^6$). The sugar from a sugar cube dissolved in 730,000 gallons (2.7 megaliters) of water (enough to fill a ship) would be in a concentration of *1 part per billion* (ppb, $1:10^9$).

ple died in 1991 from a cholera outbreak in Peru.[7] In the same year in the United States, about 25 cases of cholera were reported. Experts concluded that chlorine added to water improves safety, in part by preventing cholera. But some people are concerned that chlorine in water combines with organic compounds to form potentially hazardous products, resulting in an increased risk of cancer. Some experts suggest a risk of up to 700 cases of cancer each year in the United States.[8] So should we chlorinate or not? Science may solve our dilemma soon–in France a way to sterilize water without the use of chlorine is showing some promise.[9] Returning to the woman in Figure 5-10, she is probably relieved that the river still provides water and has probably never heard of chlorine or its risks. In summary, depending on your location

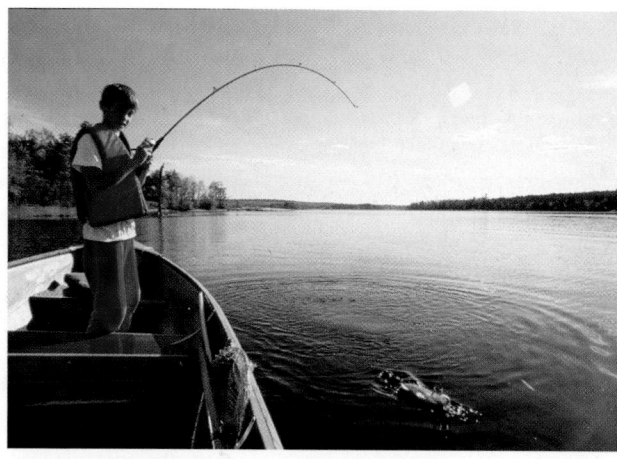

Figure 5-11. Rivers and lakes are not only sources of drinking water but also provide food and recreation.

in the world, chlorine provides relative safety from death from cholera, with a smaller risk of death from cancer.

Safety of water is a major area of public health concern and a fascinating area of study. Regrettably, we cannot spend longer on this topic except to touch on another major problem usually transmitted through water–the so-called "Legionnaires' disease." It got this name because of the deaths of a number of American Legion members attending a convention in Philadelphia a number of years ago but has since been found in other places. Domestic drinking water is thought to be a major cause of the problem[10] and moisture in air conditioning systems a significant means of transmittal of the microorganism.

Is bottled water safer and healthier than domestic tap water? About 25% of bottled water in the United States is processed tap water, which does not make it any healthier, safer, or purer than water from your tap. Some bottled water is high in sodium and does not have added fluoride.

■ Water in foods is important for quality and preservation

Water in food increases palatability by moistening the food and by dissolving sugars. When some foods take up too much moisture, they may become soggy, or they may cake and/or lose crispness. Water present naturally in foods can vary widely–plums and prunes are good examples.

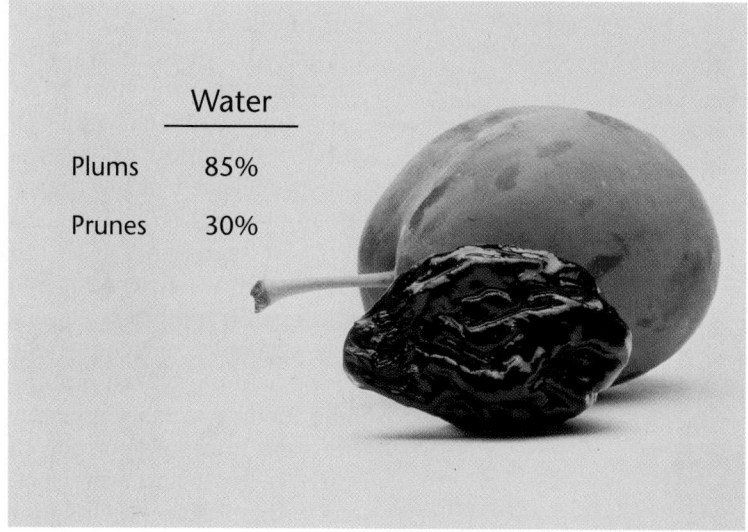

	Water
Plums	85%
Prunes	30%

Figure 5-12. If you dry a plum, you produce a prune by reducing the water content from 85 to 30%.

Food scientists are interested in the water activity (a_w) of food because a minimal amount of water is needed for the growth of microorganisms and for chemical reactions to occur. If the amount of water in a food is decreased to a minimal level, the food's shelf life is increased–we saw earlier that drying has been used to preserve food since earliest times. Water activity is a measure of the availability of water. The maximum value is 1.0. Most bacteria cannot grow at an a_w below 0.9; yeasts cannot grow below 0.85 or molds below 0.7. Let's take a look at the a_w of some foods (Table 5-1).

Table 5-1. Water Activity (a_w) of Some Foods

Food	a_w
Liver sausage	0.96
Marmalades	0.8–0.9
Salami	0.8–0.9
Honey	0.8
Dried fruits	0.7–0.8

Now let's link observations made in most kitchens to the information above on a_w values–microbial problems may occur with liver sausage, and molds can grow on some dried fruits and marmalades after a given time at room temperature. Foods with an a_w between 0.2 and 0.4 have the greatest storage stability and need no preservatives against microbial or chemical spoilage. Dehydrated foods have an a_w less than 0.6, so the amount of spoilage is low. Foods with a_w between 0.6 and 0.9 are called intermediate moisture foods (IMF). These need preservatives or special storage to prevent microbial spoilage. Decreasing a_w values to increase the shelf life of a food can be done by additives such as table salt, sugar, glycerol, and sorbitol; these are called *humectants*. But have you noticed a potential problem with these humectants? They affect the taste of a food and therefore may not be practical for commercial use.

"As weak as water" or "as dull as dishwater" are phrases you may have encountered in conversation. Food scientists no longer see water as weak or dull. They have discovered exciting new possibilities for various behaviors of water in food.[11]

Microwave heat causes water molecules to rotate back and forth on their axes, thus creating heat. Water causes many tiny "explosions" when it is exposed to sonic (sound) energy, thereby changing the texture of a food. Surface hydration allows water molecules to "stick" to another molecule–we learned earlier that 60 water molecules become attached to a hemoglobin molecule. Surface hydration "greases" molecules so that they slip past each other with "ball-bearing" effects. Food scientists use this property of water to design low- or no-fat foods. That is why water is becoming everybody's favorite fat replacer, as we shall see in Chapter 7. A debate rages as to whether water can also become "sticky" or "glassy" within a food, when it is least mobile. Learning more about this form of water will help food processors prevent deterioration in food quality such as when the food components become rubbery or crystalline. In summary, the water content and water activity of foods present many opportunities, challenges, and problems for the food industry.

Humectants: Substances that absorb moisture. They can be used to maintain the water content of foods such as bakery goods.

■ There is more to drink than just water

Caffeine

Think beyond the numbers on caffeine in Figure 5-13–coffee is what usually comes to mind when caffeine is mentioned.

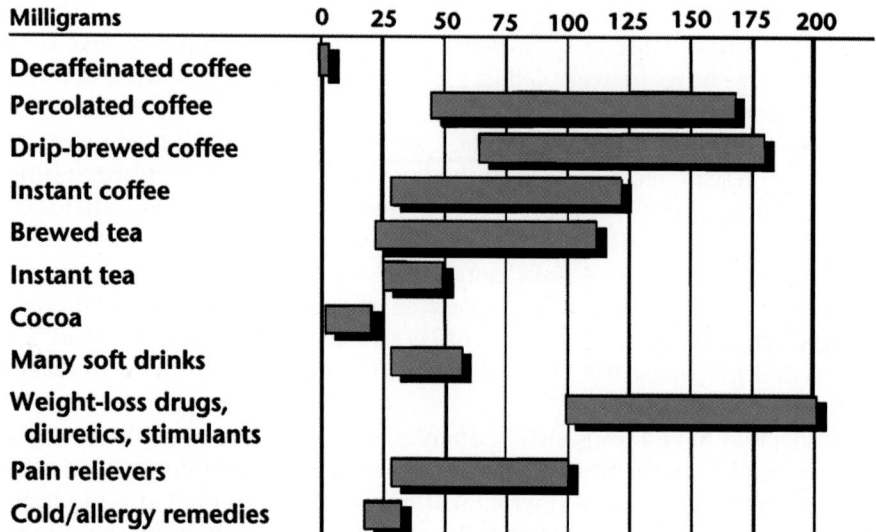

Figure 5-13. Caffeine is not only in coffee—it is also in tea, cocoa, many soft drinks, and many medications.

It is little wonder that most of us are not very good at knowing how much caffeine we consume per day.[12] North Americans consume about 227 milligrams of caffeine per day–the equivalent of over two cups of brewed coffee. The same amount of caffeine can be obtained from just over five 12-ounce cans of most soft drinks or from about six cups of tea. Caffeine intake from various over-the-counter medications may be significant for some people.

Coffee and caffeine have had their share of negative press. The data above on the caffeine content of beverages and medications were obtained from *The New York Times* (October 15, 1992), which ran a subheading entitled "Many fail to connect the brew with the blues." They refer to a study showing that caffeine withdrawal symptoms include headaches, drowsiness, fatigue, decreased performance, and in some cases, nausea and vomiting.[13] With such a collection of ailments, it is not surprising that caffeine has had a lot of media attention.

Caffeine, classified as an *alkaloid* drug, is a mild stimulant and diuretic. So why are nutritionists interested in coffee and tea consumption? After all, these are pleasant ways to increase fluid intake. Coffee adds a little potassium and niacin to the diet, and tea has a high fluoride content. Added milk offers protein, sugar, calcium, and vitamin D and is an inexpensive source of energy. But tea may present problems, especially for peo-

Alkaloids: Specific nitrogen-containing compounds of plant origin, such as found in potatoes and tomatoes. Alkaloids used in medicine include morphine and quinine.

Tannins: Specific chemicals present in teas and unripe fruits; used to clarify beers and wines. Also called tannic acid.

ple with low iron intake, because it is high in *tannins*. Iron binds with tannins to form an insoluble complex in the GI tract. In this bound form, the iron is unavailable for absorption and is excreted in the feces. This has nutritional implications if the amount of tea consumed is high, especially for female athletes. Here's why–women of childbearing years are more susceptible to iron deficiency because of blood loss during menstruation. Iron is part of the hemoglobin molecule in red blood cells. Consuming large amounts of tea (including iced tea) may decrease the absorption of iron, making it unavailable to form hemoglobin. Then the ability to take oxygen from the lungs to every cell in the body is decreased, resulting in lower athletic performance.

Some controversial issues about caffeine consumption remain. A Canadian researcher summarized the latest research on caffeine by stating that certain types of coffee brew may increase serum cholesterol, that relationships between caffeine and coronary heart disease are unresolved, and that no strong evidence links caffeine intake to various cancers. We are cautioned, however, that a "cup of coffee" means many things to different people. The source and type of coffee and the methods of roasting the beans and preparing the brew all may differ, making it difficult to detect correlations with diseases.[14]

Herbal teas have a long history of giving refreshment to people throughout the world. In recent times, the FDA has taken a cautious attitude relative to the consumption of herbal teas because some ingredients and their effects on the human body are unknown. Canada has banned the sale of 57 herbs and required warning labels on five others. The best summation of possible health risks from drinking herbal tea was given by an FDA staff person who said that it might be best to play safe and heed an old saying about those who gather wild mushrooms:

> There are old mushroom hunters. And there are bold mushroom hunters. But there are no old, bold mushroom hunters.[15]

Soft Drinks

Think about these numbers.

- There are 10 teaspoons of sugar in one can (12 ounces) of regular soda.
- Males average about two cans a day, females one and a half cans.
- A higher percentage of 12–29 year olds than of any other group drink regular soda.

Soft drinks are important contributors to fluid intake, but be careful–know your soft drinks if you are counting calories. Ten teaspoons of sugar in each can of soda pop translates into 150 calories. So you are counting calories and watching your body weight? Here is what 150 calories mean in the battle to control body weight. It takes about 3,500 calories to gain 1 pound of body fat. Divide this number by the 150 calories in each can of soda to get the number of cans needed to give 3,500 calories–24 cans of soda. At the level of consumption of sugared soda described above, it takes just 12 days for a young man and 18 days for a young woman to put on one pound of extra body fat. This assumes that food intake and energy expenditure are constant during this period–almost an impossibility in our active lives. We will revisit this important topic in Chapter 11. The good news is that when you reverse the above example, you can lose one pound of body fat by going without the sugared sodas over the same 12–18 days. All of this math juggling is eliminated if you drink diet soda, which has only one calorie per can. Better still, drink water, which has no calories and costs nothing.

Fruit Juices and Fruit Drinks

Are fruit juices and fruit drinks the same, or are we playing with words again? The answers are: no, juices and drinks are not the same in nutritive value, and yes, word games may mislead consumers. Fruit drinks are typically lower in nutrient content than fruit juices–compare the amount of some minerals and vitamins in grape juice and grape drink (Table 5-2).

The numbers speak for themselves, but consumers have been fooled in the past. Criminal prosecutions were brought against people who sold colored sugar water labeled as fruit juices or drinks. The new labeling laws discussed in Chapter 4 help the consumer by requiring explicit definitions of the percentage of juice in juice-containing beverages and clearer naming of these various beverages.

Table 5-2. Minerals and Vitamins in Two Types of Beverages

	Calcium (mg)	Potassium (mg)	Niacin (mg)	Folate (µg)	Vitamin B-6 (mg)
Grape juice	22	334	0.66	7	0.16
Grape drink	3	13	0.07	1	0.02

Is the current craze of making drinks by juicing fruits and vegetables the secret to better nutrition? Articles in magazines and newspapers and infomercials on television suggest that it is the way to better nutrient intake, to less stress on the digestive system, to a longer life with younger skin, less acne, fewer migraines, and no bleeding gums. Some have even claimed that juice will cure impotency, prostate problems, weak nails, hair loss, and much more. Common sense suggests that it makes little or no difference in nutrition or health whether fruits and vegetables are juiced or eaten whole, as long as the juice contains dietary fiber. In Chapter 4 we saw the importance of fruits and vegetables in a healthy balanced diet. Eat or juice your fruits and vegetables if you wish, because they are nutritious either way, but don't expect the medical miracles promised by the juicer salespeople.

Soups

Processors race one another to get soups for the health-conscious on the market

is how an article in a food industry trade journal starts. Think about the nutrition, health, and convenience messages on the labels of the soups you can see in your local supermarket. "Low sodium" is important because many soups are high in sodium; some of that sodium comes from the flavor-enhancer called monosodium glutamate (MSG). "Ultra Slim-Fast" gets the idea across that there are fewer calories in this product. "Healthy Request" and "Ready to Serve" emphasize that soups can be nutritious, healthy, and convenient in our busy lives. "Healthy Choice" again emphasizes health.

Watch for increased emphasis on the health and nutritional value of soup. Food scientists are formulating soups with less sodium and fat by using fat substitutes and salt-sparing ingredients–yeast extracts, natural (yeast-based) flavorings, nucleic acids, hydrolyzed vegetable protein, and flavors similar to those of fats.

Alcohol

Alcoholism: A primary, chronic disease evidenced by continuous or periodic excessive consumption of alcoholic beverages with genetic, psychosocial, and environmental factors influencing its development and manifestations.

Alcohol intake is a nutritional problem. *Alcoholism* is defined as

a primary, chronic disease with genetic, psychosocial, and environmental factors influencing its development and manifestations . . . .[16]

We have previously discussed alcohol as a toxin to the human body and seen what it can do to a developing fetus. However, most people probably do not consider that alcohol is a nutritional problem for them because they drink alcohol, if at all, in moderate amounts. "Moderate" alcohol intake is defined as one or two drinks daily. But this is too vague because whiskey has a much higher alcohol content than a similar amount of beer. Furthermore, people differ widely in their response to alcohol. In any case, even moderate drinkers should know the nutritional implications of drinking alcohol.

Alcohol and calories

Consider this–alcohol contains calories (1 gram = 7 calories) and little, if any, of other nutrients. Drinking alcoholic beverages provides calories to the body, but most drinks have no protein, vitamins, or minerals. This is important information because alcoholics and other heavy drinkers may consume more than 50% of their daily caloric intake as alcohol. This means that great care must be taken to see that the other 50% of calories comes from foods of high nutrient density, which is frequently not the case with heavy drinkers. Americans who consume alcohol (but are not alcoholic) get an average of about 10% of their total daily caloric intake from alcohol. Intake may range from less than 5% for moderate drinkers who drink about seven drinks per week to about 20% for drinkers consuming about 25 drinks per week.[17] A standard drink contains about 12 grams of alcohol, as may be found in 1.5 ounces of 80-proof spirits, a 5-ounce glass of wine, or a 12-ounce glass of beer.

High caloric intake from alcohol creates another problem in that some people tend to eat more food when consuming moderate to high amounts of alcohol. This deposition of body fat can result in obesity unless the person exercises appropriately. One thing to remember about caloric intake from alcohol is that it adds to the calories provided by dietary carbohydrates, lipids, and proteins. Put another way,

> alcohol may not appear as a layer floating at the top of a drink, but metabolically, it is nevertheless more like oil than like sugar.[18]

Alcohol decreases the absorption and metabolism of some nutrients

Alcohol decreases the absorption of folate, thiamin, and zinc, and also of pyridoxine (vitamin B-6) and biotin in heavy drinkers only. It *increases* the absorption of the metal cadmium, an environmental pollutant. Within the body, cadmium and alcohol combine to interfere with the metabolism of both zinc and copper. Alcohol also alters the metabolism of folate, pyridoxine, vitamin A, and selenium. The negative effects of alcohol on absorption and metabolism of nutrients are summarized in Figure 5-14.

Notice that the process is a vicious cycle of harmful events. Let's follow these events in a "hard drinker" who pours glass after glass of liquor into the gut (stomach and intestines). The nutrients listed above are poorly absorbed from the gut. Further malabsorption is produced by the frequent diarrhea suffered by many heavy drinkers. This increases maldigestion and malabsorption of nutrients from the gut as well as having negative effects on the liver's ability to metabolize nutrients. The diagram also shows a direct negative effect on both the gut and liver because alcohol is also a toxin. Death from cirrhosis of the liver is often related to amount of alcohol intake (Figure 5-15, next page).

Nutrition therapy can help in the recovery from alcoholism

Nutrition therapy includes diet modifications that result in a more nutritious diet, as well as individualized nutrition counseling sessions. Recovering alcoholics who receive nutrition therapy have lower intake of sugar, less alcohol craving, and significantly greater nutrient intake than those who don't receive it. Also, a greater number abstain from alcohol afterward.[19]

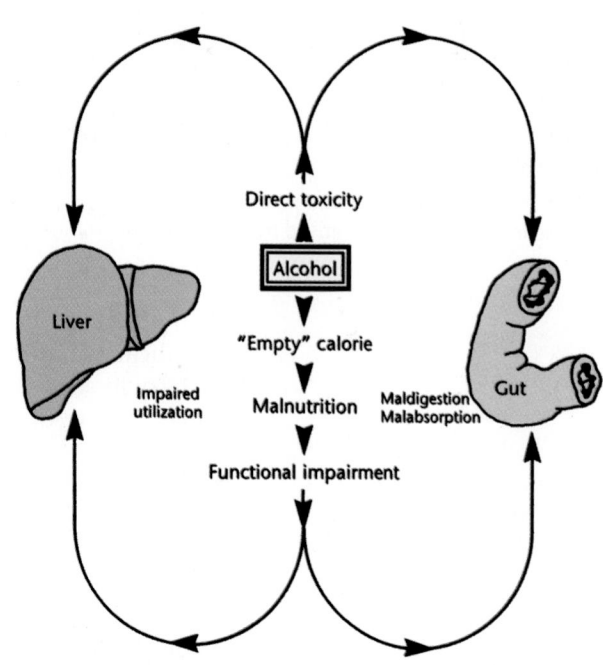

Figure 5-14. Alcohol is a toxin that must be removed from the body by the liver. It interferes with the digestion and absorption of nutrients from the gastrointestinal tract. Because the body obtains energy and no other nutrients from alcohol, malnutrition is common among long-term heavy drinkers.

Alcohol and coronary heart disease

Scientists and the media have been fascinated by recent research suggesting that moderate drinkers, especially wine drinkers, may have a lower risk of coronary heart disease than do nondrinkers. Other research shows that exercise prevents heart disease. Put these two pieces of information together and you arrive at the rather unscientific advice of one humorist that

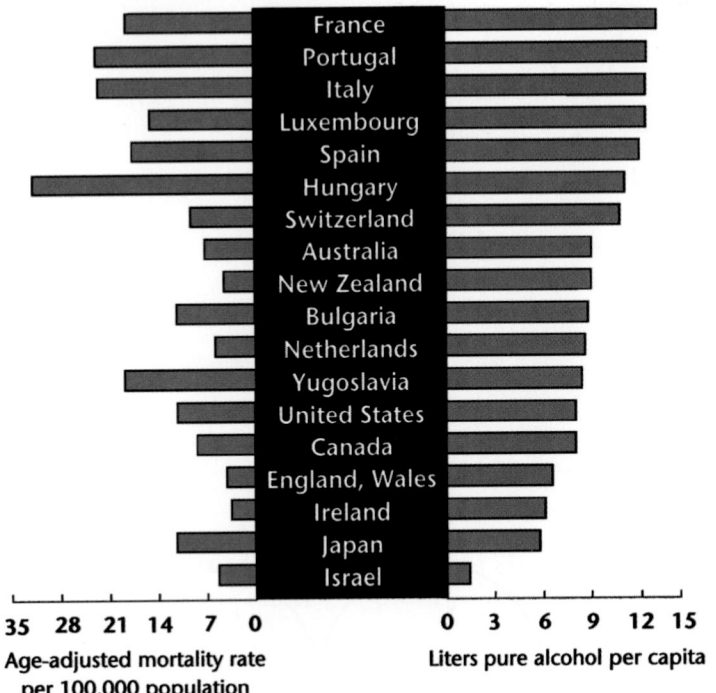

France
Portugal
Italy
Luxembourg
Spain
Hungary
Switzerland
Australia
New Zealand
Bulgaria
Netherlands
Yugoslavia
United States
Canada
England, Wales
Ireland
Japan
Israel

35 28 21 14 7 0

**Age-adjusted mortality rate
per 100,000 population**

0 3 6 9 12 15

Liters pure alcohol per capita

Figure 5-15. Relationship between per capita alcohol consumption and the death rate from liver disease caused by alcohol abuse in different countries.

the best way to protect your heart is to jog between pubs! Recent evidence does suggest that *moderate* alcohol intake (one to two drinks per day) is protective against coronary heart disease–moderate drinkers may have a lower risk than either teetotalers or heavy drinkers.[20]

Alcohol and brain damage

"Alcohol can damage the brain in many ways," warns the National Institute on Alcohol Abuse and Alcoholism. Alcohol-related brain damage in the United States accounts for about 10% of cases involving inability to remember recent events and to learn new information.

■ People are different– Effect of alcohol on nutritional status

Nutrition and other health problems are frequently confounded in alcoholics because some smoke, some have higher caffeine intake, and some may take drugs. The impact of heavy drinking on medical condition varies among people. For example, 90–100% will have fatty livers, whereas only 10–20% will have cirrhosis. Fatty liver is reversible if a person abstains from alcohol; cirrhosis is irreversible and is usually fatal.

Bulimia is a nutrition-related problem that is associated with high rates of alcoholism. We will discuss bulimia in detail in Chapter 13. Briefly, it is an eating disorder characterized by craving food and preoccupation with binge eating, loss of control during binges, and following binges with purging, usually by inducing vomiting or by the excessive use of laxatives.

Alcoholics are about 35 times more likely than nonalcoholics to use cocaine. Recent findings suggest that cocaine and alcohol combine in the body to form a more lethal drug.[21] Alcoholics are also more likely to abuse sedatives, opiates, hallucinogens, stimulants, and marijuana.

The combination of alcohol intake and drug abuse (either street drugs or pharmacologic ones) can have deadly consequences. Figure 5-16 shows what happens.

A moderate intake of alcohol (Figure 5-16A) is absorbed from the blood and taken to the liver, where the enzyme alcohol dehydrogenase converts it into another biochemical called acetaldehyde. This is the first step in the breakdown of alcohol to carbon dioxide, water, and energy. Drugs are detoxified by liver *microsomes* into less harmful metabolites.

A high intake of alcohol means that microsomes take up the overflow

Bulimia: An eating disorder involving consumption of large quantities of food at one time (bingeing), followed by purging from the body by vomiting, use of laxatives, or other means.

Microsomes: Microscopic particles from the endoplasmic reticulum (a connecting network within cells).

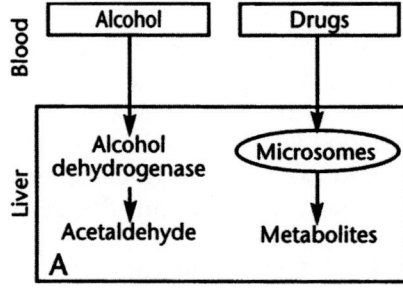

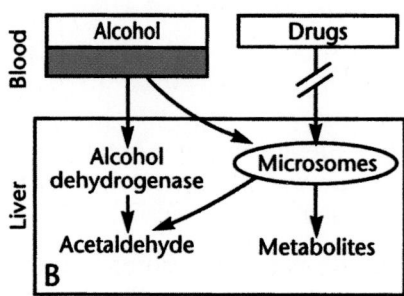

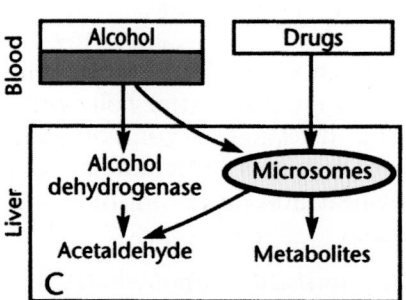

Figure 5-16. Metabolism of alcohol and of prescription and over-the-counter drugs in the liver. A, moderate intake of alcohol and drugs. B, high alcohol intake but no drug intake. C, high intake of alcohol plus intake of drugs.

from the enzyme alcohol dehydrogenase, which is working at full capacity (Figure 5-16B). Since no drugs were taken with the alcohol, the consequences to the body are not as severe as when large amounts of alcohol and drugs are both taken (Figure 5-16C). In that case, the alcohol competes with the drugs for detoxification by the microsomes. This means that the drugs remain in the body for a longer time before detoxification. The effects of this can be deadly. The best advice is: if you drink, do so in moderation, and *never* combine alcohol and drugs.

■ Food science in action–Brewing

Beer production is an example of food science in action. Beer was first made before 4000 B.C. in a region now part of Iraq and Iran, using a process that has not changed much since then.[22] This is where a can of beer begins–with barley and hops, the basic ingredients of beer (Figures 5-17 and 5-18).

Beer production begins when barley germinates after being steeped in water for one or two days. The sprouting barley is then left in a warm damp place for two to six days. This process is called malting. The sprouted grains develop enzymes that hydrolyze stored starch in barley into maltose and glucose. The resulting *malt* is then heated to destroy some of the enzymes, with the remaining enzymes continuing the breakdown of starch to sugar. The malt is then steeped again in water to soak out sugars, amino acids, and minerals. Malt wort is the name of this liquid, which is boiled to inactivate any remaining enzymes. *Hops* are added to give a bitter flavor and to inhibit the growth of bacteria. The wort is cooled and a *yeast*, usually *Saccharomyces cerevisiae*, is added. The whole mixture is fermented for about one week. It is not stirred, so the yeast rapidly exhausts all the oxygen in the mixture. The population of yeasts now grows without oxygen and in so doing ferments sugars in the wort to alcohol and carbon dioxide. The yeast settles out during a storage period and is removed. The beer is then ready for drinking.

Malt: Grain that has been moistened, sprouted, and then dried under controlled conditions, containing a mixture of starch breakdown products, mainly maltose (malt sugar). Prepared from barley or wheat.

Hops: Dried flowers of a perennial plant containing bitter resins and essential oils used in brewing.

Yeasts: Organisms used in brewing, wine-making, and baking. Rich in B-complex vitamins. Grouped with the fungi, although they are unicellular.

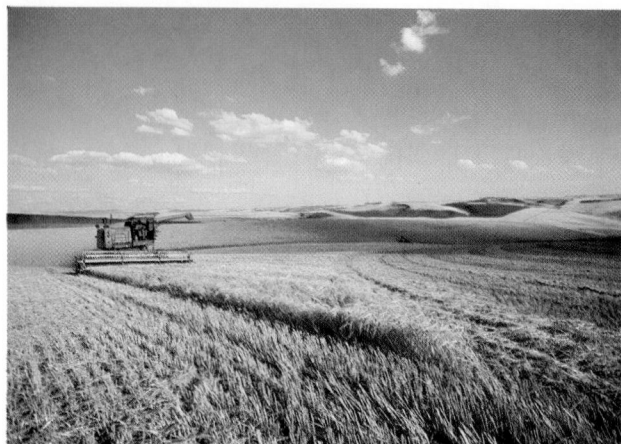

Figure 5-17. Barley is a key ingredient in beer and some other alcoholic drinks.

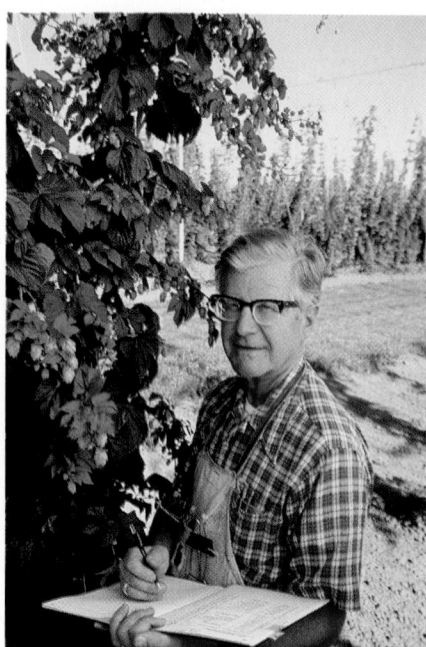

Figure 5-18. Hops are added in beer making to give a bitter flavor and to inhibit the growth of bacteria.

Wine is produced by a yeast fermentation of the sugars in grapes, but the process does not involve malting, as beer does.

A parting word on alcohol–don't assume that the alcohol used in food preparation all evaporates off. There is increased use of wines, liqueurs, and distilled spirits (brandy, whiskey) in preparing sauces, main dishes, and desserts. Alcohol is used sometimes to substitute for heavy creams. A study showed that between 4 and 85% of the alcohol was retained in the food.[23]

■ Now you know

- Oral rehydration therapy using a mixture of sugar, salt, and clean water effectively prevents dehydration from diarrhea.

- Fetal alcohol syndrome, the leading known cause of mental retardation in the United States, is caused by too much alcohol intake by the mother during pregnancy.

- Adult bodies contain about 12 gallons of water, which is essential for many vital body functions, including digestion, absorption, and transportation of nutrients; excretion of waste; control of body heat; and cushioning of tissues.

- Water of metabolism is produced in the breakdown of energy nutrients–carbohydrates, lipids, and proteins.

- Some people need increased fluid intake. They are women who are pregnant or lactating; infants; people who are vomiting or have diarrhea or fever; the elderly; people with kidney disease or on high-protein diets; people doing hard physical work; those in hot weather; air travelers; and athletes.

- Acidity in foods and the body results from hydrogen ions (H^+), is measured by pH, and is controlled by buffers.

- Edema is an accumulation of excess fluid in tissues.

- Water normally contains useful chemicals such as calcium and other minerals and added fluoride, and it *may* also contain harmful substances such as nitrates, lead, microorganisms, and organic chemicals.

- The water activity (a_w) of foods results from (but is not the same as) their moisture content and is an important determinant of their likely shelf life and other properties.

- Caffeine's role in coronary heart disease is still controversial.

- Soft drinks may be major contributors to sugar intake. Making a distinction between fruit juices and fruit drinks is important for optimizing nutritional content.

- Alcohol is a toxin, has 7 calories per gram, decreases the absorption of some nutrients, and can cause liver cirrhosis. Excess intake is a factor in coronary heart disease, and the combination of alcohol and drugs can be lethal.

- Beer is produced from cereals, usually barley with added hops.

Further Reading

1. Streissguth, A. P., and others. Fetal alcohol syndrome in adolescents and adults. *Journal of the American Medical Association* 265:1961, 1992.
2. Neeser, M., and others. "Thirst strike": hypernatraemia and acute perennial failure in a prisoner who refused to drink. *British Medical Journal* 304:1352, 1992.
3. Rand, R. P. Raising water to new heights. *Science* 256:618, 1992.
4. Ershow, A. G., and others. Intake of tapwater and total water by pregnant and lactating women. *American Journal of Public Health* 81:328, 1991.
5. Jones, J. M. *Food Safety*. Eagan Press, St. Paul, Minnesota, page 4, 1992.
6. Kross, B. C., and others. The nitrate contamination of private well water in Iowa. *American Journal of Public Health* 83:270, 1993.
7. Glass, R. I., and others. Epidemic cholera in the Americas. *Science* 256:1524, 1992.
8. Anonymous. Of cabbages and chlorine: Cholera in Peru. *Lancet* 340:20, 1992.
9. Patel, T. Water without the whiff of chlorine. *New Scientist*, page 19, November 7, 1992.
10. Stout, J. E., and others. Potable water as a cause of sporadic cases of community-acquired Legionnaires' disease. *New England Journal of Medicine* 326:151, 1992.
11. Best, D. New perspectives on water's role in formulation. *Prepared Foods* 162:59, August, 1992.
12. Bergman, E. A., and others. Caffeine knowledge, attitudes and consumption in adult women. *Journal of Nutrition Education* 24:179, 1992.
13. Hughes, J. R. Clinical importance of caffeine withdrawal. *New England Journal of Medicine* 327:1160, 1992.
14. Stavric, B. An update on research with coffee/caffeine. *Food and Chemical Toxicology* 30:533, 1992.
15. Snider, S. Beware the unknown brew: Herbal teas and toxicity. *FDA Consumer* 25(4):30, 1991.
16. Morse, R. M., and others. The definition of alcohol. *Journal of the American Medical Association* 268:1012, 1992.
17. Lands, W. E. M. A summary of the workshop "Alcohol and calories: A matter of balance." *Journal of Nutrition* 123:1338, 1993.
18. Flatt, J. P. Body weight, fat storage, and alcohol metabolism. *Nutrition Reviews* 50:267, 1992.

19. Biery, J. R., and others. Alcohol craving in rehabilitation: Assessment of nutrition therapy. *Journal of the American Dietetic Association* 91:463, 1991.
20. Jackson, R., and others. Does recent alcohol consumption reduce the risk of acute myocardial infarction and coronary death in regular drinkers? *American Journal of Epidemiology* 136:819, 1992.
21. Randall, T. Cocaine, alcohol mix in body to form even longer lasting, more lethal drug. *Journal of the American Medical Association* 267:1043, 1992.
22. Michel, R. H., and others. Chemical evidence for ancient beer. *Nature* 360:24, 1992.
23. Augustin, J., and others. Alcohol retention in food preparation. *Journal of the American Dietetic Association* 92:486, 1992.

Do the foods in the picture on the left contain sugar? Which glass on the right contains fiber?

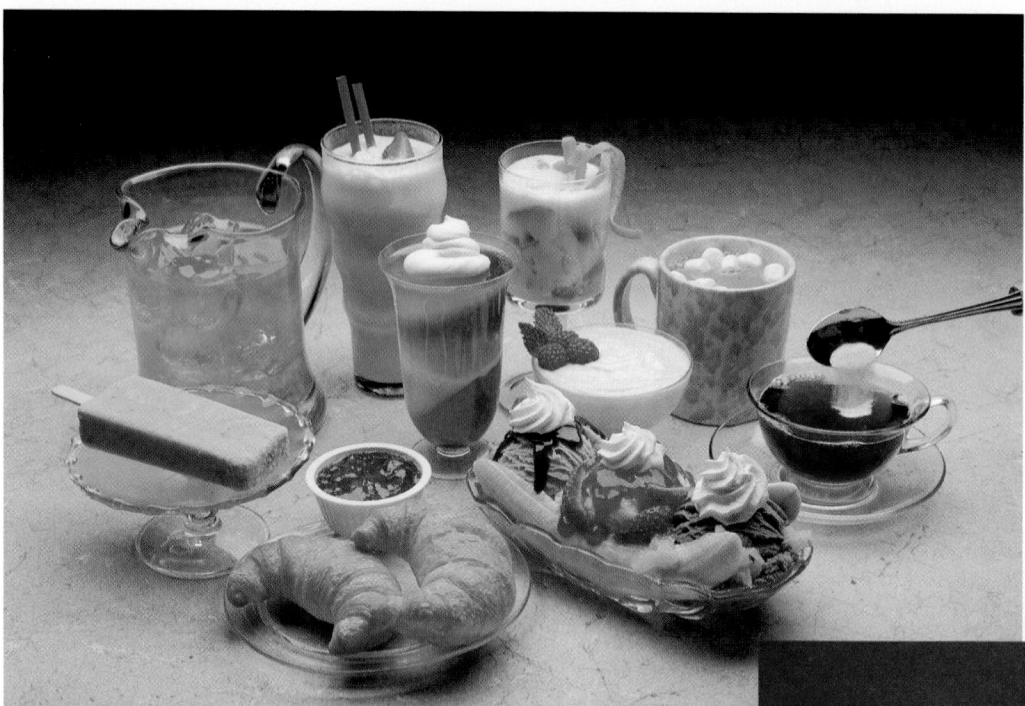

Figure 6-1. Artificial sweeteners are used in place of sugar in these and many foods and drinks.

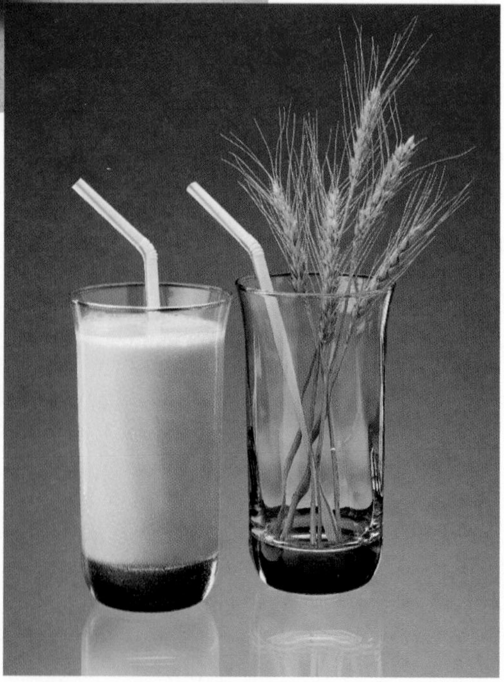

Figure 6-2. Plant foods in the diet are our normal source of fiber. However, various illnesses require it to be consumed in liquid form. Research on the chemistry of fiber has permitted the production of fiber drinks.

Carbohydrates–Cereals, Milling, and Baking

■ Carbohydrates in our lives–Some confusion and misinformation about their nutritional value

Not long ago it was impossible to get low- or no-calorie foods and drinks that still gave you the sweet taste of sugar, and most people did not know that *fiber* is a nutritional component. Now there is a parade of products made with sugar substitutes, and patients can drink their fiber. The caption on Figure 6-2 when it was used as an advertisement in a medical journal was: "Now your patients can drink their fiber while getting the extra nutrition they need." "Sugar-free," "diet," "low-calorie," and "fiber" are words that sell food and drink. This is one reason for some confusion and misinformation about carbohydrates, which are defined broadly as sugars and starches. Consumer information is not helped by books critical of sugar, with attention-attracting titles such as *Sugar Blues* and *Sweet But Dangerous*. These imply that sugar is the villain among carbohydrates. Consumer information also is not helped when some food companies attempt to hide the sugar content in foods such as some breakfast cereals and desserts. Let's look briefly at how carbohydrates influence our diet, health, and general living. We will use information from previous chapters to help in the discussion.

- We consume much more refined sugar and much less starch than our hunter-gatherer ancestors did. High-starch foods–bread, cereal, rice, and pasta–are at the base of the Food Guide Pyramid, which recommends that we eat 6–11 servings per day (see Chapter 4). On the other hand, sugar is at the apex of the pyramid, along with fats and oils, all of which we are advised to use sparingly. This is correct advice, but not necessarily easy to implement. Sugar occurs naturally in some foods, and it is added to others in manufacture because of its important func-

Fiber: Collective term for indigestible or partially digestible structural parts of plants.

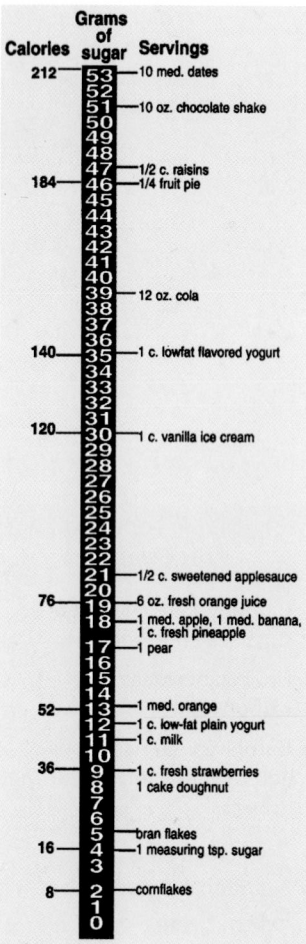

Figure 6-3. Calories from sugar and grams of sugar per serving of commonly eaten foods. The sugar in foods such as dates and raisins occurs naturally, whereas sugar is added to pies, chocolate shakes, and some other foods in this figure.

Dental caries: Tooth decay.

tional properties–as a preservative and for its sensory properties, including the production of a caramel aroma.

- High-carbohydrate foods are the most abundant, inexpensive, and readily available foods that people can eat. Think of carbohydrate-rich foods such as bread, pasta, corn, wheat, rice, and potatoes.

- Sugar may make food more palatable and may reduce calories if it replaces fat, because it contains 4 calories per gram versus the 9 calories per gram that fat contains. It may also serve as a preservative in certain foods by reducing their water activity (see Chapter 5).

- High amounts of sugar are found "hidden" in some foods such as peas, bananas, peaches, honey, sherbet, fruit pies, fruit canned in heavy syrup, low-fat fruit yogurt (not low-fat plain yogurt, which has zero sugar), and some fruit drinks (see Chapter 4). It is a natural component of other foods such as dates and raisins. The sugar content of some foods may surprise you (Figures 6-3 and 6-4).

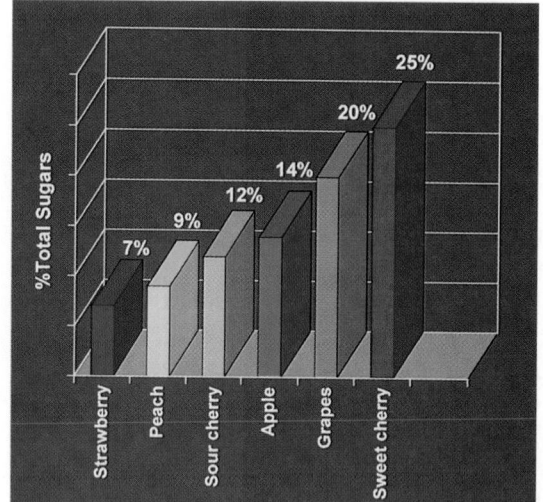
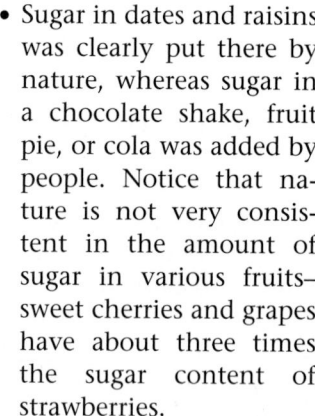
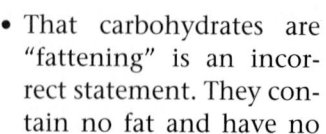

Figure 6-4. High end of the range of the sugar content of selected fresh fruits. Note the wide variation.

- Sugar in dates and raisins was clearly put there by nature, whereas sugar in a chocolate shake, fruit pie, or cola was added by people. Notice that nature is not very consistent in the amount of sugar in various fruits–sweet cherries and grapes have about three times the sugar content of strawberries.

- That carbohydrates are "fattening" is an incorrect statement. They contain no fat and have no mysterious "fattening factor." Think of what we do to some foods high in carbohydrates–we soak them in fat. Remember the differences in fat content between a raw or baked potato and French fries or between bread and a bologna and cheese sandwich. We should not blame only carbohydrates if our body fat is increasing. We gain weight when the intake of energy (calories) from all food–carbohydrates, lipids, and proteins–and from alcohol is greater than the energy expended in exercise and in meeting the energy needs of staying alive (breathing, heart function, body heat, etc.). We will examine the details of this delicate balance in Chapter 11.

- *Dental caries* can be due to many factors, including the fermentation of sugar and other carbohydrates in the mouth. Sticky foods are among the biggest culprits.

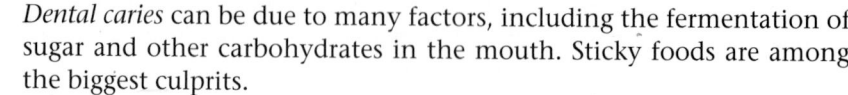

- Starchy foods are reported to help marathon runners and participants in other endurance sports (see Chapter 12).

- Fiber-rich foods in the diet may help prevent certain cancers and also constipation (fiber is referred to as nature's laxative). Also, some forms of fiber may lower serum cholesterol levels.

- There is *no* evidence showing that sugar promotes hyperactivity in children, criminal behavior,[1] or *hypoglycemia*,[2] despite reports in the media to the contrary. Perhaps a writer in the *New York Times* (October 28, 1992) best summarized the advice of experts on regulating sugar intake by children,

  > . . . portraying sugar and candy as the forbidden fruit sets the stage for a behavioral explosion when children are finally given the green light on days like Halloween.

  This statement allows us to note two universal observations in most issues in nutrition. First, many dietary and environmental factors are usually responsible for a specific outcome. Second, food and nutrient intake in moderation over a long period is always the safest bet.

- Sugar does not cause diabetes or coronary heart disease.[2]

It is time to collect our thoughts on all of the above and to see how well they fit into the following observation on sugar by John Yudkin of the University of London, England:

> Probably no single food commodity on the world market has been subjected to so much politicking as sugar. The study of this universally popular food is the province of the historian, economist, demographer, geographer, anthropologist, and sociologist, as well as the clinician and scientist.

His statement summarizes a recurring theme in this book–much of the excitement and fascination of nutrition results from the involvement not only of nutrition scientists and medical experts, but also of social scientists and food scientists and of chemical engineers who are involved in processing and fabricating new foods.

In this chapter, we study carbohydrates by looking through the professional eyes of people who produce, process, and study carbohydrates. We will also see how consumers use information on carbohydrate products. This same format is also used in our next two chapters on lipids and proteins.

Hypoglycemia: An abnormally low level of blood glucose (hypo = under, glyc = sweet, emia = blood).

■ Carbohydrates are sugar, starch, fiber, and more

Chemists' and Biochemists' View

A proper understanding of how any nutrient behaves in food and how it is used by the human body requires at least a brief look at the chemistry of the nutrient. Let's see how chemists and biochemists explain the chemistry of carbohydrates.

Think beyond the drawings in Figure 6-5. What do the three chemical structures have in common? What are the differences among them?

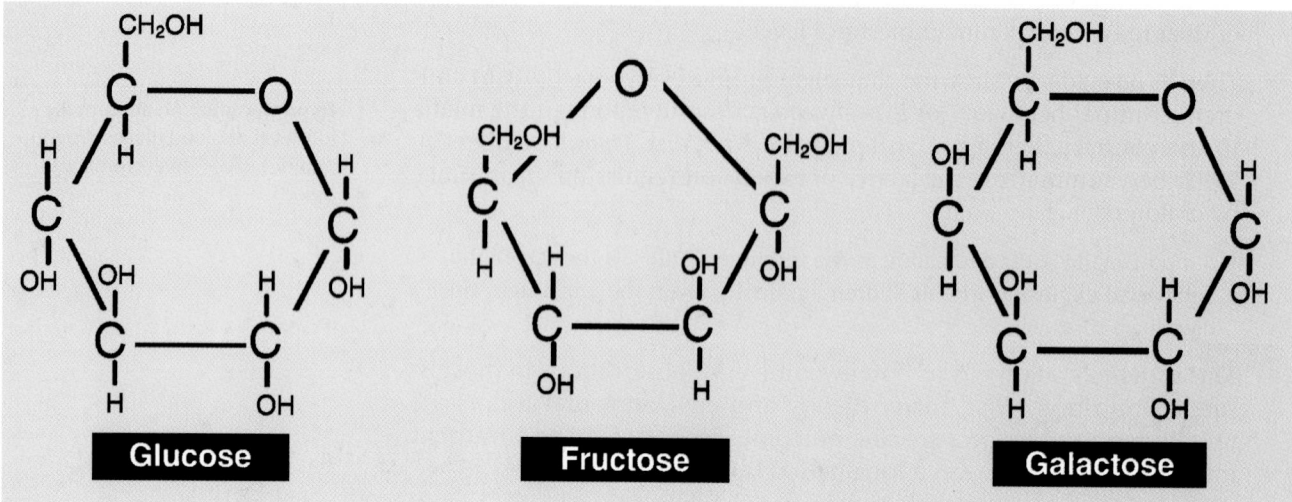

Figure 6-5. Structure of three monosaccharides–glucose, fructose, and galactose. Slight variations in the location of the atoms make each of the molecules different.

Glucose, fructose, and galactose are common monosaccharides, the "building blocks" of the carbohydrates. Notice that these monosaccharides have six carbon, six oxygen, and 12 hydrogen atoms with the general formula $C_6H_{12}O_6$. What makes glucose, fructose, and galactose different from one another is the orientation of certain oxygen and hydrogen atoms attached to the carbon atoms. These small differences in structure are sufficient to cause large differences in certain of their properties, as we will see below.

Knowledge of the structure of glucose allowed the development of chemical methods of analysis showing that glucose is present in foods in varying amounts (for instance, in fruits, vegetables, honey, and maple sugar). We also get glucose from the breakdown of starch and other carbohydrates, as well as from some amino acids. Biochemists were able to determine that glucose is the essential carbohydrate for our bodies (see Table 1-4). It is the prime fuel for the brain and nervous system. Put briefly, glucose is the primary fuel to perform any body function, in the course of which the glucose molecule is broken down to liberate energy, carbon dioxide, and water (Figure 6-6).

Nutritionists and biologists may speak of our bodies as burning carbohydrates, lipids, and proteins to provide energy. The term "burn" in this case does not mean that a flame is ignited within you, but rather that the chemistry involved is similar to that of burning fuel in a fire–oxygen (the air that you breathe) is needed to keep the fire lit; energy is produced (allowing you to run, walk, etc.); and heat is liberated (body heat).

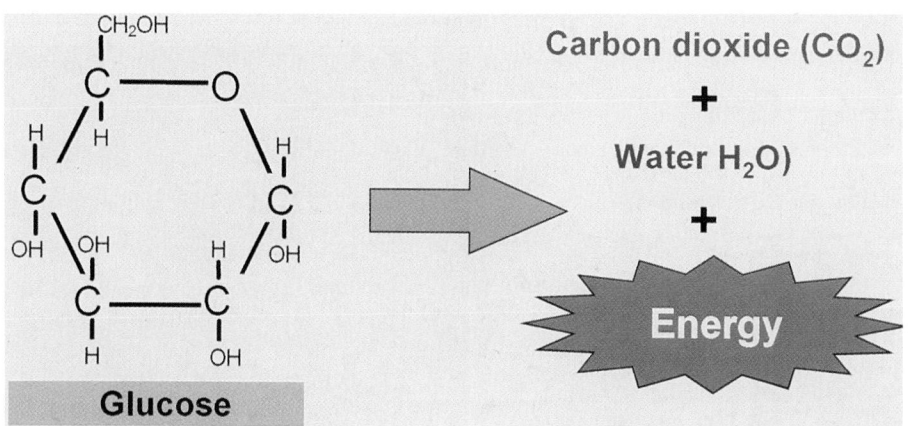

Figure 6-6. Cells metabolize glucose to produce energy, and the hydrogen, oxygen, and carbon atoms are converted into water and carbon dioxide.

Joining two monosaccharides together produces a *disaccharide* with the elimination of one molecule of water. For instance:

$$C_6H_{12}O_6 + C_6H_{12}O_6 = C_{12}H_{22}O_{11} + H_2O$$

Add up all of the carbons, hydrogens, and oxygens on both sides of the equation, and you find that they balance. Three important disaccharides each consist of two monosaccharides thus joined:

Glucose + fructose = Sucrose
(table sugar) + water

Glucose + galactose = Lactose
(milk sugar) + water

Glucose + glucose = Maltose
(in germinated seeds) + water

The original linking of monosaccharides to make sucrose and maltose is done by plants; lactose is produced by mammals. Table sugar presents a pretty picture to the chemist–tiny electrical fields surround the glucose and fructose units that combine to make up sucrose.

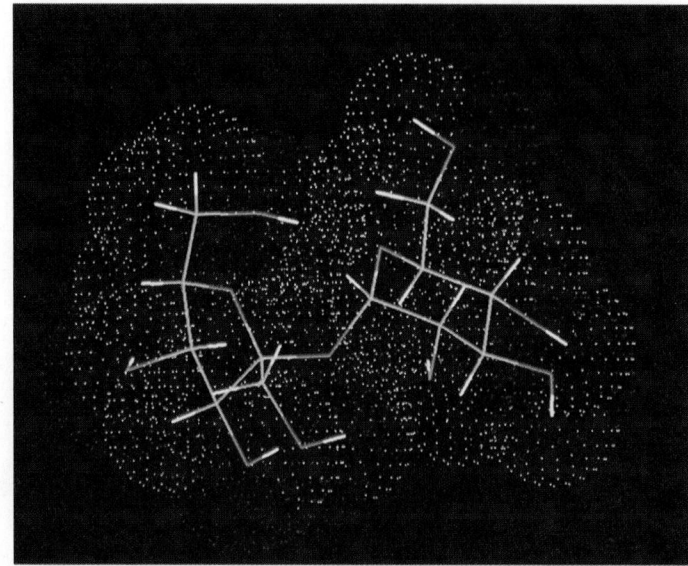

Figure 6-7. Tiny electric fields surround the atoms in the glucose and fructose that combine to form the sucrose molecule.

The combination of hundreds of glucose molecules produces a *polysaccharide*, also known as a complex carbohydrate. Starch (Figure 6-8) is such a polysaccharide, created by the linking together of glucose molecules.

Nutritionists are interested in starch because individual glucose molecules are liberated from it during digestion, making it an excellent dietary source of glucose, the essential carbohydrate.

Disaccharide: Two monosaccharides linked together; includes sucrose, lactose, and maltose.

Polysaccharide: Many glucose units joined together; starch and glycogen are the best known.

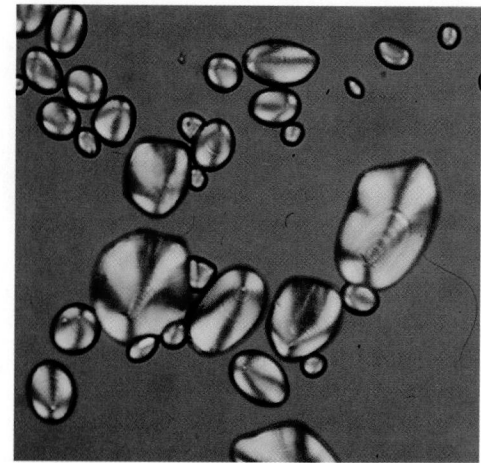

$$G–G–G–G–G–G–_n$$

$$
\begin{array}{l}
G–G–G–G–G–G–_n \\
\quad\quad\; G–G–G–G–G–_n \\
\quad\quad\quad\quad\quad G–G–G–_n
\end{array}
$$

Figure 6-8. Left, starch is composed of hundreds of glucose molecules. The starch in straight chains is called amylose (top), and in branched chains it is called amylopectin (bottom). The *n* at the end of the chain can represent a few more or up to hundreds more glucose molecules. Right, polarized potato starch, as seen under a microscope.

Glycogen: Storage form of carbohydrates in humans and animals; a branched polysaccharide with many glucose units linked together.

Cellulose: A straight-chain polysaccharide found only in plants; it forms supporting structures for plants.

Starch granules in bread and other starchy foods look like the image on the computer screen in Figure 6-9 when they are under a powerful microscope. This granular structure is disrupted by heat and stirring in food processing and during digestion, and enzymes then hydrolyze the starch to glucose, which is absorbed into the blood. Surplus glucose in the body can be converted either into body fat or into *glycogen*, which is stored in the liver and muscles. Glycogen is identical to starch in the way the glucose molecules are linked together; in fact, an old term for glycogen was "animal starch."

Cellulose, the polysaccharide that constitutes the cell walls of plants, is made up of glucose molecules linked together in a different way than starch molecules are. The digestive systems of cattle contain bacteria that are capable of breaking the links between the glucose units in cellulose. The glucose units liberated by this bacterial action are absorbed by the animal. But your digestive system cannot do this, which is why cattle can digest grass and you cannot. Cellulose thus behaves like other components of fiber in the diet of humans, passing through the GI tract undigested.

The reasons for interest in various forms of carbohydrate are summarized in Table 6-1.

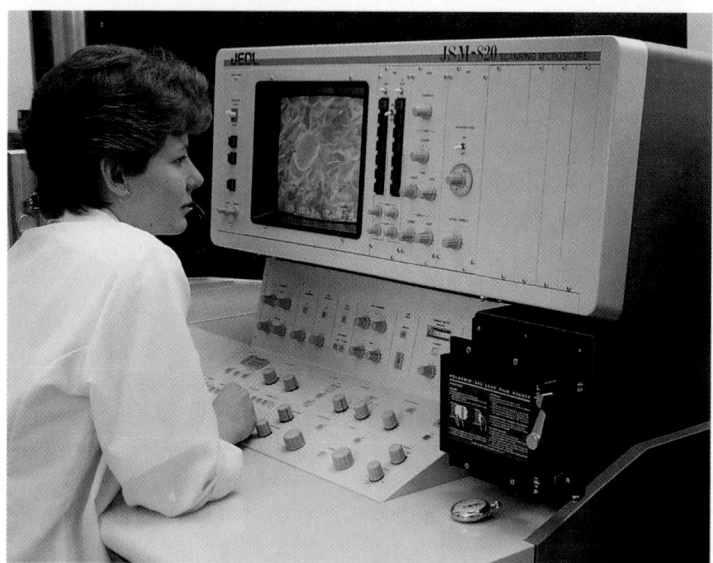

Figure 6-9. Starch can be studied with a computer to determine how it will perform in different foods. For example, starch is added to many foods as a thickening agent.

Table 6-1. Carbohydrates: Types and Importance

Carbohydrate	Description
Monosaccharide	
Glucose	Blood sugar, essential carbohydrate; main source of energy for brain and nerves; excreted in the urine by diabetics
Fructose	Sweeter than sugar
Galactose	Part of lactose (milk sugar)
Disaccharide	
Sucrose	Table sugar (beet or cane); found in fruits and vegetables
Lactose	Sugar in milk; poorly digested by some people
Maltose	In germinating seeds; important in brewing
Polysaccharide	
Starch	Excellent source of glucose
Cellulose	Part of a group of chemicals called "fiber"
Glycogen	Storage form of carbohydrate in liver and muscles in humans and animals

Farmers' and Plant Scientists' View

These people see carbohydrate-rich foods as the most important foods with which to feed the world's people and animals. Cereal grains are the major carbohydrate-rich foods. They are corn, rice, wheat, barley, millet, rye, sorghum, and oats. In addition, the carbohydrate sugar comes from cane and beet. Potatoes are rich in starch and may be a major food in the future to prevent hunger in a world with a rapidly growing population.[3]

Why is the process shown in the diagram in Figure 6-10 called the most important chemical reaction in nature?

Carbohydrates are produced in plants by a process called *photosynthesis*, which uses solar energy, water, and carbon dioxide. Without photosynthesis, people could not live on earth–we must be fed from complex foods already made by nature. We can eat plants (cereals, vegetables, and fruits) or we can consume meat and milk from animals that eat grass and other vegetation. All of these plants depend on a green pigment called *chlorophyll* to make starch out of simple ingredients–water from the soil, carbon dioxide from the air, and energy from the sun. This is how a botanist has described photosynthesis:

> Life depends on photosynthesis; chlorophyll has been referred to as the green blood of the earth.

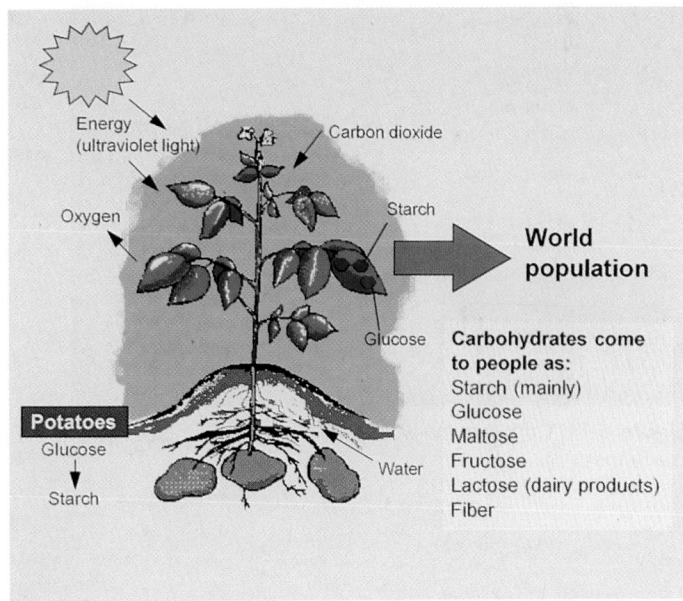

Figure 6-10. The most important chemical reaction in nature–photosynthesis. Glucose (and starch) is formed from energy from the sun, water, and carbon dioxide. This provides the plant food for animals and humans.

Photosynthesis: Manufacture of glucose from water, carbon dioxide (from the air), and energy (from the sun).

Chlorophyll: Green coloring matter found in all plants; involved in the manufacture of foods for the plant.

Environmentalists' View

Environmentalists are interested in the reported decrease in yields of corn, wheat, and other crops with high carbohydrate content because of air pollutants, including ozone and sulfur dioxide.[4] Ozone depletion in the atmosphere is partly the result of our dependence on fossil fuels to drive our cars and planes and our use of ozone-depleting refrigerants. Ethanol is a more environmentally friendly fuel additive used in some gasoline, and it can be made from grains, particularly corn. But what has this to do with nutrition? Plenty, if you consider that corn is one of the cheapest and most versatile foods available for feeding a world that has a large number of hungry mouths, with more being added each minute. We have some important choices to make, all with nutritional implications.

Think beyond the picture in Figure 6-11 to the many uses competing for this nutritious food–corn.

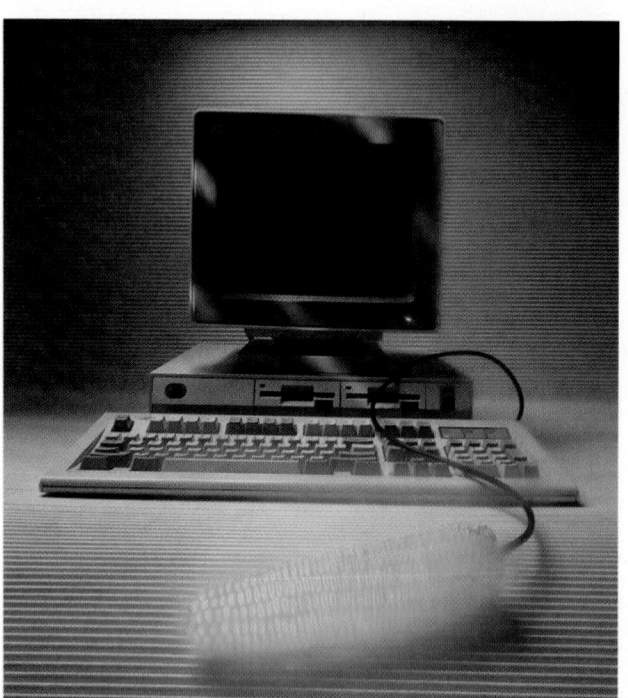

Figure 6-11. Corn has many uses as a food and, increasingly, many industrial uses.

About eight billion bushels of corn are produced each year and are shared by people, beasts, and industry. The USDA says that the corn produced in the United States is distributed in the way shown in Table 6-2.

Is it in the global interest to continue feeding cereal grains to cattle to produce meat and milk? This is an issue with enough conflicting concerns and interests to fill an entire book. Some concerns are based on sound scientific evidence, others on either incomplete studies or on emotions. The information presented here is a brief synopsis of different views as seen by different scientists and other interested groups. Most of the issues are complex and defy simple answers. You will probably have to make choices on these issues at some time in your life.

The latest data from the USDA and the World Bank indicate that 70% of the grain produced in the United States and 33% of that produced in the world is fed to livestock, primarily cattle. Animal scientists inform us that it takes about 7 pounds of grain (mainly cereal, with some soy) to produce 1 pound of beef, whether it be hamburger or the most expensive beef cuts. About 3 pounds of grain produce 1 pound of pork. The feeding of cereal grains to cattle instead of to humans is of concern to environmentalists, who consider this to be a waste of food. Many contend that it is a luxury we can no longer afford because of the number of hungry people in the world and because of the environmental pollution associated with intensive cattle raising.

There are several counterarguments to this position. One is that only some grains are suitable for human consumption, and the grains not consumed by people are fed to meat-producing animals. Thus, some grain may go to waste if it is not fed to animals. A further argument is that animals raised for meat provide a "nutritional insurance policy" against crop failures. Recent advances in biotechnology promise that the amount of grain required to supply a given amount of pork can be reduced by up to 25% by using *somatotropins*, growth hormones that can be fed to swine. Of course, many people are not happy with even the possibility of hormones produced by biotechnology in their meat (see Chapter 2). Many are unaware that hormones normally produced by the animal are present in all meat with no known harmful effects to the health of people.

Grains are the major source of food for billions of present and future people. But the present problem of feeding the hungry people of the world is an economic and political problem as well as an agricultural one. At the individual level, we are advised to have more cereal than meat in our diet–cereals are at the base of the Food Guide Pyramid, whereas meat is higher in the pyramid, mainly because of its fat content. But meat is an excellent source of protein, iron, zinc, and several vitamins, as we shall see shortly. Whether to eat meat or grains is a choice you have to make daily. Like most decisions in nutrition, it is not a simple one.

Table 6-2. Distribution of Corn in the United States

Percent of Crop	Use	Comments
0.2	Seed	High-yielding and disease-resistant seeds are planted each year to make new seed.
1.4	Food	North Americans eat relatively little whole-kernel or processed corn.
1.8	Starch	Used mainly as a thickener in foods and in industrial products
3.7	Alcohol	Used to make alcoholic drinks and as a fuel additive in gasoline
5.8	Sweeteners	Corn syrup has replaced sugar in many sweet drinks and snack foods.
45.0	Animal feed	Cattle, swine, and poultry consume large amounts.
17.0	Exports	Canada and the United States are major exporters of corn.
26.0	Ending stocks	Corn held in reserve at year's end as a buffer against bad crops in the next year

Viewpoint of Nutritionists, Dietitians, Nurses, Medical Doctors, and Physiologists

The people listed above have many interests in carbohydrates. Let's start with why fiber is important in the diet.

What fiber is

Carbohydrate-rich foods are at both ends of the Food Guide Pyramid (see Chapter 4). High fiber content is one of the reasons why bread, cereal, rice, and pasta are at the base of the pyramid, especially if eaten "whole" (unrefined). But the general public needs more education about fiber. We seem to be reasonably successful at identifying foods high in fiber but not those low in fiber, and we do not seem to know much about the role of fiber in the body.[5] Figure 6-12 shows the sources of *dietary fiber* in the typical diet of adult women in the United States.

Somatotropin: A growth hormone.

Dietary fiber: Collective term for the structural parts of plants that are not digested by humans.

Dietary fiber is not found in animal products–meats, dairy products, eggs, fats–or in sweets or beverages. The fiber that the figure shows coming from these groups was contributed by grain products or vegetables added to them.

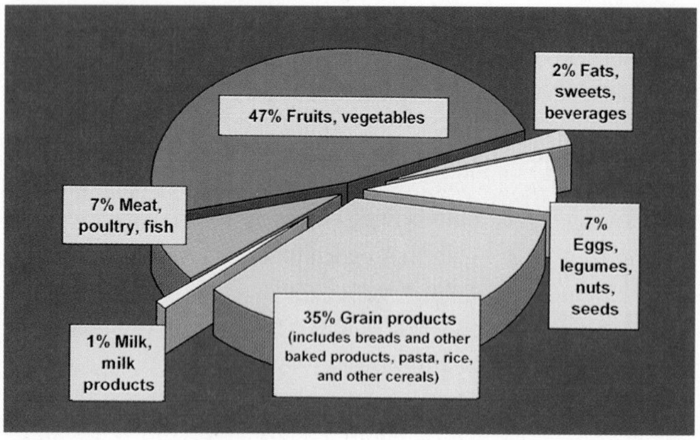

Figure 6-12. Sources of dietary fiber for women. All of us rely on plant foods, and some animal foods with added plant material, for our fiber intake.

Lignin: A noncarbohydrate associated with carbohydrates in cell walls of plants

Insoluble fiber: Sometimes called roughage; includes cellulose, lignin, and some hemicellulose.

Hemicellulose: Complex carbohydrates found together with cellulose and lignin in plant cell walls. Most gums and mucilages belong to this group of compounds.

Soluble fiber: Consists of pectins, gums, mucilages, and some hemicelluloses; constitutes about one-third of the total fiber in typical diets.

Pectins: A soluble fiber that provides firmness in plants by cementing the cell walls together; used as a setting agent in jellies and jams, an emulsifier in ice cream, and an antistaling agent in cakes. Fruits rich in pectin include plums, apples, and oranges.

Gums: Substances that can disperse in water to become viscous; used to stabilize emulsions such as salad dressings and processed cheese and as a thickener in foods. Gums used by the food industry may be extracted from certain seeds, sap of some plants, or seaweeds, or the gums may be synthetic.

Mucilages: Viscous products of some plants.

Viscosity: The property of a liquid that makes it resistant to flow. (For instance, syrup is more **viscous** than water and therefore flows more slowly.)

These numbers are worthy of closer inspection because of the importance of fiber. Unfortunately, some of the terminology on fiber is inconsistent. A term coming into general usage is "dietary fiber," which includes all naturally occurring plant material and chemically modified fiber in processed foods; both are resistant to digestion in the human GI tract. Described another way, dietary fiber is a non-starch polysaccharide plus *lignin*.

Dietary fiber consists of insoluble and soluble fiber. *Insoluble fiber* includes cellulose, lignin, and some *hemicelluloses*. Sometimes called "roughage," it remains almost intact as it passes through the entire GI tract. The highest concentrations of insoluble fiber are found in mature fruits and vegetables–broccoli, green beans, brussels sprouts, cabbage, radishes, green peppers–and in bran breakfast cereals and whole-grain breads.

Soluble fiber includes *pectins*, *gums*, *mucilages*, and some hemicelluloses. These tend to form a gel when they are in contact with water. This increases the stickiness and *viscosity* of the partially digested food in the stomach. About one-third of the total fiber in a typical diet is soluble fiber. This fiber speeds the passage of waste through the colon and is broken down by bacteria in the colon to produce fatty acids, which can be absorbed into the body.[6] Foods high in soluble fiber include beans, peas, prunes, corn, carrots, cauliflower, nuts, bananas, apples, oats, and barley.

Put in general terms, the insoluble fiber cellulose could be likened to the scaffolding of a cell, and the soluble fibers such as pectin and the hemicelluloses are a kind of biological glue to cement cells together. We still have much to learn about plant cells. It seems that cell wall structure differs among plant species and also differs during normal development within one species.[6]

Health professionals are interested in fiber for several reasons, which are discussed in the next few pages.

Action of fiber in the gastrointestinal tract

The brief summary of the effects of dietary fiber in the GI tract in Table 6-3 will give a better understanding of the issues to follow.

Effect of fiber on intestinal bacteria. Until recently, it was assumed that fiber passed through the GI tract unchanged and was excreted in the feces. However, it seems that the microorganisms we discussed in Chapter 3 digest and ferment a small amount of fiber (see step 1 in Figure 6-13 on the next page).

One expert on fiber states that each of us has about 400 bacterial species doing this work in our GI tract. What is fascinating is that the bacterial species you have are probably not exactly the same as the ones I have.[6] Bacteria in our GI tracts generate hydrogen (more from disaccharides than from other carbohydrates) and ferment pectins, gums, and modified starches to fatty acids. Tests to determine the amount of hydrogen and *methane* exhaled in the breath give a good indication of which sources of fiber are in the diet.

Methane: A colorless and odorless gas produced by the fermentation of waste matter in the GI tract.

Fiber as a laxative. Constipation is often corrected by increasing fiber intake, especially bran. We saw in Chapter 5 how fiber, being hydrophilic, binds water to increase the water content of the feces. This increases the urge to defecate.

Irritable bowel syndrome is a condition linked to stressful living, resulting in alternating diarrhea and constipation, abdominal cramps, bloating, and flatulence. A high-fiber diet frequently corrects these problems.

Diverticular disease, which occurs in many older adults, is the result of protrusions or swellings in the muscular wall of the colon.[7] The swellings arise from increased pressure applied in defecating when constipated, and they can become inflamed or burst. Symptoms include constipation, abdominal discomfort, *flatulence*, and mucous and blood in the feces. Diets high in fiber are considered beneficial in preventing the constipation that may cause diverticular disease.

Delayed gastric emptying is not fully understood. We do know that certain sources of dietary fiber such as pectins and gums slow the digestion and absorption of carbohydrates and fats.[8] They do this by interfering with digestive enzyme activity, by increasing the viscosity and volume of the intestinal contents, and by binding fat.

Table 6-3. Effects of Fiber in the GI Tract

Site	Activity
Mouth	Stimulates saliva; makes food more chewy
Stomach	Dilutes contents, pectin prolongs storage of partially digested food
Small intestine	Dilutes contents; delays absorption of nutrients due to interference with digestive enzymes; some dietary minerals not absorbed because of binding to fiber
Large intestine	Dilutes contents; bacterial action ferments some fiber; traps water
Stool	Softens; prevents constipation and hemorrhoids

Flatulence: Gas production in the GI tract. Undigested sugars serve as substrates for intestinal bacteria, which produce methane, carbon dioxide, and hydrogen.

Fiber and serum cholesterol levels

Persons with high blood cholesterol levels may have it lowered by diets high in soluble fiber from such sources as guar gum, pectin, *psyllium*, beans, barley, and oats, but insoluble fiber seems to have no such effect. Reduction is seen as a beneficial effect in the control of coronary heart disease. Fiber is thought to bind bile acids, resulting in their excretion from the body. Since bile acids are needed for the digestion and subsequent absorption of fat (including cholesterol) from the GI tract into the blood,

Psyllium: (Pronounced "sillium.") A grain similar to oats, corn, and wheat, grown mainly in India; its husk is a soluble form of fiber.

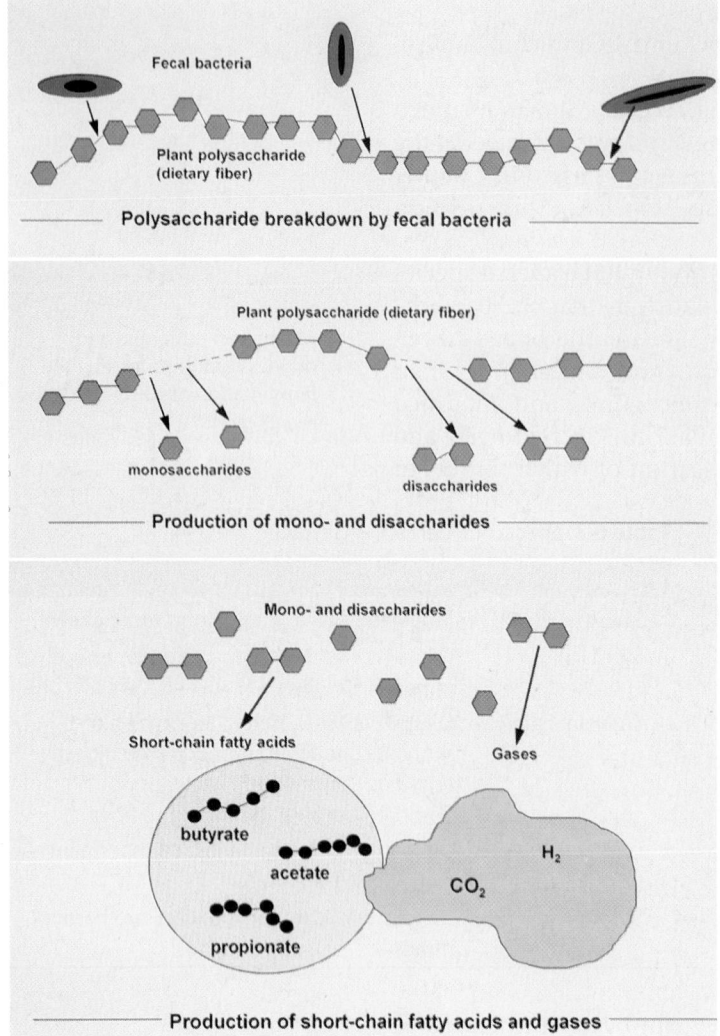

Figure 6-13. Scheme of the breakdown of polysaccharides. The gastrointestinal tract contains bacteria that digest and ferment some dietary fiber (step 1). Fiber is broken down into monosaccharides and disaccharides (step 2). Bacteria convert the monosaccharides and disaccharides into short-chain fatty acids and the gasses carbon dioxide and hydrogen (step 3).

In vitro: "Vitro" is Latin for "glass"; therefore, the term means literally "in the test-tube." In contrast, **in vivo** means "in life" or "in the living body of a plant or animal."

Phytic acid: An organic acid in cereals, especially bran, dried legumes, and some nuts.

their loss results in less dietary fat and cholesterol being absorbed into the blood.

Fiber and obesity

Explanations abound as to why a high fiber intake may be useful in the treatment of obesity. Fiber is a bulking agent that tends to give a full sensation after eating. Since fiber is mostly nondigestible, it also contributes little or nothing in caloric intake. Another explanation is that high-fiber foods take longer to chew, and their bulk may slow emptying of the stomach. It is when the stomach is distended that a full sensation is achieved. Despite these hypotheses, the conclusion from most well-conducted experiments is that fiber is not very effective as a weight-reducing agent.

Dietary fiber can have negative effects on the body

GI tract side effects can occur when a person with a low fiber intake suddenly increases fiber intake significantly–bloating, diarrhea, flatulence, and cramping are common. These symptoms disappear when fiber intake is reduced. Excessive fiber intake can even block the esophagus, stomach, or small intestine in extreme conditions, especially in the elderly and the very ill. Remember to always have adequate fluid when fiber intake is high. The reason is that fiber binds water. If fluid is not taken, fiber will draw water from the intestinal fluids. This could be a problem if young children are allowed to consume large amounts of dry breakfast cereal high in fiber as a snack food.

Mineral deficiencies. Fiber has been shown to bind a number of minerals in *in vitro* studies. Diets high in fiber are also high in *phytic acid*, which binds some minerals such as iron, zinc, and calcium and makes them nutritionally unavailable. However, this binding of minerals may not be very harmful for people consuming the typical North American or European diet. Even consumers of high-fiber diets show no widespread symptoms of severe deficiency problems with iron, zinc, or calcium. These include our ancestors, who generally consumed diets even higher in fiber than we do, strict vegetarians, and people living in most developing countries and consuming a traditional diet.[9] Nevertheless, the message bears repeating– moderation in intake of a balanced diet is what is best.

Failure to thrive. Most parents want their children to receive a healthy diet. They don't want them to eat foods of low nutritive value that might lead to obesity, coronary heart disease, and other diet-related problems later in life. To avoid these problems, parents may place their children on high-fiber, low-fat, and low-calorie diets. But, because children need more nutrients to grow, these restricted diets may lead to failure to thrive, resulting from malnutrition.

In summary, the hazards of a high-fiber diet are minimal if the diet is well balanced in all other nutrients. The recommended intake of fiber is between 20 and 35 grams per day. To get the recommended amount, one can use sources of fiber that also help to keep down the intake of fat and calories, as shown in Table 6-4.

Diabetes

Diabetes affects about 11 million Americans. It is a complex disease involving dietary and nondietary factors, which are discussed in more detail in Chapter 14. In brief, carbohydrates, especially dietary fiber, are important in the control of diabetes. An understanding of how the body deals with carbohydrates in nondiabetic people allows a better appreciation of the dietary and nondietary changes required of diabetics.[10] Figure 6-14 shows what happens to dietary glucose immediately after a person eats a meal and 6–12 hours later.

Table 6-4. Alternatives to Increase Fiber Intake While Minimizing Fat

Instead of This	Try This
Potato chips	Popcorn
Mashed potatoes or french fries	Baked potato in the skin
White rice	Brown rice
Refined cereals	Whole grain cereals
White bread	Whole wheat bread or rolls
Bread crumbs	Wheat or oat bran

In normal healthy people, the large increase in glucose in the blood after a meal triggers the pancreas to secrete insulin, one of the hormones that controls the level of blood glucose. This control is achieved when glucose is taken up by the liver, where it is stored as glycogen. The liver is remarkable because it can also make glucose from noncarbohydrate sources such as glycerol, which is a part of fat molecules; lactate, a chemical produced in the breakdown of carbohydrate, fat, and some amino acids; and the amino acids alanine and glutamine. Glucose also goes to other parts of the body. The brain is always well served with glucose, its primary fuel for energy. Muscle is another major user of glucose, and that will be important to remember when we look at carbohydrate intake by athletes (Chapter 12).

In those with diabetes, insulin either fails to work or is not secreted in amounts sufficient to remove the high amount of glucose in the blood after a meal. Dietary glucose that should have gone to the cells to provide energy is still circulating in the blood. The kidneys are working at maximum capacity cleaning incoming blood. The diabetic's blood has more glucose than the kidneys can filter, and some glucose that should be in the cells has nowhere to go except into the urine. That is why diabetics excrete large amounts of glucose in the urine. If left unchecked, this loss of glucose can result in shock and later in a deep coma and death.

The loss of glucose can be controlled by the injection of insulin and/or

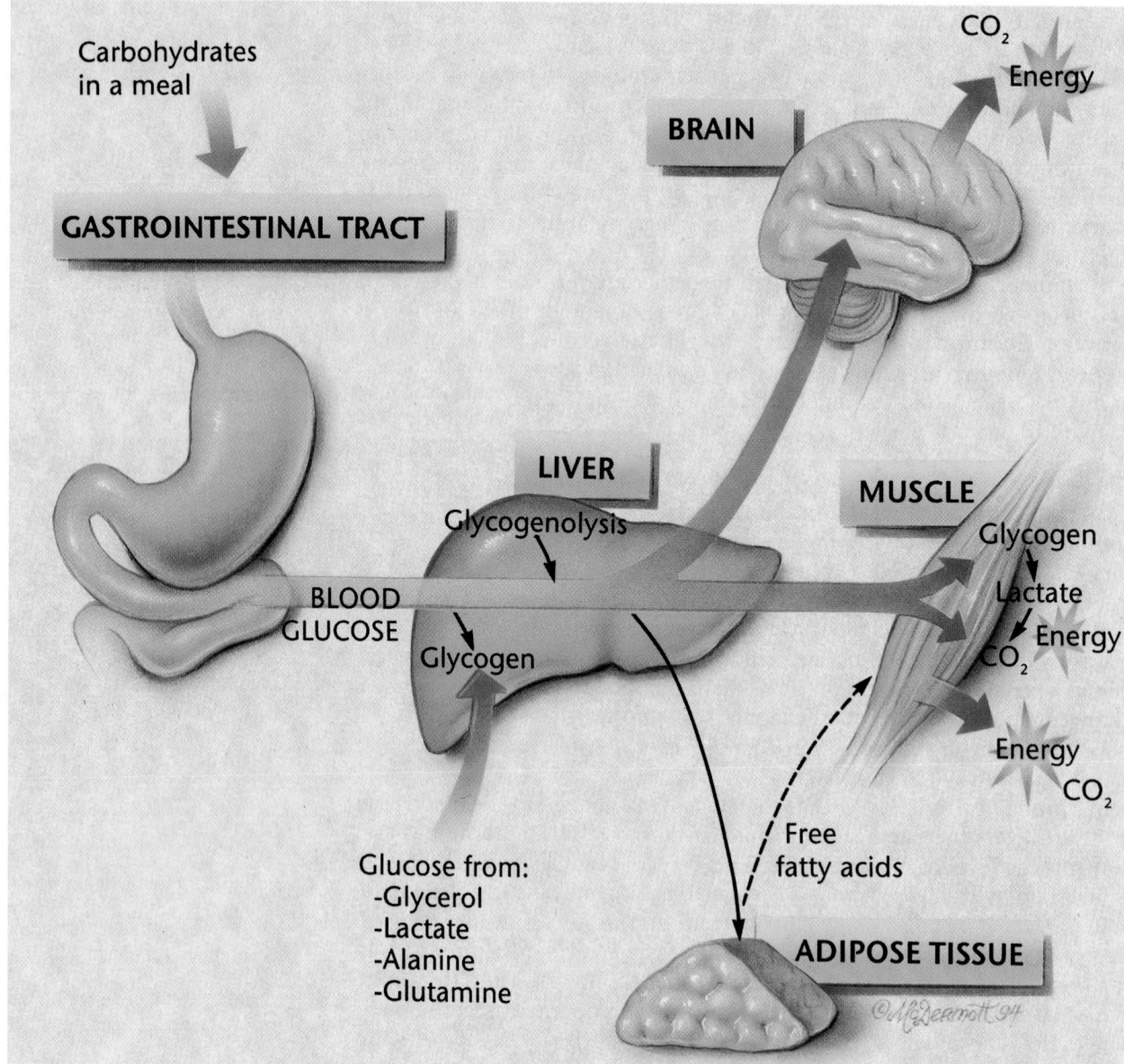

Figure 6-14. The glucose pathway. Left, immediately after a meal. Carbohydrates from the meal are digested into monosaccharides, of which glucose is the most important. After absorption into the blood stream, glucose may be stored as glycogen in the liver and muscle or used for energy by muscles and the brain. Glucose can also be formed in the body from glycerol (part

by dietary control. Limitations should be placed on eating foods that give rapid rises in blood glucose–sugar and sugar-containing foods such as candy, ice cream, and fruit. Dietary starch is not as great a problem as the simple sugars because more time is required to liberate the hundreds of individual glucose molecules that make up a molecule of starch. Diets high in fiber and in complex carbohydrates decrease the amount of glucose in both the blood and the urine. Soluble fibers such as pectin and guar gum

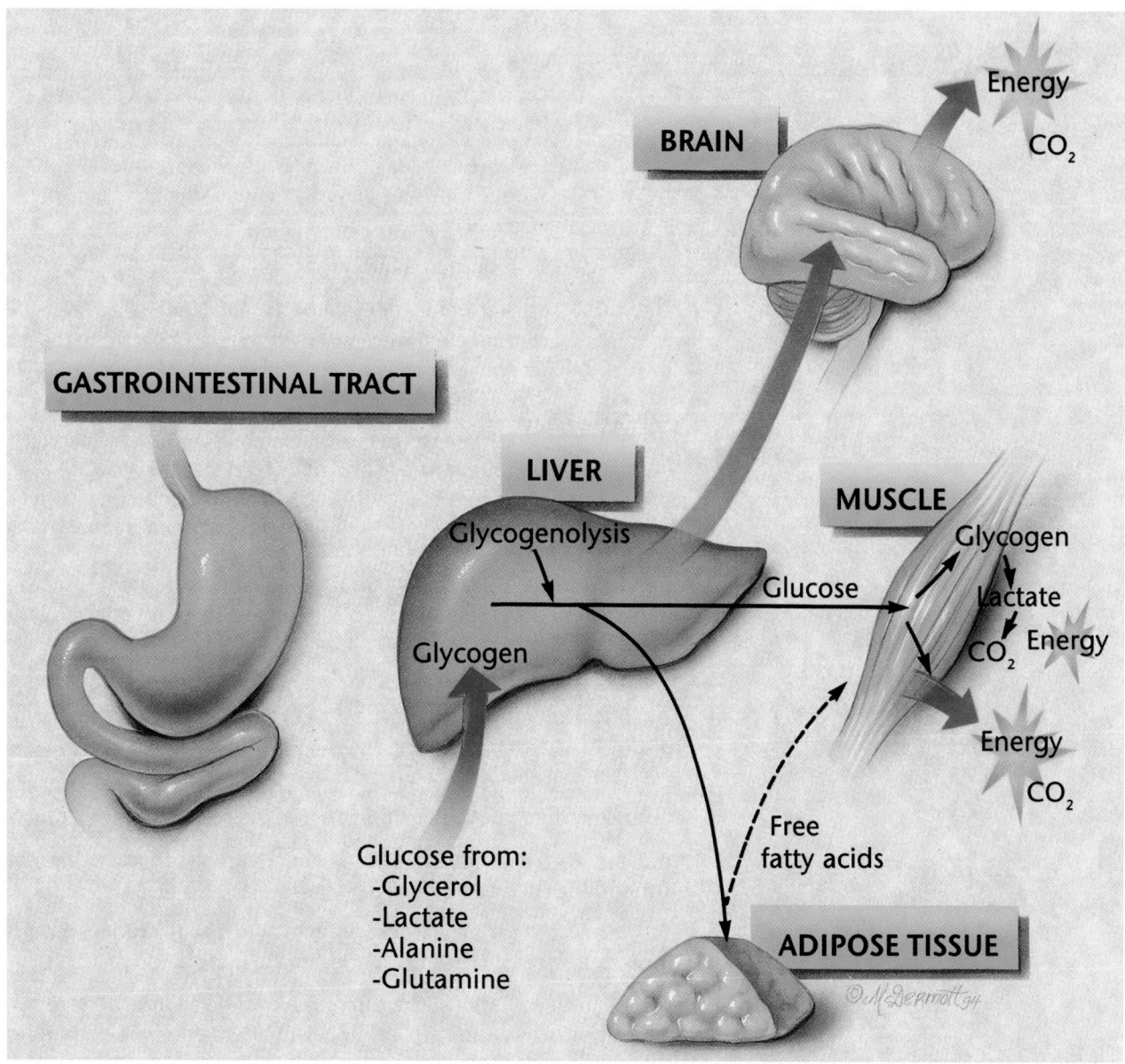

BRAIN

Energy

CO_2

GASTROINTESTINAL TRACT

LIVER

Glycogenolysis

Glucose

MUSCLE

Glycogen

Lactate

CO_2 Energy

Glycogen

Energy

CO_2

Glucose from:
-Glycerol
-Lactate
-Alanine
-Glutamine

Free
fatty acids

ADIPOSE TISSUE

©McDermott 94

of fat), lactate, and the amino acids alanine and glutamine. Some glucose is converted into fat (adipose tissue). Supplying the brain with glucose is essential. On the right, 6–12 hours after a meal. The supply of glucose from the GI tract to the liver has stopped. Less glucose goes to the muscles so that the brain can be supplied.

do this best. It is thought that soluble fibers delay absorption of nutrients from the small intestine. This delays the metabolism of carbohydrate, so less glucose is absorbed into the blood and less insulin is needed. Different foods have varying effects on the increase in blood glucose levels after a meal. The *glycemic index* is a measure of this effect (Table 6-5)–foods with low values produce the least increase in blood glucose levels after the food is eaten. These are obviously the preferred foods for people with diabetes.

Glycemic index: A scale identifying the rate and extent to which various foods influence blood glucose concentration.

Table 6-5. Glycemic Index Values for Certain Foods

Food	Glycemic Index
Glucose	100
Cornflakes	80
White rice	72
Potatoes	70
White bread	69
All bran	51
White spaghetti	50
Oatmeal	49
Peas	47
Whole-meal spaghetti	42
Baked beans (canned)	40
Lentils (similar to peas, beans)	29
Soybeans	15

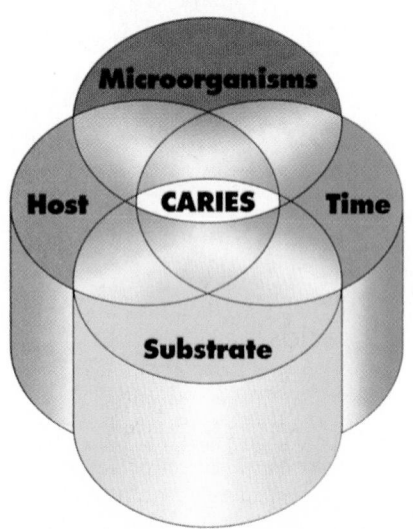

Figure 6-15. Dental caries may occur when four conditions exist simultaneously—a substrate (usually sugar or starch), a host (tooth), microorganisms on the surface of the tooth, and sufficient time for the bacteria to act on the sugar or starch.

Dentists' View

Dentists are interested in carbohydrates because of reports linking sugar intake to dental caries. A Sugars Task Force created by the FDA in the mid-1980s reported that

> evidence exists that sugars as they are consumed in the average American diet contribute to the development of dental caries.

The report concludes that

> other than the contribution to dental caries, there is no conclusive evidence that demonstrates a hazard to the general public when sugars are consumed at the levels that are now current and in the manner now practiced.

This translates to mean that there is no linkage between normal sugar intake and obesity, coronary heart disease, diabetes, hyperactivity, or criminal behavior. So, let's concentrate on the relationship between sugar intake and dental caries.

Four conditions must exist simultaneously in order for caries (tooth decay) to develop: a host tooth, a sugar substrate, microorganisms, and sufficient time.

Experts conclude that certain factors are important in dental caries.

- The physical properties of the food, especially stickiness, contribute to caries development, but the amount of sugar in the food is not critical.

- All sugars can cause caries, including cooked starch.

- Snack foods have high capacity to cause caries if they are high in fermentable sugars and cooked starch.

- Fluoride added to the water supply, to toothpaste, and to mouth rinses helps to reduce dental caries in the population.

Severely undernourished children have delayed tooth development and ultimately suffer from higher incidences of caries than do healthy children of the same age.[11]

Food Scientists' and Food Engineers' View

People who apply science to food take high-carbohydrate foods from the field and process them into more convenient forms for our busy lifestyles or convert them into ingredients that increase the palatability, texture, keeping quality, and nutritional value of food. Look at what is done to corn, for instance. Food scientists extract corn starch, which, when added to food, provides energy for the consumer and gives texture and consistency to the food. When starch is heated in water and cooled, it forms gels and pastes, which are useful properties in some foods. Corn syrups are formed by partial hydrolysis of starch to glucose, also known as dextrose. These sugars are not as sweet as sucrose (table sugar). Increased sweetness can be achieved by enzymatically converting a corn syrup containing mostly glucose into *high fructose corn syrup (HFCS)*. Such sweeteners have replaced sucrose in a variety of foods and in most soft drinks. Perhaps our most visible contact with corn products is in ready-to-eat breakfast cereals. Corn is also used in grits, porridge, tortillas, tamales, dumplings, and snacks.

High fructose corn syrup (HFCS): Glucose syrups containing more than 40% fructose.

Wheat is the main ingredient in pasta, which has been produced since earliest times in the Middle East and has developed over the centuries as a staple food in Italy. Pasta is now a popular food in the United States, in part because of the recent emphasis on increasing carbohydrate intake.[12] It is considered beneficial in managing diabetes (because of its low glycemic index value).[13] The food processor can form pasta into interesting shapes. Food scientists are developing instant pasta and shelf-stable microwavable fresh pasta so that we can prepare pasta quickly in our busy lives. Nontraditional pastas are being developed from rice, potato flour, corn, and legumes.

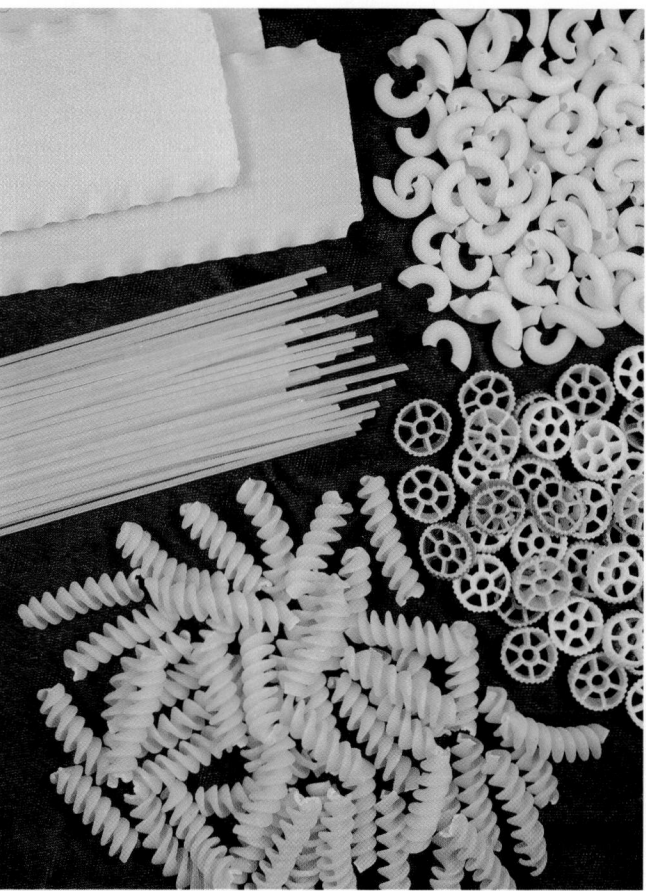

Fiber is added to foods because of its role in the total diet. It is added also in the manufacture of certain foods because its physical properties allow it to emulsify, suspend, increase water retention, increase freeze-thaw stability, control weeping of fluid from a food, and add body and texture to a food. Chemists are learning about the subtle differences among fibers obtained from oats, barley, rice, soy, psyllium, legumes, sugar beet, cottonseed, and fruit. This should result in even more interesting foods in the future.

Don't rule out sugar yet as an ingredient in processed food. A recent symposium on new perspectives on sugar highlighted new uses for sucrose in controlling the mobility of water within a food and thus preventing spoilage, new uses in chocolate and sugar confectionery, and new combinations with other substances.[14] It

Figure 6-16. Pasta, which has been produced since ancient times, is increasing in popularity in many countries.

seems that food scientists are becoming more interested in incorporating sugar into foods at a time when nutritionists want its consumption reduced (see the Food Guide Pyramid in Chapter 4).

Not all sugar substitutes are free of calories. All of the following add to caloric intake: honey, dextrose (another name for glucose), maple and corn syrups, fructose (levulose or fruit sugar), *sugar alcohols*, and high-fructose corn syrup.[15] These names are not uncommon on food labels. However, it is in the area of intense or artificial sweeteners that the greatest advances have been made. Table 6-6 lists nonnutritive and high-intensity sweeteners.

Sugar alcohols: Better known to us on food labels as mannitol, xylitol, and sorbitol, which are absorbed more slowly than most other sugars.

Table 6-6. Artificial Sweeteners

Sweetener	Sweetening Power (relative to sucrose)	Regulatory Status
Aspartame	160–220	Approved
Acesulfame K	200	Approved
Cyclamate	30	Banned in the United States, approved in Canada
Saccharin	300	Allowed in the United States by Congressional moratorium

The last word is given to James Giese, who summarized a conference on sweeteners by saying that consumers feel there is no such thing as a free lunch–that is, you cannot have sweetness without calories. They may be partly right in that the functional properties and taste profile of sucrose are difficult to replace. He does end on an optimistic note:

> . . . alternative sweeteners are useful in certain applications, and, although costly and tedious, the extensive safety and toxicological testing they undergo ensures their safe use in foods.[16]

Biotechnologists' View

These scientists are improving techniques that promise greater yields and better utilization of carbohydrate-rich foods (as well as other foods) in the future. The properties they are developing include increased resistance to insects, weeds, and diseases; improved resistance to environmental stresses such as drought, cold, salt, and environmental toxins; improved efficiency in photosynthesis; and increased protein and amino acid content. The potato chips in Figure 6-17 may not look any different from those you can buy in the store. But these may be the chips of the future. Biotechnologists have produced potatoes higher in starch, which means that there will be less fat in the potato chips you buy.

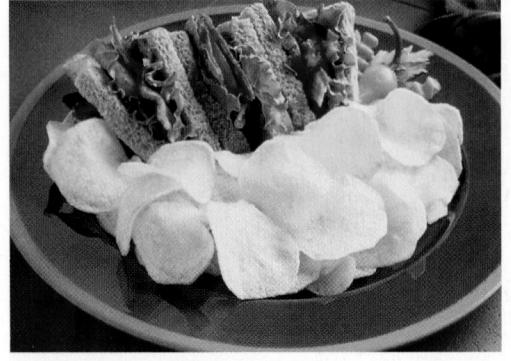

Figure 6-17. Appearances can be deceiving. These potato chips contain less fat and more carbohydrates than conventional potato chips because of the application of techniques in biotechnology to potatoes.

Toxicologists' and Food Safety Experts' View

The people who work at keeping our food safe see carbohydrates as presenting no great problems from toxic agents. Unproven or undocumented concerns about carbohydrates arise sometimes in the media. For example, modified starch was a concern recently, not because of toxicity as such but because of its use in commercial baby foods. Modified starch is produced when the properties of starch are improved or "tailored" by either chemical or physical means to meet a particular application in a food. The questions raised in the media centered on the digestibility of modified starch and the availability of energy for the baby. However, studies showed that modified starch is fully digested and that the glucose from this form of starch is fully available to provide energy for the infant. Both the National Academy of Sciences and the Committee on Nutrition of the American Academy of Pediatrics confirmed that modified starches are safe[17]–but there were many worried people for a few years.

New noncaloric sweeteners usually cause some safety concerns, due in part to our lack of understanding of the physiology and psychology of sweet taste. A wide variety of chemicals provide a sweet taste, including glucose, sucrose, fructose, and other carbohydrates; some proteins; and some amino acids linked together, such as the amino acids aspartic acid and phenylalanine in aspartame. (In contrast, a salty taste is easier to understand because only two chemicals are known to give a true salt sensation, sodium chloride–table salt–and lithium chloride.) Most artificial sweeteners have had either real or perceived safety problems. However, the safety of aspartame for use by normal healthy humans is endorsed by the American Medical Association, the American Diabetes Association, the American Academy of Pediatrics, and the American Dental Association. It is safe for the fetus at current levels of intake, and it does not promote tooth decay. People with *phenylketonuria (PKU)* must monitor their intake of phenylalanine, one of the two amino acids that constitute aspartame; hence a label warning is required. Look at a can of diet cola and you will see the warning "Phenylketonurics: Contains phenylalanine." Other sweeteners on the market such as acesulfame-K and the sugar alcohols are also considered safe.

Phenylketonuria (PKU): Genetic defect in which the essential amino acid phenylalanine is incompletely metabolized, causing brain damage and mental retardation. May be prevented by strict limitation of dietary phenylalanine.

These sweeteners are nonessential food additives, even though they are important to people with diabetes, who cannot sweeten food any other way. However, if all diet products were removed from the market and replaced by the calorie-bearing ones, obesity might be an even greater health problem than it is now. Balance that with the slight risk that might result from consuming the national average intake of artificial sweeteners, and you have another interesting choice to make.

Many people like the taste and the color of *caramel* that is found in many foods–baked goods, sauces, canned meats and stews, soft drinks, and alcoholic beverages. Caramel is formed when sugars or starch are heated in the presence of acid or alkali–sometimes described as burning sugar. Caramel color is the most widely used food color. Many different types of caramel are available because there are many options about ingredients and about method of manufacture. Most caramel colorants have 50% digestible carbohydrate, 25% nondigestible carbohydrate, and 25% polycyclic aromatic hydrocarbons (PAH). The PAHs are produced when organic matter is burned; this includes charcoal-grilled foods. Their threat to human health is unknown, although some reports have indicated that they are carcinogenic. No known health hazard is associated with caramel colorants.[17]

Caramel: Brown material formed by heating carbohydrates in the presence of acid or alkali.

Food Aid and Famine Relief Workers' View

These people see carbohydrate-rich foods as the most effective way to distribute relief food to starving people. This is because 1) they are easy to store and transport, 2) they are usually more readily acceptable to people than foods of animal origin, 3) they quickly correct problems caused by the deficient intake of energy, and 4) they are less expensive than protein-rich foods. But history teaches us an important lesson–we must not take for granted that starving people in other countries will have the facilities to prepare an unusual food or the inclination to eat it. This was seen in the 1840s in Ireland when a million people starved to death because of a dis-

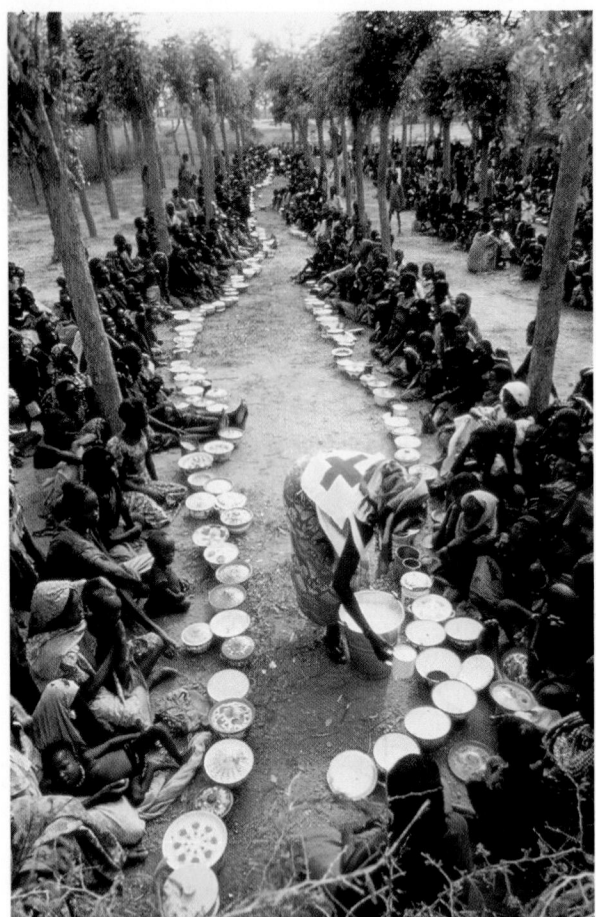

Figure 6-18. In times of food shortage, people must eat food where they find it, or be fed by relief agencies. Food aid is frequently high in carbohydrates.

ease that afflicted their main food source, the potato. Corn was one of the main relief foods in that famine. It meets all of the criteria for food aid listed above. The corn shipped into Ireland, however, was raw, hard, and unground. Such a grain needs prolonged boiling to soften it or must be milled, neither of which the typical poor households were equipped to do. Corn cooked by government agencies involved in famine relief met the food needs of only a small proportion of the population.

Economists' View

Economists regard most carbohydrate-rich foods as inexpensive and therefore suitable for extensive use in famine relief and in food assistance programs in developed countries.

Psychologists' and Behavioral Scientists' View

In spite of some claims that carbohydrates cause abnormal behavior in people, these professionals do not see carbohydrates that way. Little or no experimental evidence links sucrose or other carbohydrates with carbohydrate craving, food addiction, saccharophobia (fear of sugar), or criminal behavior.[1] In fact, researchers at the Massachusetts Institute of Technology have presented evidence that sugar has a calming effect. In their study, sugar, pasta, and bread had a sedative effect on the nervous system of human subjects. This observation is under further investigation.

Sports Physiologists', Athletic Coaches', and Athletes' View

People involved in sports understand that glycogen is the preferred storage fuel for muscles and that a diet high in carbohydrate is needed to synthesize glycogen after exhausting exercise. Many marathon runners practice carbohydrate (or glycogen) loading, which we will examine in detail in Chapter 12. Stored lipid and protein are the secondary sources of fuel for muscles.

■ People are different–Lactose content is a reason why some people cannot digest milk

Most adult people in the world have problems in digesting lactose, the disaccharide in milk. The exceptions live in central and northwestern Europe and in those parts of Africa with a long history of dairy farming. The descendants of people from these areas now living in other countries are also free of the problem. People in North America with potential problems in tolerating lactose are Native Americans, Asians, African-Americans, Hispanics, Jews, and people of Middle Eastern origin, who frequently exhibit lactose intolerance or lactase deficiency.

This intolerance occurs because the lactose molecule is too large to squeeze through the intestinal wall to move directly from the intestine into the blood. Instead, the enzyme *lactase* is secreted in the small intestine to break the linkage between the glucose and galactose units that form lactose. Both of these monosaccharides are then absorbed into the blood for transportation to the liver. Everyone is born with sufficient lactase to digest the lactose in breast milk and in cow's milk. The problem begins when the child is about five or six years of age because the initial concentration of lactase fails to increase with increasing food intake. The person may suffer from diarrhea, pain, bloating, flatulence, nausea, and sometimes vomiting. This is caused by the action of intestinal bacteria on the undigested lactose. Milk is therefore not consumed widely by teenagers and adults in populations with a high incidence of lactase deficiency because of the gastrointestinal distress they experience.

Many lactase-deficient people can tolerate modest amounts of lactose-containing foods without much difficulty–up to 250 milliliters of milk (about 1 cup). Although lactose is found only in dairy products, many other foods made with dairy products contain it also. The list in Table 6-7 shows that a wafer cookie bar, doughnuts, breakfast bars, and even the bread roll we put a hamburger into all contain at least some lactose because dairy products are part of their ingredients. Whey, which is high in lactose, is a by-product of cheese making and is used as an ingredient in some foods. People who are lactase-deficient should read food labels to see whether foods contain whey.

If you suffer from lactose intolerance or lactase deficiency, here are ways you can still keep dairy products in your diet.

Lactase: Intestinal enzyme that digests lactose by splitting it into glucose and galactose.

Table 6-7. Lactose Content of Foods

Food	Percent (grams per 100 grams of edible portion)
Pasteurized, processed cheese food, American	9.7
Ice cream, vanilla	7.4
Milk shake, vanilla	5.0
Milk	4.9
Wafer cookie bar	4.9
Chocolate drink prepared with milk	4.1
Yogurt, low-fat, plain	3.7
Sugar-coated chocolate disks	3.7
Cream	2.8
Milk, acidophilus	2.6
Doughnuts	1.8
Cheese, cream	1.7
Breakfast bar	1.0
Rolls, hamburger	0.9

- Drinking milk with a meal reduces the possibility of gastrointestinal disturbances.

- Notice above that most cheeses have less lactose than milk. Swiss and cheddar have the lowest lactose content of all cheeses.

- Yogurt is usually well tolerated by people with lactose intolerance. A half-cup serving of ice cream is usually well tolerated.

- Lactose-reduced milk is available at some supermarkets. This has about 70% less lactose than regular milk.

Protein and B-Complex Vitamins in the Wheat Kernel

Endosperm contains about
83% of the kernel
70–75 % of the protein
43% of the pantothenic acid
32% of the riboflavin
12% of the niacin
6% of the pyridoxine
3% of the thiamin

Bran contains about
14.5% of the kernel
86% of the niacin
73% of the pyridoxine
50% of the pantothenic acid
42% of the riboflavin
33% of the thiamin
19% of the protein

Germ contains about
2.5% of the kernel
64% of the thiamin
26% of the riboflavin
21% of the pyridoxine
8% of the protein
7% of the pantothenic acid
2% of the niacin

Bran: Outer layers of cereal grain; largely removed in milling to make white flour or white rice; contains fiber, vitamins, and iron.

Germ: The sprouting part of a cereal grain. In wheat, it is rich in thiamin, riboflavin, and vitamin B-6 and contains most of the fat in the grain; is separated along with the bran during milling to make white flour.

- You can add the enzyme lactase to a glass of milk. Wait a short while for the enzyme to break the lactose into glucose and galactose.

■ Nutrition in action–Milling and baking

Milling

Milling is the conversion of wheat into flour and rough or brown rice into white rice. Nutritionists are interested because parts of the grain are removed during milling, thereby reducing the nutritive value of the whole grain. The diagram in Figure 6-19 shows the parts of the wheat kernel.

Bran and *germ* are removed from the wheat kernel when it is milled to make flour for some cereal products, including white bread. These two parts of the kernel contain many important nutrients (see margin list). Since large portions of the vitamins and minerals in the bran and germ are removed during milling, certain nutrients are added back to the refined flour. This enrichment of white flour and bread was first mandated by the federal government in 1941. Millers and bakers were required by law to ensure that thiamin, riboflavin, niacin, and iron were added as part of the campaign during World War II to combat the malnutrition identified in young men enlisting in the armed forces.[18] Some people feel that it is a sad commentary on modern society that we take nutrients out of flour during milling and add them back into flour during baking. However, as a result of enrichment, many vitamin deficiencies have virtually disappeared in the United States and also in other countries.

In the past, white bread was associated with wealthy people, and whole grain or brown bread was "peasant food." Recently whole-grain bread, made from flour that still contains the bran and germ, has increased in popularity.

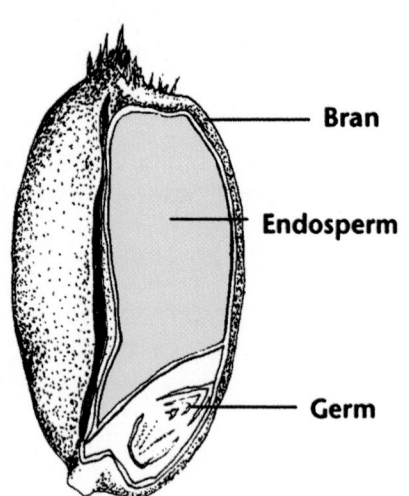

Figure 6-19. A kernel of wheat–an excellent source of nutrients.

Baking

Commercial baking provides many items in our diet–bread and rolls, cakes, cookies, and crackers. With usually only slight variations in ingredients and/or baking methods, we get many ethnic, regional, or novelty baked goods, including native flat breads and pita (pocket) bread (both originally from the Middle East), pizza dough, bagels, English muffins, doughnuts, pretzels, pies, and pastries, including croissants and "Danish" rolls. Breads from many different cultures are available.

Successful baking requires extensive scientific knowledge because each of several areas of science has an influence on the quality of the final baked product. The entire baking process requires an understanding of food science and the physical chemistry of the various nutrients. Bakers must understand carbohydrates because starch and sugar contribute to structure and flavor, fats and oils because they provide tenderness and shortness to the baked product, and proteins because they provide the structure and texture of dough and baked goods. Bakers must also understand enzymes, which break down the starch in wheat; yeasts, which form carbon dioxide; and molds and bacteria, which provide the enzymes to break down starch. In addition, bakers need to know when and how to add seven groups of ingredients important in baking–wheat flour, other flours, sugars and syrups, shortenings, eggs and egg products, dairy products and blends, and water. A close inspection of this list shows why some baked goods were among the foods already listed as containing lactose, and the presence of eggs is why cholesterol is listed for some bakery products.

Enzymes are important in baking because they improve flour quality, retard staling, improve dough, and increase efficiency in the utilization of doughs to make cookies, biscuits, and crackers. Enzymes also improve the color of the crust and the quality of high-fiber baked goods, and they reduce the phytate content in whole-grain baked goods. This last function has direct nutritional implications because phytate binds calcium, iron, and zinc in foods, making them unavailable to the body. Most of the enzymes used in baking come from fungi and bacteria–another example of how helpful bacteria are in food science and in nutrition.

Staling is the loss of freshness in bread that includes toughening of the crumb and general firming in texture, with a resulting loss of aroma and flavor. It is not necessarily re-

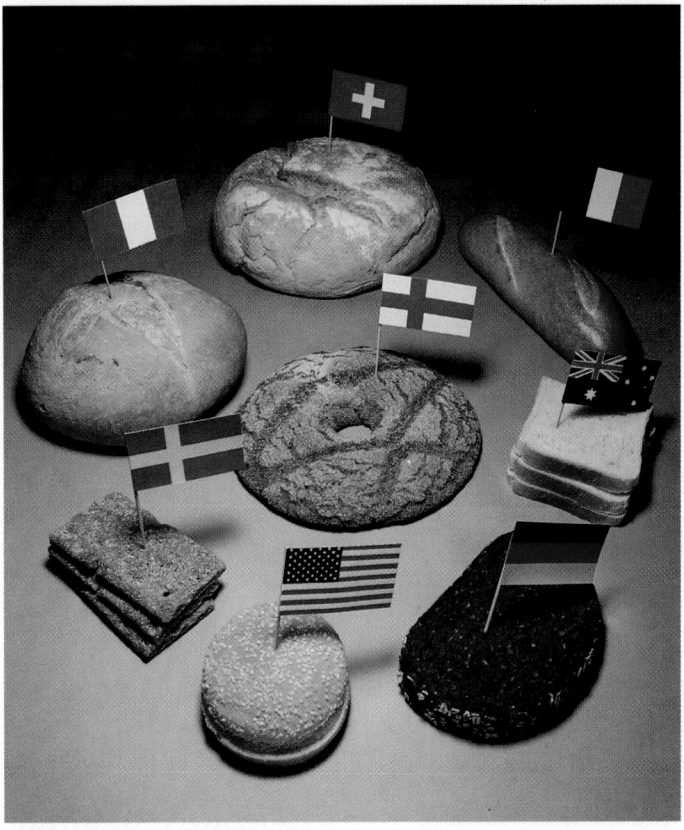

Figure 6-20. Bread takes many interesting forms around the world. In addition to these forms, you may have eaten tortillas from Mexico, pita from the Middle East, naan from India, or African sponge bread.

lated to the loss of moisture from the product. About 3–5% of all baked goods produced in the United States are lost to staling each year–this loss is valued in excess of $1 billion. The nutritional implications of this loss are significant because baked goods are nutritious foods, are acceptable to most peoples irrespective of race or religion, and are easily transported and prepared.

Ready-to-eat breakfast cereals are another form into which cereal products can be baked. Such cereals comprise a huge market and a significant source of nutrients for many people in industrialized countries. Results of a supermarket survey reveal some interesting numbers–152 different ready-to-eat breakfast cereals were found, with 32 making a statement on the front of the package that they contain fiber.[19] These figures emphasize the size of this market and its influence in nutrition. "No salt added" or "low sodium" were on 23 labels. "No added sugar" and "no preservatives" were listed 12 and 10 times, respectively. But that is not all–statements such as "all natural," "no artificial colors," "no artificial flavors," "no artificial sweeteners," "no added fat," "no cholesterol," and "naturally low in cholesterol" were used on some products. The message from this long list is clear–cereal producers go to great efforts to distance the product from some of the real or perceived villains in nutrition we have met so far: sugar, cholesterol, fat, additives, and salt. It is also an interesting example of why the new labeling laws regulating nutrition claims to the consumer are so necessary. (Of course, cereal producers are not the only food manufacturers who use their labels to make nutrition statements.)

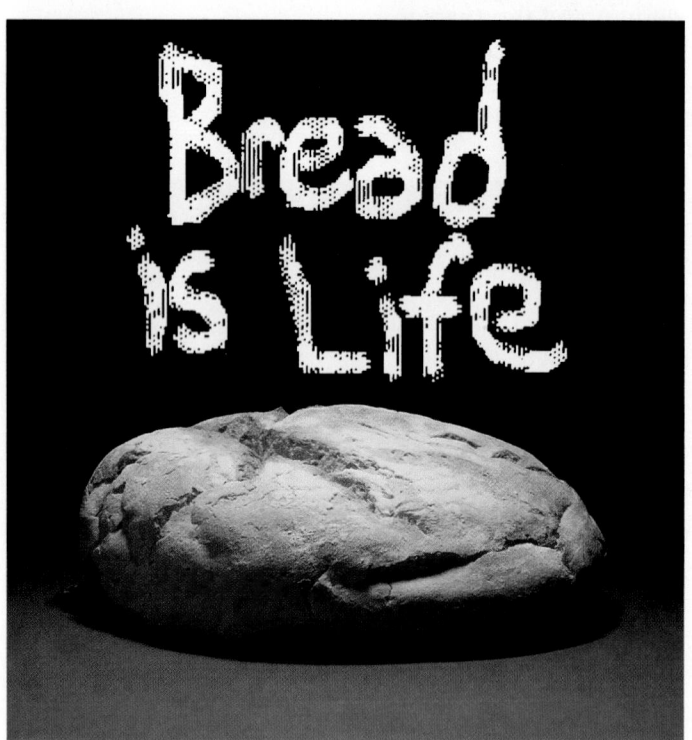

Figure 6-21. Bread, in its many forms, is the staple food for much of the world and is an important contributor of nutrients to the diet.

Finally a word about the words used to describe the cereals we have examined. What is called "corn" in the United States is called "maize" in most of the rest of the world. In other English-speaking countries "corn" refers to the most common cereal grain, or to any cereal grain. When "corn" is mentioned in the Bible, it usually means barley (which, by the way, is "korn" in Scandinavia). In England "corn" usually refers to wheat; in Scotland it usually refers to oats. With this international verbal confusion, we leave the carbohydrates and move on to the lipids.

■ Now you know

- We consume more sugar and less starch and fiber than our ancestors did.

- Carbohydrate-rich foods include bread, pasta, corn, wheat, rice, potatoes, and sugar.

- Sugar and sweeteners make food more palatable for many people.

- Sugar is a natural component of many foods.

- Carbohydrate-rich foods in moderation are no more fattening than other foods.

- Dietary fiber may help prevent colon cancer and reduce blood cholesterol.

- No scientific evidence links sugar to hyperactivity or to criminal behavior.
- Carbohydrates are classified as monosaccharides, disaccharides, and polysaccharides. Glucose, a monosaccharide, is the carbohydrate used directly by the human body. Glycogen is the storage form of glucose.
- Plants produce glucose by photosynthesis.
- Feeding cereal grains to cattle to produce meat is the basis for a substantial portion of the agricultural economy in the United States and some other countries but is seen by some environmentalists as a waste of food and a cause of pollution.
- Dietary fiber is a group term for cellulose, hemicellulose, lignin, pectin, and gums.
- Dietary fiber consists of soluble and insoluble substances not digested by enzymes in the GI tract. It reduces constipation, assists in maintaining a healthy GI tract, and may delay gastric emptying. Very high fiber intakes cause abdominal distress, bind some minerals, and may cause failure to thrive in young children.
- In diabetes, glucose that should have gone to cells is left in the blood because of insufficient insulin. The effects of diabetes can often be controlled by diet.
- Sugar is related to dental caries, especially if the sugared food is sticky.
- Nonnutritive sweeteners (aspartame, acesulfame K, and saccharin) give a sweet taste but few or no calories.
- Carbohydrates present no major toxicological problems.
- Carbohydrate-rich foods are useful in famine relief.
- No evidence shows sugar to be a cause of diabetes or coronary heart disease.
- Lactose intolerance or lactase deficiency affects primarily people of non-northern European origin. Ingestion of milk and some other dairy products can cause gastrointestinal distress.
- Milling removes some nutrients, but flour is typically enriched by the replacement of these nutrients.
- Many items in our diet are baked goods–bread and rolls, cakes, cookies, and crackers. Baking is a technology with input from many branches of science.

Further Reading

1. Robinson, J., and Ferguson, A. Food sensitivity and the nervous system: Hyperactivity, addiction and criminal behaviour. *Nutrition Research Reviews* 5:203, 1992.
2. Szepesi, B. Carbohydrates. In: *Present Knowledge in Nutrition*, 6th ed. M. Brown, editor. International Life Sciences Institute, Washington, DC, page 47, 1990.
3. Niederhauser, J. S. The role of the potato in the conquest of hunger and new strategies for international cooperation. *Food Technology* 46:(7):91, 1992.

4. Heck, W. W., and others. Air quality and the productivity of crops and forests. In: *Agriculture and the Environment: The 1991 Yearbook of Agriculture*, page 107. Superintendent of Documents, U.S. Government Printing Office, Washington, DC, 1991.

5. Sobal, J., and Cassidy, C. M. Public perceptions of fiber in foods. *Ecology of Food and Nutrition* 26:303, 1991.

6. Eastwood, M. A. The physiological effect of dietary fiber: An update. *Annual Review of Nutrition* 12:19, 1992.

7. Jones, D. J. Diverticular disease. *British Medical Journal* 304:1435, 1992.

8. Schneeman, B. Nutrition and gastrointestinal function. *Nutrition Today* 28(1):20, 1993.

9. Walker, A. R. P., and others. Fiber, phytic acid, and mineral metabolism. *Nutrition Reviews* 50:246, 1992.

10. Dinneen, S., and others. Carbohydrate metabolism in non-insulin-dependent diabetes mellitus. *New England Journal of Medicine* 327:707, 1992.

11. Anonymous. Nutritional status and dental caries. *Nutrition Reviews* 49:158, 1991.

12. Giese, J. Pasta: New twists on an old product. *Food Technology* 46(2):118, 1992.

13. Duxbury, D. D. Fiber: Form follows function. *Food Processing* 54(3):44, 1993.

14. Five papers from a symposium entitled "New Perspectives on Sucrose." *Food Technology* 47(1):130, 1993.

15. Greeley, A. Not only sugar is sweet. *FDA Consumer* 26(3):16, 1992.

16. Giese, J. H. Alternative sweeteners and bulking agents. *Food Technology* 47(1):114, 1993.

17. Jones, J. M. *Food Safety*. Eagan Press, St. Paul, MN, 1992.

18. Sebrell, W. H. A fiftieth anniversary–Cereal enrichment. *Nutrition Today* 27(1):20, 1992.

19. Reineccius, G. A. Ready-to-eat breakfast cereals. *Cereal Foods World* 35:339, 1990.

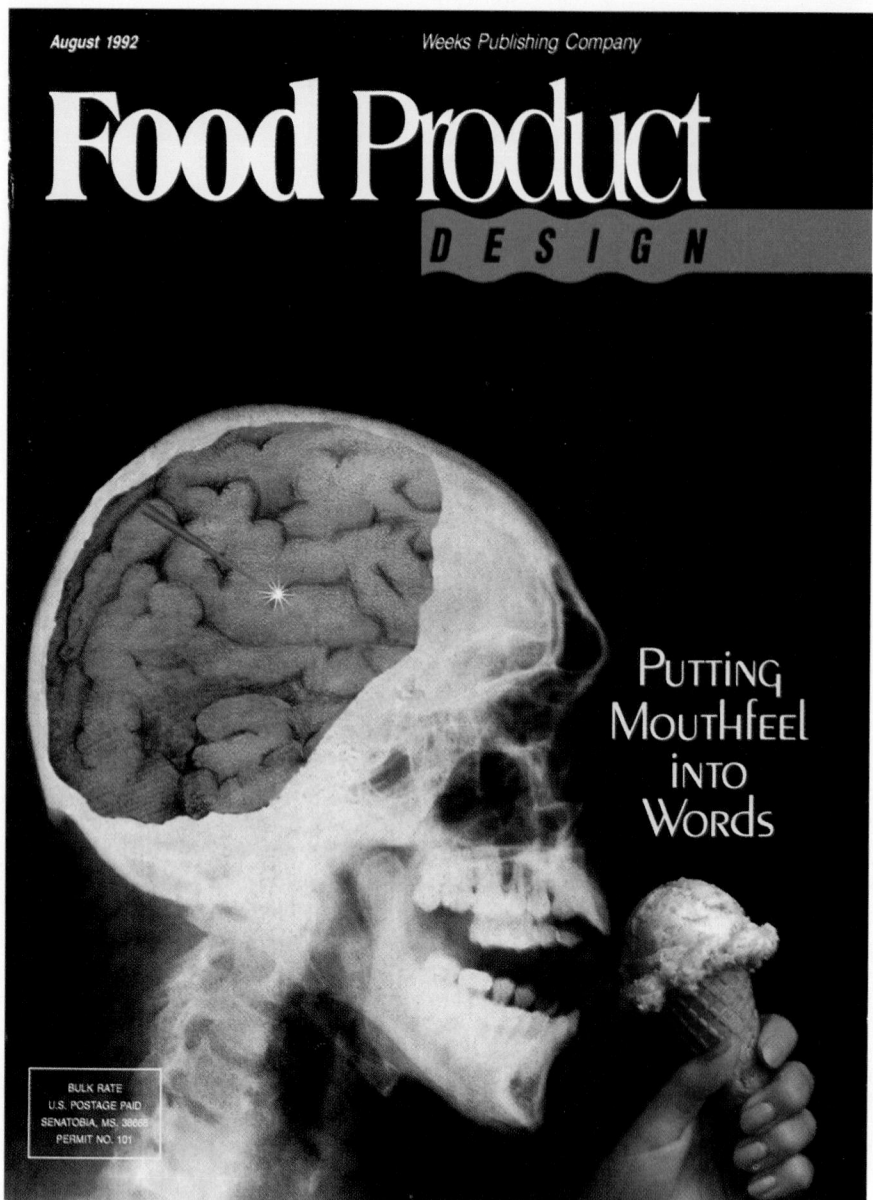

Figure 7-1. The taste and mouthfeel that we associate with ice cream result from the brain reacting to the attributes of fat in the ice cream. But new products made with fat substitutes also cause the brain to register the taste and mouthfeel of fat.

Lipids–Fats, Oils, and Fat Substitutes

■ Lipids in our lives–Essential, misunderstood, but too much may be harmful

The most important part of your sensory apparatus is your brain. It measures the taste, smell, and mouthfeel of all of the food and drink you consume. When you eat an ice cream cone, it registers the creamy mouthfeel and fatty taste of the ice cream. In recent years, food scientists, chemists, and psychobiologists have created fat substitutes that create a similar response in the brain and give the taste and mouthfeel of fat without containing the high number of calories associated with fat.

People enjoy foods containing fats (lipids) because of the sensory experiences that fat provides–it makes food flavorful, creamy, juicy, smooth, firm, tender, or rich. We need some fat in our diet, but a problem in many countries, including the United States, is that we consume too much of it.

Let's take a closer look at an ice cream cone. Assume that it is a rich vanilla, a cup of which contains about 24 grams of fat, which contribute 216 calories out of a total of about 350 calories in the ice cream. The percent calories from fat in this ice cream is thus over 60% (216 ÷ 350). It has been recommended that we consume diets with no more than 30% of calories from fat. Take a quick trip back to Chapter 4 to refresh your memory on foods high in fat.

Do people crave fatty foods, and, if so, why? These questions are receiving extensive research. We know that overweight people prefer foods high in fat and carbohydrates. This is caused by high levels of *endorphins*, which are chemicals made in the brain. They are important appetite stimulators that especially increase our liking for fatty foods. The hunt is on by drug companies for chemicals that will neutralize the effects of endorphins, thereby reducing the craving for fatty foods. Some limited success has been achieved with experimental animals given drugs such as naloxone. Much time, effort, and money is being spent in trying to get a safe drug to decrease fat intake.

Endorphins: Chemicals produced by the brain to stimulate appetite and to control pain.

Adipose tissue: Tissue in which fat is stored.

However, there is much more to fat in the body than the *adipose tissue* that many people want to get rid of. Lipids are one of the energy nutrients, without which our bodies could not function. In this chapter, we will follow the fats in foods as they are put to use by the body.

■ Lipids have many important functions in the body

The most efficient energy source in the body is fat

Animals, including humans, use fat as their main energy source because it allows them to carry their energy reserves around with them. In contrast, plants don't have the energy requirement for movement, so they store energy as carbohydrates. All of this is explained by looking at a few numbers. Fat provides two and one-quarter times more energy than the same weight of carbohydrate or of protein (nine calories per gram as contrasted with four per gram), making fat a very efficient source of energy. To get the same amount of energy as provided by fat, we would have to walk around with much more stored carbohydrate (or protein, which is a poor source of energy, as we will see in Chapter 8). Furthermore, carbohydrates stored in the body require additional water, which adds further to body weight. Fat is insoluble in water and is stored in fat droplets.

The human race could not have survived without body fat as a source of energy. The luxury and pleasure of eating ice cream and many other contemporary foods were not available down through the ages. People went hungry in periods between harvests or from one hunting season to another, and body fat reserves were broken down to provide additional energy for survival. Women normally have more body fat than men. This was good in times past because it assured a greater body reserve of energy during food shortages and famines. In this way, the gender more important for survival–the female–survived to reproduce future generations. This observation is borne out in current famines in Africa and was borne out under starvation conditions in the concentration camps in World War II, where more women than men survived. In our well-fed and leisure-loving society, this excess body fat is probably an unnecessary reserve of energy.

The lower limit for body fat in healthy adult men is about 5%. This is the amount of body fat in most world-class marathon runners. In women, menstruation and conception do not occur if body fat is below a certain amount; the exact amount is controversial because of inadequate methods of measuring body composition. Extreme body fat losses occur in severe famines and in starvation, severe illness, and situations when individuals purposely deny themselves food, either because they have eating disorders or because they are in training for an athletic event. In these cases, the body has a safety mechanism to prevent the additional energy demands of pregnancy and lactation, and it is evidently mediated by the amount of body fat. Recent evidence suggests that obese women also have difficulties with menstruation and in becoming pregnant.[1]

Cell membranes contain a number of different lipids

Membranes are the gatekeepers to cells, and lipids are an important part of membrane structure. They serve as *phospholipids* by combining with phosphorus, as *glycolipids* ("glyco" comes from the Greek word for "sweet") by combining with carbohydrates, and as cholesterol, which is a *sterol*. About half of the molecules in an average membrane are phospholipids (Figure 7-2).

Phospholipids are arranged in membranes so that the water-seeking (hydrophilic) phosphate "heads" point toward both the watery exterior and interior of the cell. The water-avoiding (hydrophobic) lipid "tails" are buried in the middle of the membrane. Why is all of this detail important to nutritionists? Nutrients must enter and waste must be excreted through the membrane. It is also the barrier that may or may not be crossed by drugs and toxins. Another reason is that membranes are rich sources of cholesterol. Membranes get much of their rigidity from cholesterol, which thereby performs the same role in animal cell structure as cellulose does in plant cell structure (see Chapter 6). Cholesterol is manufactured within the membrane, and additional amounts are brought there in the blood.

Phospholipid: A lipid substance containing phosphorus and fatty acids; lecithin is a good example.

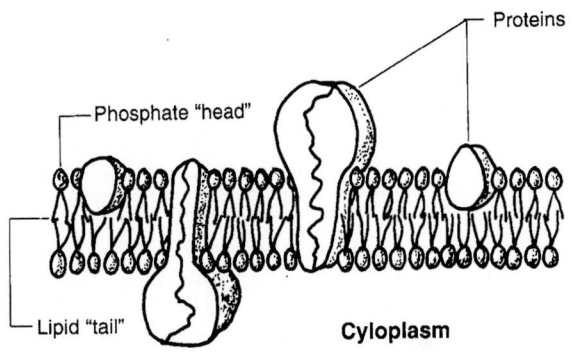

Figure 7-2. The membrane on the surface of a cell consists of a double layer of lipids interspersed with protein molecules. Membranes play many roles, including keeping the cell intact and controlling which chemicals enter and leave it.

Nerves have lipids in their structure

The brain is the processing center for messages transmitted by nerves throughout the body. The brain in the picture in Figure 7-1 is busy receiving many messages on the delights of eating ice cream. A network of nerves throughout the body allows various sensations to be collected and recorded in the brain. An important part of the nerve structure is the *myelin sheath* that surrounds nerve fibers. Important components of myelin include cholesterol, phospholipids, glycolipids, and fatty acids. Recent evidence suggests that some fatty acids are vital in the fetal development of the brain and *vascular system*.[2]

Lipids insulate the body

Body temperatures are kept within a normal range partly by the effective insulation provided by the fat layer under the skin (subcutaneous fat). This is a useful feature in cold climates but can be uncomfortable for obese people in very hot climates.

Important body organs are protected by fat

Fat provides a cushion around important organs in humans and animals–kidneys, heart, and reproductive organs.

Lipids are part of prostaglandins

Prostaglandins are called "local hormones" because they are made in the tissue in which they act. They are produced in all parts of the body and are

Glycolipid: Fatty acids combined with a carbohydrate; found mainly in the myelin sheath around nerve fibers.

Sterol: One of the group of lipids that includes vitamin D, cholesterol, and male and female sex hormones.

Myelin sheath: The covering around nerves; consists of fatty acids, cholesterol, phospholipids, and glycolipids.

Vascular system: The heart, blood vessels, lymphatic system, and their parts considered collectively.

Prostaglandins: "Local hormones" made in all tissues in the body. Involved in contraction of the uterus during labor, in the control of inflammation, and in blood pressure maintenance.

involved in the contraction of the uterus during labor, in the control of inflammation and headaches, and in blood pressure maintenance. This type of local activity makes the prostaglandins different from other hormones; insulin, for example, is secreted by the pancreas but acts on many tissues in the body.

■ Lipids in foods perform many useful functions

Dietary guidelines, the Food Guide Pyramid, and various other recommendations all emphasize restriction of dietary fat to 30% of total calories or less (Chapter 4). Foods with moderate to high fat contents are found in the following groups–baked goods, salad dressings, dairy products, meat and meat products, frozen desserts, frostings and fillings, sauces, gravies, and soups. It seems that we cannot escape eating fat in our diet. This is partly because some foods have hidden fat. We can avoid eating visible fats such as those in meats, oils, and some dairy products such as butter. However, it is usually impossible to cut off or separate the fat in baked goods, some salad dressings, frozen desserts, frostings and fillings, and sauces, gravies and soups.

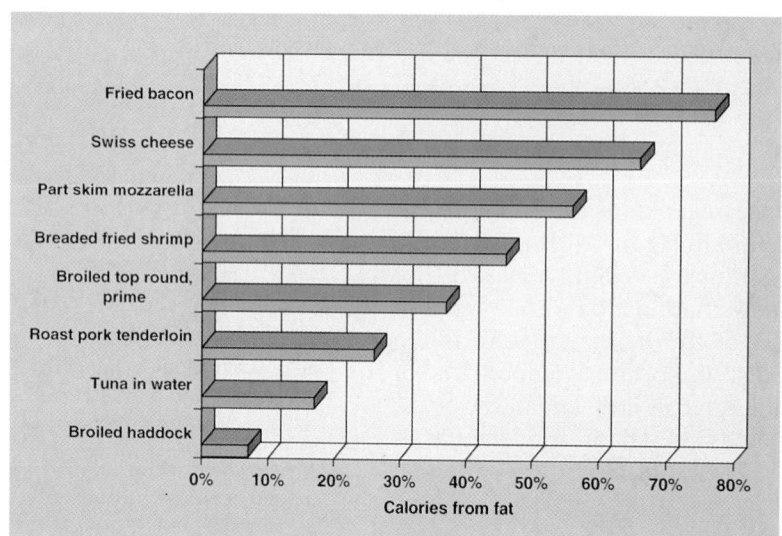

Figure 7-3. Percent calories from fat in major protein sources. Some foods high in protein are also high in fat.

Think beyond this information. Do you see some of your favorite foods in Figure 7-3?

Unfortunately, many of the major protein sources in our diet are also high in fat. In Chapter 8, we will see that people enjoy high-protein foods for a variety of reasons. Fat comes with the protein if care is not exercised in the selection and preparation of the food.

Lipids are the source of the essential fatty acids

We must have some fat in our diet to ensure the intake of the *essential fatty acids (EFAs)*. The EFAs are called essential because our bodies cannot make them; thus, it is essential that they be provided in the diet. About 40 fatty acids occurring in food and in our bodies are considered nonessential because the body can synthesize them. Linoleic acid was long considered the only EFA. It is a polyunsaturated fatty acid found in a number of plants, vegetable oils, lean pork, and eggs. Scientists now suspect that another group of polyunsaturated fatty acids is essential also. This includes alpha-linolenic acid, found in most vegetable oils, and its more polyunsaturated "cousin," docosahexaenoic acid, found in seafood.[3] A varied diet with plenty of plant foods should provide sufficient amounts of EFAs to avoid deficiency symptoms.

Essential fatty acids (EFAs): Fatty acids that are not synthesized in the body and must be provided in the diet to maintain health. These are linoleic acid, alpha-linolenic acid, and docosahexaenoic acid.

Dietary lipids are a source of energy

Lipids contain two and one-quarter times more energy than either carbohydrates or proteins. This makes them a concentrated energy source. It also may cause health problems if people do not exercise enough to burn off the additional calories consumed in the diet. Extra fat accumulates in the body, causing overweight and obesity.

In Chapter 4, we examined some foods high in fat. Here we look at an important set of numbers–the amount of fat and the percentage of total calories coming from fat in a number of fast foods.

Notice in Table 7-1 how some foods with the same *number of calories* from fat have significantly different values when fat is expressed as a *percentage of total calories*. For example, a burrito, an apple turnover, fried chicken, and french fries all have 126 calories from fat. But the burrito and the turnover both have 33% of total calories coming from fat, whereas the percent calories from fat is 53% for the fried chicken and 49% for the French fries.

Fat-soluble vitamins are carried by lipids

The fat-soluble vitamins–A, D, E, and K–are carried by lipids in plant and animal foods. The body needs fats in order to absorb these vitamins, which are stored with the fat in the body.

Palatability of food is increased by lipids

Taste, aroma, and texture or juiciness are covered by the term "palatability." Most of us love what fat does to our food, so we find it difficult to follow dietary recommendations to reduce fat intake. It is fat that gives meat most of its juiciness. Regular hamburger has about 30% fat. Meat with 5% fat is available and may be healthier, but it lacks juiciness and taste. Fat has a great ability to absorb fat-soluble flavors–pure fat itself is almost tasteless.

Table 7-1. Fat in Traditional Fast Foods

Fast Food Item	Calories from Fat	Fat as Percent of Total Calories
Bacon cheeseburger	252	55
Fish sandwich	243	50
Cheeseburger	135	42
Burrito	126	33
Fried chicken, 3 ounces	126	53
French fries	126	49
Turnover, apple	126	33
Pizza, pepperoni, one slice	108	35
Hamburger	99	35
Taco	90	52
Pizza, cheese, one slice	81	28
Chili, 1 cup	81	35
Shake, vanilla, 10 ounces	72	17

Lipids increase the satiety value of a meal

Lipids increase satiety, the full feeling after eating. Movement through the GI tract is slower for lipids than for carbohydrates or proteins, which is why some good weight-reducing diets do include fat. This may seem odd, because of the higher caloric content of fat, but another factor is at work here–a full-feeling stomach may help people to reduce their food intake. However, athletes are advised to monitor their fat intake before an event, because performance is usually sluggish when the stomach is still full of food.

■ Lipids as studied by different professions

The many functions of lipids (fats, oils, and waxes) in the human body and in food are studied by various professionals.

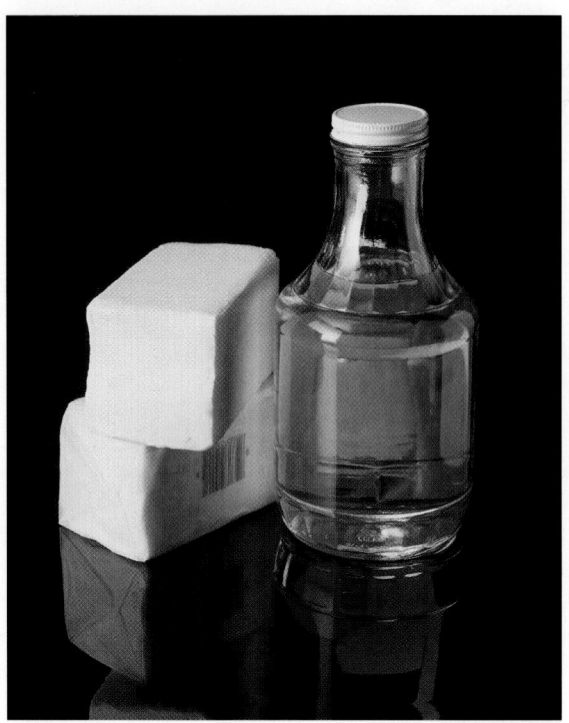

Figure 7-4. Dietary lipids are mainly in the form of fats and oils.

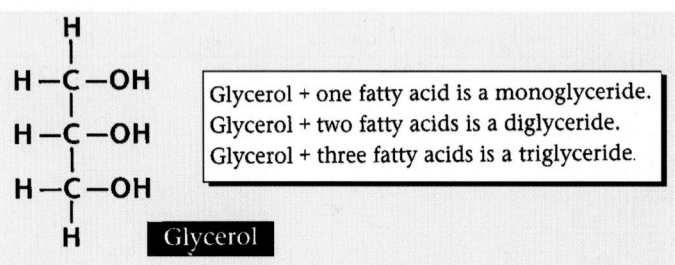

Glycerol + one fatty acid is a monoglyceride.
Glycerol + two fatty acids is a diglyceride.
Glycerol + three fatty acids is a triglyceride.

Glycerol

Figure 7-5. The chemical structure of a glycerol molecule, made up of atoms of carbon, hydrogen, and oxygen. When glycerol is combined with one, two, or three fatty acids, it forms a mono-, di-, or triglyceride, respectively.

Coronary heart disease (CHD): The most common type of heart disease, caused by narrowing of the arteries that feed the heart.

Chemists and Biochemists

Chemists and biochemists provide information important to nutritionists on the chemical structures of different fats and oils. Lipids are made up of carbon, hydrogen, and oxygen atoms that have combined to form fatty acids. Over 40 different fatty acids are found in nature. Sometimes they are free, but usually they are combined with the organic alcohol glycerol, forming a large number of different combinations in our bodies and in food (Figure 7-5).

Nutritionists are most interested in triglycerides because over 90% of the lipids in food and in the human body are triglycerides. (When we mention fat in food or in the body, we are mostly talking about triglycerides.) Serum (blood) triglyceride levels are good indicators of the amount of fat in the blood. In some research, positive correlations were noted between high levels of serum triglycerides and *coronary heart disease (CHD)*. We will review this after we look at the structure of fatty acids.

Fatty acid molecules consist of chains of carbon atoms of varying lengths having an acidic group (–COOH) at the end of the molecule. Hydrogen atoms are bound to the carbons along the chain. Chemists refer to short-, medium-, and long-chain fatty acids. Short-chain fatty acids are of little interest to nutritionists except that butyric acid (with four carbon atoms) is in high concentration in butter. Medium-chain fatty acids contain 8–12 carbon atoms and account for 10% of the lipid in our food. The most abundant fatty acids, and the ones most important in nutrition, are long-chain fatty acids consisting of 14, 16, 18, and 20 carbon atoms.

Stearic acid (Figure 7-6) is an 18-carbon fatty acid present in most animal and vegetable fats in triglyceride form. It is a saturated fatty acid, which means that all carbons are saturated with hydrogen and no more hydrogen can be added to the molecule.

If you remove two hydrogens from a fatty acid, a monounsaturated fatty acid is obtained. Figure 7-7 shows the structure of oleic acid, an 18-carbon monounsaturated fatty acid found in most triglycerides. It is by far the most plentiful of the unsaturated fatty acids and is in high concentrations in these fats:

Human fat	Margarine	Peanuts
Avocados	Almonds	Lard
Olive oil	Cooking oils (especially canola oil)	

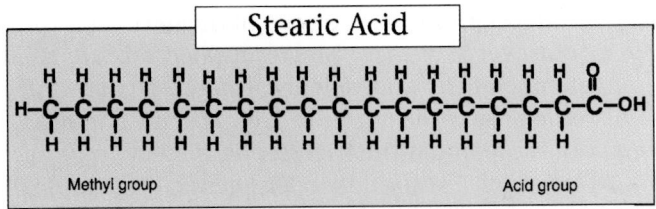

Figure 7-6. Stearic acid is a long-chain saturated fatty acid that is present in most animal and vegetable fats in the triglyceride form.

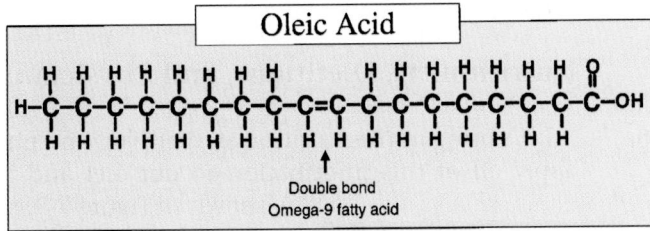

Figure 7-7. Oleic acid is a long-chain, monounsaturated fatty acid (it has one double bond between two carbon atoms).

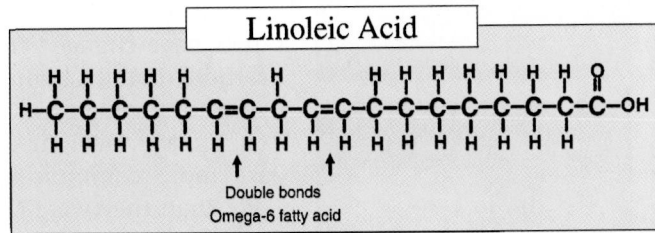

Figure 7-8. Linoleic acid is a long-chain polyunsaturated fatty acid that is essential in the diet. It has two double bonds between carbon atoms.

Removal of at least two more hydrogen atoms produces a polyunsaturated fatty acid. An example (Figure 7-8) is the 18-carbon linoleic acid, mentioned earlier as an essential fatty acid, which is found in triglycerides of:

Safflower oil	Peanut oil	Sunflower oil
Soybean oil	Walnuts	Cottonseed oil
Sesame oil	Soft margarine	

The omega-3 (or ω-3) fatty acids are polyunsaturated acids that have been much in the news lately because they may be beneficial against CHD and other illnesses.[4] An important omega-3 polyunsaturated fatty acid with 18 carbon atoms and three double bonds is alpha-linolenic acid, which was mentioned above as a newly designated essential fatty acid. It is present in high amounts in the triglycerides of plant seed oils and to a lesser extent in leafy vegetables and animal fats. Another omega-3 fatty acid is docosahexaenoic acid, found mainly in lipids in fish.

Good sources of linoleic acid, an essential fatty acid:

- Whole wheat
- Corn
- Soybeans
- Peanuts
- Avocado
- Pork (lean only)
- Egg

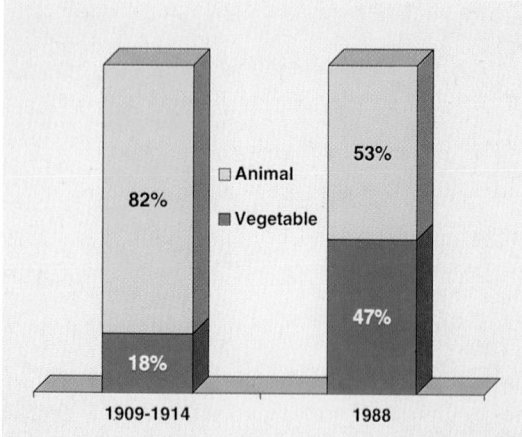

Figure 7-9. Types of fat in the U.S. food supply in the early and late 20th century.

A few physical properties of the fatty acids can be seen in our everyday lives. Most saturated fats are solid at room temperature, and polyunsaturated fats are soft or liquid. The greater the degree of fatty acid unsaturation, the softer or more liquid the triglyceride is likely to be at room temperature. Exceptions to this general rule are palm oil and coconut oil, which are highly saturated yet soft at room temperature. Take beef from the refrigerator and squeeze some of the fat between your fingers–it is fairly solid. Squeeze fish fat, and you will find it squishy because it is higher in unsaturated fatty acids.

Nutritionists, Dietitians, and Physicians

Let's bring in the nutritionist, dietitian, and physician to apply all of this information to our diet and health. As shown in Figure 7-9, the typical diet in the United States has changed considerably in its sources of fat since the early 1900s.[5] These changes have occurred in many countries as diets have changed from high-carbohydrate to high-fat foods. Some of the high-protein, high-fat foods shown in Figure 7-3 are more common in today's diet than they were at the turn of the last century.

The most recent values for fat intake can be further subdivided by degree of unsaturation (Figure 7-10).

Notice in Figure 7-10 how foods from animals provide about 60% of the saturated fat in our diet. This includes fat from meat, poultry, fish, and dairy products. More than 40% of the monounsaturated fatty acids come from meats and dairy products, but fats and oils are the single largest contribu-

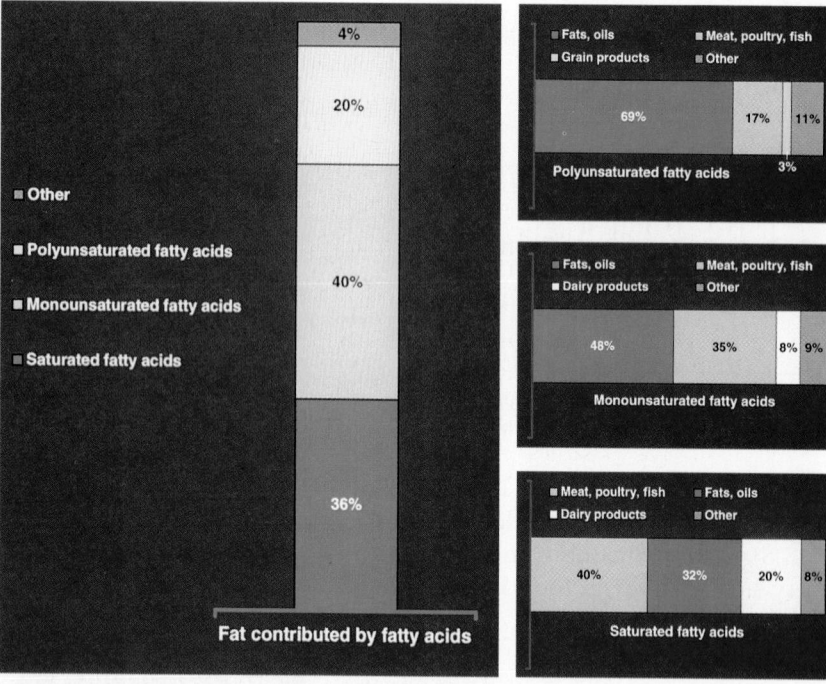

Figure 7-10. Fat contributed by different kinds of fatty acids in the U.S. food supply (left) and the sources of polyunsaturated, monounsaturated, and saturated fatty acids (right). Note that plant foods provide most of the polyunsaturated fatty acids and foods of animal origin provide most of the saturated ones.

tor in this group. Vegetable oils provide by far the greatest amount of polyunsaturated fatty acids, as the manufacturers of vegetable cooking oils and margarine are constantly reminding us. Notice the small amount of polyunsaturated fatty acids in meats, with none listed for dairy products. At first glance this may seem odd because the plant diet of farm animals is high in unsaturated fat. However, these ruminant animals have bacteria in their GI tracts and their own enzyme systems to convert mono- and polyunsaturated fatty acids into the saturated form. This process of *hydrogenation*, whereby hydrogen atoms are added at the double bonds, increases the degree of saturation and thereby the hardness of the fat. Food scientists use this process industrially to harden fats for different foods. On a package of margarine, the phrase "partially hydrogenated" comes before the name of one or more ingredients. We will see later the practical and health consequences of hydrogenation.

Fats and oils from common plants and animals vary considerably in their fatty acid composition. We will refer to Figure 7-11 again as we see how different professions use information about lipids and their constituent fatty acids.

Cholesterol is also a lipid, although it has a chemical structure (Figure 7-12) totally different from those of the fatty acids. It is perhaps the best known of the lipids because of many reports linking high levels of cholesterol in the diet and in blood with CHD. Cholesterol is found only in foods of animal origin.

Since cholesterol has such a negative image in advertisements and labels ("no cholesterol," "cholesterol-free," and "low cholesterol"), many people are surprised to learn that the liver and intestines synthesize about 75% of the cholesterol in the human body. We need cholesterol to give rigidity to membranes and to synthesize vitamin D in the body. It is an important component of bile acids and is involved in

Hydrogenation: Treatment of liquid oils with hydrogen to saturate some double bonds in the fatty acid chains, which increases the melting point and hardens the fat. Cottonseed, corn, and sunflower are among the oils commonly hydrogenated for use in margarine and cooking fats.

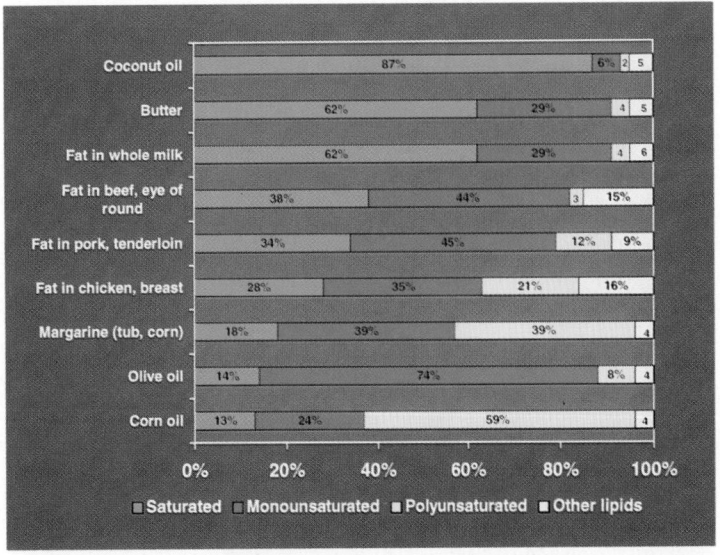

Figure 7-11. Types of fatty acids in various foods. Notice that foods from animals are usually the highest in saturated fatty acids. However, coconut oil also has a high content of these fatty acids. Saturated fatty acids may increase blood cholesterol levels in some people.

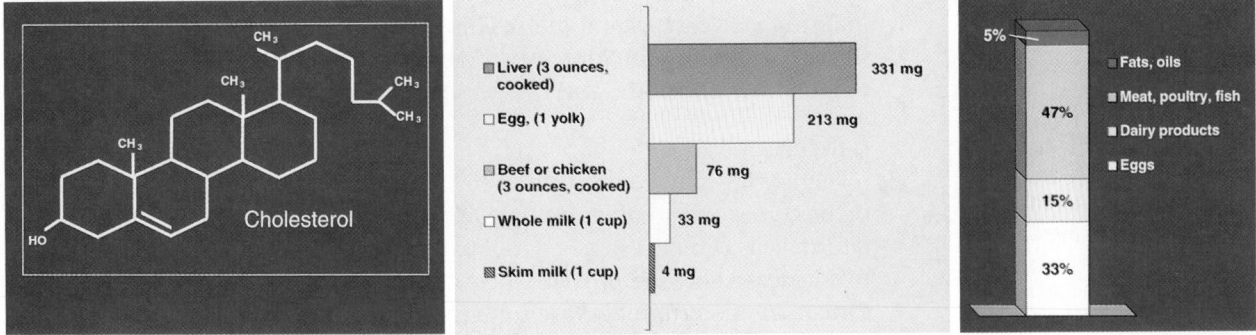

Figure 7-12. Left, the chemical structure of cholesterol is different from that of other lipids. Each of the hexagon-shaped rings has carbon atoms at each of the points. (The carbons are not shown here for simplicity's sake.) Middle, cholesterol is found in varying amounts in different foods. Right, sources of cholesterol in the U.S. food supply. Note that cholesterol in the diet comes from foods of animal origin only.

the synthesis of the steroid hormones, including the female and male sex hormones.

The work of chemists and biochemists contributes greatly to our understanding of the role of lipids in health and disease. These scientists studied proteins combined with lipids (lipoproteins) and determined their structure. Nutritionists and medical doctors took this chemical information and found that high levels of lipoproteins in blood may be deposited in major blood vessels, resulting in CHD.[6] But lipids are of great interest for other health reasons also,[4] as suggested by the photo in Figure 7-13.

Think beyond the picture. Is fat a tornado destructive to our health?

The answer should be familiar by now–it depends on the amount and type of fat consumed. What follows is a brief review showing that fatty acids can have both positive and negative effects on health problems–positive in terms of lowering blood pressure, inflammation, and infection and of assisting the immune system–and negative because there seems to be an association between certain dietary fats and some cancers, kidney disease, non-insulin-dependent diabetes, obesity, and CHD.

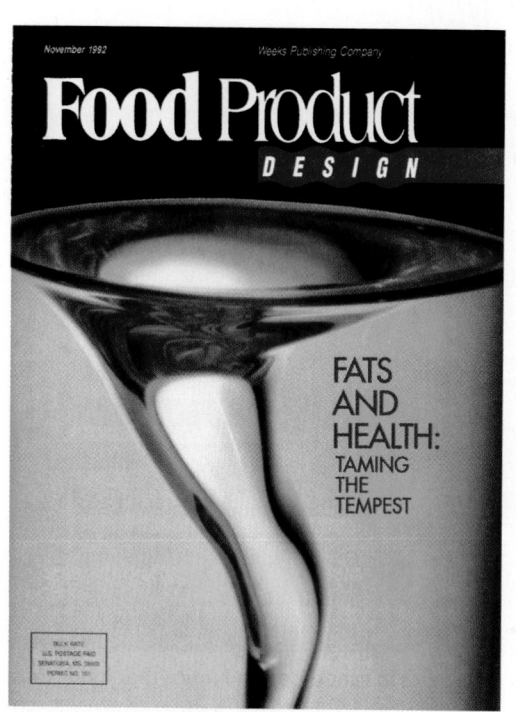

Figure 7-13. This journal for people who develop food products used a "tornado" to introduce its issue on fats.

Blood pressure

Blood pressure may be lowered by polyunsaturated fatty acids. Linoleic acid decreases *systolic and diastolic blood pressure* in males and females with mild-to-moderate hypertension (high blood pressure). The amount needed to achieve this is 6–10% of total caloric intake. This is considerably higher than the usual intake of 5% or the minimum level of 1% of total calories from linoleic acid, below which deficiencies of linoleic acid occur.

Obesity

Obesity develops and/or is maintained in some people consuming high-fat diets. The emphasis must be on the words "some people" because other people can achieve weight maintenance on high-fat diets. This suggests that a complex interrelationship exists among the sensory properties of fat, the metabolic effectiveness of fat within the body, and the genetic background of the person.[4]

Cancer

Dietary fat may be a causal agent in several kinds of cancer.[4] This statement comes from epidemiologic, clinical, and experimental studies. High fat intake is thought to be related to cancer of the colon, the pancreas, and to a lesser extent the prostate. Relationships between fat intake and breast cancer are uncertain and are undergoing further investigation. Such studies are complicated because of the many other variables in the diet that may be related to cancer, including overall caloric intake and energy expenditure.

Systolic and diastolic blood pressure: The pressure existing in the large arteries at the height of the pulse wave. High blood pressure exists when persistent systolic and diastolic blood pressures are above 140 and 100 millimeters of mercury, respectively. Blood pressure reports give systolic pressure as the top number and diastolic pressure as the bottom number.

Diabetes and kidney disease

Non-insulin-dependent diabetes and kidney disease may be related to high dietary fat intakes. Non-insulin-dependent diabetes occurs more frequently in obese than in nonobese people.[4]

Non-insulin-dependent diabetes: A disorder in which adequate amounts of insulin are produced by the pancreas but the insulin is not used normally.

Infections and immunity

Infections are increased and immunity decreased when diets are deficient in essential fatty acids. However, high concentrations of fat also tend to suppress immune functions. Marine fish oils may be protective against infections as well as inflammation in some tissues.[7] Fatty acids are thought to act on the immune system by altering cell membrane structure and function and by changing fatty acid metabolism. Much more remains to be learned in this area.

Coronary heart disease

Cholesterol and the amount and type of fat are among several risk factors in CHD. The other risk factors (cigarette smoking, high blood pressure, diabetes, obesity, being male, and having a family history of CHD before age 55) will be examined in detail in Chapter 14.

Lowering high blood cholesterol levels reduces the risk of CHD by slowing the rate of buildup of fatty deposits in the walls of arteries.

Some studies show that, for adults with high blood cholesterol levels, each 1% reduction in total cholesterol level results in a 2% reduction in the number of heart attacks.[8] This means that if the population in general, and especially men with risk factors for heart disease, reduced serum cholesterol levels by 15%, CHD risk would decrease by 30%. According to the American Society for Clinical Nutrition, results of studies such as these indicate that the incidence of CHD will be substantially reduced if blood choresterol levels are reduced by diet or, if necessary, by drugs.

Given the importance of these findings, let's examine the factors influencing your blood cholesterol levels.

- **Diet** has the largest effect on blood cholesterol level among the factors you can control. Saturated fat increases blood cholesterol more than anything else you eat. Dietary cholesterol has a lesser effect, produced through different physiological mechanisms.[9] Changing to a low-fat, low-choles-

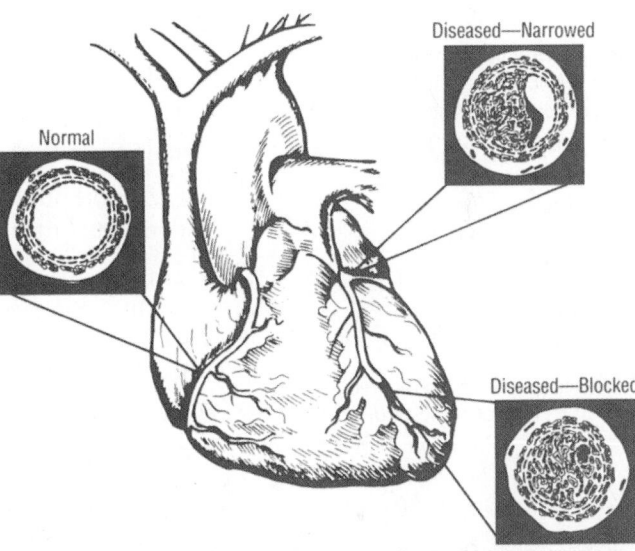

Figure 7-14. Front view of the heart, showing cross sections of the arteries. Cholesterol becomes part of a fatty deposit called plaque that blocks the arteries, thus producing coronary heart disease (CHD).

Table 7-2. Factors That Increase the Risk of Developing Coronary Heart Disease (CHD)[a]

Controllable	Uncontrollable
High blood pressure	Gender
High blood cholesterol	Heredity (family history of CHD)
Smoking	Age
Obesity	
Physical inactivity	
Diabetes	
Stress[b]	

[a] These are not all of the causes of CHD. Even with none of these risk factors, a person might still develop the disease.
[b] Scientists still do not know exactly how stress is involved in heart disease.

Foods high in saturated fat include:

Some cuts of:	Butter
Beef	Milk and cream
Lamb	Cheese
Pork	Lard
Chocolate	Palm oil
Peanut butter	Coconut oil

High-density lipoprotein (HDL): A lipoprotein with a high protein content; considered the "good" type of cholesterol.

Lipoprotein (a): A genetic variant of low-density lipoprotein (LDL).

Low-density lipoprotein (LDL): A lipoprotein with a high cholesterol content; considered the "bad" type of cholesterol.

terol diet is the best way to control blood cholesterol. Drugs can be used under medical supervision but may have troubling side effects.

- **Body weight** has an influence on serum cholesterol levels;[10] most overweight people can reduce cholesterol levels by losing body weight.

- **Physical activity and exercise** help control body weight, lower blood pressure, and may increase the level of *high-density lipoprotein (HDL)*, the "good" type of cholesterol.

- **Genetic factors** are important because of an inherited tendency for high blood cholesterol levels in some people. If this is the case in your family, then your parents, children, brothers, and sisters should have their blood cholesterol levels checked.[8] Researchers are beginning to use gene therapy to control inherited high blood cholesterol levels.

New genes delivered to her liver have significantly lowered the life-threatening cholesterol levels of a 29-year-old Canadian woman

says a report published in the *Journal of the American Medical Association*. The report continues:

. . . the woman has severe familial hypercholesterolemia, the rare disease in which the liver lacks the receptor for low-density-lipoprotein (LDL) and is therefore incapable of clearing the "bad" form of cholesterol from her blood.[11]

New evidence also suggests that a high blood level of *lipoprotein (a)*, a genetic variant of *low-density lipoprotein (LDL)* (the "bad" cholesterol), is another risk factor in coronary heart disease.[12]

- **Gender/age** is an important factor influencing blood cholesterol levels, as seen in Figure 7-15. CHD is the leading cause of death and disability for both men and women in the United States.[8] About one out of five men and one out of 17 women will have symptoms of heart disease before the age of 60. Blood cholesterol levels begin to rise at age 20. An important change occurs in women after the menopause–blood cholesterol levels rise to a level higher than in men. Oral contraceptives and pregnancy increase blood cholesterol in some women. These elevated levels should return to normal within 20 weeks after the birth of the child.

- **Alcohol** in moderate amounts has a positive influence on blood cholesterol by increasing HDL cholesterol. Media publicity about the "French paradox" attracted attention to the argument that the French people on average eat a diet high in fat, including saturated fat–plenty of butter, cheese, and meats–which they wash down with generous amounts of red wine. Yet the French have lower rates of CHD than do North Americans. Researchers at the University of California, Davis may have an answer.[13] Alcohol content may not be the sole

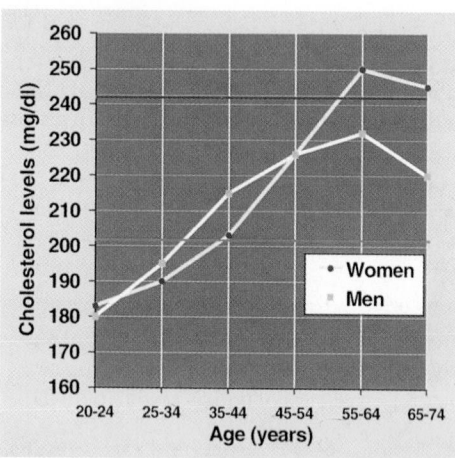

Figure 7-15. Mean total cholesterol levels of men and women. Your blood cholesterol level increases as you age, regardless of the diet you consume. Levels above the red line are dangerous. Note that women after menopause have higher blood cholesterol levels than do men of the same age.

explanation; *phenolic compounds* in the wine may inhibit the oxidation of LDL. This puts them in the class called antioxidants, which are of increasing importance in nutrition, food science, and food safety. Accordingly, we will return to antioxidants in more detail later.

- **Stress** is reported to raise blood cholesterol levels, but other associated factors may be responsible. In times of stress, people may eat more foods that are high in saturated fat and cholesterol.[4] Cholesterol reductions can be achieved by modest increases in meal frequency without an increase in caloric intake.[14] Stressed-out people should take time out more often to eat smaller amounts of food as snacks.

Phenolic compounds: Compounds combined with phenol, which is a relative of benzene.

Terms such as HDL and LDL, which arose in the discussions above, are summarized in Figures 7-16 and 7-17.

Farmers and Plant and Animal Scientists

These people have a significant impact on the amount and type of fat in our foods.

The fat content of meat-producing animals has decreased significantly over the years (Figure 7-18). Much of this change was brought about by genetic selection of animals for more muscle (lean) and less fat. The fat and cholesterol content and the fatty acid profile of meat are influenced by a wide range of inputs on the farm and in the kitchen. On the farm these include species, age, gender, breed, body type, nutrition, and management (whether range-fed or feedlot-fed), while in the kitchen the method of cooking the meat may change the fat content considerably. The amount and type of fat in milk is more difficult to change genetically. If changes can be made, they will probably come through biotechnology.

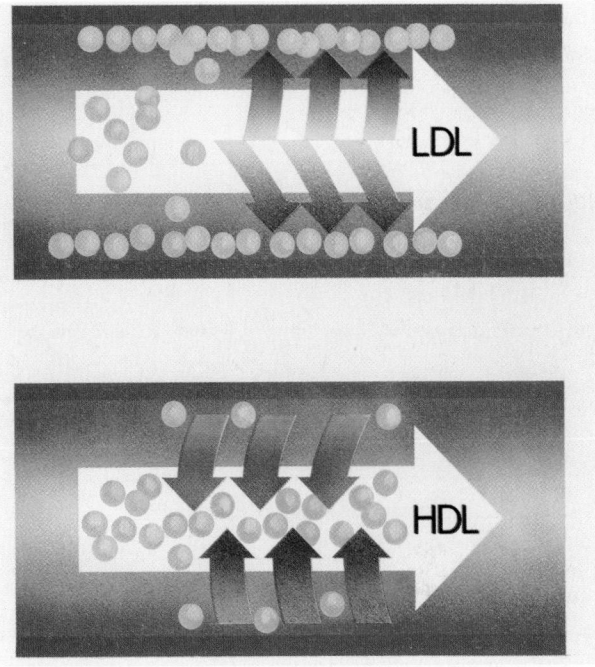

Figure 7-16. Low-density lipoprotein (LDL) delivers cholesterol to the arteries. High-density lipoprotein (HDL) delivers cholesterol to the liver, where it is metabolized.

Plant scientists can genetically engineer oil-producing plants to change the amount and the type of unsaturated fatty acids.[15] Plants have multiple genes for fatty acid synthesis and so can be manipulated easily to improve the plant's nutritional quality. All of this information is translated by the farmer into decisions about which oil-producing plants are most profitable to grow. Oilseeds, especially canola, soy, safflower, and sunflower, meet consumer health demands for plant oils with low saturated fat. To the plant geneticists and food technologists goes the credit for the incorporation of canola and sunflower oil into many foods. Rapeseed was the predecessor crop to canola. It was high in a toxic fatty acid called erucic acid, which caused damage to heart muscle. Through genetic selection, the erucic acid was essentially removed, producing canola, from which a safe oil is extracted. Higher concentrations of oleic acid (Figure 7-7) were bred into

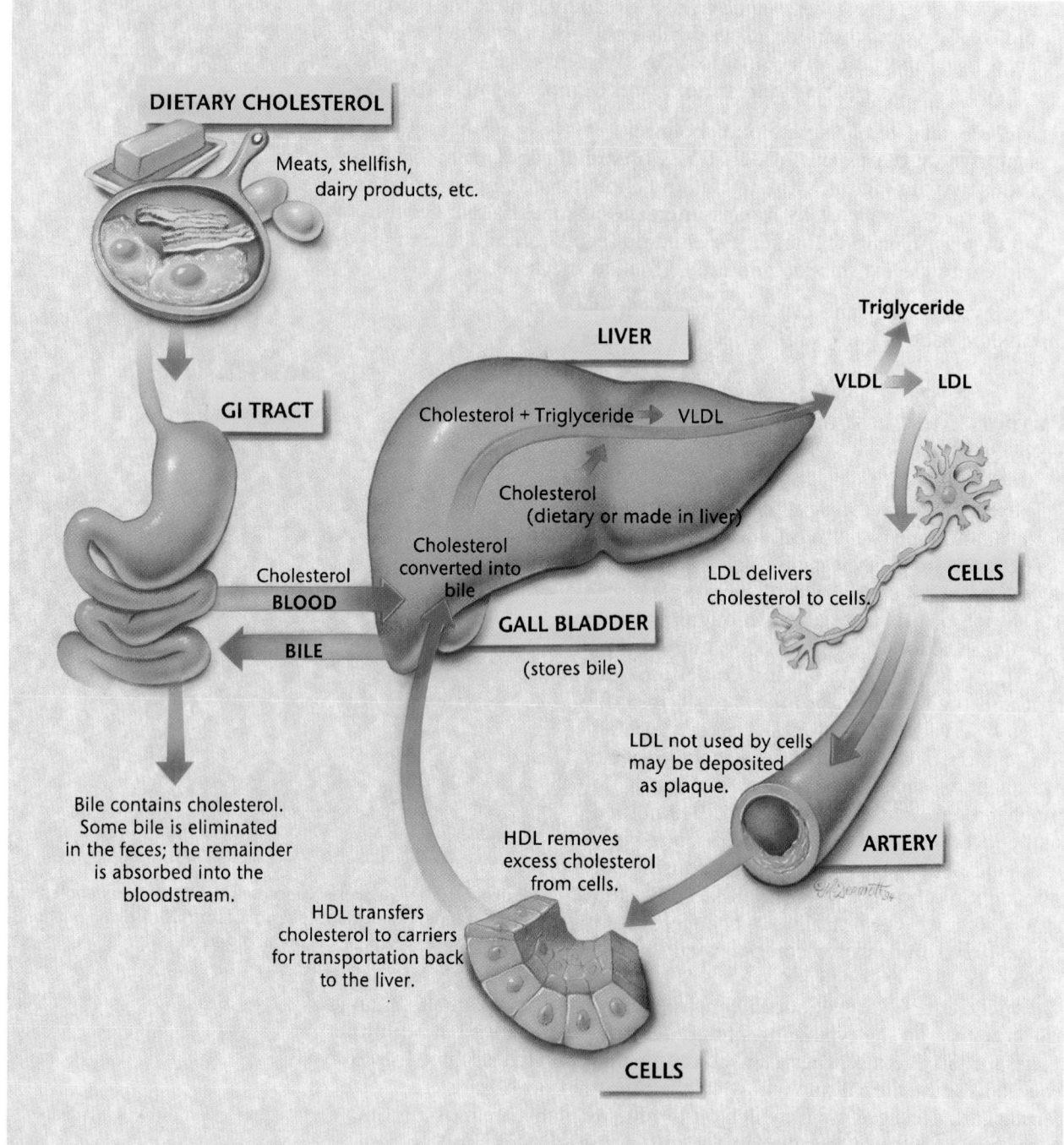

Figure 7-17. The travels of low-density lipoprotein (LDL) and high-density lipoprotein (HDL). Some cholesterol in the body comes from the diet, passing through the GI tract and into the blood, where it goes to the liver. Other cholesterol is manufactured in the liver. Together with triglyceride, the cholesterol forms very-low-density lipoprotein (VLDL). In the blood stream, the triglyceride is separated off, leaving LDL, which carries cholesterol to the cells. As it passes through the arteries, some of the LDL is deposited on the cell walls and builds up as plaque, which inhibits the flow of blood. The HDL removes excess cholesterol from the cells and facilitates its transfer back to the liver, where it is converted to bile. The bile may be stored in the gall bladder or may return to the GI tract, where some of it is eliminated in the feces, thus removing cholesterol from the body. This diagram shows why HDL is considered the "good" cholesterol and LDL the "bad" cholesterol.

sunflower seeds, which allows sunflower seed oil to withstand higher cooking temperatures.

Environmentalists

Some environmentalists consider most animal production a misuse of food, especially corn, and a cause of harm to the environment. Among the arguments presented is that the conversion of corn into body fat in meat animals is wasted effort. This fat is usually trimmed from meat before consumption. The *Wall Street Journal* took this line of reasoning a step further a few years ago by reporting a description of the environmental consequences of human obesity that was made by scientists at the University of Illinois:

> . . . if the 110 million adult Americans who are overweight would slim down and stay slim, the energy that would be saved in planting, cultivating, harvesting, processing, transporting, selling, storing, and cooking the food that now keeps them plump would more than supply the annual residential electrical requirements of Chicago, Boston, San Francisco and Washington.

Excess fat in the body or fat trimmed and discarded from meat is a waste with environmental impact. This fact should be balanced against the nutritional importance of appropriate amounts of meat in the diet and against the economic and political impact of farmers and meat processors on local and national economies.

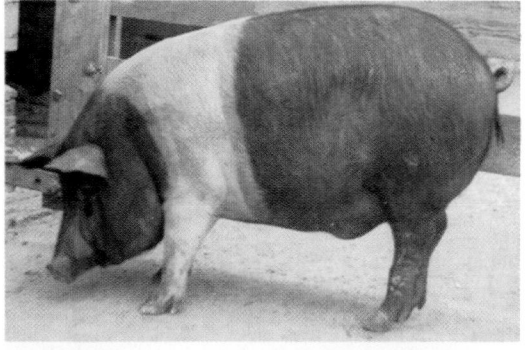

1940'S HOG

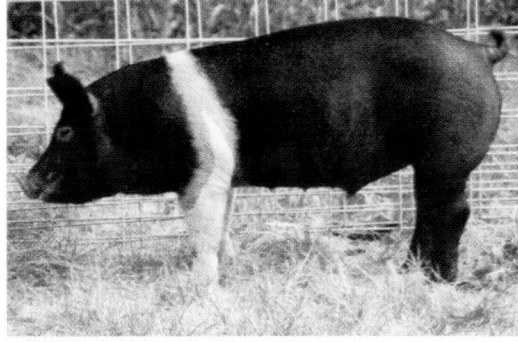

1990'S HOG

Figure 7-18. Genetic selection has played a big part in producing pigs with less fat than pigs had 50 years ago.

Food Service Managers and Chefs

These people have a difficult time responding both to dietary recommendations and consumer demands. Governmental and health professionals recommended reductions in total fat intake, so food service managers responded with low-fat menu options. But, some consumers seem to be tiring of these options and are buying high-fat items in increasing quantities. "Fast-food restaurants have gone off their diet" is how an article in the *Wall Street Journal* (August 23, 1993) introduces this latest trend. It continues,

> while burger joints still cater to the health-conscious with salads and a few other lean selections like baked potatoes, their menus are increasingly filled with grease-laden sandwiches.

Low-fat eating options are still available. A report published by the American Dietetic Association gives some good advice for consumers of various traditional ethnic foods. Here are some of the main points.[16]

Miso: A food paste originally made in Japan by fermenting moldy rice with soybeans and salt.

- **Japanese dining** presenting traditional foods offers many low-fat selections. Many low-fat dishes feature vegetables and small portions of chicken, seafood, and beef. Lean ingredients are used to make glazes and sauces. Tempura foods should be avoided or eaten sparingly because they are battered and fried.

   Low-fat choices include *miso* and bean soups, most combinations of grilled meats and seafood, teriyaki chicken, sukiyaki, udon (noodles), steamed rice, and rice noodles.

- **Indian dining** is mainly vegetarian because of the influence of Hinduism, the major religion in India. Dishes usually consist of plenty of spicy vegetables, brown rice, and low-fat sauces made with yogurt. Chicken is the favorite meat. Some dishes have coconut milk or cream, which is high in saturated fatty acids, and *ghee*, which is a type of butter fat used in India.

Ghee: Clarified butter fat made by heating and separating the water; made from milk of cow, buffalo, goat, or sheep; does not become rancid as rapidly as butter; popular in India.

   Low-fat choices include lentil and chickpea curries, chicken and vegetables, basmati rice, raita (cucumber and yogurt sauce), naan (baked unleavened bread), and fruit and vegetable chutneys.

- **Chinese dining** is a mixture of high-fat and low-fat dishes. High-fat foods include some stir-fry dishes and all deep-fat fried meats, especially in sweet and sour dishes.

   Low-fat choices include hot-and-sour soup, wonton soup, chicken chow mein, chicken or beef chop suey, stir-fry meat with vegetables (usually small amounts of meat are in these dishes), steamed rice, and fortune cookies.

- **Mexican dining** may have several high-fat foods–cheese, sour cream, and guacamole–which might accompany low-fat foods such as beans, corn, tomatoes, and tortillas. Lard is often used to fry tortilla shells and beans.

   Low-fat dining includes salsa, gazpacho, red beans and rice, soft chicken tacos, taco salad without the fried shell, chicken and rice, fajitas, and burritos.

- **Italian dining** is healthier if you substitute red sauce for white sauce (cream) on the pasta. Control fat intake by avoiding the many fried dishes, olive oil, cheese, and fatty meats like sausage.

   Some low-fat suggestions include minestrone, bread sticks, pasta with red sauce, veal picata, and chicken or veal cacciatore.

For more common individual foods, we are advised to follow the recommendations in Table 7-3 to change our diets from high-fat to low-fat foods.

Food Scientists

Food scientists make important contributions to the composition of fat in foods. Some people think cooking food does not involve science, but it does.

Table 7-3. High-Fat Foods and Low-Fat Substitutions

High-Fat Food	Low-Fat Food	High-Fat Food	Low-Fat Food
Whole milk	Skim milk	Fried eggs	Poached or baked eggs
	Buttermilk	Hot dogs and	Chicken
	Nonfat powdered milk	hamburgers	Skewered shrimp
Bacon	Chicken	on a cookout	Broiled fish
	Canadian bacon	Peanut butter and	Turkey breast
Bologna, frankfurter,	Chicken or turkey	jelly sandwich	Chicken
sausage	Lean, thinly sliced beef		Water-packed tuna
Avocado	Cucumber		Crabmeat or shrimp salad
	Zucchini		Low-fat cheese
	Lettuce	Fast food bought in a	Pack a homemade meal of
Creamy or high-fat	Low-fat cheese	restaurant on a long car	lean broiled chicken, fruits,
cheeses	Cottage cheese	trip	and raw vegetables
Ice cream	Ice milk	Cream pie	Unfrosted cake, made with less
	Frozen low-fat yogurt		fat than the recipe calls for
Nuts	Fruit or vegetable snack	Potato chips	Raw vegetables
	Dry cereal		Whole-grain crackers
	Popcorn		Pretzels
Hot fudge sundae	Frozen yogurt or ice milk	Breakfast sausage	Toast with cottage cheese
	with sliced or crushed fruit	Whipped cream	Whipped evaporated skim milk
Ground beef	Extra lean or lean beef or		(bowl and beaters must be
	poultry with all fat trimmed		thoroughly chilled)
Fatty pork, spare rib,	Well-trimmed lean pork	Oil or mayonnaise	Tomato sauce
ground pork	(leg, ham, picnic)	dressing on cold pasta	Yogurt laced with herbs
Sour cream	Low-fat yogurt	salad	
	Imitation sour cream	Chocolate	Candy (if you must have it)
Regular salad dressing	Reduced-calorie salad dressing		that contains no chocolate
	Vinegar		Sweet wafers made with no fat
	Lemon juice	Hot chocolate or	Hot chocolate or chocolate milk
Cream	Skim milk	chocolate milk	made with skim or low-fat milk
	Evaporated skim milk	(made with whole	Strawberry or raspberry syrup
Liver	Lean meat	milk)	mixed into skim or low-fat milk
	Chicken		Hot or cold lemonade
	Fish		Fruit juice
	Veal		Skim milk "blenderized" with
	Low-fat cheese		raw fruit such as bananas or
			strawberries

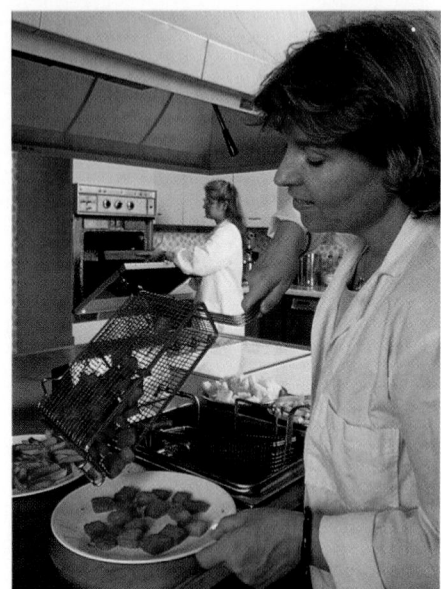

Figure 7-19. Much research is conducted to find the most effective ways to prepare low-fat dishes.

Emulsion: Mixture of two immiscible compounds such as oil and water, where one is dispersed in the other in the form of fine droplets. They stay mixed because of the presence of an **emulsifying agent**. These include gums, egg yolk, albumin and casein (both proteins), and lecithin. Emulsifying agents are used in margarine, ice cream, and salad dressing.

Lipophilic: (literally, "lipid-loving") Having the ability to combine with lipids.

Trans and cis fatty acids: Fatty acids with the same molecular and structural formulas but existing in different geometric forms. The *cis* form is the natural form and can be metabolized by the body. *Trans* forms are suspected of being involved in coronary heart disease.

Lipid oxidation: The process that makes fat rancid, producing off-odors and off-tastes in foods.

Think beyond Figure 7-19 to get a sense of the chemistry and nutrition involved in cooking.

The fat you decide to put in the pan when you cook involves both chemistry and nutrition. Refer back to Figure 7-11 to get information on the fatty acid composition of a number of cooking oils and margarine. Just 50 years ago, these choices would not have been available to you. For example, soybean oil was rarely added to food then, yet today it is the major edible oil in the United States. Food chemists were able to preserve its flavor and prolong its shelf life. Many other foods also are different now than they used to be. Fat content is reduced in beef patties and in sausages by using proteins and carbohydrates such as starches, fibers, and gums as additional ingredients. The cholesterol content of eggs can be lowered by food processing technology.

Food scientists have an interesting physical problem to contend with in foods–how to get fat and oil to mix with water so that we don't see globs of fat or layers of oil when we use the food. There are two types of *emulsions* in food: oil-in-water, as found in milk, mayonnaise, salad dressing, gravy, cream soups, and ice cream, and water-in-oil, as found in margarine, butter, and egg yolks. Emulsifiers have one part of the molecule that is hydrophilic and another part that is hydrophobic and therefore, *lipophilic*. *Emulsifying agents* include lecithin, gums, egg yolk, alginates, casein, and glycerol monostearate, among others. They are used in baking to help incorporate fat into the dough and to keep the crumb soft.

Our bodies make emulsifiers also. Bile is manufactured in the liver to act as an emulsifier in the digestion of dietary fat in the GI tract.

All of these examples are success stories. Not so successful from a health perspective is the hydrogenation of liquid oils by the addition of hydrogen atoms to double bonds, thereby increasing the degree of saturation. Hydrogenation hardens the fat (i.e., increases the melting point) and is applied frequently to vegetable oils used in the manufacture of margarine, cookies, and cakes. It is not uncommon to see the term "partially hydrogenated" on food labels. Problems arise because of the fatty acids formed by hydrogenation; some have a *trans* rather than the normal *cis* spatial alignment of the carbon chain. Nutritionists are interested in these because the consumption of *trans* fatty acids may contribute to the occurrence of CHD.[17] This does not mean that we should eliminate from our diets foods containing partially hydrogenated fat, but it is yet another example of the value of a varied diet.

Lipid oxidation is a process that makes fat rancid, thus decreasing shelf life because of off-odors and off-tastes in foods. It occurs most frequently in foods high in polyunsaturated fatty acids. Lipid oxidation is reduced by storing food for only short periods before consumption; by storing food away from air; by hydrogenating the fat, thereby reducing the degree of unsaturation; and by the use of antioxidants such as tocopherols (vitamin E) or BHT and BHA. It is common to find BHT or BHA listed on food labels as a preservative because they can serve as an antioxidant for the vitamin A present as well as for the fatty acids, thus preventing rancidity. Many oils contain naturally occurring tocopherols and so have their own built-in antioxidant. Fish oil seems to be very susceptible to oxidation even in the presence of antioxidants.[18]

Food Safety and Food Toxicology Experts

These people are concerned about a number of potential health problems associated with lipid oxidation, as well as with excessive and prolonged use of antioxidants. The emphasis should be on the word "potential" because the chemistry involved is complex.

> Investigation of toxicities of individual dietary lipid oxidation products is complicated by the incomplete knowledge of their interactions within foods

is how one researcher describes the present state of knowledge.[19] Lipid oxidation products are thought to cause coronary heart disease. The antioxidants BHT and BHA may cause liver damage, and there is conflicting evidence on whether they are cancer-causing. Regulatory agencies have various antioxidants under observation. At the levels used in foods and in normal intakes, BHT and BHA are considered safe. Should we stop using antioxidants? This is another case in which the risks must be weighed. If no preservatives were used and the fat were allowed to become oxidized (rancid), people would avoid the food because of the bad taste and odor. Also, some oxidation products are toxic.

Economists

Economists are interested in lipid nutrition because of the cost of ingredients to manufacture foods such as margarine or cookies. The final selection of a vegetable oil is likely to be made more on the basis of cost than of nutritional concerns. In least-cost formulation, food manufacturers use the least expensive available component of a food. This is why the source of plant oils may change from time to time on labels on margarine and other foods.

Medical economists are interested in the fat-cholesterol-heart disease debate because of the cost of cardiovascular disease care in the United States ($109 billion in 1992–over four times the cost of the food stamp program). About one-third of the 1.5 million U.S. heart attack victims each year die. The cost and effectiveness of cholesterol screening and other preventive measures for the entire population is being questioned. Of special concern is the lack of information on cholesterol treatment of women, children, young men, and the elderly upon which to do a cost-effectiveness analysis for the entire population.[20]

■ The consumer and the scientists

Consumers must sift through much information about the health benefits and health concerns regarding dietary lipids. They need to examine

Lecithin: A phospholipid consisting of glycerol, fatty acids, phosphoric acid, and choline; common in many foods such as soybeans, peanuts, and corn.

statements by nutrition experts carefully before accepting them. Application of "thinking beyond" the statement or problem will certainly assist us in asking the correct questions and evaluating answers. We have met several examples in which nutrition experts have insufficient information to make a final statement on an issue or where experts disagree on the interpretation or application of research findings. And consumers are also exposed to information from less creditable sources. Perhaps the best example is *lecithin*. Would you be interested in lecithin if promised that it would slow aging, improve memory, assist in losing weight, and lower serum cholesterol? Too good to be true? Unfortunately, yes, but some consumers are unaware of the following information. Lecithin is common in many foods such as soybeans, peanuts, and corn. It is used by the food industry as an emulsifier and as an anti-spattering agent in frying fats. Despite popular belief, lecithin is not absorbed intact from the GI tract. It is a phospholipid and is digested into its components–glycerol, fatty acids, phosphoric acid, and choline. Lecithin is an important part of cell membranes, but the body contains the components of lecithin and can make what it needs by combining them. This is another example of how an understanding of the chemistry and physiology of a compound can enable a consumer to save money and also avoid possible health problems and certain disappointments.

■ People are different–Response to dietary lipids varies among people

"Normal plasma cholesterol in an 88-year-old man who eats 25 eggs a day" is the title of a research paper in the *New England Journal of Medicine,* a highly respected medical journal.[21] If you apply all of the information in this chapter, you will understandably respond, "Surely this must be wrong." The man consumes an enormous amount of cholesterol each day–the Dietary Guidelines recommend a total daily intake of cholesterol equivalent to the amount of cholesterol in one egg. We are told that he has eaten this number of eggs for many years for psychological reasons. The article explains why he is free of all signs and symptoms of CHD. For one thing, he inefficiently absorbs cholesterol from his GI tract so that most of this huge amount of cholesterol is excreted in his feces. Also he converts a lot of cholesterol into bile acids, thus making it unavailable to be deposited in the arteries. He also does not synthesize much cholesterol, and the excretion of cholesterol-containing bile is increased, thus removing cholesterol from the body. In summary, he is a lucky fellow in avoiding coronary heart disease and a good example of how people respond differently to nutrients and other substances in the diet.

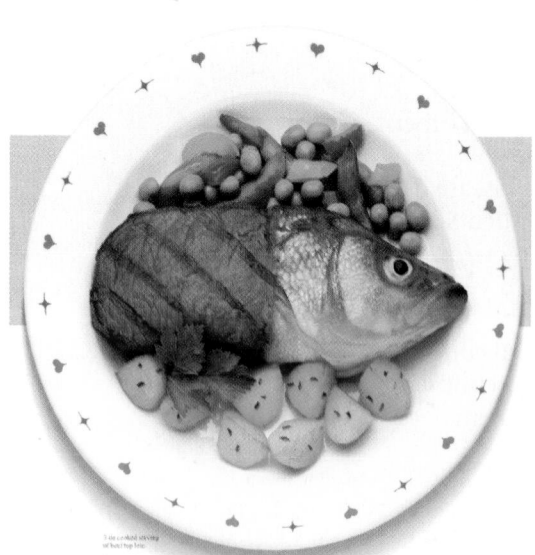

Figure 7-20. Reasonable amounts of fish and lean meat contribute important nutrients to the diet.

Think beyond Figure 7-20. Can you eat from both sides of the plate and be healthy?

Both the American Heart Association and the National Cholesterol Education Program recommend up to 6 ounces per day of lean meats, poultry, or seafood. This amount is based on the evidence we have examined about relationships between lipids and CHD. It would be a mistake, however, to conclude that lipids are the only factors associated with CHD. A statement from the National Institutes of Health recognizes that people can be exposed to other risk factors, including differences in lifestyle, obesity, cigarette smoking, and sedentary lifestyle.[22] Thus, diet and weight control, exercise, and smoking cessation are the primary emphases for the control of CHD.

■ Nutrition in action–Low-fat, no-fat, and light foods

"Are all those 'light' foods just a passing fad?" is the heading of an article in the *New York Times* (March 31, 1993). "Light foods" here refers to low-fat and no-fat foods. The answer may be surprising, "Surveys show that sales are light, too." Light foods are created from fat substitutes or fat mimics. Let's see what those are.

Fat substitutes give all or most of the functional properties of fat–appearance, texture, flavor, mouthfeel–without the caloric price we pay for real fats, which is 9 calories per gram of fat. This is done with some clever chemistry. The following is a list of current and proposed ingredients for fat substitutes.[23]

Carbohydrate- and protein-based materials:
    Modified glucose *polymers* (polydextrose)
    Modified corn, potato, rice, and tapioca starches
    Gums and *algins*
    Cellulose derivatives
    Microencapsulated proteins
Lipid-based materials:
    Fatty acid *esters* of sugars and sugar alcohols (sucrose polyesters)
    Various glyceryl esters
    Branched triglyceride esters
    Specific naturally occurring lipids (including jojoba oil)
Polyglycerol esters

Figure 7-21 shows what one of the best known of the fat substitutes looks like.

Think beyond the picture. What characteristics of the material make it look like fat?

There is no fat here, but the texture of fat is produced when spherical particles of hydrated protein roll over one another. The protein sources in this case are from egg white and milk protein. This is how fat substitutes deliver lower calories to the body. Most of the carbohydrate- and protein-based material listed above, as

Polymers: Compounds formed by the combination of two or more molecules of the same substance, in this case many molecules of modified glucose.

Algins: Substances found in many seaweeds; form viscous solutions; hold large amounts of water and are useful as thickeners and stabilizers in foods such as ice cream and synthetic cream.

Esters: Compounds produced from the combination of organic acids and alcohols. For example, acetic acid combined with ethyl alcohol gives ethyl ester. Fats are esters because of the combination of fatty acids with glycerol, which is a type of alcohol.

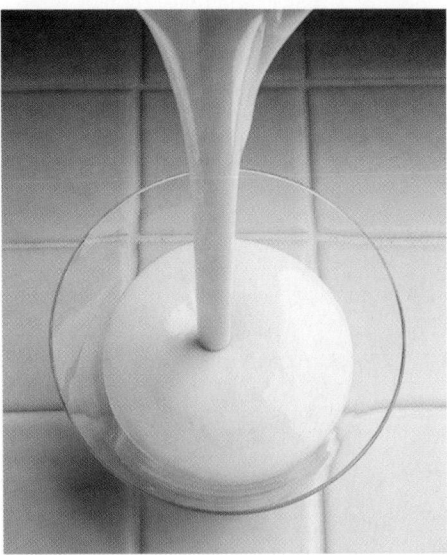

Figure 7-21. It looks like fat, it pours like fat, it has the texture of fat, but it is not fat. Simplesse is a fat substitute made from proteins.

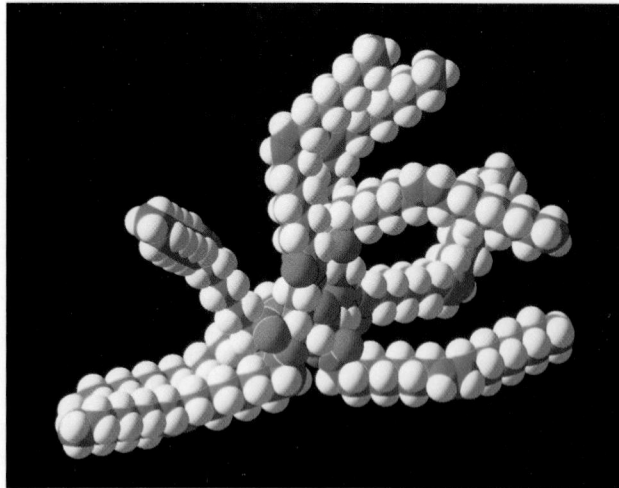

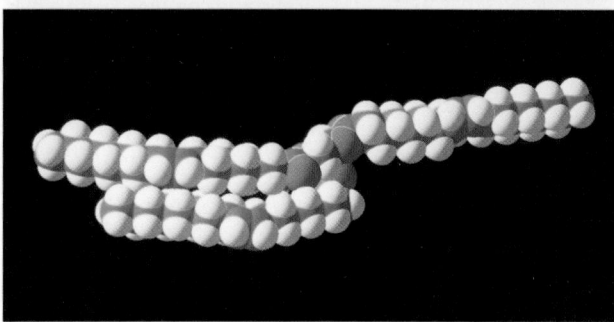

Figure 7-22. Top, molecular model of olestra, a fat substitute with the physical characteristics of fat. Bottom, molecular model of a triglyceride (glycerol plus three fatty acids) found naturally in food. Enzymes in the body can digest the triglyceride but cannot digest olestra because of its different physical structure. Thus, olestra is not absorbed into the body, and the calories associated with fat are not absorbed. However, the person eating olestra has the sensation of eating fat in the food.

well as the polyglycerol esters, are partially or fully digested in the GI tract and absorbed. Because carbohydrates and proteins have less than half of the caloric content of fat and because of the water included in the particles, such products provide less than one-fifth of the calories in the equivalent amount of fat. The gums and cellulose derivatives go largely undigested, and so they provide few or no calories to the body.

Chemists have been innovative in making a lipid-based fat substitute with a chemical structure (Figure 7-22, top) that resembles the structure of a triglyceride (Figure 7-22, bottom). The difference is the larger molecular size of the fat substitute, which resists digestion and thus is excreted in the feces. There is some concern that this may result in reduced absorption of some fat-soluble vitamins and in possible diarrhea.[23]

Observing the future development of the fat substitute market should be interesting because it has great economic potential, but many questions remain to be answered. More information is needed from testing low-fat diets for the elderly, children, and women. We need to know whether at these critical parts of the life cycle the digestive system is altered radically by a high intake of fat substitutes. If so, this may reduce the availability of other nutrients to the body. Then there are the unresolved issues in the fat-cholesterol-CHD debate. Fat substitutes have as their largest target market the people concerned about CHD. We saw that the factors affecting this disease involve not only diet (including lipids) but nondietary factors also. The contributions of each of these factors, both singly and in combination, to diseases such as CHD are not definitively known. Until more answers are available, it is prudent to follow the recommendations of credible national and professional organizations.

Regulatory agencies are monitoring the health benefits of fat substitutes.[24] People consume foods with fat substitutes to reduce their intake of fat and calories from fat. But we do not know yet whether people who consume high amounts of fat substitutes actually decrease their fat and calorie intake. Many may compensate by increasing total food intake.

So far we have looked at substances that manufacturers can use instead of fat. Other ingenious ways to lower fat in foods are attempted. Water is added, but this may cause undesirable microbial action requiring additional preservatives. Air is sometimes added to puff up foods on the assumption that increased bulk dilutes the fat content. The low-calorie margarine products in Table 7-4 contain less fat and more water than butter or regular margarine.

The literature seems unified in the view that no perfect fat substitute has been discovered yet. Let's end with the consumers' view:

> The potential market for good-quality products incorporating a fat substitute is high . . . . lower-fat products currently available on the marketplace are not completely meeting consumer demand.[25]

It seems fair to say that much work remains to be done–and it will be, because of the number of dieters (Figure 7-23) in the United States.

■ Now you know

- People have strong sensory preferences for foods high in fat.

- Fat is the most efficient energy source in the body.

- There is a lower limit to body fat, below which menstruation and conception do not occur.

- Lipids are important in the structure and function of cell membranes.

- Nerves have lipids in their structure.

- Lipids insulate the body and protect important body organs.

- Lipids are part of prostaglandins–hormone-like chemicals assisting in the contraction of the uterus in labor, control of inflammation, and maintenance of blood pressure.

- Lipids in foods provide the essential fatty acids, are a source of energy, carry the fat-soluble vitamins, add palatability to food, and increase the satiety value of a meal.

- Lipids are classified as mono-, di-, and triglycerides, and fatty acids are classified as saturated, monounsaturated, and polyunsaturated.

- Foods of animal origin are highest in saturated fatty acids, and foods from plants are highest in polyunsaturated fatty acids.

- Cholesterol is found only in foods of animal origin; about 75% of the cholesterol in the human body is synthesized by the body.

- Polyunsaturated fatty acids may lower blood pressure.

- High-fat diets may contribute to obesity.

- Fat is suspected as a causal agent of some cancers.

- Non-insulin-dependent diabetes and kidney disease may be related to high dietary fat intake.

Table 7-4. Butter Versus Margarine

Product (1 tbsp)	Fat (grams)	Calories
Butter	11	100
Butter-margarine blend	11	100
Stick, tub, or liquid margarine	11	100
Whipped margarine	7	66
Diet margarine	6	50
Spread	6–7	50–75

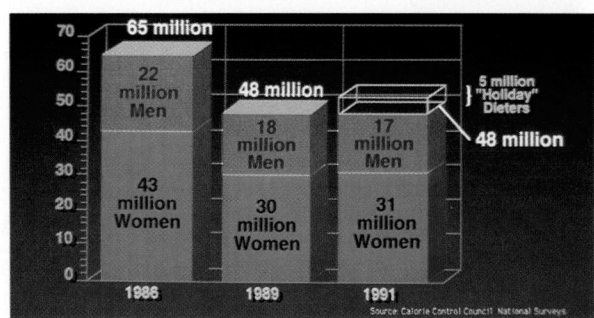

Figure 7-23. Even though the number is decreasing, millions of people still diet to remove unwanted body fat.

- Deficiency of essential fatty acids leads to increased infections and decreased immunity.

- Cholesterol and the amount and type of fat are two of several risk factors in coronary heart disease.

- Farmers and plant and animal scientists have decreased the amount and improved the type of fat in foods.

- Some international and ethnic dining includes low-fat foods.

- Fat is incorporated into processed foods with emulsifiers. Hydrogenation, *trans* fatty acids, and lipid oxidation may present health problems.

- Fat substitutes reduce fat and caloric intake, but the perfect fat mimic has not been found yet.

Further Reading

1. Zaadstra, B. M., and others. Fat and female fecundity: Prospective study of effect of body fat distribution on conception rates. ***British Medical Journal*** 306:484, 1993.
2. Crawford, M. A. The role of dietary fatty acids in biology: Their place in the evolution of the human brain. ***Nutrition Reviews*** 50(4)(Part II):3, 1992.
3. Connor, W. E., and others. Essential fatty acids: The importance of n-3 fatty acids in the retina and brain. ***Nutrition Reviews*** 50(4)(Part II):21, 1992.
4. Beitz, D. C., and others. ***Food Fats and Health.*** Council for Agricultural Science and Technology, Ames, Iowa, 1991.
5. Raper, N. R., and others. ***Nutrient Content of the U.S. Food Supply, 1909–1988.*** Home Economics Research Report No. 50. U.S. Department of Agriculture, Washington DC, 1992.
6. Lawn, R. M. Lipoprotein(a) in heart disease. ***Scientific American***, 266(6):54, 1992.
7. Ross, E. The role of marine fish oils in the treatment of ulcerative colitis. ***Nutrition Reviews*** 51:47, 1993.
8. U.S. Department of Health and Human Services, Public Health Service, National Institutes of Health. ***So You Have High Blood Cholesterol . . .*** NIH Publication No. 92-2922, 1992.
9. Mott, G. E., and others. Dietary cholesterol and type of fat differentially affect cholesterol metabolism and atherosclerosis in baboons. ***Journal of Nutrition*** 122:1397, 1992.
10. Roncari, D. A. K. Obesity and associated apolipoprotein abnormalities: Relation to coronary heart disease. In: ***Cholesterol and Coronary Heart Disease: The Great Debate***. P. Gold and others, eds. Parthenon Publishing Group, Park Ridge, New Jersey, page 151, 1992.
11. Randall, T. First gene therapy for inherited hypercholesterolemia a partial success. ***Journal of the American Medical Association*** 269:837, 1993.
12. Scanu, A. M. Lipoprotein(a): A genetic risk factor for premature coronary heart disease. ***Journal of the American Medical Association*** 267:3326, 1992.
13. Frankel, E. N., and others. Inhibition of oxidation of human low-density lipoprotein by phenolic substances in red wine. ***Lancet*** 341:454, 1993.
14. Edelstein, S. L., and others. Increased meal frequency associated with decreased

cholesterol concentrations: Rancho Bernardo, CA, 1984–1987. *American Journal of Clinical Nutrition* 55:664, 1992.

15. Ohlrogge, J., and others. Plant fatty acid biosynthesis and its potential for manipulation. In: *Biotechnology and Nutrition*. D. D. Bills and S.-D. Kung, eds., Butterworth- Heinemann, Boston, page 365, 1992.

16. Callahan, M. *Skimming the Fat: A Practical Food Guide.* The American Dietetic Association, Chicago, page 12, 1992.

17. Willett, W. C., and others. Intake of *trans* fatty acids and risk of coronary heart disease among women. *Lancet* 341:581, 1993.

18. Gonzalez, M. J., and others. Lipid peroxidation products are elevated in fish oil diets even in the presence of added antioxidants. *Journal of Nutrition* 122:2190, 1992.

19. Kubow, S. Lipid oxidation products in food and atherogenesis. *Nutrition Reviews* 51:33, 1993.

20. McBride, P. E., and Davis, J. E. Cholesterol and cost effectiveness: Implications for practice, policy, and research. *Circulation* 85:1939, 1992.

21. Kern, F., Jr. Normal plasma cholesterol in an 88-year-old man who eats 25 eggs a day: Mechanisms of adaptation. *New England Journal of Medicine* 324:896, 1991.

22. NIH Consensus Development Panel on Triglycerides, High-Density Lipoprotein, and Coronary Heart Disease. Triglyceride, high-density lipoprotein, and coronary heart disease. *Journal of the American Medical Association* 269:505, 1993.

23. Mela, D. J. Nutritional implications of fat substitutes. *Journal of the American Dietetic Association* 92:472, 1992.

24. Vanderveen, J. E., and Glinsmann, W. H. Fat substitutes: A regulatory perspective. *Annual Review of Nutrition* 12:473, 1992.

25. Bruhn, C. M., and others. Consumer attitudes and market potential for foods using fat substitutes. *Food Technology* 46(4):81, 1992.

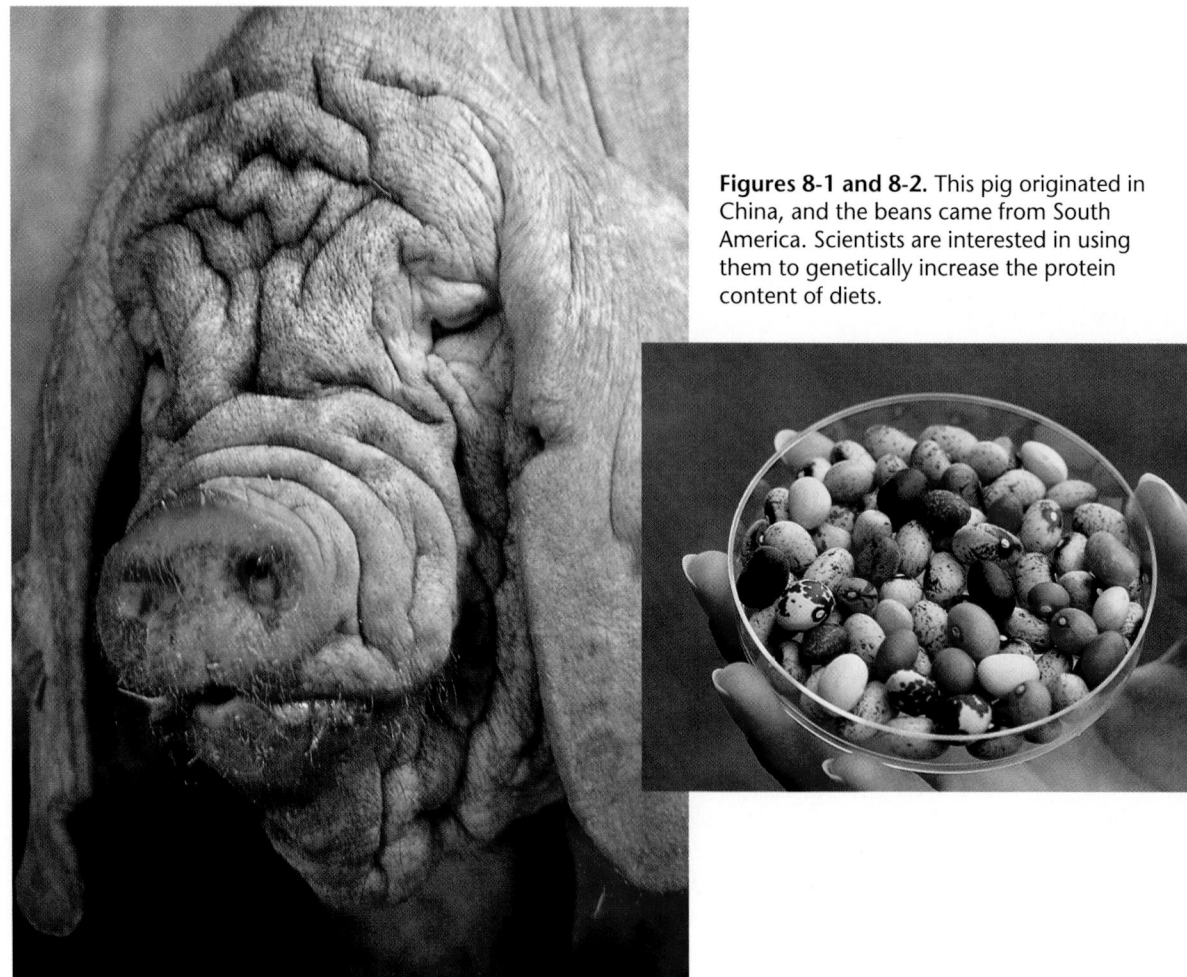

Figures 8-1 and 8-2. This pig originated in China, and the beans came from South America. Scientists are interested in using them to genetically increase the protein content of diets.

## CHAPTER 8

Proteins–Meat, Fish, and Other Protein Sources

■ Proteins in our lives–"Protein" means "of prime importance"

If "protein" means "of prime importance" in the Greek language, why are two seemingly odd photographs introducing such an important nutrient? It is because both pork and beans are good sources of dietary protein. Other good protein sources are eggs, beef, poultry, fish, milk and other dairy products, and nuts. Scientists at the USDA are studying this breed of pig and these beans (called nuñas, pronounced *noon-yahs*) as possible dietary protein sources of the future.

The pork and beans photographs also illustrate a number of points about dietary protein. First, we don't all consume the same high-protein foods, for a variety of reasons. Second, the search for suitable sources of protein is worldwide and ongoing. Third, pure protein foods don't exist, only protein-rich foods. Meat, fish, eggs, and beans all contain other nutrients such as vitamins, minerals, fat, and carbohydrate.[1] Discussing carbohydrates in Chapter 6 was easy because sugar and starch, which you can buy in stores, are almost pure carbohydrate. Vegetable oils and a lump of fat on a piece of meat are almost all lipid. But think about protein–can you buy pure protein in a store? No, although pure protein (such as the milk protein casein) is added to some foods during manufacture. Protein is thus represented in our diet by foods high in protein but not by pure protein foods.

Proteins are "of prime importance" because they are found everywhere in nature–in humans, animals, plants, and microbes. They are in every cell in the human body, where they are involved in the growth and maintenance of the body and in the regulation of many functions in cells. They also provide energy for the body in emergencies such as starvation, extreme dieting, and the wasting produced by diseases such as cancer. Without various body proteins, we could not survive. For example, muscle proteins allow skeletal muscles to contract and relax, thereby allowing the body to move; cardiac muscles pump blood from the heart; and muscles in

Collagen: An insoluble protein that gives rigidity to cells and tissues; found in skin, bone, ligaments, and cartilage.

Peptide: Two or more amino acids joined together. It may be part of a protein.

Peptide bond: The chemical link between amino acids in a peptide or protein; forms the backbone of protein molecules.

the gastrointestinal tract squeeze the feces toward expulsion from the body. All enzymes are proteins, and they are involved in almost every metabolic activity in the body. The specific chemical properties of the proteins *collagen* and elastin are essential for the "scaffolding" that gives cells, tissues, and the entire body a rigid structure.

Consuming enough protein may be a matter of life and death during famines and also a day-to-day problem in many developing countries. Mortality is usually high for people on very low-protein diets because the antibodies that protect the body from infections are proteins. Low levels of antibodies expose undernourished children, in particular, to infections that could lead to death. In contrast, many people in developed countries have no problem with consuming twice the RDA for protein. Some people are fascinated with amino acids and protein and have even higher intake in the form of supplements for body building, mood control, and other real or imagined functions of protein.

■ Proteins are studied by different professions

Chemists–Studying Protein Structure and Function

Understanding how proteins function in living cells requires knowledge of their structure. Imagine the structure of protein as a giant beaded necklace with each bead an amino acid and the thread linking the amino acids together as the *peptide bond*. The structure of proteins may be straight-chained and fibrous, as in hair or blood-clotting proteins, thereby giving them rigidity. Proteins may also be coiled and globular, as in some of the blood proteins. This shape allows the large protein molecules to squeeze through tiny blood vessels in the body. Using the necklace analogy, it is equivalent to the string of beads being clumped in a knot.

Chemists and biochemists can represent the structure of different protein molecules as shown in Figure 8-3 (all are at the same magnification).[2] These illustrations represent chains of amino acids linked together by peptide bonds. Size and shape differ from one protein to another because of the number and type of amino acids and their location in the molecule. Proteins are considered to be small when they have 125–150 amino acids joined together; large proteins can have over 5,500 amino acids in their molecule.[2] Chemists use these differences in size as one way to separate different proteins.

Notice how proteins have different activities in the body. Hemoglobin and myoglobin transport oxygen

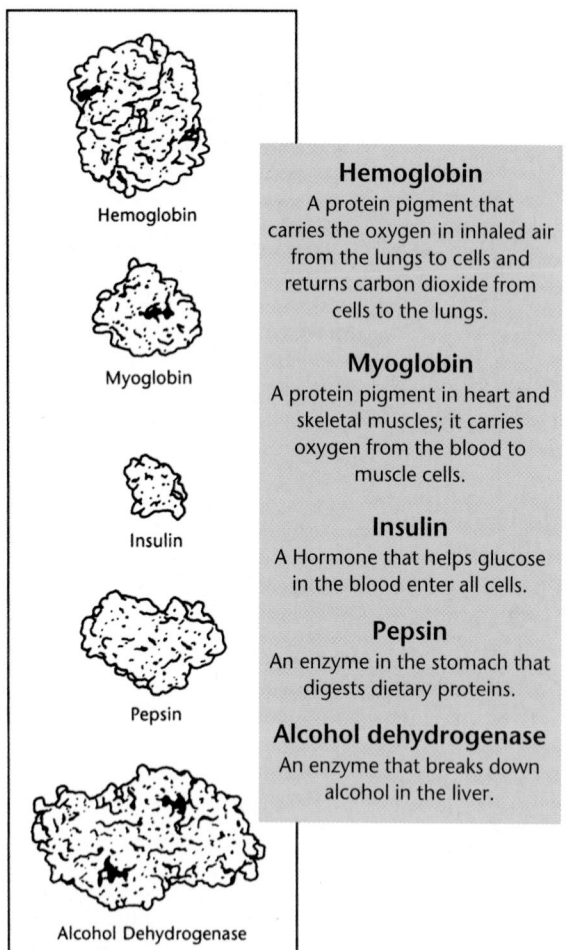

Hemoglobin
A protein pigment that carries the oxygen in inhaled air from the lungs to cells and returns carbon dioxide from cells to the lungs.

Myoglobin
A protein pigment in heart and skeletal muscles; it carries oxygen from the blood to muscle cells.

Insulin
A Hormone that helps glucose in the blood enter all cells.

Pepsin
An enzyme in the stomach that digests dietary proteins.

Alcohol dehydrogenase
An enzyme that breaks down alcohol in the liver.

Figure 8-3. Amino acids combine to form three-dimensional protein structures. Shown here are proteins of interest to nutritionists.

and carbon dioxide and belong to the group called functional proteins. Insulin is a hormone that is a protein, although not all hormones are proteins. Pepsin and alcohol dehydrogenase are enzymes–the thousands of enzymes in our bodies and in animals, plants, and microbes are all proteins.

Amino acids

Amino acids contain carbon, hydrogen, and oxygen, and in this respect they resemble carbohydrates and lipids. But all amino acids also have nitrogen in their structure, and three amino acids have sulfur. Figure 8-4 shows the general structure for *all* amino acids.

The –NH_2 amino group gives amino acids their name. There are 20 different amino acids, of which nine are called *essential amino acids*; these are not made in sufficient amounts in the human body and must be provided in the diet. Biochemists have determined how nonessential amino acids are made from other chemicals in the body.

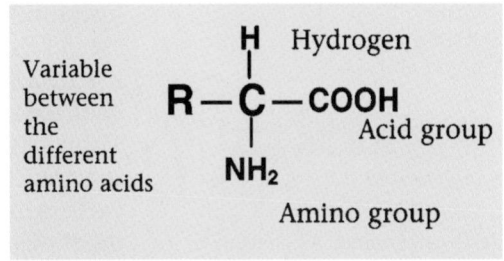

Figure 8-4. General structure of an amino acid. Like carbohydrates and lipids, it contains carbon, hydrogen, and oxygen. In addition, an amino acid contains nitrogen.

Essential amino acids: Amino acids that must be provided by the diet because they cannot be synthesized in the body at a rate sufficient to meet the body's requirement for growth and maintenance.

Nitrogen-fixing bacteria: A special type of bacteria; forms nodules in roots of legumes (beans, peas, and lentils) that "fix" or convert nitrogen from the air. This nitrogen is available to the plant for conversion into amino acids.

Table 8-1. Essential and Nonessential Amino Acids

Essential	Nonessential
Lysine	Alanine
Tryptophan	Arginine
Phenylalanine	Aspartic acid
Methionine	Cysteine
Leucine	Cystine
Isoleucine	Glutamic acid
Threonine	Glutamine
Valine	Glycine
Histidine	Proline
	Serine
	Tyrosine

Amino acids are the major source of nitrogen for the human body. Small amounts of nitrogen are also found in nucleic acids (DNA and RNA) and in the B-complex vitamins (thiamin, riboflavin, niacin, vitamin B-6, pantothenic acid, biotin, folacin, and vitamin B-12). Plants usually have little problem getting enough carbon, hydrogen, and oxygen to make amino acids and other nutrients containing these elements. However, getting sufficient nitrogen to make amino acids may be a problem in certain parts of the world. The soil may lack nitrogen, and nitrogen fertilizers may be too expensive for local farmers. There is increasing interest in *nitrogen-fixing bacteria*, which attach to the roots of plants such as those in the bean family, including soybeans. They give roots the appearance shown in Figure 8-5.

The white nodules attached to the roots contain the nitrogen-fixing bacteria. The plant and bacteria work in cooperation. Bacteria utilize or "fix" nitrogen from the air, converting it to another form of nitrogen, which is then transferred to the plant for incorporation into amino acids.[3] Plant proteins are synthesized from the amino acids, which in turn become protein sources in the diets of animals and humans.

DNA controls the unique sequence of amino acids in each protein. All proteins are made from only 20 different amino acids. Here is an il-

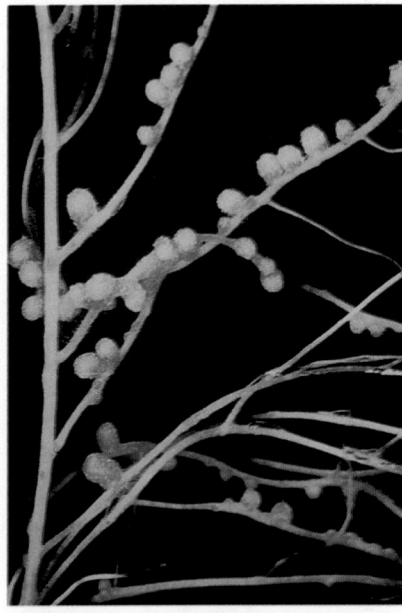

Figure 8-5. Nitrogen-fixing bacteria are white nodules on the roots of plants of the bean family, including soybeans. These bacteria obtain nitrogen from the air and incorporate it into the plant, thus lessening the need for nitrogen from the soil.

lustration of this–think of each letter in the words "seed," "seek," "seem," "seen," "seep," "seer" as an amino acid and the word as a protein. See how the meaning changes significantly when only one letter in each word is changed. Amino acids have exactly the same relationship to proteins. Think of the great number of combinations of the 20 different amino acids that can be made, and you will see why thousands of different proteins exist in nature. However, if DNA misplaces one amino acid in the hundreds of amino acids in a single protein, the protein is changed, which may cause major health problems. An example is *sickle cell anemia*, which occurs relatively frequently among people of African descent. Hemoglobin's ability to deliver oxygen to cells and to remove carbon dioxide from cells is reduced when just one amino acid (glutamine) is replaced by another amino acid (valine) in the hemoglobin structure. The disease may even be fatal.

Sickle cell anemia: A hereditary form of **anemia** with abnormally shaped red blood cells caused by an amino acid alteration in hemoglobin. Decreases the capacity to deliver oxygen to cells and to remove carbon dioxide.

Farmers and Plant and Animal Scientists–Producing High-Quality Protein Foods

Think beyond this photograph in Figure 8-6.

Nutritionists are interested in farming because this is where the food chain begins and because farm productivity determines the availability and cost of nutrients. Foods high in protein include meat, fish, poultry, eggs, dairy products, nuts, and legumes (including soybean and other beans, garden peas, and lentils). Nutritionists are also interested in how farmers may adopt new scientific

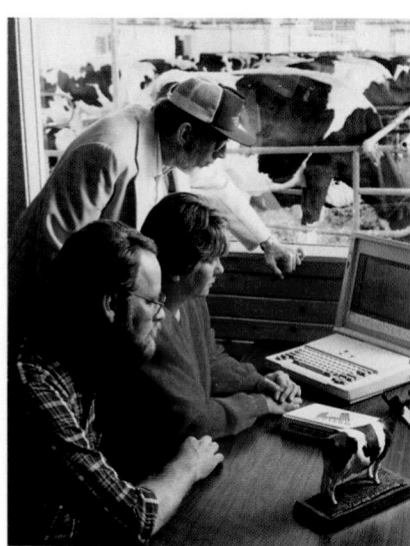

Figure 8-6. Food production on modern farms is both a science and a business.

advances in genetics, genetic engineering, and biotechnology. Each of these factors is important in determining the quantity and quality of protein and other nutrients we consume. Americans now consume more protein from animal sources than they did in the early 1900s.

Many factors have influenced the present consumption pattern for protein. Increased efficiency in farming has resulted in decreases in food costs. Improved storage and delivery systems for foods have allowed better distribution of high-protein foods such as meats, fish, and dairy products–all foods that spoil easily unless refrigerated or dried. Consumer preference for protein increases as people become more wealthy. But health-conscious con-

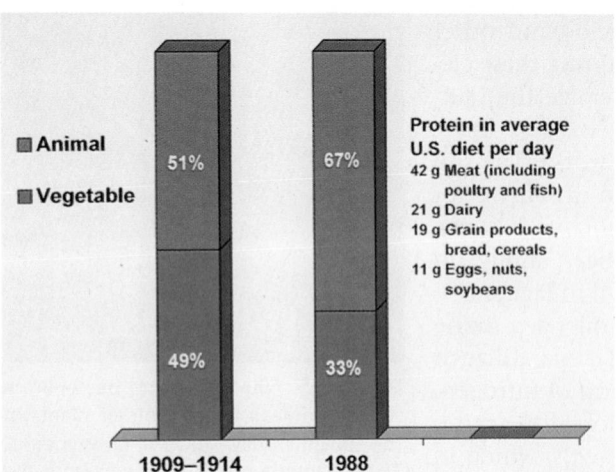

Figure 8-7. We consume more animal protein now than people did in the early 1900s. Meat, poultry, and fish are the highest contributors of dietary protein.

sumers want protein-rich foods with less fat. This is why the consumption of beef and whole milk is decreasing and that of poultry, fish, and low-fat milk and other dairy products is increasing.

Some consumers have questioned certain actual or potential methods of food production. In Chapter 2 we dealt with the issue of pesticides in the production of plant foods. Another issue is the ethics of animal agriculture. This is complicated by different interpretations of scientific facts, by economic considerations, and by emotional responses. A USDA scientist has stated that

> the future course of animal agriculture may be determined more by the ethics of animal use than by technology.[4]

The debate revolves around views ranging from a belief at one extreme that humans have unlimited rights over animals to a belief at the other extreme that animals are naturally entitled to the same rights as humans. It is not the function of this book to arbitrate between these positions but rather to recognize the nutritional implications of each. A potentially great impact on nutrient intake could result from controversies over the degree of hardship to animals from intensive livestock and poultry production (so-called "factory farms"), the ethics of genetic engineering, the necessity of using animals in laboratory research, the use of pesticides to kill insects, and even whether meat should be part of the human diet at all.

Couple this situation with an increasing demand for food to meet a rapidly expanding global population. Protein may be the nutrient that most limits population because of the difficulty of producing protein-rich foods from animals (especially in tropical countries), the high cost of protein-rich foods, and problems with their preservation and distribution, especially in developing countries. With all of these issues to consider, you can see why nutritionists have great interest in what is happening on the farm.[5]

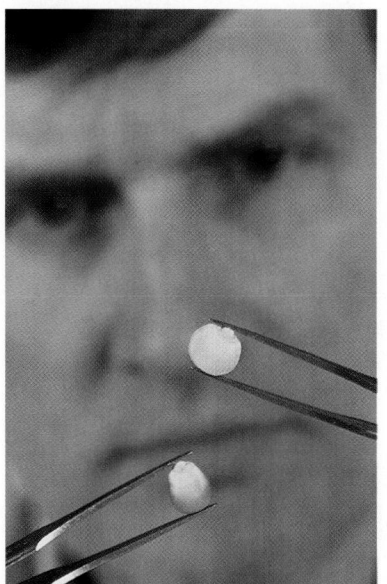

Figure 8-8. The two grains of corn may look the same, but nutritionally they are different. The top grain is high in lysine, an essential amino acid that normally occurs in low amounts in cereals. Geneticists have played an important role in improving the lysine content of corn.

Geneticists–Great Advances but Possible Future Problems

More nutritious food can be produced by improved farming methods, but the greatest advances may come from genetic engineering.[5] Genetics has already produced advances that benefit nutrition. We will look at a few examples of how protein nutrition has been improved.

The two grains of corn in Figure 8-8 look the same, but the nutritional im-

Limiting amino acid: The essential amino acid in a protein that is in the smallest amount relative to dietary needs. Lysine is the limiting amino acid in cereal proteins, and the sulfur amino acid methionine is the limiting amino acid in most animal and vegetable proteins.

pact of the top grain is significantly greater, especially in developing countries. It has a higher concentration of the essential amino acid lysine. To understand the significance of this, we return to the list of essential amino acids in Table 8-1. These are the amino acids that cannot be made by the body at a rate that will meet the body's demand for protein for growth and maintenance. Lysine is at the top of the list of essential amino acids. Consuming enough lysine is not a problem for most people in developed countries (including the United States), who consume a mixed diet of both plant and animal foods. However, in developing countries, most people are dependent on foods from plants because of the scarcity and cost of meat animals. Usually the cereal grains form the most plentiful crop. The problem is that lysine is the *limiting amino acid* in cereal grains. "Limiting" means that this is the essential amino acid that occurs in the lowest concentration relative to metabolic requirements. So people who are dependent upon cereals (rice, corn, barley, etc.) for protein may not get enough lysine. Genetic alterations increasing the concentration of lysine can have significant nutritional impact, especially for people in periods of increased nutrient demand, such as infancy, childhood, pregnancy, lactation, and recovery from illness or starvation.

The Green Revolution in the 1970s was a series of scientific discoveries that increased the total yield of protein-rich plant foods in many countries.[5] However, scientists are cautious about predicting further success in the genetic manipulation of plants, according to an article in the *Economist* (June 12, 1993).

> Of all living creatures, plants have proved the most resilient to the tamperings of genetic engineers. That is because they are so good at adapting themselves.

The nutritional implications of this statement are significant for the future; we may not be able to improve the nutritional quality of plants any further.

Genetic selection of farm animals has increased their efficiency in producing meat with more lean and less fat, has improved milk yields, and has brought about greater resistance to disease. Further increases in the amount of protein and other nutrients from these sources may be limited because of technical difficulties. Also, an ethical question was posed by a British scientist:

> . . . we must also question our right to manipulate the nature and quality of life of animals which have the capacity to perceive not only visceral sensations, such as hunger and pain, but also some higher concepts such as pleasure and frustration.[6]

This is just a glimpse of both sides of some difficult issues. They are presented here without judgment because volumes have been written on them and the debate is ongoing. They do serve to remind us that the future production of protein-rich foods through genetic manipulation is determined both by technical advances and by societal attitudes. Nutritionists are concerned about the outcomes, and all of us have choices to make as individuals that should be made unemotionally on the basis of scientific facts.

Biotechnologists–Cautious Optimism for a Positive Impact on Protein Nutrition

We saw in Chapter 1 how some techniques in biotechnology have existed for thousands of years. Recent advances in biotechnology also have an impact on nutrition. For instance, many changes in proteins (and other nutrients) have been made by methods involving *recombinant DNA (rDNA)*, gene transfer, embryo manipulation and transfer, plant regeneration, tissue culture, and bioprocess engineering.[7] Meat quality has been improved and better food ingredients are made through enzymes generated by biotechnology.

Recombinant DNA (rDNA): DNA altered to produce a slightly different protein from that produced by the unaltered form.

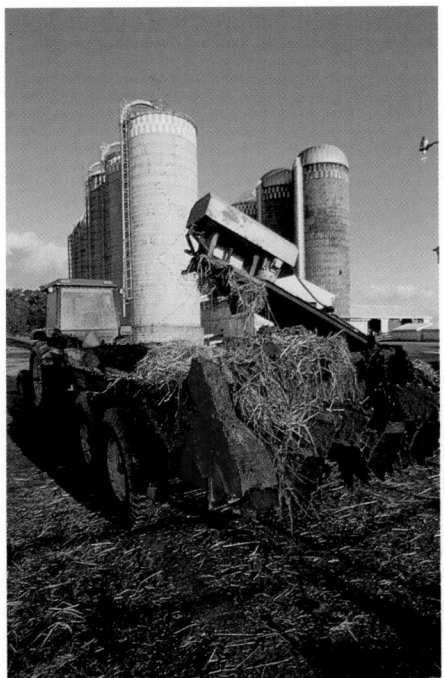

Figure 8-9. Environmental damage may be a consequence of producing some high-protein foods. Manure can cause problems with odor and with runoff into rivers and streams, thus causing water pollution.

Environmental Scientists–Pollution May Be Caused by Intensive Animal Production

Think beyond this picture in Figure 8-9. Why is manure discussed in a nutrition book?

Why not? Even a winner of the Nobel Prize for Chemistry writes about it in a discussion on science and food production![5] There is little dispute that animal products make important contributions to our diet.[1] But production of the high-protein animal foods–meat, dairy products, eggs–results in manure being produced in large amounts. The corn silos in the background of the photograph illustrate the cycle between corn, meat, and dairy products. In traditional farming, some of the corn is fed to the animals, and the stalks are used for bedding. The resultant manure is spread on the land to prevent soil erosion and to fertilize the soil with the nitrogen, potassium, and phosphorus it contains. This cycle has been practiced for centuries, but modern intensive methods of raising meat animals create new problems with the disposal of manure. Animals raised in indoor feed lots stand on slats through which their feces drop. These are washed away by large volumes of water to huge lagoons for storage. The first problem is the amount of water used, since water is a nutrient in short supply in many areas (Chapter 5). The second is that the chemicals in manure may seep into the soil and pollute groundwater and rivers, causing problems with the drinking water supply and creating a hazard for fish and other life in rivers. This manure is not recycled back to the land. Another way of handling the manure is to pile it into mountainous heaps. Transporting it to enrich the land is usually too expensive, and odor from these manure piles or lagoons may be a problem for neighbors. Animal scientists are working on these problems in the context of "waste management." We should be aware of these issues involved in providing animal sources of dietary protein.

Food Scientists–Using Proteins to Make Food More Acceptable

Dipeptide: Two amino acids joined by a peptide bond.

Sulfites: Chemicals widely used as preservatives in fruit juices and syrups, on fruits, and in sausage, beer, and wine. They give an unpleasant taste to food. Are driven off by boiling or cooking.

Food scientists can make some foods more palatable by using the individual or combined chemical and physical properties of proteins. For example, some amino acids have either sweet or bitter tastes; the intense sweetener aspartame is a *dipeptide*, a combination of aspartic acid and phenylalanine. Amino acids combined with other chemicals give a meat-like aroma and flavor. The ability of proteins to bind water is important in sausage manufacture, and the foaming and whipping properties of proteins are used in certain foods. Some plant proteins such as soy can be textured into fibers that can be compressed to produce a fabricated meat analog referred to as textured vegetable protein. In many foods, amino acids can combine with carbohydrates such as glucose to give the brown color and aromas characteristic of roasting, baking, grilling, and frying. Food scientists also devise methods of processing and preparing food that maximize the nutritive value of protein.

A cut apple exposed to the air turns brown after a while and is not as appealing to eat as when it was freshly cut. Scientists at the USDA are using a soybean protein solution to produce films, coatings, and other plastic-like products into which an apple can be dipped (Figure 8-10). The result is that the apple does not brown, and the nutrients in the apple, plus the small amount of protein from the soy film, can be consumed with no waste and no damage to the environment.

Enzymes have been used since ancient times to make bread, cheese, beer, and other fermented products and to tenderize meat. Only recently, however, have we understood how they function. The technology and economics of enzyme use are becoming more attractive to food manufacturers. Among other reasons is consumer resistance to having "chemicals" used in food production. Although enzymes are chemicals, they are from natural sources, frequently from microorganisms.[8] Using enzymes instead of "chemicals" may produce fewer by-products, and the chemical reactions may be easier to control. For example, a bacterial enzyme may replace *sulfites* as a dough conditioner in bakery goods. Sulfites in food products can create allergic reactions in some people, especially those with asthma, and this is of concern to the FDA. Using an enzyme eliminates this problem. Enzymes also

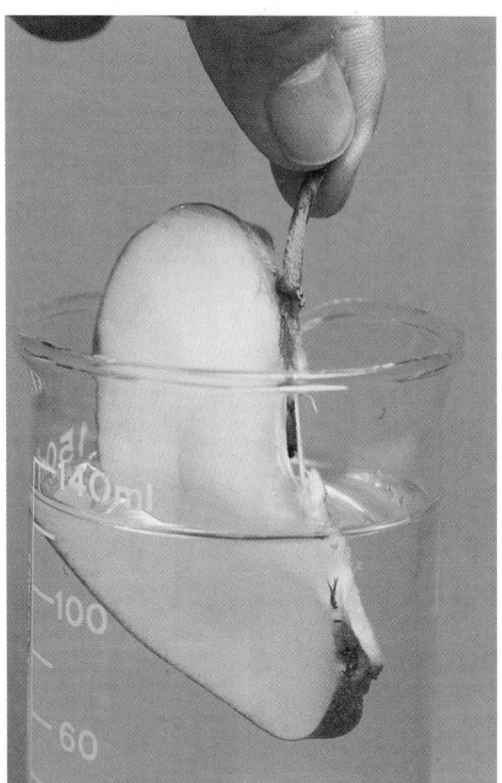

Figure 8-10. Food scientists have discovered that some proteins in liquid form can be used to coat cut pieces of food to prevent damage from air. This cut apple will not become brown because the film of protein protects the cut surface from the air.

play an important role in dealing effectively with food processing wastes by changing them into more usable components.[9] Economic use of such wastes makes food more affordable and may prevent environmental damage.

Many innovative uses are made of proteins and amino acids. For example, the solubility of peptides allows them to be used as a source of proteins in infant and baby foods, special dietetic products, and sports drinks. The protein gelatin is also used creatively in confectionery, meat canning, jelly powder, and pharmaceutical capsules. Gelatin is extracted from cattle bones, hide pieces, and pork skins.

Much of our food is heated, and in this process the proteins in the food may be *denatured*. The presence of heat, acid, salt, or mechanical action can cause the structure of food proteins to unfold because of breaks in the linkages joining the various strands of amino acids. This change, usually irreversible, makes the proteins less soluble and more viscous. This is what happens when eggs are heated. It also occurs when salt is added during cheesemaking and when eggs are whisked.

Denatured protein: A protein in which the molecular structure has been modified so that its properties and biological activity are destroyed or diminished.

Some food processing procedures may affect the body's utilization of proteins and amino acids.[10] Acid, alkali, or heat treatment may destroy some essential amino acids or decrease the digestibility of proteins. Lysine is an essential amino acid that is damaged by heat. This may be a problem in areas where protein intake is marginal and people are dependent on cereals for protein, since, as we saw above, lysine is already the limiting amino acid in cereals.

Economists–Protein-Rich Foods Are Usually Expensive

Protein is a limiting nutrient for many people because of its high cost in comparison to carbohydrate-rich foods. People who may have low protein intake include the elderly, single-parent families, the homeless, and others with low incomes. The cost of providing a given amount of protein varies among different foods and within some categories of food. Take time to do some price comparisons in your local supermarket, looking at the cost of protein in your favorite foods. Read the label for the protein content per serving, the number of servings in the package, and the price. Compare the costs of different foods when standardized for 100 grams of protein. Here is an example from a high-fiber breakfast cereal:

- Grams of protein per serving, 4
- Servings in the package, 11
- Purchase price in the store, $2.59
- Therefore, 44 grams of protein costs $2.59.
- 100 grams of protein costs $5.89.

Poverty in developing countries makes it difficult for many people, especially children, to meet their protein intake requirements.

The U.S. market for amino acids is large–over $600 million per year. Most of these amino acids are added to food and feed for humans and animals and are made by new production technologies, including biotechnology and fermentation processes. Some amino acid supplements are consumed by people who falsely believe that they help in building muscle.[11] Other amino acids are made for the food flavor market. Glutamic acid is incorporated into the flavor-enhancer monosodium glutamate (MSG), and aspartic acid and phenylalanine are combined to form the artificial sweetener called aspartame.

Physiologists–Digestion and Absorption

Plants and animals use the 20 different amino acids to manufacture specific proteins for various activities. Plant and animal foods have few naturally free amino acids (those not joined together by a peptide bond), so the chains of amino acids in proteins must be broken in the digestive system. The free amino acids can then be absorbed into the blood to be transported to every cell in the body. Figure 8-11 shows what happens to dietary protein.

Digestion

Proteins are broken into individual amino acids or into di- or tripeptides by enzymatic hydrolysis. Some of this occurs in the acidic medium of the stomach, with *pepsin* playing an important part. Digestion of the remaining protein fragments and absorption of the resulting amino acids occurs in the small intestine. Di- and tripeptides are broken into individual amino acids as they cross into the blood through the wall of the intestine. All amino acids in the blood are free and are taken to the liver, where one of three things can happen to them.

1. They may form part of the amino acid pool in the liver (Figure 8-11a). This pool is not very large. It is used if amino acids must be exported from the liver to other tissues such as muscles, kidneys, and pancreas.

2. They may be used to synthesize proteins (Figure 8-11b). Some of these proteins are used by the liver; others are exported to the tissues. For example, the liver synthesizes the protein albumin and other blood proteins for export to the blood.

3. Excess amino acids are broken down by the liver (Figure 8-11c). The amino (NH_2) group, when released from an amino acid, is transferred to form part of the nitrogen-containing chemical called *urea*. It is taken by the blood to the kidney and is excreted in the urine. This is an important mechanism for getting rid of unwanted nitrogen, which could be toxic to the body if not excreted. The carbon skeleton from the dismantled amino acid is used to synthesize glucose or fatty acids. The liver can store the glucose as glycogen and the fatty acids as triglycerides.

The digestion of protein has important nutritional implications. First, severe undernutrition interferes with the digestion and absorption of proteins. Second, there are circumstances in which the function of a specific protein (such as the hormone insulin) is not maintained when it is ingested and passed through the digestive system. If insulin is taken orally, its structure is broken in digestion, thereby depriving it of all hormonal activity. The body then uses the amino acids from insulin in the same way as those from other dietary proteins–it synthesizes them into one or more of the hundreds of different proteins in the body. Therefore, some diabetics must inject insulin directly into the blood.

Pepsin: An enzyme secreted in the stomach to digest dietary proteins.

Urea: Waste nitrogen excreted in the urine. Formed by the liver and excreted by the kidneys.

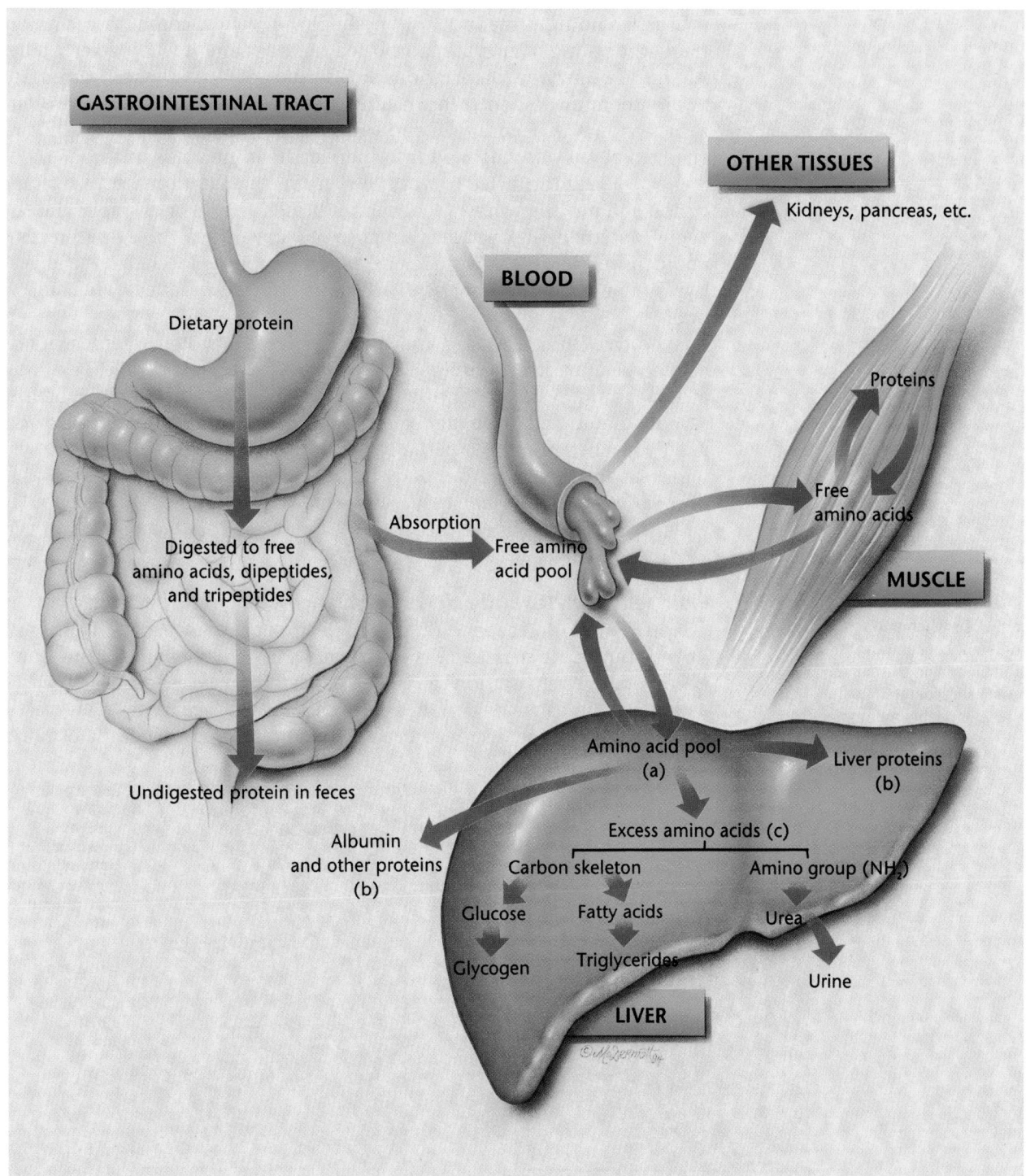

Figure 8-11. Metabolism of protein. Dietary proteins are digested in the gastrointestinal tract, and the amino acids are absorbed into the blood. There they form a pool of free amino acids (amino acids that are not joined by peptide bonds). The blood distributes free amino acids to all tissues, especially muscles, where they are built up into proteins. The liver has a free amino acid pool (a), which can be converted into liver proteins (b) or made into albumin and other proteins and exported to the blood (b). Excess amino acids have their carbon portion converted into glucose or fatty acids, and the amino group (NH_2) is converted into urea for excretion in the urine (c).

Understanding protein digestion should prevent a common consumer fraud–the selling of enzymes purported to be of benefit when taken orally. After these enzyme preparations are swallowed, exactly the same fate awaits them as described for insulin. The shape and size of the two enzymes shown in Figure 8-3, and of any other enzyme taken orally, are changed as they are digested into individual amino acids in the GI tract. Some people are attracted to worthless enzyme preparations because of nutrition and health promises that cannot be delivered. For example, the enzyme superoxide dismutase is supposed to slow down the aging process, and pepsin and other digestive enzymes are supposed to help your digestive system, but none of these will have any special effect when taken orally.

Hydrolyzed proteins, also known as predigested proteins, represent another type of worthless commercial preparation for most people. Let's look at how an impressive scientific term misleads some consumers. Proteins, carbohydrates, and lipids are hydrolyzed during normal digestion. Do you need your dietary protein partially hydrolyzed to "save" the digestive system wear and tear? No. Your body hydrolyzes protein when needed and it does so at no additional cost! The term "hydrolyzed" became popular when hydrolyzed protein was used in some weight-reducing diets in the 1970s and 1980s.

Osmotic pressure: Pressure that develops when two solutions of different concentrations (such as the blood and the extracellular fluid) are separated by a semipermeable membrane (such as the wall of the blood vessel).

Fluid, electrolyte, and acid-base balance

Proteins help to regulate fluid and electrolyte balance in body tissues. This is important because cells must have a certain level of fluid to function properly. Dehydration causes cell damage, and excess fluid also causes a problem. Fluids are held in the cells by *osmotic pressure*. When the level of protein in the blood decreases because of a protein-poor diet, the osmotic

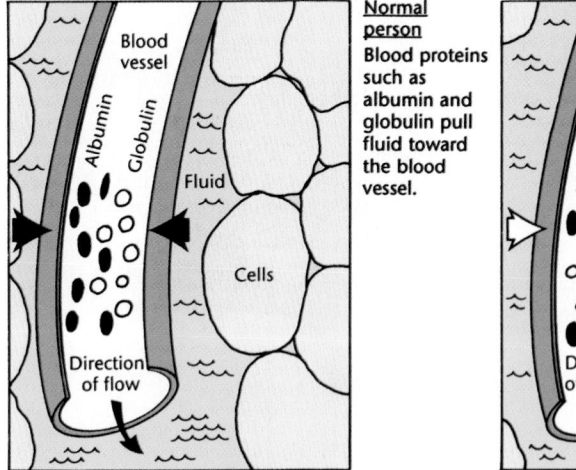
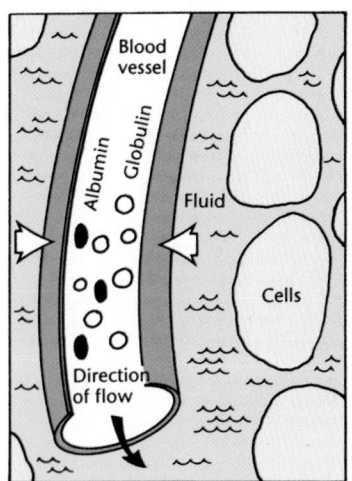

Figure 8-12. Fluid behavior in a normal person (left) and a person with edema (right). In a healthy person, osmotic pressure pulls fluid from the extracellular space into the blood vessel. Severe undernutrition may reduce the level of the blood protein albumin. This decreases the osmotic pressure, and so fluid is not pulled toward the blood vessel. It accumulates in the extracellular space, resulting in edema.

pressure also decreases, resulting in the accumulation of fluid that is called edema (Figure 8-12). Children with certain types of protein-energy malnutrition exhibit edema, especially in the arms, legs, and face (see Figure 5-8). It disappears when protein intake is improved.

Electrolyte balance is maintained in part by cell proteins. Sodium is kept outside of cells in the extracellular space, while potassium stays within cells. This balance is important for the functioning of nerves and muscles (including heart muscle), and for the integrity of red blood cells. Proteins also act as buffers to maintain the acid-base balance (see Chapter 5) and keep the pH at the proper level. Inactivation of enzymes caused by wide swings in pH within cells could be fatal.

Biochemists–Studying the Link Between Protein Metabolism and Nutrition

Body proteins include all enzymes, some hormones (such as insulin), antibodies, and proteins with other chemicals joined to them such as hemoglobin and myoglobin. Biochemists study the metabolic pathways by which body proteins are synthesized and broken down. The diagrams in Figure 8-13 show the metabolic pathways used by the body in dealing with amino acids between meals, after an overnight fast, or when food intake is severely reduced because of prolonged starvation from famine, an eating disorder, a severe weight-loss diet, or cancer and other illnesses.

Between meals, tissues such as the brain and liver rely mainly on glucose for energy. In addition, fat stored in adipose tissue provides free fatty acids to the liver and muscles to be broken down for energy (Figure 8-13A). In this way, the body's stores of carbohydrate and fat are said to have a "sparing effect" on body protein and amino acids–they do not have to be used for energy. When you wake up in the morning, some free amino acids in your muscles were used for energy during the overnight fast (Figure 8-13B). However, this has no negative effect on muscle mass or function. It is only in extreme weight loss resulting from famine, severe illness, severe dieting, or eating disorders that significant amounts of amino acids are used for energy. In these situations, most of the energy reserves in the form of carbohydrate and fat have been used up, and the body turns to amino acids as the last resort for an energy supply (Figure 8-13C). Muscle proteins then provide amino acids to be broken down for energy. This explains why individuals with severe weight loss have lost much of their muscle mass and look like skin and bone.

The elimination of carbon dioxide and water when lipids and carbohydrates are broken down for energy presents no difficulty to the body, whereas elimination of the nitrogen from amino acids when proteins are used for energy requires an additional step. The nitrogen is used in the creation of water-soluble compounds, such as urea, which are then excreted in the urine.

In summary, proteins and amino acids are not primary energy sources and are spared so they may be involved in many vital body functions. Lipids are the most efficient energy source.

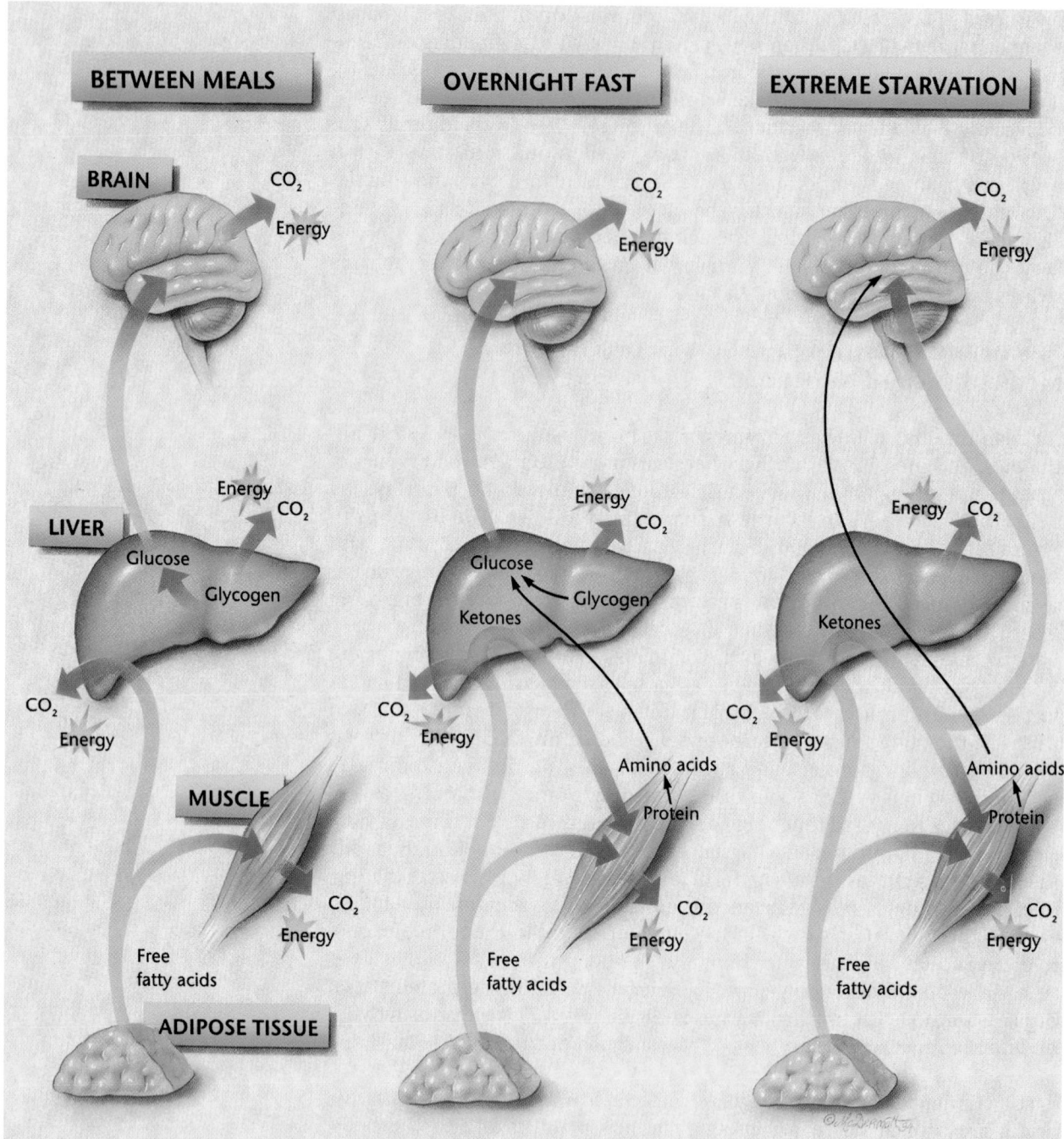

Figure 8-13. Biochemical metabolism of protein during times of no food intake. A, between meals, stored glucose and fat provide energy to muscles and brain. B, during the overnight fast, some amino acids in muscles are converted to glucose to be used for energy, especially by the brain. C, in cases of extreme starvation, much amino acid is used from the muscles, especially to fuel the brain.

Nutritionists, Dietitians, and Famine Relief Workers–Studying Body Needs for Quantity and Quality of Dietary Protein

Nutritionists are interested in the amount of essential and nonessential amino acids needed by the body at various stages of the life cycle. We know that protein is in every cell in the body; thus, it is important to know how much protein is needed for the rapid growth of youth, for pregnancy and lactation, or for the elderly. Nutritionists study how protein deficiency is measured in the body and what the best dietary sources of protein are, especially for the essential amino acids. Dietitians want to know the correct amount of protein needed by people with various illnesses and for health maintenance. For example, people recovering from surgery or from severe burns require increased protein intake to replace the protein in lost tissues. Food aid and social workers want foods with protein of high quantity and quality that are acceptable to the recipients at the least cost.

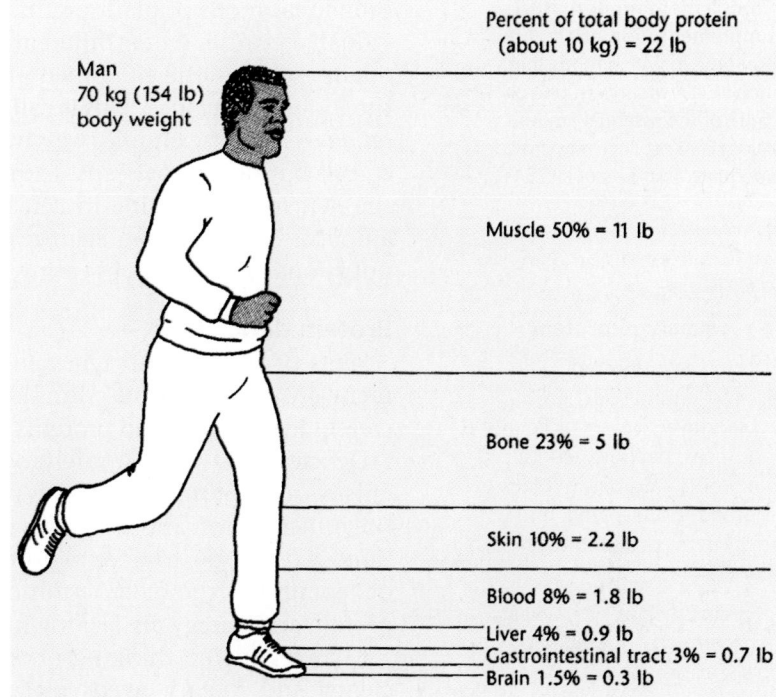

Figure 8-14. The protein content in an adult male is about 10 kilograms (about 22 pounds). Muscles have the greatest amount of protein, but all tissues have some.

Measuring protein quality

What does "high-quality protein" in a food mean? It means that the food has adequate amounts of the essential amino acids needed by the body for protein synthesis. We saw earlier that there are nine essential amino acids that cannot be synthesized by the body. The most critical of these are lysine, which is the limiting amino acid in most cereals, and methionine, which is limiting in soybeans and other plant foods. The protein quality of a food is measured by calculating the chemical score, which indicates the amount of the most limiting amino acids in comparison with a reference protein of high quality, such as those from eggs or milk. The protein quality can be tested biologically by feeding rodents the test food and measuring how these animals retain body protein and grow when compared with another group of animals fed a reference protein of high quality such as casein (a milk protein).

High-quality proteins are found in eggs, dairy products, meats, poultry, and fish. Among plants, soybeans have high-quality proteins. Average-quality protein is found in other legumes and in nuts, most grains, and vegetables. Gelatin is a poor-quality protein with a low chemical score.

In general, foods of animal origin have a higher protein quality than do

Two units of the United Nations dealing with nutrition issues–the Food and Agriculture Organization (FAO) and the World Health Organization (WHO)–issued a report in 1990 showing why adequate dietary intakes of essential amino acids (EAAs) by infants are critical. Infants require EAAs for growth and maintenance, whereas adult requirements are for maintenance only. Infants require 4.1 times more lysine, 2.5 times more methionine plus cystine, and 3.4 times more tryptophan than adults do.

Complementing or mutual supplementation effect: An outcome in which foods that individually are low in one or more of the essential amino acids (EEAs) collectively provide adequate amounts of all EEAs.

To improve the quality of protein:

combine
legumes such as black-eyed peas, chickpeas, peas, peanuts, lentils, sprouts, and beans (black, broad, kidney, lima, mung, navy, pea, and soy)

with
grains such as rice, wheat, corn, rye, bulgur, oats, millet, barley, and buckwheat.

Kwashiorkor: A form of malnutrition in infants caused by severe deficiency of protein associated with inadequate intake of energy. Symptoms include poor growth, edema, wasting of muscles, and mental apathy.

individual foods of plant origin. The emphasis here is on the word "individual" because, when different foods of plant origin are combined, the quality score of the combined proteins may be much higher than each of the individual values. This is called the *complementing or mutual supplementation effect*. For example, we saw that lysine is the limiting amino acid in cereals but not in soybeans. Eating cereals and soy on the same day allows the deficiency of lysine in cereals to be complemented by the adequate amounts of this amino acid in soybeans. This is another example of the nutritional advantages in eating a widely varied diet.

Protein deficiency

Signs of protein deficiency include stunting of growth, poor development of muscle, edema, thin and fragile hair, poor skin quality, and decreases in certain blood proteins.

Deficiency of protein rarely occurs without deficiencies of other nutrients because protein-rich foods are usually high in other nutrients such as the minerals iron and zinc. This is why the term "protein-energy malnutrition" is used now to refer to protein-poor diets ("calorie" was used instead of "energy" in the older terminology). It acknowledges the fact that both protein and energy are lacking in the diet.

Changes in the thinking of experts over the years about protein deficiency and dietary needs present a useful demonstration of how our knowledge of nutrition is modified as new information becomes available. Early knowledge of severe protein deficiency in people was provided by the pioneering work of Dr. Cecily Williams in West Africa in the 1930s. She documented the disease known as *kwashiorkor*, a form of malnutrition that was thought to result simply from lack of adequate protein. (See Figure 5-8, which shows edema, one symptom of kwashiorkor.) Between World War II and the early 1960s, high protein intake was emphasized as being beneficial to health. Since the 1970s, it has become apparent that, in severe malnutrition, dietary energy is the most limiting component. Relief efforts should concentrate on providing adequate energy intake first, followed by appropriate amounts of protein. Even kwashiorkor now is seen as the result of protein deficiency in conjunction with inadequate intake of energy.

Research in India showed that some young children had diets adequate in protein but low in energy. When their calorie gap was bridged with supplemental energy from carbohydrate and fat sources such as wheat flour, sugar, and edible oil, but with little or no additional protein, growth of these children resumed and deficiency symptoms disappeared.[11]

Recommended intake

The amounts of protein thought to be needed for growth, maintenance, and repair of tissue have been revised many times since the early 1900s.[12] Earlier recommended intake levels of dietary protein were much higher than those recommended today. Back then, not all of the essential amino acids had been discovered; the interrelationships among protein, carbohydrates, and lipids were not as well understood; and even scientists were impressed with the fact that the most productive and prosperous people were those who ate the most protein.[12] Most attention is now given to understanding dietary requirements of the elderly, especially people over 75 years of age.[13] Recommended levels of protein intake are given in the RDA table on the inside back cover of this book.

The RDA of protein for adult men and women is based on the formula of 0.8 grams of dietary protein per kilogram of body weight per day. Here's how to calculate your own RDA for protein:

- Convert your body weight from pounds into kilograms (pounds ÷ 2.2 = kilograms)

- Multiply the result by 0.8 (the recommended protein intake for adults is 0.8 grams of protein per kilogram of body weight per day). This conversion factor applies to young adult men and women.

- Compare your answer with values for your age group in the RDA table inside the back cover of this book. RDA values in the table are based on "reference" men and women with body weights of 70 and 56 kilograms, respectively. If your answer differs from the value in the RDA table, it is because your body weight is different from the "reference" weight.

Nitrogen balance

RDA values for protein are derived from *nitrogen balance* studies made on people. This method relies on the fact that all amino acids, and thus all proteins, contain nitrogen. Chemically it is difficult to measure protein and amino acids in the body but relatively easier to measure nitrogen. Amino nitrogen accounts for about 16% of the weight of proteins. Nutritionists therefore measure the amount of nitrogen in the body and multiply the answer by 6.25 (100 ÷ 16 = 6.25). A nitrogen balance study is done by measuring the nitrogen intake in food as well as the nitrogen loss. Loss in nitrogen consists of the end products of protein metabolism that are excreted in urine and sweat, plus the nitrogen in the feces resulting from nitrogen unabsorbed from the diet and dead cells from the GI tract. Other sources of nitrogen loss include cut hair and nails and the dead cells from skin and elsewhere.

Nitrogen balance studies are usually done over a 7-day period. Values change in the following situations:

- **Positive nitrogen balance:** Nitrogen intake is greater than nitrogen loss from the body. This occurs during growth and regeneration and is observed in infants, children, during pregnancy and lactation, and in recovery from starvation, burns, and severe illness.

- **Negative nitrogen balance:** Nitrogen intake is less than nitrogen loss. It occurs when people are on restrictive weight-loss diets (800 calories per day or less), are starving, suffer from anorexia nervosa, have been bedridden for long periods, or have major injuries, burns, or terminal cancer.

- **Nitrogen equilibrium:** When nitrogen intake is the same as nitrogen loss from the body, the person is said to be in nitrogen equilibrium,

Nitrogen balance: The difference between the intake of nitrogen as dietary protein and the excretion of nitrogen as urea and other waste nitrogen compounds. May be positive, negative, or in equilibrium.

Table 8-2. Digestibility of Animal and Plant Proteins

Protein Source	Digestibility (%)
Eggs	97
Wheat, refined (white flour)	96
Milk and cheese	95
Peanut butter	95
Meat and fish	94
Rice, polished	88
Wheat, whole	86
Oatmeal	86
Corn (maize)	85
Beans	78
Mixed U.S. diet	96

Cross-linking: Formation of bonds between amino acids in adjacent peptide chains.

which is the case in healthy, nonpregnant, nonlactating adults consuming a balanced diet.

Protein intake by most Americans is adequate; 14–18% of total dietary calories comes from protein, and foods of animal origin contribute about 65% of dietary protein.

Digestibility

Not all dietary protein is digested to the same extent. Differences in digestibility are due to intrinsic differences in the food proteins, including how the chains of amino acids are arranged. Tightly coiled protein molecules are more difficult to digest than are those with a more open structure that digestive enzymes can attack more easily. Cell walls around the protein in the cell may be difficult to digest. Other factors such as dietary fiber may modify protein digestion. Amino acids in foods may be *cross-linked* by certain chemical reactions, thus making the amino acid less available.

Think beyond the photograph in Figure 8-15. Why experiment with beans?

We have just seen that beans have lower digestibility than other protein-rich foods. Although the combination of essential amino acids in bean protein is good, the lower digestibility decreases their impact as a food when protein intake is marginal, especially for children. Food scientists are working with nutritionists to devise ways to improve the digestibility and palatability of beans. Think of the lower cost and greater ease of transportation and storage afforded by beans than by protein-rich foods of animal origin. Improvement of bean digestibility would make a positive impact on the availability of protein for many people.

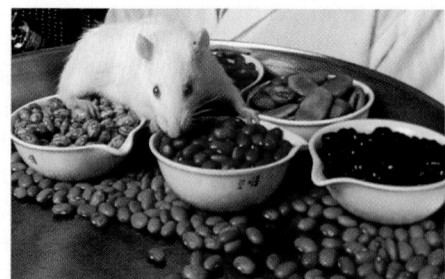

Figure 8-15. Beans are a good source of dietary protein, but humans and animals have difficulty in digesting all of the proteins in beans.

No increases in the RDA for protein are made for the stresses encountered in daily living. However, extreme environmental or physiological stresses increase nitrogen loss from the body. Surgical stress, fevers, infections, and burns result in increased loss of nitrogen through the urine, and increased dietary protein intake is needed to replace this loss. The amount of protein and the amino acid composition of the protein in premature infants also must be monitored carefully.

No known health problems arise from protein intake that is moderately above requirements, but evidence from animal studies suggests that high dietary protein intake may damage the kidneys. The National Research Council (NRC) suggests that it is prudent to maintain an upper limit at twice the RDA for protein.

Sports Physiologists–No Strong Evidence That Protein or Amino Acids Give Competitive Advantage

An adequate dietary protein intake as part of a balanced diet is essential for optimal athletic performance. Additional amino acid supplements do not make physiological or biochemical sense because the excess amino acids will be stored as fat or used for energy rather than for increasing muscle mass. However, this does not seem to prevent amino acids from being the most frequently advertised nutritional supplement in health and bodybuilding magazines![14]

Scientists are examining claims by Olympic-level athletes that a nitrogen-containing chemical called *creatine* suppresses fatigue.[15] Creatine is found in high concentration in meat. It is supposed to help transport extra energy to muscle to allow muscle proteins to continue contracting. Some evidence suggests that performance could be raised by 1–4%. This may be significant in some fast events where a few hundredths of a second can mean the difference between a gold medal and fourth place.

Creatine: A nitrogen-containing compound; an essential part of the energy release system of muscle. Present in meat and some soups.

Virologists and Immunologists–Proteins Are Important in Viruses and in the Immune System

Think beyond the picture in Figure 8-16.

You are looking at the good, the bad, and the ugly among proteins. The good protein is in the blue-colored cell. The bad and the ugly protein is in the yellow-colored AIDS virus. Viruses are described as "a piece of bad news wrapped in protein" because no known virus helps humankind. They are up to 100 times smaller than bacteria, are surrounded by a protein envelope, and cause many diseases in plants, animals, and people. Most people encounter a viral attack sometime during their lives because measles, the common cold, smallpox, poliomyelitis, *hepatitis*, and the majority of infections in the upper respiratory tract are caused by viruses. Among the problems faced by a person with the AIDS virus are problems with nutrition, including the loss of appetite and the wasting of the body. Further details on the impact of AIDS on nutrition is given in Chapter 14.

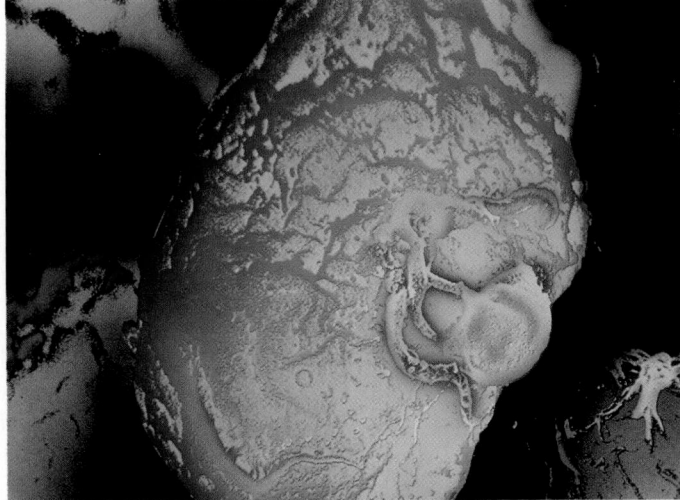

Figure 8-16. The AIDS virus and other viruses contain proteins. An AIDS virus is seen here budding from a normal cell.

Hepatitis: Inflammation of the liver caused by a virus.

Nutritional immunology or immunonutrition is a newly recognized subdiscipline.[16] Malnutrition suppresses the immune system, which increases a person's risk of getting infectious diseases such as measles, typhoid fever, or malaria. Since earliest times, people have known that many deaths during famines are due to epidemics and not to the lack of food *per se*. For example, measles in a community in an industrialized country usually causes only slight inconvenience and a few days lost from school for the children. In developing countries, in times when protein intake is low, measles is a common cause of death. Epidemiologic studies confirm that infection with malnutrition is a major cause of illness and death in developing countries, especially among children.[17] Famine relief in Somalia in 1993 prompted a report by U.S. military physicians outlining the consequences of infectious diseases in that country.[18] They stressed that children at refugee camps were malnourished and at risk of viral diseases such as measles. The elderly in all countries are more prone to infections, in part because of decreased functioning of the immune system.

Immune function is decreased when diets are deficient in iron and vitamin A, which often happens when the diets are deficient in protein. When iron-deficient individuals receive iron supplements, the severity of infection decreases. The risk of death from measles is reduced considerably when supplementary vitamin A is given to malnourished children.[19]

Microbiologists–Will Proteins from Microbes Solve the World's Protein Supply Problems?

Whether microbes can solve the protein supply problem in the human diet is a question that has been asked since the 1940s, and the answer is both "yes" and "no."[3] Yeast is a microbe that can form a nutritious food and can be grown on molasses, a waste product of sugar refining. After being harvested and dried, the resulting product has a pleasant toasted, meaty flavor. However, people in the parts of the world most in need of increasing their dietary protein intake would not accept it as a food. Yeast will also grow on petroleum, and the nasty taste in the resulting product can be removed. It has been suggested that diverting 3% of the world's oil production to produce yeast could double the world's protein supply.[3] Other protein-yielding microbes can be grown on syrup prepared from cereal starch or on natural gas. Proteins from these sources have been fed to cattle and to fish, thereby increasing protein yield from foods that are more acceptable to individuals. *Algae* such as *Chlorella* use sunlight and carbon dioxide for growth. They have a high yield per acre of a protein that is said to taste like fishy spinach. *Spirulina* grows in salty lakes, is harvested easily, and can be dried in the sun and eaten as a cookie.

So why are we not eating more protein from microbes? Most businesses are not enthusiastic because they feel people are not ready to accept protein from microbes. In addition, sophisticated technology is needed to produce and harvest them, and removal of water at the industrial production level requires technology that is both expensive and energy-consuming. Our last words on protein from microbes are quoted from an eminent microbiologist, John Postgate:

> Microbes are already established constituents of animal feeds; it is probably just a matter of time before microbes become an accepted part of the diets of ordinary people.[3]

Algae: A class of mainly aquatic plants that includes seaweeds. Derivatives of algae hold water and are used by the food industry as thickeners, stabilizers, and gelling agents.

Toxicologists–Contamination of Some Amino Acid Supplements Can Be Deadly

During the summer and fall of 1989, a mysterious illness involving muscle pain, fatigue, weakness, headache, and fever spread throughout the United States. A further symptom was eosinophilia, which is a high concentration of eosinophils (certain cells in the blood), resulting in the term *eosinophilia-myalgia syndrome (EMS)* for this condition. At least 38 deaths from heart, lung, and nerve complications resulted. Eventually it was discovered that the people had taken supplements of L-tryptophan manufactured by a particular company.[20] As a result, the FDA forced a recall on all dietary supplements of L-tryptophan; impurities in the L-tryptophan were suspected. The problem was first discovered in New Mexico, where some physicians and an alert reporter for the *Albuquerque Journal* brought the problem rapidly to public attention. The reporter won a Pulitzer Prize for his part in tracing the problem to L-tryptophan.

Tryptophan is an essential amino acid, but the animal protein in a normal American diet supplies twice the amount needed. *Vegans* can get sufficient amounts by taking plant proteins from a variety of sources.[21] Contamination of free tryptophan could be a significant problem because it is used as a drug or as a food additive in infant formulas and medical foods. Some people self-prescribe tryptophan to help themselves sleep because of its mild hypnotic effect.[22]

The following example shows how toxic levels of a normally nontoxic amino acid can build up in the body because of a defect in the functioning of one enzyme. Phenylketonuria (PKU) is a genetic disease caused by failure of the appropriate enzyme to convert the amino acid phenylalanine into the amino acid tyrosine. Dangerous levels of phenylalanine accumulate in the blood, and if PKU is not treated early, brain damage and mental retardation may occur. Early screening of infants for PKU is considered one of the successes of modern medicine.[23] Dietary treatment is by a combination of protein restriction and an amino acid supplement that contains extra tyrosine and all the essential amino acids except phenylalanine. PKU patients have generally been removed from the diet at eight years of age. The latest guidelines suggest that this dietary treatment should continue beyond eight for as long as possible, despite difficulties with compliance. Women with PKU must return to a strict diet before they become pregnant.[23] People who have PKU are advised of high phenylalanine content by special warnings on food labels. For example, diet drinks with the sweetener aspartame have this warning–Phenylketonurics: Contains phenylalanine.

Eosinophilia-myalgia syndrome (EMS): A blood disorder caused by suspected contamination of supplements of L-tryptophan. Caused muscle pain, fatigue, weakness, headache, fever, and death in a number of people.

Vegans: People who consume no foods of animal origin, as contrasted with vegetarians, who often consume dairy products and eggs.

Allergists–Allergic Reactions May Occur When Intact Proteins Are Absorbed from the GI Tract

Certain intact proteins may escape digestion in the GI tract and be absorbed into the blood, where the body considers them to be foreign proteins. Normally, intact proteins and peptides in the blood are eliminated from the body through the action of the immune system.[24] Our blood has antibodies to a wide range of dietary proteins. Antibodies are even secreted into the GI tract, thus ensuring that no intact proteins or large peptides enter the blood. Unfortunately, this system breaks down for a few people, and an allergic reaction to the foreign protein is set up. This is most likely to occur in infants, because the GI tract is not fully developed.

Allergic reactions to eggs, milk, soybean, and wheat are known. Reports from Japan indicate increasing incidence of rice-associated allergy.[25] To counteract this problem, a hypoallergenic rice in grain form has been created with almost all allergenic proteins removed. It retains half or more of the principal rice seed protein. Skin problems caused by the allergy are improved or eliminated when allergic people switch to hypoallergenic rice. This has significant nutritional implications for people who depend on a large intake of rice.[25]

Psychologists–Do Proteins Influence Behavior?

Neurotransmitters: Chemicals (30–40 different ones) produced in and released from nerves that influence the transmission of the nerve impulse.

Serotonin: An important neurotransmitter in the brain; made from the amino acid tryptophan.

Neurons: Nerve cells; involved in the transmission of nerve impulses.

Two areas of nutrition that interact with developmental and behavioral psychology are the effect of protein-energy malnutrition on brain development and the influence of amino acids on *neurotransmitters*, especially *serotonin*.

Protein-energy malnutrition has negative effects on brain development, resulting in decreased number and size of *neurons* and reduced production of neurotransmitters.[26] The brain is most vulnerable to malnutrition during periods of maximum growth in late pregnancy and in the first few months after birth. Researchers are wrestling with the question of whether the negative effect on the brain and on intellectual development is caused by a deficiency of protein, deficiencies of other nutrients in the diet, or the presence of disease and the lack of support systems encouraging development.

Neurotransmitters are affected by some diets deficient in amino acids.[26] The essential amino acid tryptophan is required to make the neurotransmitter serotonin (5-hydroxytryptamine or 5-HT). Tryptophan is in highest concentration in eggs, soybeans, milk, oatmeal, and meat. High serotonin levels induce sleep, and high-carbohydrate diets increase serotonin levels. People are sleepier after a high-carbohydrate meal than after a high-protein meal irrespective of whether it is breakfast or lunch. This seems odd because the high-protein meal would have more tryptophan than the high-carbohydrate meal. Biochemists provide an explanation. Nutrients must pass the blood-brain barrier, which controls the entry of all chemicals from the blood to the brain. This entry is selective–some nutrients pass more easily than others. Tryptophan passes easily into the brain, where it is converted into serotonin. However, when foods high in protein are eaten along with carbohydrate, other amino acids compete with tryptophan to enter the brain, and some of the tryptophan is excluded. So less serotonin is synthesized, resulting in greater alertness.

■ People are different–Vegetarianism

Some of the most famous creative and successful people have been vegetarians–the mathematician Pythagoras, the poet Shelley, the playwright George Bernard Shaw, the political activist Ghandi, and many others. Nowadays people are vegetarians for a variety of reasons.

Vegetarian diets are healthy because of their low saturated fat and cholesterol content. Vegetarians usually live healthy lifestyles, with physical activity and little alcohol consumption or cigarette smoking. Individuals consuming an uncooked vegan diet have been found to have reduced enzyme activities in fecal bacteria, which seems to reduce the risk of colon cancer.[27]

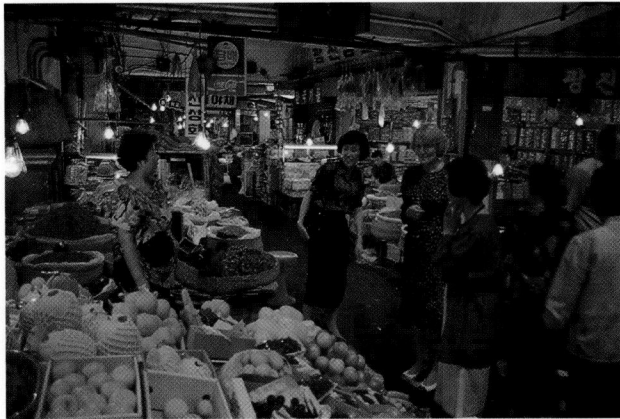

Figure 8-17. A Korean market. Great variety in plant foods is available in most markets around the world.

There are varying degrees of vegetarianism:

- semivegetarian–avoids certain types of meat, poultry, or fish.
- lacto-ovo vegetarian–eats no animal flesh but does eat eggs and dairy products.
- lacto-vegetarian–eats no animal flesh or eggs but does use dairy products.
- vegan–eats no animal flesh, eggs, or dairy products. Some vegans refuse to wear leather or woolen goods.

Vegetarians, and especially vegans, should follow the FDA recommendations on how to obtain problem nutrients.[28]

Table 8-3. Replacement of Animal Sources of Nutrients for Vegetarian Diets

Nutrients Most Likely to Be Lacking	Non-Animal Replacements
Vitamin B-12	Fortified soy milk and cereals
Vitamin D	Fortified margarine, sunshine
Calcium	Tofu, broccoli, seeds, nuts, kale, bok choy, legumes (peas and beans), greens, calcium-enriched grain products, lime-processed tortillas
Iron[a]	Legumes, tofu, green leafy vegetables, dried fruit, whole grains, iron-fortified cereals and breads, especially whole wheat
Zinc	Whole grains (especially the germ and bran), whole wheat bread, legumes, nuts, tofu
Protein	A variety of nuts, vegetables, and grains

[a] Absorption of iron is improved by vitamin C, which is found in citrus fruits and juices, tomatoes, strawberries, broccoli, peppers, dark-green leafy vegetables, and potatoes with skins.

The American Dietetic Association has the following recommendations for vegetarians:

- Minimize intake of less nutritious food such as sweets and fatty foods.

- Choose whole or unrefined grain products instead of refined products.

- Choose a variety of fruits and vegetables, including good sources of vitamin C to improve iron absorption.

- Choose cooked beans, tofu, soy milk, nuts, or seeds as a substitute for meat. (Nuts and seeds tend to be high in fat, so use sparingly if you are following a low-fat diet.)

- Choose low-fat varieties of milk products, if they are included in the diet.

- Avoid excessive cholesterol intake by limiting eggs to 3 or 4 yolks a week.

- For vegans, use properly fortified food sources of vitamin B-12, such as fortified soy milks or cereals, or take a cyanocobalamin supplement.

- For infants, children, and teenagers, ensure adequate intakes of calories and of iron and vitamin D, taking supplements if needed.

- Consult a registered dietitian or other qualified nutrition professional, especially during periods of growth, breast feeding, pregnancy, or recovery from illness.

- If exclusively breast feeding premature infants or babies beyond 4–6 months of age, give vitamin D and iron supplements to the child from birth or at least by 4–6 months, as your doctor suggests.

- Usually take iron and folate (folic acid) supplements during pregnancy.

Tasty vegetarian dishes can be arranged by using the full array of fruits, vegetables, grains, and herbs and by consulting the wide variety of vegetarian cookbooks available.

■ Nutrition in action–Meat, fish, freezing, and drying

North Americans have a high meat intake, with poultry increasing in popularity in recent years. This trend is in agreement with the Dietary Guidelines (Chapter 4).

Meat, poultry, and fish are excellent sources of good-quality protein, iron, zinc, and several of the B-vitamins. However, when shopping for meat products, it is important to be aware of the following nutrition facts:[29]

- Most processed meats such as frankfurters, sausages, salami, and liver sausage are generally high in fat and sodium.

- Chicken franks are high in fat.

- All ground beef/hamburger meat is high in fat.

- Organ meats such as liver, kidney, brains, heart, and sweetbreads are generally low in fat but high in cholesterol.

- Duck and goose are both high in fat.

- The sodium content is high in corned beef, dried beef, chicken and turkey rolls, clams, crab, herring, salmon, sardines, shrimp, tuna, anchovies (canned, smoked and dried), and other marine food. Some sodium can be removed by rinsing the fish before cooking.

- Breaded fish sticks and stuffed chicken breasts may have hidden fat.

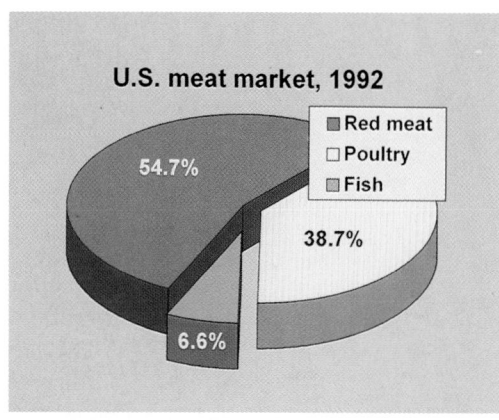

Figure 8-18. Meat, poultry, and fish are important sources of dietary protein. In the United States, sales of fish are small in relation to those of red meat and poultry.

Preparation techniques can help reduce the fat content of meats.

- Select lean cuts, trim visible fat, and cook without fat or drain fat after cooking.

- Remove the skin from poultry before cooking; this decreases the fat content by one-half.

As consumers have become more aware of fat in meat and tried to avoid it, producers have worked to reduce the fat in what they sell. Farmers may use genetic selection to grow animals with less fat. Food scientists are studying what factors produce lean meat. The amount of fat and lean is measured in carcasses to determine the influence of breed of animal, diet fed, age at slaughter, and other factors that affect the amount of fat in meat.

Incorporation of soy protein into meat products is another way in which the fat and caloric content can be reduced while traditional quality is maintained.[30]

All of the above changes in fat content in meat products are positive because of suggested correlations between meat consumption and factors that promote a healthy lifestyle, including the intake of other nutrients, even though the issue of meat consumption and health remains controversial. One study showed that individuals who ate red meat and poultry less than once per week were less likely to drink alcohol, reported more physical activity, and had diets that were higher in carbohydrates, starch, fiber, vitamins A and C, and calcium and lower in energy, fat, and protein. They also had lower body size and lower concentrations of total serum cholesterol, LDL, and triglycerides compared with individuals who consumed meat frequently.[31]

Storage and delivery of meat, poultry, and fish

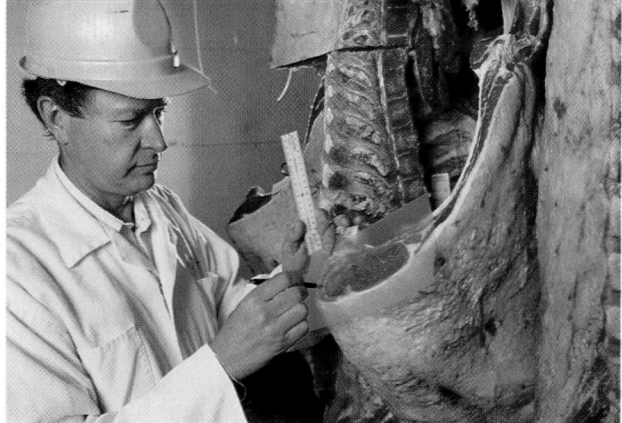

Figure 8-19. Packing company inspectors monitor the amount of lean meat (which is high in protein) to ensure that the consumer demand for more lean and less fat is met.

are difficult because of their high water content, which leads to a high ability to spoil quickly. Dried meat and fish have not been popular on a wide scale, leaving freezing as the main means of storing meats and fish.

Freezing food slows down, but does not stop, the physical and chemical reactions involved in the deterioration of food. Consumers perceive frozen food as having sensory and nutritional qualities superior to those of food preserved by other methods.[32] To achieve this high quality, the food must undergo careful pre-freezing preparation, control of the freezing process, and appropriate storage of the frozen product. Rapid freezing is the method of choice, but this is the most expensive form of freezing food.

This discussion of freezing relates to nutrition in many respects. Consumers get the high-protein foods they want, and the nutritional value is maintained. Freezing does present the problems of storage and transportation in low-income populations. In times of famine, meat is rarely used to supplement diets. Difficulties in maintaining raw meat without spoiling and the high cost of dehydration are reasons why dried milk rather than dried meat is used in famine relief.

■ Now you know

- Protein is in every living cell.

- It is the limiting nutrient in many peoples' diets, especially in developing countries.

- Proteins are needed for growth and maintenance, for regulation of cell function, and as an emergency source of energy.

- Proteins are composed of amino acids, which are joined by peptide bonds. All amino acids contain the amino group (NH_2).

- DNA controls the unique sequence of amino acids in each protein.

- Production of more food protein is influenced by genetics, biotechnology, and genetic engineering and by people's opinions about the use of farm animals for food.

- Geneticists and biotechnologists have increased the quantity and quality of protein in some crops and animals.

- Production of animal protein may involve environmental costs unless proper waste management is implemented.

- Food scientists make use of enzymes and physical changes in proteins to improve food properties. Some amino acids and dipeptides are used for their flavor properties.

- Since protein-rich foods can be expensive, intake by the poor, elderly, and homeless may be low.

- Understanding protein digestion helps consumers avoid being duped by preparations such as protein hydrolysates and partially digested protein.

- Body proteins are needed for acid-base balance and for fluid and electrolyte balance.

- Carbohydrates and lipids in the body have a sparing effect on body proteins during energy deficits.

- Proteins from a single animal source have the optimum combination of essential amino acids; combinations of plant protein sources produce the same result.

- Protein deficiency is usually seen in combination with deficiencies of other nutrients.

- The protein RDA for adult men and women in the United States is based on 0.8 grams of dietary protein per kilogram of body weight per day.

- Nitrogen balance measures the difference between the intake and loss of nitrogen. Nitrogen balance is positive during growth, negative during tissue wasting, and in equilibrium when adults consume a balanced diet.

- The average American diet gets two-thirds of its protein from animal sources and one-third from plants.

- Digestibility of food proteins varies, with eggs being among the most digestible and beans among the least.

- Proteins and amino acids offer little if any competitive advantage to athletes.

- Antibodies are proteins, and viruses have a coating made of protein. Severe protein deficiency reduces antibodies, thus increasing death from infections.

- Protein from microbial sources may be important for an increasing global population.

- Contaminants in supplements of the amino acid L-tryptophan caused a number of deaths.

- Phenylketonuria (PKU) causes brain damage and mental retardation if phenylalanine-free diets are not consumed.

- Absorption of intact proteins into the blood may set up an allergic reaction.

- Protein-energy malnutrition has negative effects on brain growth.

- The neurotransmitter serotonin is made from tryptophan and induces sleep. Meals high in protein lead to greater alertness than do high-carbohydrate meals.

- Vegetarian diets are healthy, provided a wide variety of food is consumed.

Further Reading

1. Guthrie, J. F., and Raper, N. Animal products: Their contribution to a balanced diet. *Food Review* 15(1):29, 1993.

2. Goodsell, D. S., and Olson, A. J. Soluble proteins: Size, shape and function. *Trends in Biochemical Sciences,* page 65, March 1993.

3. Postgate, J. *Microbes and Man*, 3rd edition. Cambridge University Press, Cambridge, England, 1992.

4. Wunderlich, G. The ethics of animal agriculture. *Food Review* 14(4):24, 1991.

5. Perutz, M. F. *Is Science Necessary? Essays on Science and Scientists*. Oxford University Press, Oxford, England, 1991.

6. Webster, J. Animal genetics–Of pigs, oncomice and men. *Trends in Biotechnology* 11(1):1, 1993.

7. Sanders, M. E., and others. Research needs in biotechnology. *Food Technology* 47(3):18S, 1993.

8. Penet, C. S. New applications of industrial food enzymology: Economics and processes. *Food Technology* 45(1):98, 1991.

9. Abelson, P. H. Expanding the uses of enzymes. *Science* 259:1675, 1993.

10. Friedman, M. Dietary impact of food processing. *Annual Review of Nutrition* 12:119, 1992.

11. Gopalan, C. The contribution of nutrition research to the control of undernutrition: The Indian experience. *Annual Review of Nutrition* 12:1, 1992.

12. Carpenter, K. J. Protein requirements of adults from an evolutionary perspective. *American Journal of Clinical Nutrition* 55:913, 1992.

13. Jackson, A. A. Chronic undernutrition: Protein metabolism. *Proceedings of the Nutrition Society* 52:1, 1993.

14. Philen, R. M. Survey of advertising for nutritional supplements in health and bodybuilding magazines. *Journal of the American Medical Association* 268:1008, 1992.

15. Coghlan, A. Meat extract keeps athletes' muscles working. *New Scientist,* page 7, August 8, 1992.

16. Beisel, W. R. History of nutritional immunology: Introduction and overview. *Journal of Nutrition* 122:591, 1992.

17. Chandra, R. K. Protein-energy malnutrition and immunological responses. *Journal of Nutrition* 122:597, 1992.

18. Heppner, D. G., and others. The threat of infectious diseases in Somalia. *New England Journal of Medicine* 328:1061, 1993.

19. Scrimshaw, N. S. The challenge of global malnutrition to the food industry. *Food Technology* 47(2):60, 1993.

20. Nightingale, S. L. Update on EMS and L-tryptophan. *Journal of the American Medical Association* 268:1828, 1992.

21. Herbert, V. L-tryptophan. A medicolegal case against over-the-counter marketing of supplements of amino acids. *Nutrition Today* 27(2):27, 1992.

22. Steinberg, L. A., and others. Tryptophan intake influences infants' sleep latency. *Journal of Nutrition* 122:1781, 1992.

23. Anonymous. Phenylketonuria grows up. *Lancet* 337:1256, 1991.

24. Mills, E. N. C., and others. Biochemical interactions of food-derived peptides. *Trends in Food Science and Technology* 3:64, 1992.

25. Watanabe, M. Hypoallergenic rice as a physiologically functional food. *Trends in Food Science and Technology* 4:125, 1993.

26. Venero, J. L., and others. Changes in neurotransmitter levels associated with the deficiency of some essential amino acids in the diet. *British Journal of Nutrition* 68:409, 1992.

27. Ling, W. H., and Hanninen, O. Shifting from a conventional diet to an un-

cooked vegan diet reversibly alters fecal hydrolytic activities in humans. *Journal of Nutrition* 122:924, 1992.

28. Farley, D. Vegetarian diets. The pluses and the pitfalls. *FDA Consumer* 26(4):20, 1992.

29. Finn, S., and Kass, L. S. *The Real Life Nutrition Book*. Penguin Books, New York, page 94, 1992.

30. McMindes, M. K. Applications of isolated soy protein in low-fat meat products. *Food Technology* 45(12):61, 1991.

31. Slattery, M. L., and others. Meat consumption and its associations with other diet and health factors in young adults: The CARDIA study. *American Journal of Clinical Nutrition* 54:930, 1991.

32. George, R. M. Freezing processes used in the food industry. *Trends in Food Science and Technology* 4:134, 1993.

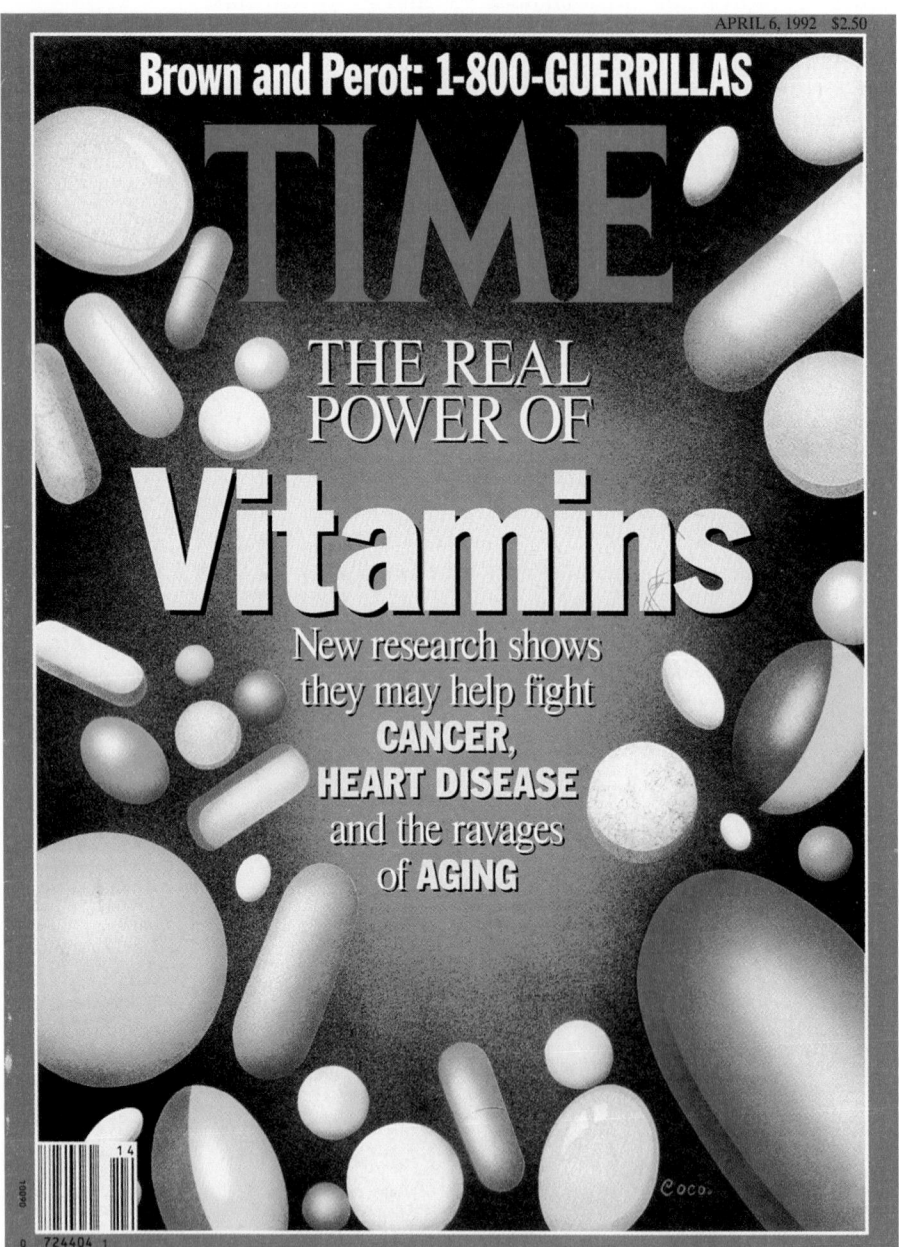

Figure 9-1. Vitamins prevent deficiency symptoms, and new evidence suggests that they many prevent certain diseases. Research is ongoing to determine how they work in our bodies.

## CHAPTER 9

Vitamins–Fruits and Vegetables

■ Vitamins in your life– How much is enough?

To consumers, seeing vitamins on the cover of a national news magazine adds to the importance of vitamins and even gives them celebrity status. Is this justified? There is much that scientists and the general public can be excited about concerning vitamins. Evidence suggests that vitamins assist in the fight against important killer diseases such as cancer and heart disease and help slow the aging process. We get these health benefits with adequate vitamin intake. Intakes are adequate for most people in developed countries, where the distresses caused by vitamin deficiencies in the past are now rare. We no longer worry much about deficiencies of vitamin D and poor bone formation, of vitamin C and bleeding gums, of thiamin and various nerve and blood dysfunctions.

Unfortunately, the news from many of the developing countries is not as encouraging. An international conference sponsored by the United Nations in 1992 set as its goal for the year 2000 the elimination of all nutritional deficiencies, especially of vitamin A. The statistics on vitamin A deficiency show that over 124 million children are estimated to be vitamin A deficient,[1] and up to half a million young children each year become permanently blind because of it. Yet for less than 25 cents per year for vitamin A supplements, the eyesight of a person can be saved. Vitamin A deficiency is responsible for about 40,000 deaths *every day* throughout the world, especially of children under age five. Many of these deaths occur because of decreased resistance to infections–we are learning that vitamin A acts as a protector against infections.

Contrast all of this with information presented by FDA officials showing that four out of 10 Americans use vitamin and mineral supplements regularly, spending over $2.7 billion on them. Vitamin and mineral supplements are the third largest over-the-counter category and the largest drug category of trade in the United States.[2]

Major Topics in This Chapter

Thirteen legitimate vitamins are known; many nonvitamins are sold as vitamins.

Vitamins are divided into fat-soluble vitamins (A, D, E, and K) and water-soluble vitamins (C and the B-complex).

■

Vitamin A deficiency is common in some developing countries; deficiencies of other vitamins may occur also.

Vitamins vary in their stability to heat, light, and air, which thus influence the level of vitamin intake.

Antioxidant properties of vitamins E and C and beta-carotene (related to vitamin A) may prevent coronary heart disease, cancer, and damage to the immune system.

■

Nutrition in Action— Antioxidants

Table 9-1. Vitamins and Nonvitamins

Type and Common Name	Also Known As
Fat-soluble	
Vitamin A (carotene is a precursor)	Retinol
Vitamin D (7-dehydro-cholesterol is a precursor)	Cholecalciferol (D-1), ergocalciferol (D-2)
Vitamin E	Tocopherols (alpha- tocopherol is the most active)
Vitamin K	Menadione
Water-soluble	
Vitamin C	Ascorbic acid
B-complex	
Thiamin	Vitamin B-1
Riboflavin	Vitamin B-2
Niacin (tryptophan is a precursor)	Nicotinic acid, nicotinamide, vitamin B-3
Vitamin B-6	Pyridoxine, pyridoxamine, pyridoxal
Pantothenic acid	
Biotin	
Folacin	Folic acid, folate
Vitamin B-12	Cobalamin
Nonvitamins	
Rutin	Lipoic acid
Bioflavinoids	Vitamin P
Para-amino-benzoic acid	PABA
Carnitine	Choline

Nonvitamins: Chemicals not meeting all criteria to be called vitamins but marketed as vitamins.

Laetrile: Sometimes called vitamin B-17; it is not a vitamin but was sold in the 1970s as a possible cancer treatment. Contains the poison cyanide.

The vitamins were discovered in the early 1900s. Clearly, before that time, people got their vitamins from the same place they had always gotten them and still get them–from food. So why the excitement about vitamins and vitamin supplements? Discovery of the vitamins involved brilliant science–several of their discoverers received the ultimate honor, a Nobel Prize. The impact of their discoveries on society was great–the prevention of eye, bone, blood, nerve, and other disorders. Out of legitimate applications of vitamins eventually there came more questionable claims. If you read some of the articles and advertisements on vitamin supplements, you may believe that they can cure all of the real and perceived ills of modern society. Let's look at the scientific facts about the vitamins so that we can put some of these claims into perspective.

Vitamins: Only Thirteen Legitimate Ones Exist

It is important that we establish which are the real vitamins and which are *nonvitamins*, substances that don't fit the definition of vitamins but are sold as vitamins to the public. The 13 vitamins and some nonvitamins are listed in Table 9-1.

The list of nonvitamins is probably incomplete because, unfortunately, it increases as new opportunities arise to cash in on people's health concerns. Some nonvitamins also drop from the list as the public becomes aware that they are worthless, even dangerous in many situations. For instance, *laetrile* was prominent in the 1970s as a possible cancer cure and was sold in some states as a vitamin. Its claim to cure cancer has long since been disproven. Laetrile is a cyanide-containing chemical extracted from apricot kernels. The cyanide was supposed to kill cancer cells; unfortunately it kills all cells and is highly dangerous in large amounts. Moreover, people using laetrile in the mistaken belief that it was curing cancer often delayed more appropriate medical treatment. Other nonvitamins promise to help you "feel good" and to cure tiredness, moodiness, and other problems–all difficult to define and measure.

Problems exist also with the vitamins because of unproven promises. For example, a multivitamin preparation that supposedly increased a child's IQ and test scores was marketed in Britain in the early 1990s. What parent could pass up such an offer? The British regulatory agencies were not impressed, and the manufacturers were found guilty of deceiving the public.[3]

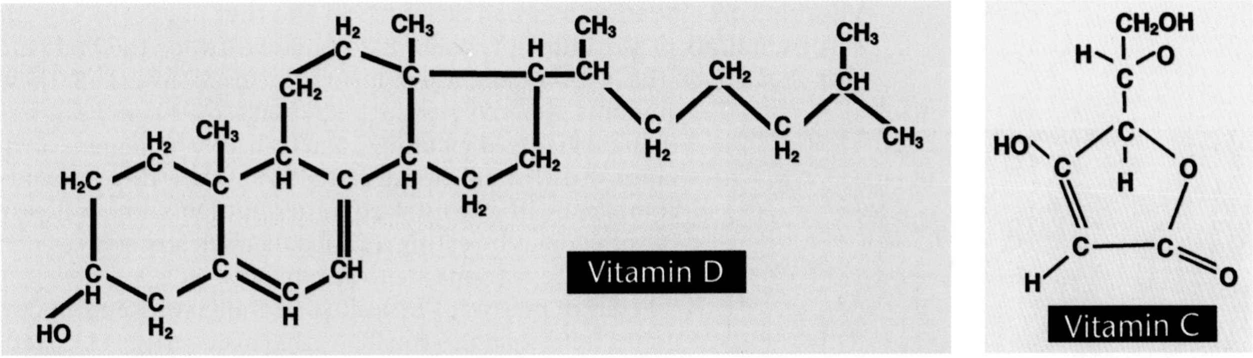

Figure 9-2. Chemical formulas of vitamins D (left) and C (right). Notice that the chemical structures of vitamins differ considerably.

So, let's get to a definition of vitamins:

> Vitamins are organic substances, required for specific metabolic functions in the body, that must be provided in small amounts in the diet.

"Vitamins are organic substances . . ."

"Organic substances" means that all vitamins contain the chemical carbon (C). (Note that this use of "organic" is different from the popular use of this word in the term "organic foods," which means food produced without the use of pesticides, additives, or chemical fertilizers.) The carbon content of vitamin D and vitamin C is obvious (Figure 9-2).

The chemical structures of vitamins D and C are completely different; in fact, there are no similarities in chemical structure among any of the 13 vitamins. The only meaningful grouping of the vitamins is based on their solubility in either fat or water, as we saw in Table 1-4. Synthetic vitamins made in a laboratory test tube have exactly the same chemical structure, crystal structure, and metabolic functions as do natural vitamins obtained from foods such as the rose hips shown on the Canadian stamp. No laboratory tests can tell us which vitamin is natural and which is synthetic. This is important because some vitamin preparations may have the image of being natural (and carry a higher price tag), but it is impossible to determine whether or not they are produced by the less expensive synthetic process.

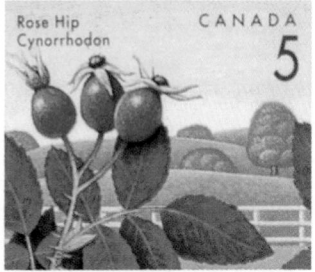

Figure 9-3. Rose hips are rich sources of vitamin C.

Vitamins are "required for specific metabolic functions . . ."

Each vitamin performs specific metabolic functions in the body (Table 9-2).

Some functions are performed by one vitamin (for example, vitamin A affects vision), but some can be performed by more than one. Antioxidant activity is performed by either vitamins E and C or by beta-carotene (a *precursor* of vitamin A).

Knowing the normal functions of a vitamin allows you to understand the disorders produced by a deficiency of that vitamin. For example, because vitamin K is involved in blood clotting, severe deficiencies of this vitamin may lead to excessive bleeding.

Precursor: A substance from which another substance is formed.

Vitamins are "needed in small amounts in the diet . . . ."

The amounts of the different vitamins recommended for the body are very small (see the RDA values listed inside the back cover). If these amounts were converted into intake over one year, less than 22 grams of vitamin C and only 0.73 milligram of vitamin B-12 would be suggested. These are tiny amounts compared with the intake of other nutrients, and it is easy to get enough by eating a varied diet. Dietary sources rich in different vitamins are shown in Table 9-3.

Most vitamins are measured in milligrams and micrograms (refer again to the RDA table inside the back cover), but there are a few important exceptions (Table 9-4).

Understanding these units of measurement is important, especially in the case of vitamin A. The concentration of this vitamin in supplements is usually given as international units (IU), whereas the scientific literature uses the more accurate unit retinol equivalent (RE). We will see the scientific justification for the use of certain measurements for vitamins A and E and niacin when we examine these specific vitamins.

■ The fat-soluble vitamins: A, D, E, and K

The fat-soluble vitamins are associated with fats and oils in foods and are digested and absorbed with lipids in the diet. They are not excreted in the urine because they are not soluble in water. This has important consequences, one

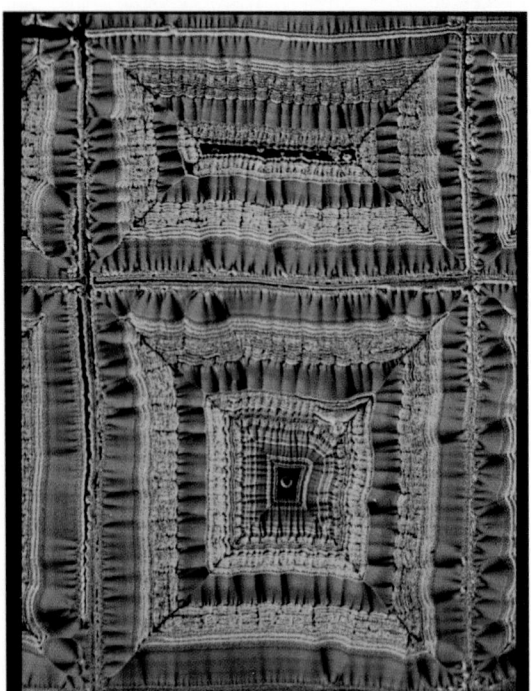

Figure 9-4. This is how chemists see crystals of vitamin C.

Table 9-2. Some Metabolic Functions of the Vitamins

Metabolic Function	Vitamins Involved
Help with release and formation of energy in the metabolism of carbohydrates, fats, and proteins	Release: thiamin, riboflavin, niacin, vitamin B-6, biotin, pantothenic acid Formation: biotin
Blood formation	Vitamins B-12, B-6, and C, folacin
Bone and teeth formation	Vitamins A, D, and C
Neuromuscular function	Vitamins A, B-6, B-12, thiamin, niacin, pantothenic acid
Maintenance of skin condition	Vitamins A, C, and B-6, riboflavin, niacin, pantothenic acid
Eye function	Vitamin A
Antioxidant activity	Vitamins A, E, and C, beta-carotene
Blood-related processes	Vitamins K (helps clotting) and E (prevents red bloods cells from breaking)
Reproduction	Vitamin A (sperm formation and maintenance of normal menstrual cycle), vitamin A and riboflavin (prevent birth defects)
Hormone formation	Vitamin A, pantothenic acid (steroid hormones), vitamin B-6 (norepinephrine and thyroxine)
Interaction with hormones	Vitamin D (calcium-regulating hormones)

of which is that they have greater storage capacity than other vitamins. This means that it usually takes longer for symptoms of deficiency in fat-soluble vitamins to occur than for symptoms of deficiency in water-soluble vitamins. Another important consideration is that excess intake of fat-soluble vitamins is stored along with fat in the body and can build up to toxic levels, whereas excess intake of the water-soluble vitamins is generally excreted in the urine. Factors interfering with the digestion and absorption of fat (malnutrition, abuse of laxatives, faulty bile production because of liver disease) also interfere with the absorption of the fat-soluble vitamins.

These general similarities in the fat-soluble vitamins are worth remembering as we look at the specific nutritional characteristics of each one.

Table 9-3. Best Dietary Sources of Vitamins

Food Group	Good Source of
Meat, poultry, fish, beans	Thiamin, riboflavin, niacin, vitamins B-6 and B-12, pantothenic acid, folacin
Milk, cheese	Vitamins A, D, B-6, B-12, riboflavin
Breads, cereals	Thiamin, riboflavin, vitamin B-6, folacin, pantothenic acid, biotin
Fruits, vegetables	Vitamins A, C, K, riboflavin, folacin
Fats and oils	Vitamins A and E

Table 9-4. Different Units of Measurement for Some Vitamins

Vitamin	Unit Used in RDA Table	Unit Used in Food Composition Tables, Vitamin Supplement Labels	Unit Used in Conversion Factors
A	RE (retinol equivalent)	IU	1 RE = 5 IU (This is an approximation because different forms of vitamin A differ in vitamin activity. The new unit—RE—accounts for this variation; IU does not.)
Niacin	mgNE (niacin equivalent)	mg	1 mgNE = 1 mg of niacin or 60 mg of tryptophan
E	mgαTE (alpha-tocopherol)	IU	No conversion factor because several forms of vitamin E are expressed in TE, but only alpha-tocopherol is expressed in IU.

Vitamin A

Think beyond the photograph in Figure 9-5. Can you see the colors on the disks?

To study vitamin A deficiency, researchers ask volunteers to sort colored disks in a dim light. If they are lucky enough to see the colors on the disks, then their intake of vitamin A is probably adequate. Many people of all ages in the world are less fortunate, especially those living in the central parts of Asia, in Africa, and in parts of Latin America, where the intake of vitamin A is low. Some people are permanently blind because of vitamin A deficiency.

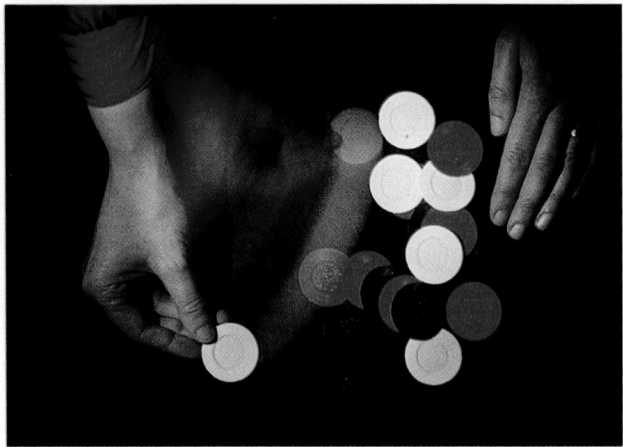

Figure 9-5. One test for vitamin A deficiency. People who cannot distinguish between colors in a dim light are deficient in vitamin A.

Epithelial cells: Layer of cells forming the epidermis, which is the external layer of skin, and the mucous membranes.

Genitourinary: Pertaining to the genitals and urinary organs.

Acne: A skin disorder consisting of pimples and inflammation.

Vitamin A was the first of the vitamins to be discovered, and our knowledge of its many functions in the body has grown in recent years.

Functions of vitamin A

Vision. Mild deficiency causes night blindness; severe deficiency causes permanent blindness.

Immune system. Vitamin A increases resistance to infections, including measles in children.[4]

Growth of cells. It is especially important in cell division and in the growth of specialized cells such as sperm.

Fetal development. Transfer of vitamin A from the mother to the fetus is vital for its normal development.

Quality of *epithelial cells*. These cells form the outer layer of cells in the skin and the mucous membranes (in the GI and the *genitourinary* tracts). Vitamin A keeps them moist; when it is deficient, they dry out and are more prone to infections. Much attention has been given to the treatment of *acne* with a drug called accutane, a chemical relative of vitamin A that is taken by mouth in capsule form. It is approved by FDA for severe acne that does not respond to other treatments. This is great, but important negative side effects may occur if accutane is used without medical supervision.[5] These effects include high risk of a deformed infant if it is taken even for short periods during pregnancy. Liver damage is another risk for all people.

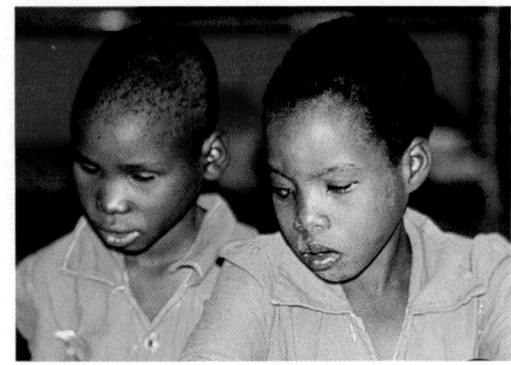

Figure 9-6. Children blinded by vitamin A deficiency.

Another chemical relative of vitamin A used against acne is Retin-A, which is applied on the skin and therefore does not have the side effects caused by accutane.

Taste and appetite. These are negatively affected by a deficiency of vitamin A because the cells associated with the taste buds and tongue become dry.

Antioxidant activity. This is the most recently discovered aspect of vitamin A and its precursor beta-carotene.[6] Antioxidants are compounds that protect other compounds from the damaging effects of oxygen. For example, vitamin A can react with oxygen to prevent it from combining with fat, which causes rancidity in foods, or from damaging the fat in membranes and other lipid-containing cell components so as to induce permanent damage. Other dietary antioxidants include vitamins E and C. Diets rich in antioxidant vitamins may be beneficial against cancer, cardiovascular disease, infectious diseases, aging, and *cataracts*. This is an impressive list, to which we will return at the end of this chapter.

Forms of vitamin A

Active forms of vitamin A, the most common of which is retinol, are found only in foods of animal origin. Plants contain precursors of vitamin A. Precursors, sometimes called provitamins, are converted into the active form of a vitamin in the body. There are about 50 different precursors of vitamin A in plants. Called *carotenoids*, these are a group of yellow and red pigments structurally related to carotene. They produce the coloring in carrots, peaches, and many other fruits and vegetables. After we eat a meal containing vitamin A precursors (carotenoids) from foods of plant origin, the carotenoids are converted into vitamin A. When you eat a carrot containing beta-carotene and a piece of meat, which contains preformed vitamin A, this is what happens (Figure 9-7).

The carotenoid beta-carotene, from the carrot, is converted in the intestinal mucosa into the active forms of vitamin A called retinal and retinol. Because beta-carotene is converted in a ratio of 6:1, it has less vitamin A activity per unit weight than the active forms. Some beta-carotene is also absorbed into the blood. Retinol, from the meat and from the conversion of beta-carotene, is carried in the blood to the liver, where it is hooked onto a protein called retinol binding protein (RBP) for transportation to the rest of the body.

Figure 9-7 shows why we refer to vitamin A concentrations as retinol equivalents (RE) rather than international units (IU). The term RE covers both the preformed and precursor forms of vitamin A.

Food sources of vitamin A

Nearly half of the total vitamin A intake in the typical U.S. diet is provided by vegetables and thus by the precursors of vitamin A.

Americans consume an average of about 1,640 RE or 8,200 IU per day, which is higher than the RDA for adults. Some Americans, including some Hispanics and children of other ethnic groups, do have low intake of vitamin A-rich foods. However, blindness due to vitamin A deficiency is rare in the United States. Dietary deficiencies in other parts of the world result mainly from low intake of foods of animal origin, as well as to lack of knowledge of how to supplement children's diets of rice, wheat, and starchy foods with foods high in beta-carotene.

Vitamin A deficiency symptoms

The health of epithelial cells is affected in vitamin A deficiency, resulting in a number of symptoms.

- **Dry, hardened skin.** This process is called *keratinization*. Vitamin A can be looked upon as a type of lubricant for the skin. When dry and hard, the skin is more vulnerable to bacterial and viral infections.
- **Night blindness.** In normal vision, *rhodopsin* (visual purple) is formed when vitamin A combines with the protein *opsin* in the *rods* (light-sensitive cells at the back of the eye). When light strikes the

Cataracts: Dimming or fuzzing of the lens in the eye, thereby decreasing vision.

Carotenoids: One of a group of pigments (such as carotene) ranging in color from light yellow to purple; widely distributed in plants.

Keratinization: Hardening of cells until they are rough and dry.

Rhodopsin (visual purple): A protein pigment involved in vision; occurs in the outer parts of the rods in the retina of the eye; important in night vision.

Opsin: A protein in the eye involved in vision.

Rods: Long slender bodies in the eye that respond to faint light.

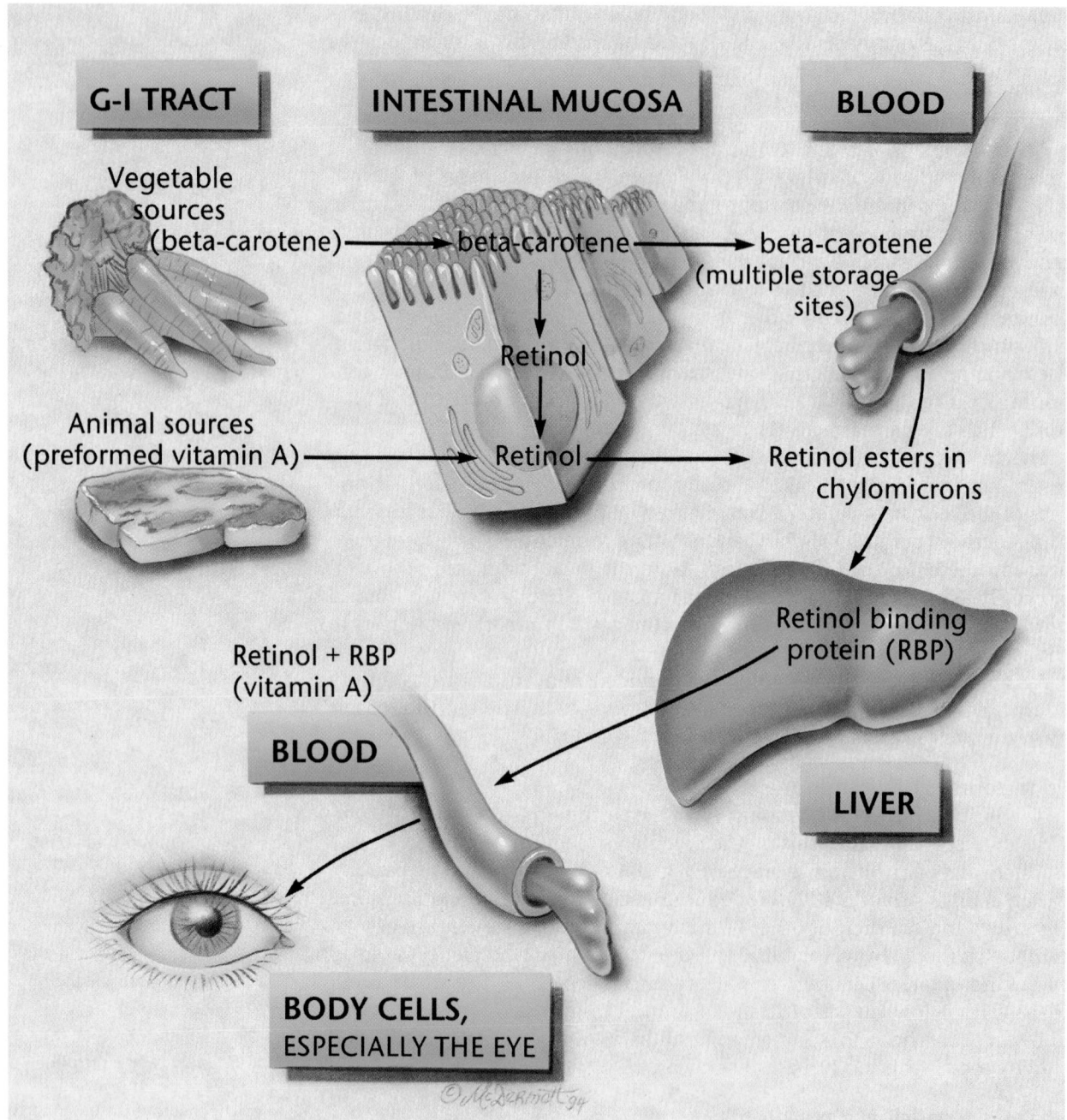

Figure 9-7. Absorption and metabolism of vitamin A and beta-carotene. Vitamin A occurs in foods of animal origin only, and beta-carotene is in foods of plant origin only. Beta-carotene is converted into retinol (an active form of vitamin A) in the intestinal mucosa. Blood takes the vitamin A to the liver, where it is combined with a protein for transportation to tissues, especially the eye.

eye, the rhodopsin breaks down and the eyes adapt to the bright light. More rhodopsin must be synthesized before the eyes can see in dim light again. If levels of vitamin A are low, the eye takes a longer time to recover from bright light. This is called night blindness. The condition could have fatal results in situations when a person faces flashing lights or must move rapidly from bright to dim lights (such as after passing an oncoming car at night in a rural area).

- **Clouding of the cornea.** Hardening of the epithelium of the eye (the cornea) is called *xerophthalmia*. It causes blindness in cases of extreme vitamin A deficiency.
- **Reduced growth in children**
- **Negative effects of protein metabolism in children**
- **Liver damage, especially in alcoholics**
- **Iron deficiency anemia**

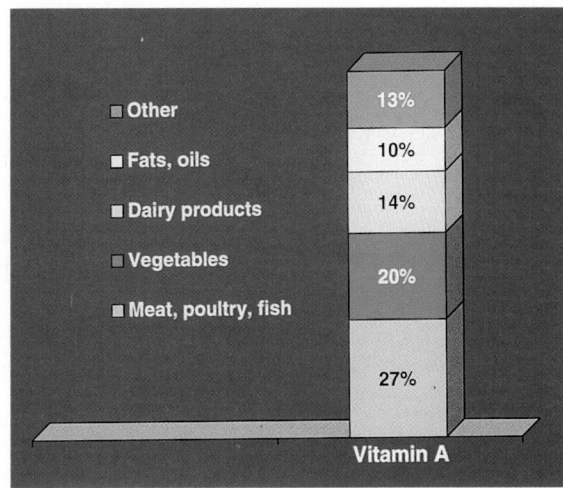

Figure 9-8. Sources of vitamin A in the U.S. food supply.

Transport of vitamin A during starvation

Figure 9-7 shows retinol binding to a protein in the liver to create *retinol binding protein (RBP)*. This is the means of transportation for vitamin A to the tissues, including the eyes. People eating a balanced diet have no problem in making this linkage of the vitamin to a protein. People who are starving for any reason–famine, political hunger strike, severe anorexia nervosa–run the risk of vitamin A deficiency, even though there may be plenty of vitamin A in the liver. Here is what happens. Vitamin A, being fat-soluble, is stored in large amounts in the liver. During starvation, very little food is taken in, and the amino acid supply to the liver is very much reduced. RBP cannot be synthesized, so those otherwise adequate amounts of vitamin A must remain in the liver. Meanwhile, the amount of vitamin A in the eye is reduced, and perhaps to levels that cause blindness. This is a good example of how adequate supplies of a nutrient may exist in a storage tissue but, because of a "transportation problem," cannot be taken to the target tissue.

Xerophthalmia: Deficiency of vitamin A that causes drying of the membranes in the eye, resulting in blindness.

Retinol binding protein (RBP): A protein synthesized in the liver to transport vitamin A to cells, including those in the eye.

Vitamin A toxicity

High intake of vitamin A may be toxic and could result in death. The maximum recommended daily intake of vitamin A for adults is 5,000–10,000 RE or 25,000–50,000 IU. There are reports of people consuming 6–24 pounds of beef liver a week; a single pound of liver, when cooked, contains 240,000 IU of vitamin A.

Symptoms of vitamin A toxicity include severe headaches, gouty arthritis with pain in the bones and joints, diarrhea and vomiting, dry skin, loss of hair, cessation of menstruation, and retardation of growth. Alcohol intake increases the toxic effects of excess vitamin A.

No evidence of toxicity from high intake of beta-carotene has been reported. The skin does become yellow–this happens to people who eat large amounts of carrots–but the condition goes away when normal intake of beta-carotene is resumed.

Vitamin D

We need vitamin D in our body for three main functions:

- to increase the mineral content of bones
- to assist in the absorption of calcium and phosphorus from the GI tract
- to assist the kidney to conserve minerals (which otherwise would be excreted in the urine and lost to the body).

Vitamin D is a curious nutrient–it is in very short supply in most foods, but deficiency is uncommon in most countries. No vitamin D of any dietary significance is found in plant foods, and even in animal foods it is limited–eggs, liver, and small fish such as sardines are the main dietary sources. This does not seem to be much of a choice because we are advised in various dietary recommendations to reduce our intake of eggs, and most people do not list liver or sardines as foods they frequently eat. On the other hand, commercial milk suppliers have a legal requirement to add vitamin D to specific foods such as milk, which thus becomes an important source of vitamin D for many people. However, not everybody can tolerate milk because of the presence of lactose. Enter a little sunshine to the rescue–vitamin D is called the "sunshine vitamin." This is one vitamin we get free. The ultraviolet rays of the sun (or even UV lamps) act on a chemical called 7-dehydrocholesterol that occurs naturally in the skin, converting it into vitamin D in the liver and kidneys.

Even this raises an interesting question: Vitamin D is made in the body and is not necessary in the diet, at least for people who get plenty of sunlight. At the start of this chapter we saw that the definition of a vitamin includes the phrase ". . . and must be provided in small amounts in the diet." Is vitamin D really a vitamin? When it was originally discovered, it seemed to meet the strict definition of a vitamin. Advances in knowledge have since revealed how the body can manufacture it. So technically it is not a vitamin. However the term "vitamin" remains, due partly to history and tradition.

The availability of vitamin D through the action of sunlight presents a problem because increasing evidence suggests a relationship between sunlight and skin cancer. Scientists assure us that, for light-skinned adults, an estimated 10–15 minutes exposure to the noonday sun twice a week is sufficient. For dark-skinned adults, more time is needed because the amount of ultraviolet light reaching the skin is reduced by dark or black skin. It is also reduced by different times of the day than noontime, air pollution, and sun-blocking lotions, so the optimum time in the sun varies for different people.

Recent evidence suggests that postmenopausal women with low vitamin D intake (100 IU per day) benefit from increasing their daily intake to 500 IU. This can significantly reduce the rate of wintertime bone loss and increase bone density in the spine.[7] Strengthening of the spine is particularly important because osteoporosis is a problem for many women after menopause, as we see in Chapter 10, where calcium and osteoporosis are discussed.

Vitamin D deficiency and bone problems

There is a relationship between the bow-legged appearance of a person with *rickets* caused by vitamin D deficiency and the term "rickety" to describe a chair or table that wobbles because of uneven legs. The disease rickets, named after the old English word meaning "to twist," is characterized by bowed legs and small lumps on the ribs, resulting in poor bone formation. Rickets was a common deficiency disease in most countries until the early 1900s. Now it is considered rare in developed countries. This is due to the addition of vitamin D to dairy products and margarine and to less air pollution. In the 1920s and 1930s, the extent of air pollution was so great in industrialized cities that the ultraviolet rays of the sun could not penetrate the industrial smog. There is some evidence that the incidence of rickets may be on the rise again. Many factors are involved–premature births, prolonged breast feeding of infants or feeding them milk not fortified with vitamin D, lack of exposure to sunlight, and the increasing popularity of vegan diets containing only plants, which provide no vitamin D, especially if exposure to sunlight is minimal.

Cultural factors may also contribute to vitamin D deficiency, as seen in the higher incidence of rickets in the children of Asian emigrants to Great Britain compared to that in the rest of the population. Many Asian emigrants are vegetarian because of their religious requirements, and thus their vitamin D intake is low. As part of their cultural practice, Asian children are completely wrapped in clothing during infancy. Finally, sunshine is frequently in short supply in the British climate anyway. All of this adds up to a higher incidence of rickets in these children. Recently, a fabric was developed that allows penetration of ultraviolet light to the skin. This may be the necessary compromise that will allow cultural practices to be preserved while decreasing the extent of rickets in this population.

Rickets is the vitamin D deficiency disease of children. When vitamin D deficiency occurs in adults, the problem is called *osteomalacia*. The loss of calcium causes the bones to be weak and brittle, and pain is common. The disorder is treated with small oral doses of vitamin D.

Prevention of vitamin D deficiency is important during all phases of the life cycle. It is important in pregnancy and lactation because of the growth of bone in the fetus and infant. Bone growth and maintenance require vitamin D in the remaining periods of life also. The elderly have particular problems because their diet is frequently low in vitamin D and they may be house-bound for long periods with no access to sunlight. Moreover, the skin of an 80-year old is only half as efficient as that of a 20-year old in converting the vitamin to the active form.

Rickets: Deficiency of vitamin D; causes softening of bones due to low calcium content.

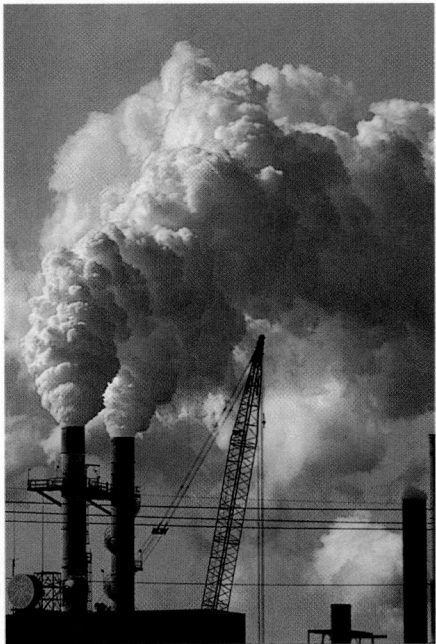

Figure 9-9. Air pollution was a major contributor to vitamin D deficiency in people in the early 1900s. This problem has been almost eliminated by better understanding of the importance of a clean environment, the various Clean Air Acts, and addition of vitamin D to milk.

Osteomalacia: Softening of bones, making them brittle; caused by a deficiency or loss of body calcium; increased by vitamin D deficiency.

Vitamin E

"A vitamin in search of a disease" was how vitamin E was once described by an expert on this nutrient. There is no known evidence of a dietary deficiency of vitamin E in humans. Yet, in the popular literature, the claims are many–vitamin E will extend your life, protect your heart, and improve your sex life. The latter claim is scientifically unproven, but it comes from the fact that the vitamin was discovered when the missing compound interfering with reproduction in rats was shown to be vitamin E. Now most interest in this vitamin involves its activity as an antioxidant, which is discussed with other antioxidants at the end of this chapter.

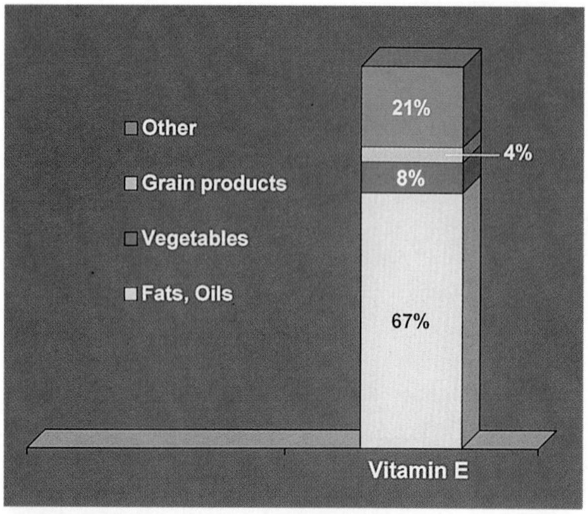

Tocopherols: Chemical name for some forms of vitamin E.

Vitamin E is a group term for the eight *tocopherols* found in plants– "tocos" comes from the Greek word meaning "offspring." Alpha-tocopherol has the highest biological activity in humans, but others are sold commercially, especially gamma-tocopherol.

Fats and oils provide most of the vitamin E in the U.S. diet. The best food sources are plant oils (soybean, cotton, sunflower) and margarines and shortenings made from those oils. Good sources of the vitamin are whole grains, nuts, eggs, leafy green vegetables, liver, and milk. Vitamin E is found in all food groups. Most eating patterns provide sufficient amounts, and deficiencies are not seen, except perhaps in a person who has difficulties in digesting and absorbing fat.

Figure 9-10. Sources of vitamin E in the U.S. food supply. Notice that vitamin E intake is highest from fats and oils.

Vitamin E protects against the harmful effects of atmospheric ozone in its role as an antioxidant.[8] A scientist who advocates the taking of vitamin E supplements justifies the recommendation because of its antioxidant activity.[9] He suggests that such high pharmacologic doses are required that it might be best to call vitamin E an antioxidant rather than a vitamin under such circumstances.

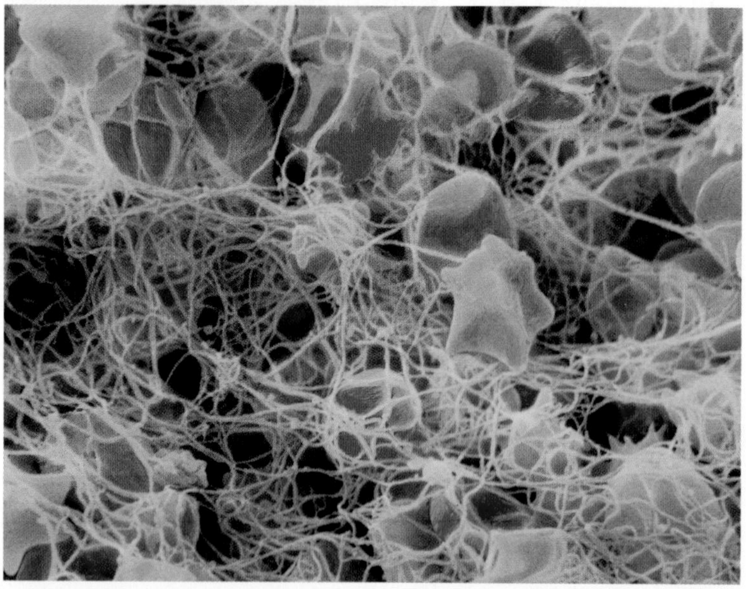

Vitamin K

The remarkable structure in Figure 9-11 could make the difference between life and death. The fibrous structures are a blood clot, and vitamin K performs a critical function in its formation. A Danish scientist discovered how vitamin K works in the mid-1930s. He gave his new discovery the name "koagulation." *Blood coagulation* is the main

Figure 9-11. A blood clot. Vitamin K is one factor essential to its formation. Deficiency of vitamin K can cause death by prolonged bleeding.

function of vitamin K in the body. It is involved in making a protein in the liver that then undergoes a series of chemical reactions in the blood, which in turn leads to a blood clot that stops bleeding.

Blood coagulation: Formation of a blood clot; stops bleeding; vitamin K is needed for coagulation.

Vitamin K is found in adequate amounts in all diets, with green leafy plants as the best sources. Other good sources include cereals, fruit, dairy products, and meat. Bacteria in the large intestine also synthesize vitamin K, which can then be absorbed into the blood.

Vitamin K deficiencies are rare in the general population. Deficiencies lead to *hemorrhages* because of the body's inability to clot blood, and death may occur. (This is not the same as hemophilia, which is excessive bleeding because of a genetic disorder in the blood clotting mechanism.) If vitamin K deficiency does occur, it usually results either from fat malabsorption or from high doses of oral antibiotics that kill the intestinal bacteria that synthesize it. A newborn infant may be deficient in vitamin K because the infant's intestinal system is sterile at birth, and intestinal bacteria cannot supply enough of the vitamin for about seven days. Thus, newborn infants are often given vitamin K immediately to prevent hemorrhaging. The practice of giving vitamin K to infants has raised a debate. An epidemiological study reported that infants given vitamin K after birth had higher incidences of cancer later in childhood. These were very preliminary data, but they prompted the following appropriate heading in an editorial in a medical journal: "Vitamin K and childhood cancer. The risk of hemorrhagic disease is certain; that of cancer is not."[10]

Hemorrhage: Abnormal bleeding.

Toxicity symptoms from excess vitamin K intake are unknown.

■ The water-soluble vitamins–Vitamin C and the B-complex

Water-soluble vitamins are less stable to heat, air, and light than are the fat-soluble vitamins, resulting in significant losses during the processing, cooking, and storage of food. Even though all are soluble in water, they have no similarities in chemical structure. They are easily absorbed from the GI tract into the blood supply. Excess intake is filtered out of the blood by the kidneys and dumped into the urine. This is the body's safety mechanism for getting rid of high vitamin intake as supplements. Because the excess is excreted in the urine, toxicity is less often encountered with them than with the fat-soluble vitamins. Many water-soluble vitamins act as *coenzymes*, mainly in energy metabolism.

Coenzymes: Substances needed to assist certain enzymes.

Vitamin C (Ascorbic Acid)

Scurvy, the deficiency disease of vitamin C, was a great problem for explorers in past centuries. It was not uncommon for a large portion of the crew to have bleeding gums, loosened teeth, anemia, and general debility at the end of a long sea voyage, and many of the crew died. Food consisted entirely of nonperishable foods that could be carried on board ships. It was not until the mid-1700s that this nutritional deficiency was corrected and long voyages became safer. A Scottish physician noticed that oranges and lemons prevented scurvy. Acceptance of sound nutrition advice was as slow then as it sometimes is now. When he finally convinced the right people of the health benefits of these fruits, the British navy began regular rations of lime juice during long voyages. To this day British people are called "limeys" in certain parts of the world. No comparable problem exists today–even the astronauts have their vitamin C-fortified drinks in space. Vitamin C is also called ascorbic acid, which means "no scurvy." This little lesson in nutrition history allows us to take away some important messages that are relevant to our own interests in nutrition. First, many excellent life-saving discoveries in nutrition were made by simple observation. No fancy instruments were needed here, just a keen eye. Second, it takes time for some recommendations in nutrition to be accepted–government agencies, the food industry, and educators all know that fact. Third, the Scottish physician used food as a medication. This is not unlike many situations today, including the use of certain foods for their antioxidant properties, as we will see at the end of this chapter. Fourth, it usually takes a long time to extract and identify the chemical responsible for the nutrition effect. In this case, the discovery of vitamin C came 200 years after people learned how to use it.

Sources of vitamin C

Human beings, primates, and guinea pigs do not synthesize vitamin C, whereas dogs, cats, and all other animals and plants do. Thus, we humans must depend on the food supply for it. In the near future, some vitamin C added to foods may be synthesized by bacteria. Using bacteria is easier and faster than other methods of synthesizing the vitamin. Big investments are involved because vitamin C sales are over $450 million per year. Some of these sales are for vitamin C as a supplement. As you read the advertisements for nutrition supplements, notice how the word "natural" is emphasized. You may be told that the product contains only the natural form of the vitamin, usually obtained from rose hips. Do not be misled into thinking that a "natural" vitamin is better than a synthesized vitamin. The chemical structure for vitamin C is no different whether it is extracted from rose hips or synthesized in the laboratory. But, according to some Japanese scientists, we may not have to depend on food or bacteria for vitamin C for much longer, because of advances in genetic engineering. The title of their chapter in the book *Biotechnology and Nutrition* has almost a science fiction ring to it: "Cloning of a gene related to the missing key enzyme for biosynthesis of ascorbic acid in humans."[11] Until we can genetically engineer this missing key enzyme, we must depend on food sources of the vitamin.

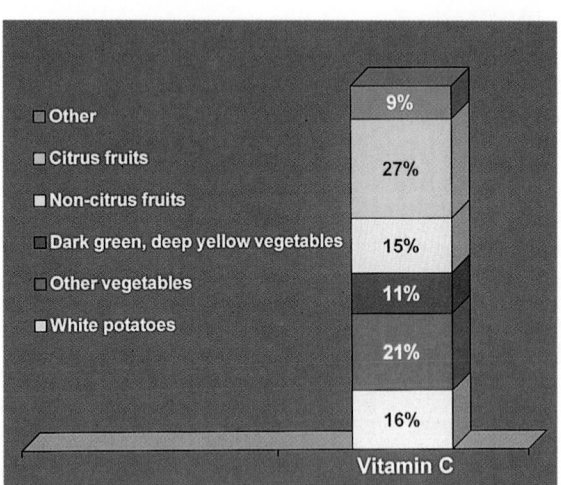

Figure 9-12. Sources of vitamin C in the U.S. food supply. It occurs in a variety of fruits and vegetables.

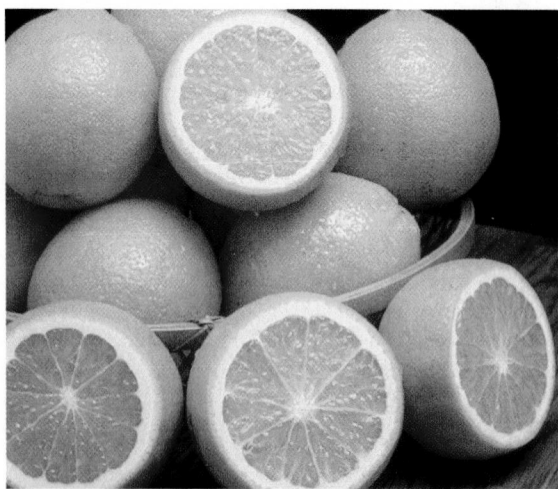

Figure 9-13. Oranges and other citrus fruits are excellent sources of vitamin C.

Fruits and vegetables are the providers of vitamin C in our diet. Because it is a water-soluble vitamin, peeling, soaking, cutting, and cooking cause some loss of vitamin C. Milk is a poor source, and liver and fish are the only other animal sources. Pasteurization of milk and other dairy products removes most of the vitamin.

Adult men and women have an RDA of 60 milligrams and a requirement of 10 milligrams of vitamin C. The requirement means that an intake of less than 10 milligrams per day over a few weeks should cause vitamin C deficiency symptoms. The RDA for cigarette smokers is set at about 100 milligrams because smoking adversely affects vitamin C metabolism in humans. Recent research suggests that smokers may need up to 200 milligrams of vitamin C to achieve the same serum vitamin C levels as those of nonsmokers.[12] Other people also thought to need an intake higher than the RDA for vitamin C include women taking oral contraceptives and people after surgery or trauma. Contrast all of these numbers with the average vitamin C intake for the average American of about 120 milligrams per day. The amounts of vitamin C in some common fruits and vegetables, especially citrus fruits, are relatively high.

Functions of vitamin C in the human body

Vitamin C influences many chemical reactions in the human body. The following list shows some of what it does.

Table 9-5. Vitamin C in Some Common Foods

Food	Amount	Amount of Vitamin C (milligrams)
Orange	1 (or ½ cup of orange juice)	86
Grapefruit	1	54
Strawberries	1 cup	26
Sweet potato, baked	1	28

- **Increases the absorption of iron.** Iron-deficiency anemia is avoided when diets are high in vitamin C because the vitamin converts iron into a chemical form more easily absorbed from the GI tract.

- **Influences serum cholesterol levels**, although its influence on lowering serum cholesterol is debated.

- **Affects the immune system.** Vitamin C makes oral tissues less permeable to bacteria and their toxic products.[13] Vitamin C also helps *leukocytes* (white blood cells) function properly. Leukocytes are important in the proper working of the immune system.

Leukocytes: White blood cells; act as scavengers in the body and thereby help to combat infection.

- **Affects the synthesis of collagen.** Collagen is the "scaffolding" that gives rigidity to cells in gums, muscles, blood vessels, bones, and cartilage. Failure to produce collagen results in weak blood vessels, muscle tissue breakdown, and an inability to make scar tissue (so wounds are slow to heal). Spongy gums are the most visible symptom of failure to produce adequate amounts of collagen.

- **Possibly affects the metabolism of drugs and toxicants by the liver.**

- **Protects DNA in sperm.** This could reduce the risk of offspring inheriting genetic faults.[14]

Vitamin C deficiency

Severe vitamin C deficiency is rare in developed countries such as the United States. Commercially prepared infant formulas in the United States are required by law to be fortified with vitamin C, and drinks such as apple juice for infants and children are also fortified. Human milk contains adequate amounts of the vitamin for the normal length of breast feeding.

Megadoses of vitamin C–Effective?

Most nutritionists are not enthusiastic about megadoses of vitamin C, which means 10 times the RDA (e.g., 600 mg) or more. The reason is that several unfavorable consequences are possible:

Gout: Metabolic disease resulting in arthritis and inflammation of the joints, usually in the knees and feet.

Hemolytic anemia: Anemia resulting from the breaking of red blood cells. Hemoglobin is liberated from the red blood cell and cannot perform its oxygen-carrying function.

- *Gout*
- Destruction of vitamin B-12 in foods
- Interference with urine tests for diabetes
- *Hemolytic anemia* among some African-Americans, Sephardic Jews, and Asian-Americans.

Rebound scurvy may result when a person moves from a very high intake to a normal intake of vitamin C. This is because the body has a defense mechanism against such high doses of the vitamin. Even the fetus has this defense mechanism if the mother is taking megadoses of vitamin C. After a return to normal levels, the defense mechanism continues to destroy the vitamin, causing a normally adequate intake of vitamin C to result in a deficiency. For example, an infant born to a mother who had megadoses of vitamin C during pregnancy now gets the vitamin from human or cow's milk, which are fairly low in the vitamin. The defense mechanism goes on working, decreasing even these low levels, and so the baby may get rebound scurvy.

Whether megadoses of vitamin C can prevent the common cold has been a "hot" topic ever since Linus Pauling published his book *Vitamin C and the Common Cold* in 1970. The verdict is still mixed. At best, persons receiving such megadoses may recover more quickly from colds than others, but they are still susceptible. In any event, we should be aware of the significant negative aspects of taking large amounts of vitamin C.[15]

Food scientists and vitamin C

Interest in the chemical properties of vitamin C has caused food scientists to find many productive uses for this nutrient. It functions both as an antioxidant and an oxidant, depending on the circumstances, to do the following:

Nitrites: Salts added to foods such as bacon to prevent botulism. Nitrosamines, which are carcinogens, are formed when nitrites combine with amines in the stomach and also during cooking.

- Maintain quality, color, and freshness in a variety of products made from fruits, vegetables, meats, and seafoods
- Slow the development of unpleasant odors in seafoods, oils, fats, and dairy products
- Inhibit the development of nitrosamine (a carcinogen) when *nitrites* are added to meat
- Improve bread dough and increase loaf volume.

B-Complex Vitamins Deal with Energy, Metabolism, and Oxygen

The functions of the B-complex vitamins and the specific vitamins that perform them can be grouped as follows:

- **Energy release**–thiamin, riboflavin, niacin, pantothenic acid, and biotin
- **Energy formation**–biotin
- **Protein and amino acid metabolism**–vitamin B-6
- **Delivery of oxygen to cells**–folacin and vitamin B-12.

All of these vitamins are essential in all cells during the process of obtaining energy from lipids, carbohydrates, and proteins. Here is how you use them whenever you exercise. They function as coenzymes to assist the many enzymes needed for the process that produces energy, carbon dioxide, and water.

What quantities of these vitamins are needed to release energy in cells? The RDA tables inside the back cover show RDA values for thiamin, riboflavin, and niacin for all age groups and the Estimated Safe and Adequate Daily Dietary Intakes (ESADDI) for biotin and pantothenic acid. Table 9-6 shows the RDA values for adult women and men aged 19–24 years.

Notice how small amounts produce dramatic effects in energy release. The recommended intake for young women is lower than that for young men. The reason for this is the lower caloric intake of women, with lower total energy expenditures and therefore lower requirements for these vitamins to act as coenzymes for energy release. Our knowledge of biotin and pantothenic acid is incomplete, so only ranges of values can be given for adults. These are 30–100 micrograms for biotin

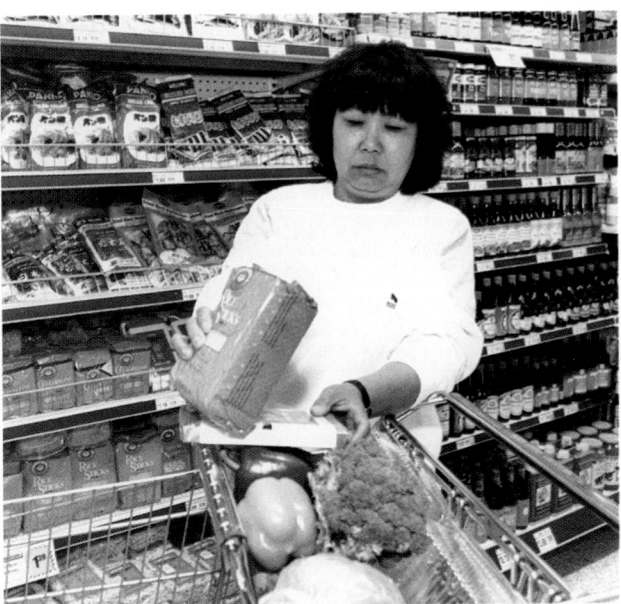

Figure 9-14. B-complex vitamins are in plentiful supply in many of the foods in this woman's shopping basket. Good food choices should remove the necessity for most people to buy supplements to prevent vitamin deficiencies.

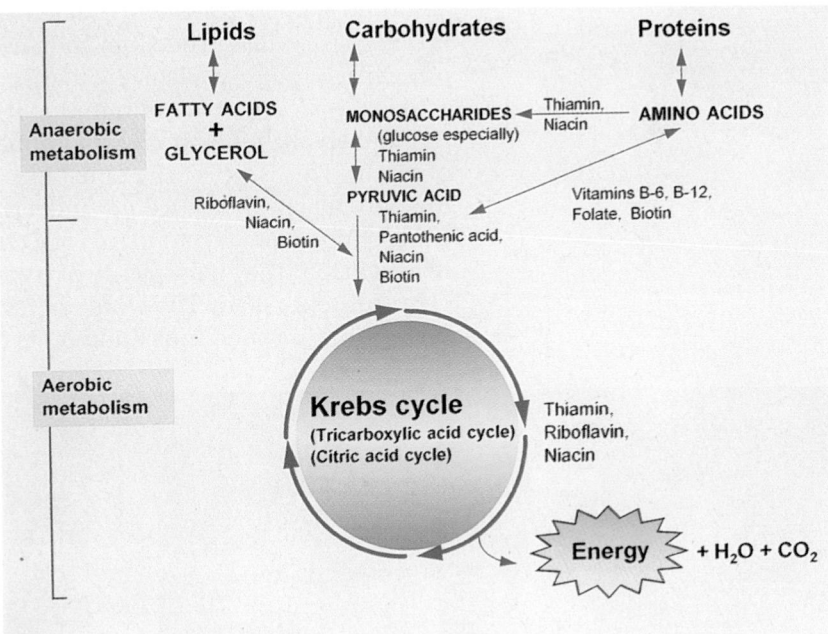

Figure 9-15. The role of vitamins in the metabolism of lipids, carbohydrates, and proteins. Specific vitamins act as coenzymes during the process of converting the energy nutrients into carbon dioxide, water, and energy.

and 4–7 milligrams for pantothenic acid. Some research suggests that riboflavin requirements of older women (50–67 years) increase with exercise training.[16]

When dietary intake of these vitamins is low, the coenzymes are not formed to maximum levels. Enzyme reactions are then not at maximum rate, and your athletic performance is also not at its maximum level.

Fortunately, many foods high in energy are also high in these nutrients. Exceptions are the low-nutrient, calorie-dense foods such as sugar, honey, fats, and oils.

Thiamin. Grain products are rich in thiamin, much of it added after milling to replace what is lost during milling. Meats are good sources of the vitamin, with pork having about three times as much as beef.

Riboflavin. If dairy products are a part of your diet, you should not have a problem with riboflavin intake. All dairy products are rich sources of this vitamin. However, ultraviolet light can destroy much of it. Milk today, packaged in plastic or paperboard containers, has much more riboflavin than in the past when it was delivered in glass bottles. Then it frequently remained on a doorstep steeped in sunshine. Meat and grain products are also good sources of riboflavin.

Niacin. Meats provide nearly half, and grain products one-third, of the niacin intake of the people of the United States. Some niacin in plant foods is bound in a form that is unavailable for absorption from the GI tract of humans. For example, the bound niacin in corn is made more available for absorption when corn is pretreated with lime water–this is done in the making of tortillas. The Hopi Indians in the southwestern United States make niacin more available by roasting the corn in hot ashes.

Niacin is a curious vitamin in that it can be formed from the amino acid tryptophan–60 milligrams of tryptophan can be converted into 1 milligram of niacin. This is where the term "niacin equivalent" comes from; measuring only niacin intake would underestimate total intake by omitting the contribution from tryptophan. For example, milk and eggs contain very little niacin, but they have plenty of tryptophan to offset that lack.

Pantothenic acid. The word comes from the Greek meaning "from all sides." This is a good indication of its dietary availability–it is found in ad-

Table 9-6. RDA Values for Some Vitamins

Vitamin	Women[a]	Men[a]
Thiamin	1.1 mg	1.5 mg
Riboflavin	1.3 mg	1.7 mg
Niacin	15 mgNE	19 mgNE

[a] Aged 19–24 years.

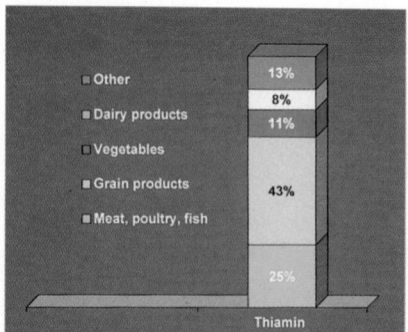
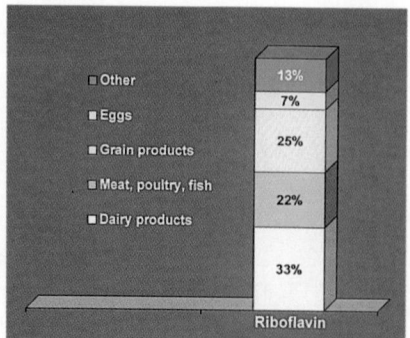
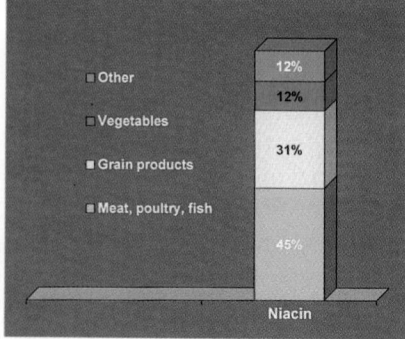

Figure 9-16. Sources of thiamin, riboflavin, and niacin in the U.S. food supply.

equate amounts in many foods, and deficiencies are rare. Pantothenic acid is a key coenzyme in the conversion of pyruvic acid into the chemical at the beginning of the Krebs cycle (Figure 9-13). This moves the breakdown of glucose, some amino acids, and fatty acids from the *anaerobic* to the *aerobic* phase of energy metabolism. It is in the aerobic phase that most energy is produced. Hence, pantothenic acid is a key vitamin in the production of energy in your cells.

Biotin. The best dietary sources of biotin are liver, egg yolk, soy flour, cereals, and yeast. Meats and fruits are poor sources. Information on biotin in food tables is incomplete, so biotin intake is seldom measured in dietary surveys of the population. Biotin is also synthesized by bacteria in the intestine, but our information on the bacterial contribution to our biotin intake is also incomplete. This may sound as though biotin is a neglected vitamin. Not so; because biotin is very widespread in food, deficiencies are rare. As a result, nutritionists turn their attention to studying its metabolic effects, which have more practical applications.

Deficiencies in energy-release vitamins

The same wide variety of foods contain the five vitamins discussed above. Thus, when people are deficient in one of these vitamins, they are likely to be deficient in all five, although this is rare in developed countries.

Thiamin. The story of how thiamin was discovered through observations on thiamin-deficient chickens is an interesting one. In Southeast Asia in the early part of the century, a new cook at a hospital used whole-grain unpolished rice instead of the usual polished rice. One of the doctors noticed that chickens feeding on the leftover rice from the hospital had lost the weakness in their legs that had been present when they were eating polished rice. He went on to define thiamin as a new vitamin and collected a Nobel Prize in 1929 for his work, which all began by watching chickens.

Thiamin deficiency causes adverse changes to the nervous and cardiovascular system. The name for its symptoms is *beriberi* (meaning "I can't, I can't"). These include loss of reflexes, mental confusion, paralysis, irritability, edema (wet beriberi), wasting of muscles (dry beriberi), and heart failure. Alcoholics tend to have the highest incidence of thiamin deficiency in industrialized countries. Alcohol interferes with thiamin absorption, and prolonged deficiency produces brain damage. Furthermore, alcoholics may get over half of their total caloric intake from alcohol, resulting in a generally poor diet as well as a low thiamin intake.

Riboflavin. Deficiency signs include skin changes, cracks at the corners of the mouth, and anemia.

Niacin. *Pellagra* is the name of niacin deficiency; it causes the three D's: diarrhea, dermatitis, and *dementia*–and possibly a fourth D, death.

Pellagra causes the tongue to be frequently scarlet in appearance and extremely painful. Think about how a deficiency of niacin, which causes this painful tongue, may quickly lead to many other nutrient deficiencies because of difficulties in eating.

Pantothenic acid and biotin. No known deficiencies have been named or even reported for these two vitamins.

Anaerobic: ("without oxygen") Not requiring oxygen.

Aerobic: Requiring oxygen.

Beriberi: Deficiency of thiamin, producing edema, cardiovascular changes, muscle weakness, nerve degeneration, and loss of appetite.

Pellagra: Deficiency of niacin resulting in the three D's— diarrhea, dermatitis, and dementia (and in several cases, death).

Dementia: Irreversible mental degeneration, including loss of memory.

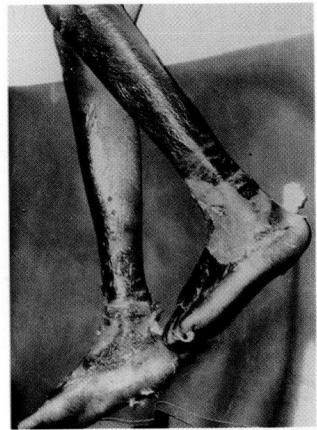

Figure 9-17. Skin changes in pellagra. These are reversible when niacin intake is adequate.

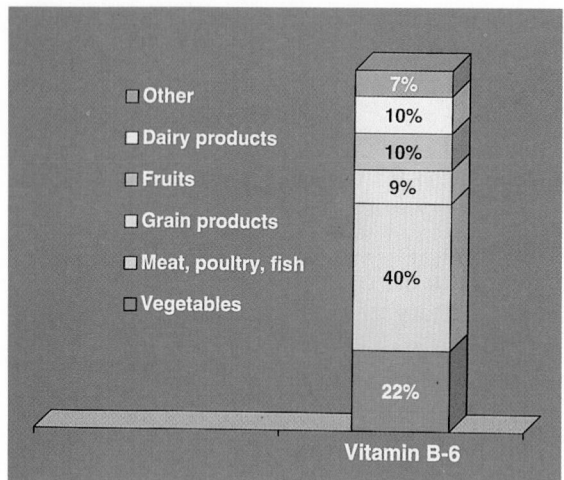

Figure 9-18. Sources of vitamin B-6 in the U. S. food supply.

Vitamin B-6

This vitamin consists of three chemically, metabolically, and functionally related forms–pyridoxine, pyridoxal, and pyridoxamine. It acts as a coenzyme in the metabolism of protein and essential and nonessential amino acids and is involved with the conversion of tryptophan to niacin. It could be called a busy coenzyme because it is involved with over 60 different enzymes. The RDA for vitamin B-6 increases when dietary protein increases. The extra protein recommended for pregnancy should be accompanied by extra amounts of this vitamin.

Meats are the best source of vitamin B-6 in the U.S. diet, followed by vegetables. Some people have low intake, especially college students and teenagers. Several drugs, including penicillin and estrogens, can interfere with its activity. Women who are taking estrogen for osteoporosis should be aware of this negative effect on vitamin B-6. Some evidence suggests that 50 milligrams of vitamin B-6 per day may relieve premenstrual tension, but more study is needed in this area. Excessively high intake can be dangerous also. One woman consumed 125,000% of the RDA for vitamin B-6 for four months, which produced defects in nerve function–an unsteady walk, numbness of the feet, and clumsiness of the hands–so one should beware of too high an intake. Deficiencies of vitamin B-6 are rare and usually occur in association with deficiencies of other B-complex vitamins. Deficiency symptoms include convulsions, dermatitis, and anemia. In infancy, deficiency can lead to nerve disorders.

Folacin and Vitamin B-12

Folacin is also called folate or folic acid, and vitamin B-12 is called cobalamin because it contains the cobalt atom in its structure. These two vitamins work together in several important areas:

- In the development of red and white blood cells
- In RNA and DNA formation. Folacin and vitamin B-12 are involved in cell division at critical periods of growth.
- In the conversion of certain amino acids to other amino acids.

The recommended intake of each of these vitamins is tiny, but the impact of a deficiency in them is considerable.

Folacin is widely distributed in foods, with green leafy vegetables, legumes, liver, and some fruits being excellent sources. This vitamin has a chemical structure that makes it very difficult to measure. In some foods, folate is affected by the presence of substances that make it unavailable for absorption.

Folacin deficiency causes people to be weak, pale, tired, and forgetful. Pregnancy and adolescence increase the requirement for it. Also at risk of

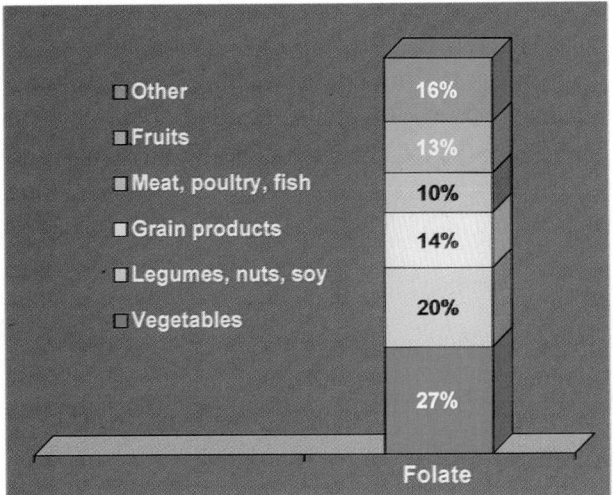
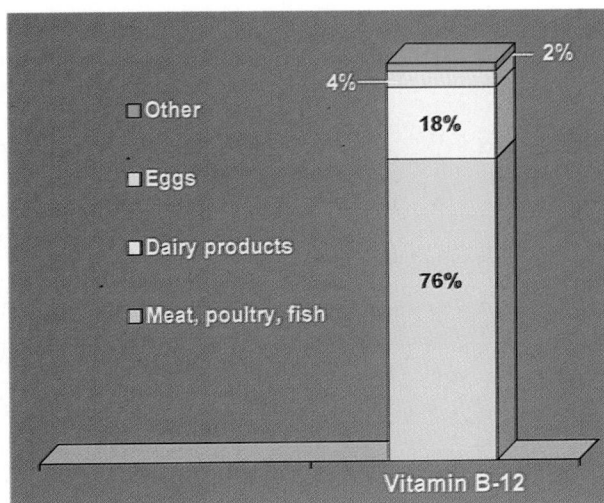

Figure 9-19. Sources of folate (left) and vitamin B-12 (right) in the U.S. food supply.

deficiency are people who take drugs to control cancer, *malaria*, and *epilepsy*.

Think about the implications of the sources of vitamin B-12. It is in highest concentration in meats, with dairy products the next best source. This situation may present a problem for vegans, who do not consume any foods of animal origin, unless they are very watchful of their diet. Seaweed is a good source of the vitamin, but the much-promoted *Spirulina* may be a poor source. The best sources of vitamin B-12 for vegans are fermented soy and cereal products such as tofu and tempeh because bacteria in these foods contribute to the intake of the vitamin.

Infants and children of vegans may require vitamin B-12 supplements. Another group of people may have more than normally adequate diets and yet be deficient in this vitamin. This is because vitamin B-12 requires a protein called the *"intrinsic factor"* to carry it from the GI tract into the blood. The intrinsic factor may be lacking because of a genetic defect or because of the surgical removal of the part of the GI tract involved in vitamin B-12 digestion and absorption. People with this problem must receive the vitamin by injection at regular intervals.

Deficiency symptoms of vitamin B-12 include nerve disorders, especially of the spinal cord. This results in altered movement, numbness in the limbs, and possibly mental disturbances. *Megaloblastic anemia*, which occurs if the red blood cell is large but not fully developed, interferes with the delivery of oxygen to cells. Fortunately, this condition is reversible.

Vitamin B-12 is red. It has no known toxicity symptoms when consumed in megadoses. For this reason, some doctors give it as a placebo. It is used also by some health-promoters, who sell it in the form of oral tablets, gels that are placed inside the nose, or other forms.

The greatest interest in these vitamins in recent years concerns the positive role of folacin in reducing the incidence of neural tube defects, including *spina bifida*,[17] which are the most common major birth defects in the

Malaria: An infectious disease that affects red blood cells; has negative effects on the digestive and nervous systems; transmitted by mosquitoes, especially in equatorial parts of the world.

Epilepsy: A condition characterized by disturbed brain function, usually with convulsions.

Spirulina ("blue-green manna"): A type of algae supposed to contain vitamin B-12 and to depress appetite. There is no evidence for these claims.

Intrinsic factor: A substance synthesized in the GI tract that assists in the absorption of vitamin B-12.

Megaloblastic anemia: Anemia in which red blood cells are large, underdeveloped, and have reduced oxygen-carrying capacity.

Spina bifida: Birth defects in the spine resulting in a tumor and deformity.

United States and other countries. Genetic factors play a role in causing them, but environmental factors may also be involved. Neural tube defect can be reduced dramatically when women take multivitamin or folacin supplements during the first six weeks of pregnancy. Nevertheless, high incidences of the defect occur among poor people. These results raise the concern that an important group of U.S. women do not receive sufficient folacin to minimize their risk of a defective pregnancy.

■ Vitamins vary in their stability

Some not too robust vitamins are fragile to heat, light, and/or air:

- **Heat:** Vitamins A, D, E, C, B-6, thiamin, riboflavin, folacin, and pantothenic acid
- **Light:** Vitamins A, D, E, K, B-6, riboflavin, and folacin
- **Air:** Vitamins A, D, E, C, B-12, thiamin, and folacin.

These losses can be large for some vitamins during cooking of food and canning of vegetables and fruits.

These numbers tell their own story–don't overcook the vegetables if you want to maximize vitamin intake. Your food will contain more vitamins if it is cooked for shorter times, at lower temperatures, and with a minimum amount of water. Canned foods have been heated and so have less vitamin content than frozen foods because of the lack of stability of some micronutrients to heat. Canned vegetables that are stored for several years have an additional vitamin loss of about 20%. But we should not play with numbers too much. What's important is how much of the vitamin is left after cooking or canning. For example, pork loses about half of its thiamin content after normal cooking, but it is still an excellent source of thiamin even with only 50% of the vitamin remaining.

In general, foods have the highest concentration of vitamins if eaten raw. Since that is not possible for many foods, then cooking in the least amount of water for the shortest time at the lowest possible temperature is

Table 9-7. Maximum Loss from Cooking

Vitamin	Loss (%)
A	40
D	40
E	55
K	5
C	100
Thiamin	80
Riboflavin	75
Niacin	75
B-6	40
Biotin	60
Pantothenic acid	50
Folic acid	100
B-12	10

For the most vitamins in cooked food, use

- the least water
- the shortest time
- the lowest temperature.

Table 9-8. Vitamin Losses Through Processing or Canning of Vegetables

Processed Product	Vitamin Losses, as Percent of Freshly Cooked and Drained Product				
	A	B-1	B-2	Niacin	C
Frozen product[a] (cooked and drained)	12[b] 0–50[c]	20 0–61	24 0–45	24 0–56	26 0–78
Sterilized product[d] (drained)	10 0–32	67 56–83	42 14–50	49 31–65	51 28–67

[a] Asparagus, lima beans, green beans, broccoli, cauliflower, green peas, potatoes, spinach, brussels sprouts, and baby corn-cobs.
[b] Average values
[c] Range.
[d] The same as for note a, except for broccoli and brussels sprouts. Values for potato include the cooking water.

the next best alternative. Finally, the best recipe for avoiding deficiencies of any nutrient is to eat as varied a diet as possible.

■ Nutrition in action–Antioxidants

Antioxidants in foods are defined by the FDA as preservatives that specifically retard deterioration, rancidity, or discoloration due to oxidation. Oxidation occurs in fatty acids in foods when oxygen is added to unsaturated sites in fatty acid molecules. Helpers in this process include oxygen, light, heat, some pigments, alkaline conditions, and the degree of unsaturation of a compound. For example, polyunsaturated fatty acids are more prone to lipid oxidation than are monounsaturated fatty acids (see the fatty acid structures in Chapter 7).

Oxidation in food results in fat becoming rancid, with resulting off-odors and off-flavors. The food is usually wasted, and if it is eaten, some potentially toxic products of oxidation are consumed.

Oxidation of lipids in the body also causes considerable damage, including damage to membranes, increased probability of coronary heart disease, altered platelet functions, damage to the immune systems, DNA *mutations*, and other changes.[18]

Nutritionists and food scientists are very interested in antioxidants because they prevent this deterioration in food quality and damage to cells in the body. They act like the buffers we discussed in Chapter 5 by reacting with an oxidizing agent, usually oxygen. After the oxygen molecule has been joined to the antioxidant, it is not free to react with an unsaturated fatty acid, and so it can no longer cause oxidation. It is not uncommon to see either BHT or BHA listed on a food package. Their antioxidant properties lengthen the shelf life of the food. Other chemicals with antioxidant properties include the tocopherols (vitamin E) and ascorbic acid.

The body has its own system of protective antioxidant mechanisms. These are listed here because you will probably be reading much information about them in the near future.

Mutation: Changes in DNA structure so that the normal genetic message is usually not transmitted.

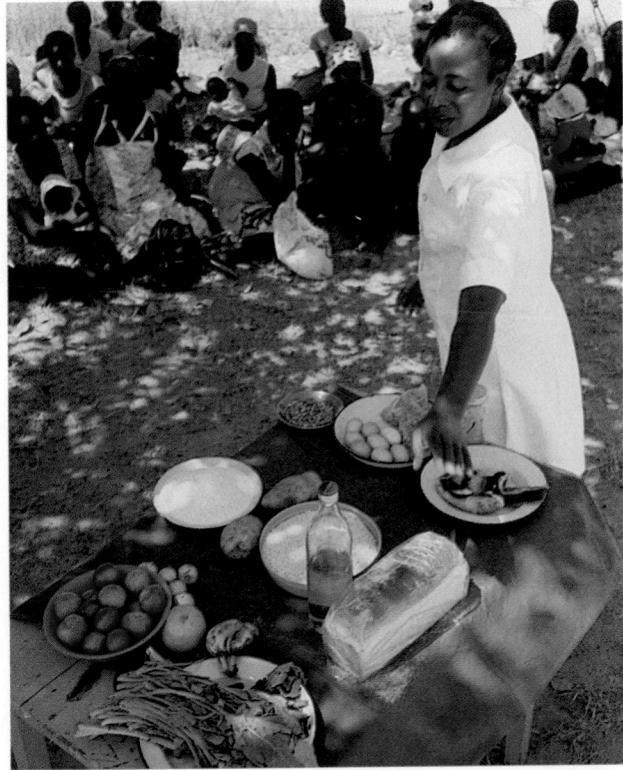

Figure 9-20. Foods from all over the world contain antioxidants.

- **Preventive antioxidants:** Enzymes (superoxide dismutase, catalase, and glutathione peroxidase)
- **Primary antioxidants:** Alpha-tocopherol (vitamin E), phenolics, flavonols, catechins
- **Complementary agents:** Vitamin C, beta-carotene, retinoids (related to vitamin A)

We learned earlier that vitamin C protects lipids in the body from oxidative damage.[19] This includes protection for the immune system and protection against cancer-causing agents. Foods containing vitamins E and C are protective against cardiovascular disease and cataracts. Much research is in progress on how these antioxidants slow the aging process. Researchers at the USDA Human Nutrition Research Center on Aging at Tufts University in Boston find that diets rich in antioxidant vitamins may be important in maintaining optimal health by reducing the incidence of some age-related health problems–arthritis and wound healing are two examples. Vitamin E is suggested as an important protective antioxidant for elderly people.[20]

Sports physiologists and athletes are interested in the antioxidant nutrients because oxidative damage occurs in tissues (especially muscle, liver, and blood) during exercise. The amount of damage depends on exercise intensity and training state. Some evidence suggests that dietary vitamins E and C may be protective against such damage, but further studies are needed.[21] This is a very active area of research, and much more remains to be learned about the mechanisms by which the three nutrients vitamins E and C and beta-carotene perform their protective antioxidant functions.

■ Now you know

- Deficiencies of some vitamins (vitamin A, for example) are common in certain parts of the world.

- Thirteen legitimate vitamins are known, but many nonvitamins are sold as vitamins.

- Vitamins are defined as organic substances that are required for specific metabolic functions in the body and that must be provided in small amounts in the diet.

- Vitamins are divided into the fat-soluble vitamins (A, D, E, and K) and the water-soluble vitamins (C and the B-complex vitamins).

- The main functions of the fat-soluble vitamins include: for vitamin A, vision and the immune system; for vitamin D, bone formation; for vitamin E, antioxidant properties; and for vitamin K, blood coagulation.

- The main functions of the water-soluble vitamins include: for vitamin C, protection of gums and soft tissue and antioxidant functions; for thiamin, riboflavin, niacin, biotin, and pantothenic acid, coenzyme activity in energy metabolism; for vitamin B-6, amino acid and protein metabolism; for folacin and vitamin B-12, coenzymes and cell growth.

- Vitamins vary in their stability to heat, light, and air. Heating and canning of vegetables and fruits result in vitamin losses. But concentrations of vitamins remaining in many foods are such that they are still good sources of vitamins. Eating raw food or minimally heated foods is preferable to minimize vitamin loss.

- Antioxidant properties of vitamins E and C and beta-carotene are important in preventing damage to membranes and the immune function, DNA mutations, and coronary heart disease.

Further Reading

1. Humphrey, J. H., and others. Vitamin A deficiency and attributable mortality among under-5-year-olds. ***Bulletin of the World Health Organization*** 70(2):225, 1992.

2. Bender, M. M., and others. Trends in prevalence and magnitude of vitamin and mineral supplement usage and correlation with health status. ***Journal of the American Dietetic Association*** 92:1096, 1992.

3. Dyer, C. Intelligence claims for vitamins may breach Trade Descriptions Act. ***British Medical Journal*** 304:337, 1992.

4. Ross, A. C. Vitamin A status: Relationship to immunity and the antibody response. ***Proceeding of the Society for Experimental Biology and Medicine*** 200:303, 1992.

5. Willis, J. L. Acne agony. ***FDA Consumer*** 26(6):23, 1992.

6. Canfield, L. M., and others. Carotenoids as cellular oxidants. ***Proceeding of the Society for Experimental Biology and Medicine*** 200:260, 1992.

7. Anonymous. Preventing wintertime bone loss: Effects of vitamin D supplementation in healthy postmenopausal women. ***Nutrition Reviews*** 50:52, 1992.

8. Pryor, W. A. Can vitamin E protect humans against the pathological effects of ozone in smog? ***American Journal of Clinical Nutrition*** 53:702, 1991.

9. Horwitt, M. K. Data supporting supplementation of humans with vitamin E. ***Journal of Nutrition*** 121:424, 1991.

10. Hull, D. Vitamin K and childhood cancer. ***British Medical Journal*** 305:327, 1992.

11. Nishikimi, M., and others. Cloning of a gene related to the missing key enzyme for biosynthesis of ascorbic acid in humans. In: ***Biotechnology and Nutrition***. D. D. Bills and S.-D. Kung, editors. Butterworth-Heinemann, Boston, page 315, 1992.

12. Schectman, G., and others. Ascorbic acid requirements for smokers: Analysis of a population survey. ***American Journal of Clinical Nutrition*** 53:1466, 1991.

13. Goldschmidt, M. C. Reduced bactericidal activity in neutrophils from scorbutic animals and the effect of ascorbic acid on these target bacteria in vivo and in vitro. ***American Journal of Clinical Nutrition*** 54:1214S, 1991.

14. Bradley, D. An orange a day helps to keep the sperm OK. ***New Scientist*** 133(1812):20, 1992.

15. Hemila, H. Vitamin C and the common cold. ***British Journal of Nutrition*** 67:3, 1992.

16. Winters, L. R., and others. Riboflavin requirements and exercise adaptation in older women. ***American Journal of Clinical Nutrition*** 56:526, 1992.

17. Willett, W. C. Folic acid and neural tube defects: Can't we come to closure? ***American Journal of Public Health*** 82:666, 1992.

18. Kinsella, J. E., and others. Possible mechanisms for the protective role of antioxidants in wine and plant foods. ***Food Technology*** 47(4):85, 1993.

19. Frei, B. Ascorbic acid protects lipids in human plasma and low-density lipoprotein against oxidative damage. ***American Journal of Clinical Nutrition*** 54:1113S, 1991.

20. Meydani, M. Protective role of dietary vitamin E on oxidative stress in aging. ***Age*** 15:89, 1992.

21. Witt, E. H., and others. Exercise, oxidative damage and effects of antioxidant manipulation. ***Journal of Nutrition*** 122:766, 1992.

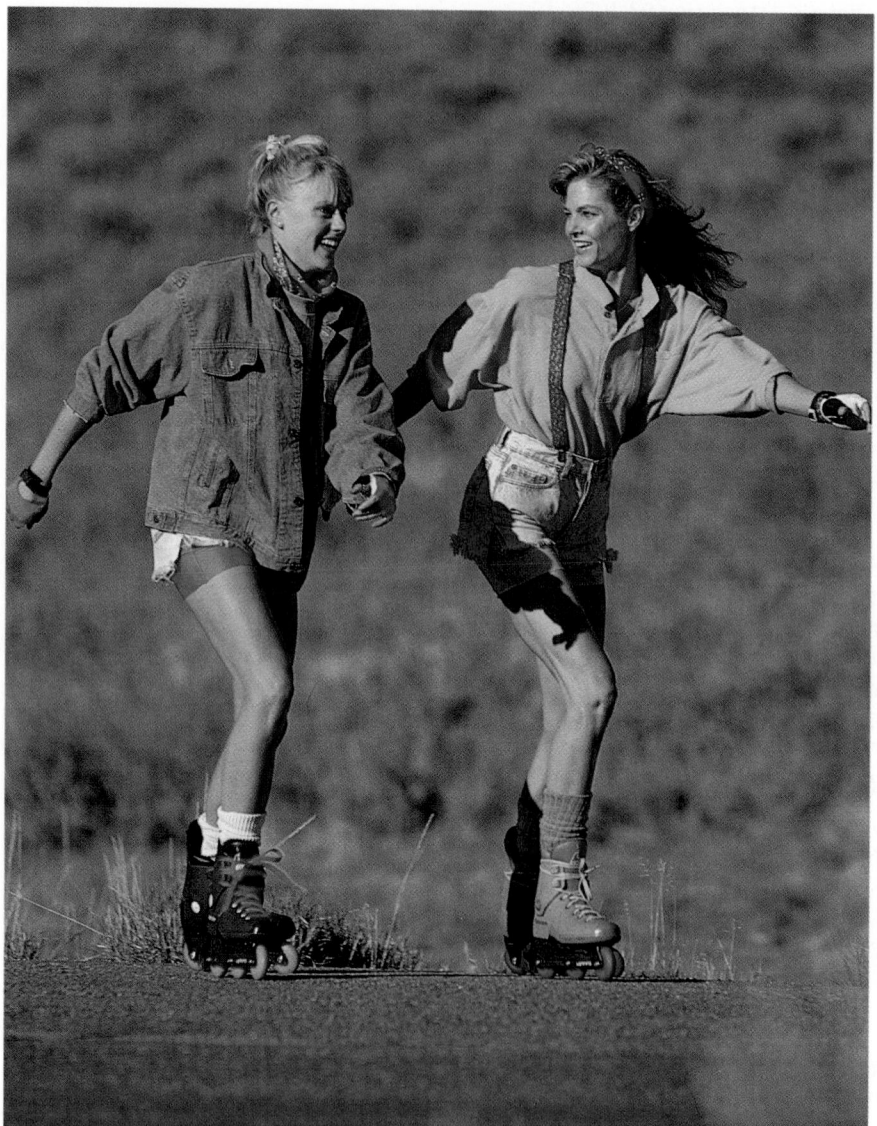

Figure 10-1. Active bodies need minerals, which assist the functioning of body tissues, such as muscles and blood, and the release of energy from the energy nutrients.

Minerals–Dairy Products

■ Minerals in our lives–Many functions are vital

We saw in earlier chapters that individuals, such as those in the picture, could not perform physical activity without an adequate dietary intake of energy from carbohydrates, lipids, and proteins, as well as a supply of B-complex vitamins to assist in energy metabolism. Some minerals interact in all of these activities. This last group of nutrients is vital for health and for many body processes. Mineral functions in the body are summarized in the overview of nutrients in Table 1-4. In most activities, the mineral works in combination with compounds synthesized from other nutrients. For example, iron is combined with the protein globin to form hemoglobin, without which these young women could not be enjoying this activity.

Minerals Perform Many Important Functions in the Body

- **Oxygen-carrying capacity: iron.** Muscles cannot work for prolonged periods without oxygen. Reduced capacity to deliver oxygen seriously hinders muscles from performing at maximum work capacity. Iron-containing hemoglobin in the blood carries oxygen from the lungs to all cells in the body.

- **Muscle-nerve function: sodium, potassium, calcium, magnesium, and chloride.** Nerves stimulate muscles to contract and relax, thus producing strength for physical activity. These minerals are vital in the transmission of the electrical impulses that initiate and maintain the contraction and relaxation of muscles.

- **Enzyme activity: phosphorus, magnesium, iron, zinc, selenium, manganese, copper, and molybdenum.** The functioning of hundreds of enzymes in the body depends on various minerals. Many of these enzymes are involved in energy metabolism.

- **Glucose metabolism: chromium.** Chromium is a mineral much discussed in the media. It is important in glucose metabolism and thus in

Major Topics in This Chapter

Different minerals perform important body functions including oxygen transport, nerve-muscle function, enzyme activity, energy metabolism, formation of some hormones, water balance, acid-base balance, and the growth of tissues.

Adequate mineral intake can be a problem, especially for teenage girls, premenopausal women, and the elderly.

Deficiencies of some minerals may have physical, psychological, and/or economic costs.

■

Macrominerals (needed in highest amounts by the body) are calcium, phosphorus, sodium, potassium, chloride, magnesium, and sulfur. Nutritionally important microminerals include iron, zinc, iodine, selenium, fluoride, and copper.

■

People Are Different–Clay eating and lead contamination of food and drink

Nutrition in Action–Minerals and dairy products

energy metabolism. When dietary intake of chromium is low, a diabetes-like syndrome exists.[1]

- **Thyroid hormones: iodine.** Iodine-containing thyroid hormones are important in energy regulation. Dietary deficiency of iodine causes decreased production of thyroid hormones, resulting in decreased energy production.

- **Body-water balance: sodium, potassium, and chloride.** The distribution of fluids between the cells and the space around them is regulated by these ions (see Chapter 5). Edema results from an alteration in body-water balance. Excessive use of diuretics can lead to damaging changes in the level of these ions in the body.

- **Acid-base balance: sodium and potassium phosphate and bicarbonate.** Maintaining pH within correct ranges is important for the normal functioning of enzymes (see Chapter 5). Sodium and potassium phosphate and bicarbonate, as well as proteins, act as buffers in preventing wide swings in pH values in cells and in the blood.

- **Bones: calcium and phosphorus.** Calcium and phosphorus, and the proportions of each, determine bone strength. Osteoporosis is the loss of bone mass resulting from the loss of calcium. This results in increased incidences of bone fracture, especially in postmenopausal women.

- **Tendons: sulfur.** Tendons, which hook muscles to bones, have a high concentration of proteins rich in sulfur-containing amino acids.

Table 10-1. Mineral Content in the Body of a 70-Kilogram Adult Male[a]

Mineral	Symbol	Amount (grams)
Calcium	Ca	1,100
Phosphorus	P	500
Potassium	K	140
Sulfur	S	140
Sodium	Na	100
Chloride	Cl	95
Magnesium	Mg	19
Silicon	Si	18
Iron	Fe	4.2
Fluorine	F	2.6
Zinc	Zn	2.3
Copper	Cu	0.07
Manganese	Mn	0.01
Iodine	I	0.01

[a] Values for adult women are about 25% less because of the smaller body size of women.

The power, grace, and elegance of human motion in sporting events, dance, gymnastics, and other activities result from careful coordination of input from many nutrients, among which individual minerals have an important role to play. But minerals also play roles in which they coordinate with other nutrients. For example, blood clotting requires not only calcium but vitamin K and a number of specific proteins. Hair strength is affected by the sulfur in sulfur-containing amino acids. Strong teeth are dependent upon calcium, phosphorus, and fluoride. And in the stomach, chloride combines with hydrogen to produce hydrochloric acid, which is important in the digestion of food.

Minerals are important in our lives, but the small amount we have in our bodies surprises some people. Fourteen minerals totaling 2,121 grams (76 ounces or 4¾ pounds) can be found in an adult male weighing 70 kilograms (154 pounds).

Even smaller amounts of nickel, vanadium, and arsenic occur in the body and yet are considered essential. But isn't arsenic a poison? Yes, in large amounts, but tiny amounts must be supplied in the diet because arsenic is required for the metabolism of some sulfur-containing amino acids and their metabolites.

Compare the concentration of various minerals in the body with each other and with the list of their functions. Notice that although iron is vital for the delivery of oxygen to cells, its concentration in the body is low relative to that of other minerals such as calcium or phosphorus. The amount of a mineral in the diet and the importance of its functions are not always proportional.

Recommended Dietary Intake Levels of Specific Minerals Are Not Proportional to Their Functional Importance in the Body

The RDA table at the back of this book shows that tiny amounts of some minerals are recommended in the diet. For example, calcium, phosphorus, and magnesium are recommended in the highest amounts, followed by iron and zinc. All of these are measured in milligram amounts. Concentrations of iodine and selenium are measured in micrograms, which are each one-thousandth of a milligram. Minerals are categorized as *macrominerals*, those that are recommended in amounts greater than 100 milligrams per day, and *microminerals*, or trace elements, which are recommended in amounts less than 20 milligrams per day. The concentration of macrominerals in food and their functions in the body are mostly well understood. Less well understood are the microminerals, and experts argue about whether other minerals should be added to the essential list. Perhaps this is to be expected, in view of the tiny amounts measured. The total amount of trace elements in the body of an adult is about one ounce. Some trace elements are measured in nanograms–a nanogram is one billionth of a gram, or one twenty-eight billionth of an ounce. Specialized instruments are required to measure these tiny amounts.

Macrominerals: Minerals recommended in amounts greater than 100 milligrams per day. They are calcium, phosphorus, sodium, potassium, chloride, magnesium, and sulfur.

Microminerals: Also called trace elements. Minerals recommended in amounts less than 20 milligrams per day. They include iron, zinc, iodine, selenium, fluoride, and copper.

How Do Nutritionists Learn About Minerals?

Research with experimental animals provides most of our information about mineral requirements for humans.[2] The importance of nickel, molybdenum, and arsenic was learned from animal research. Feeding diets deficient in certain minerals allows the scientist to determine the effects of the deficiency in various tissues. Most of these experiments cannot be performed on people for ethical reasons, so observations made from animal experiments are applied to people. Other important information on the role of minerals in human nutrition is obtained from observations on the diet composition of economically important animals such as swine, beef, and poultry and from diet formulations for pets.

Diet surveys of mineral intake by certain parts of a population are done frequently. Such surveys have shown that certain groups in the United States have a low intake of particular minerals (Table 10-2).

The reasons for low intake of specific minerals include lack of knowledge about foods rich in minerals, lactose intolerance (causing some groups to have low intake of calcium-rich dairy products), and economic shifts resulting especially in lower intake of foods rich in iron and zinc. Good sources of iron and zinc are more expensive–meats, for example. Therefore, people on low incomes and the elderly are most affected.

Table 10-2. Population Groups in the United States with Low Intake of Certain Minerals

Group	Calcium	Magnesium	Iron	Zinc	Copper	Manganese
6- to 11-month-olds					x	
2-year-olds			x	x	x	
Girls 14–16 years old	x	x	x	x	x	x
Boys 14–16 years old				x	x	
Women 25–30 years old	x		x	x	x	
Men 25–30 years old					x	
Women 60–65 years old	x			x	x	
Men 60–65 years old					x	

Deficiencies and Excesses of Minerals Inflict Costs

Physical costs

Much physical pain is caused by deficiencies and excesses of specific minerals. Deficiency of these minerals leads to these results:

- **Calcium**–broken bones, especially in the elderly
- **Magnesium**–*neurological disturbances*
- **Iron**–inadequate pregnancy weight gain[3]
- **Iron, copper, or iodine**–physical weakness
- **Fluoride**–tooth decay
- **Selenium**–muscle pain
- **Potassium, magnesium**–heart failure.

Neurological disturbances: Dysfunction of the nervous system.

Excesses are also a problem.

- **Sodium**–hypertension, a factor in coronary heart disease
- **Iron**–increased risk of heart attacks.

Psychological costs

Many physical costs also have a psychological component. The following results of deficiency can affect a person's mental and emotional well-being.

- **Iron, iodine, or copper**–reduced physical activity
- **Zinc**–impaired sexual development
- **Iodine**–decreased mental and physical growth. *Cretinism* causes mental retardation and dwarfism. It occurs in infants born to mothers deficient in iodine during the first trimester of pregnancy.

Cretinism: Severe mental and physical retardation of infants caused by iodine deficiency during pregnancy.

Economic costs

Most physical and psychological costs also result in economic costs. Here are the outcomes of deficiency:

- **Iron**–decreased capacity for physical work. This can have severe economic and nutritional implications for low-income people, especially in developing countries. Mental development of anemic children is decreased.
- **Calcium**–osteoporosis, leading to bone fractures. This has implications in work performance and in health costs, especially for the el-

derly. Osteoporosis affects about 24 million people in the United States, mainly post-menopausal women, and causes about 1.3 million fractures per year. The annual cost of treating patients with osteoporosis ranges from 7 to 12 billion dollars.[4]

- **Iodine**–decreased quality of life, productivity, and educational achievements. These effects are prevalent especially in parts of Africa, Asia, and Latin America.

Good physical performance is important for economic and psychological well-being. The ability to earn sufficient income to feed adequate diets to families is critically important. In many countries, people are paid by the amount of work done rather than by an hourly rate, causing reduced work performance to have severe economic consequences.

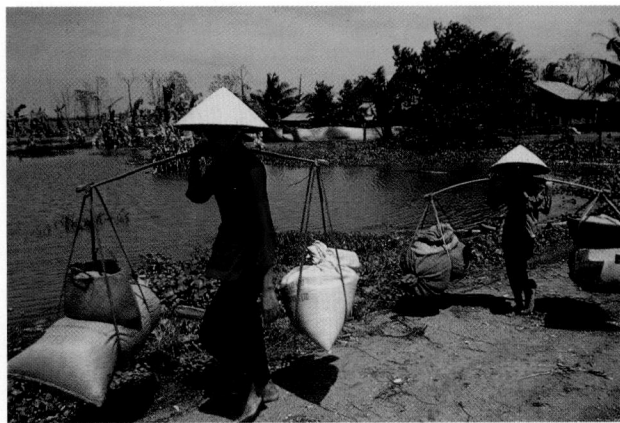

Figure 10-2. Both macro- and microminerals are needed to keep the body in good condition so that it can work or play.

■ Macrominerals

The macrominerals are calcium, phosphorus, sodium, potassium, chloride, magnesium, and sulfur. Attention in the popular press is directed mainly to calcium because of the importance of osteoporosis and to sodium because of its relationship to hypertension in some people.

Calcium and Phosphorus

Figures 10-3 and 10-4 probably sum up much of the interest in calcium. Osteoporosis is a major health problem with significant economic costs. The weakening of bones, leading to increased bone fractures in the elderly, is seen in Figure

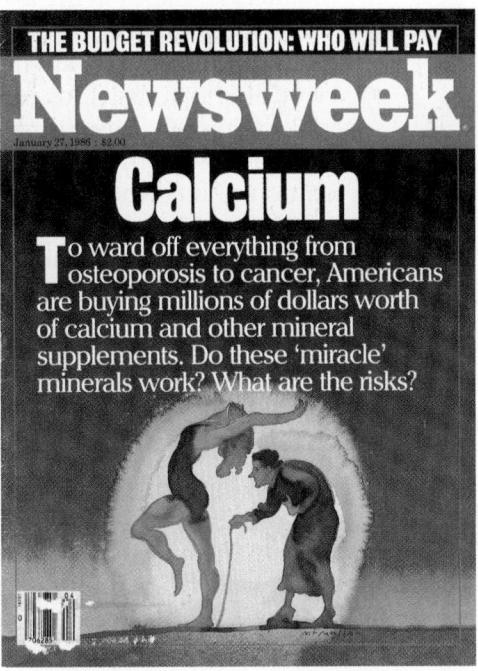

Figure 10-4. Calcium is a topic in the news because of its role in preventing osteoporosis and other diseases.

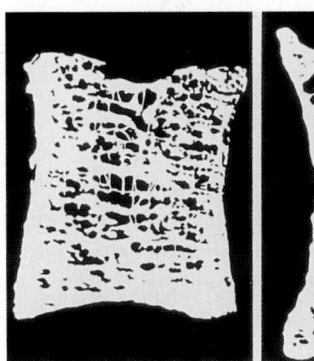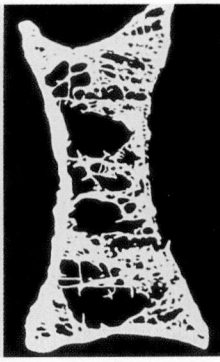

Figure 10-3. Bone from a normal person (left) and thinner bone from a person with osteoporosis (right).

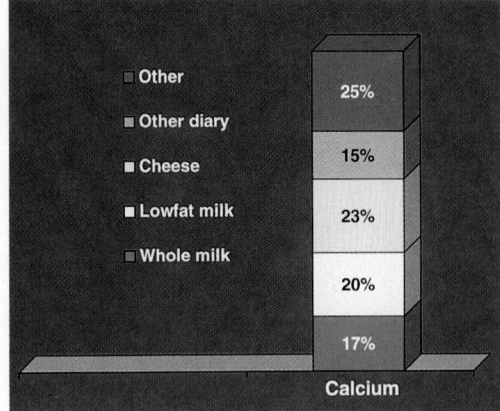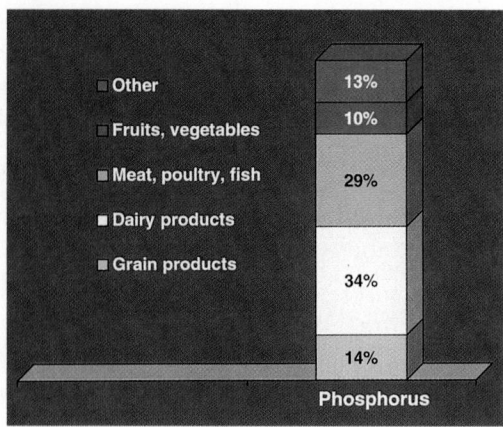

Figure 10-5.
Sources of calcium (left) and phosphorus (right) in the U.S. food supply.

Good sources of:

Calcium	Phosphorus
Milk	Milk
Cheese	Cheese
Yogurt	Yogurt
Eggs	Meat
Tuna	
Peanut butter	
Beans	

Hydroxyapatite: The hard substance between cells in bones and teeth consisting of calcium, phosphorus, hydrogen, and oxygen.

10-3. Adequate calcium intake throughout life is important. Figure 10-4 raises a familiar dilemma in nutrition: Do these supplements work–and are there any risks in taking them? The major sources of calcium and phosphorus in the typical U.S. diet are shown in Figure 10-5.

Notice that dairy products (cheese, low-fat milk, and whole milk) provide 75% of the total calcium intake. In the "other" category are leafy green vegetables such as broccoli, kale, and collard, calcium-precipitated tofu, calcium-fortified foods, and soft bones of fish such as sardines and salmon. Since most of these foods are not regular menu items for many people, attention must be paid to calcium intake if the intake of dairy products is low. Water is a variable source of calcium, and some antacids are calcium salts.

Phosphorus sources are much more varied in the diet, and dietary deficiencies of it are rare. An exception is small, premature infants fed human milk exclusively. These infants need more phosphorus than is contained in human milk for the rapid rate of bone formation they require. Another exception results when people consume large amounts of antacids containing aluminum hydroxide. This aluminum salt binds phosphorus in the GI tract, making it unavailable for absorption.

Calcium and phosphorus are the most abundant minerals in human beings (see Table 10-1). More than 99% of the calcium and 85% of the phosphorus are in bones and teeth. Bone also contains important amounts of magnesium, iron, and zinc. It is made up of canals, through which pass blood vessels that bring nutrients to the bone cells and nerves. *Hydroxyapatite* is the hard substance between cells in bones and teeth; it consists of a combination of calcium, phosphorus, hydrogen, and oxygen. The protein collagen acts as the "scaffolding" to hold the hydroxyapatite in place. Bone is a living tissue, increasing in length and width during growth and continually being broken down and rebuilt, even in the elderly.

The 1% of calcium and 15% of phosphorus occurring in soft tissue have many important functions. Calcium in the soft tissue is used for:

- Blood clotting
- Activation of some enzymes
- Excitation of nerves and muscles. Nerves are excited by the passing of an electrical signal along nerve fibers. The signal passes to mus-

cles, which then contract. If this process does not happen, nerves and muscles cannot work. The heart is the most important muscle in our body.

- Stimulation of some hormone secretions
- Control of calcium-deficiency hypertension in at-risk populations.[5] These include African-Americans, Japanese, alcoholics, diabetics, salt-sensitive individuals, pregnant women, and the elderly.

This seems to be a lot of work for 1% of body calcium! But 1% is all that is needed. The body has an effective way of maintaining blood and cell calcium at this level. Bones are the great reserve of calcium, and two hormones make sure that the level of calcium outside the bones remains at 1%. *Parathyroid hormone* (or parathormone) removes calcium from storage in bones when blood calcium is low. *Calcitonin* removes calcium from blood when levels are too high and returns it to the bones. This system of checks and balances ensures a stable level of blood calcium for delivery to cells. Recent evidence from the Harvard Medical School seems to explode the myth that a high intake of calcium leads to formation of insoluble deposits in soft tissue. Investigators found that high dietary calcium intake *decreases* the risk of kidney stones.[6] All of this evidence seems to point to a low risk of health complications when calcium supplements are used responsibly. The phosphorus level in the body is not controlled by hormones. There is less likelihood of phosphorus deficiency because of the wide distribution of phosphorus in foods.

The RDA for both calcium and phosphorus for men and women over 25 years of age is 800 milligrams. The daily intake of Americans averages 890 milligrams for calcium and 1,540 milligrams for phosphorus.

Phosphorus functions as:

- Part of the nucleic acids, DNA and RNA
- Part of the adenosine triphosphate (ATP) molecule, which is a storage form of energy in cells
- Part of phospholipids
- A coenzyme for some enzymes.

Because of the importance of these functions, the quality of life, and even life itself, depends on an adequate supply of calcium and phosphorus in the diet.

Absorption and utilization of calcium

Figure 10-6 shows how calcium is absorbed from the GI tract and transported by the blood to bones and all the cells in the body, while unabsorbed calcium is excreted in the feces. Calcium in the body may be excreted in urine and sweat.

An individual is in calcium balance when calcium intake from the diet approximately equals calcium excretion from the body. In positive calcium balance, intake exceeds excretion so that calcium is retained in the body; in negative calcium balance the converse is true.

Positive calcium balance is helped by vitamin D and the lactose in dairy products. They assist calcium absorption from the GI tract into the blood supply. Since calcium is absorbed in its ionizable form, easily soluble calcium salts are more bioavailable.

Parathyroid hormone: A hormone secreted by the parathyroid gland located close to the thyroid gland in the neck; moves calcium from bone to blood when blood levels of calcium are low.

Calcitonin: A hormone from the thyroid gland that decreases high blood calcium levels by depositing the extra calcium in bones.

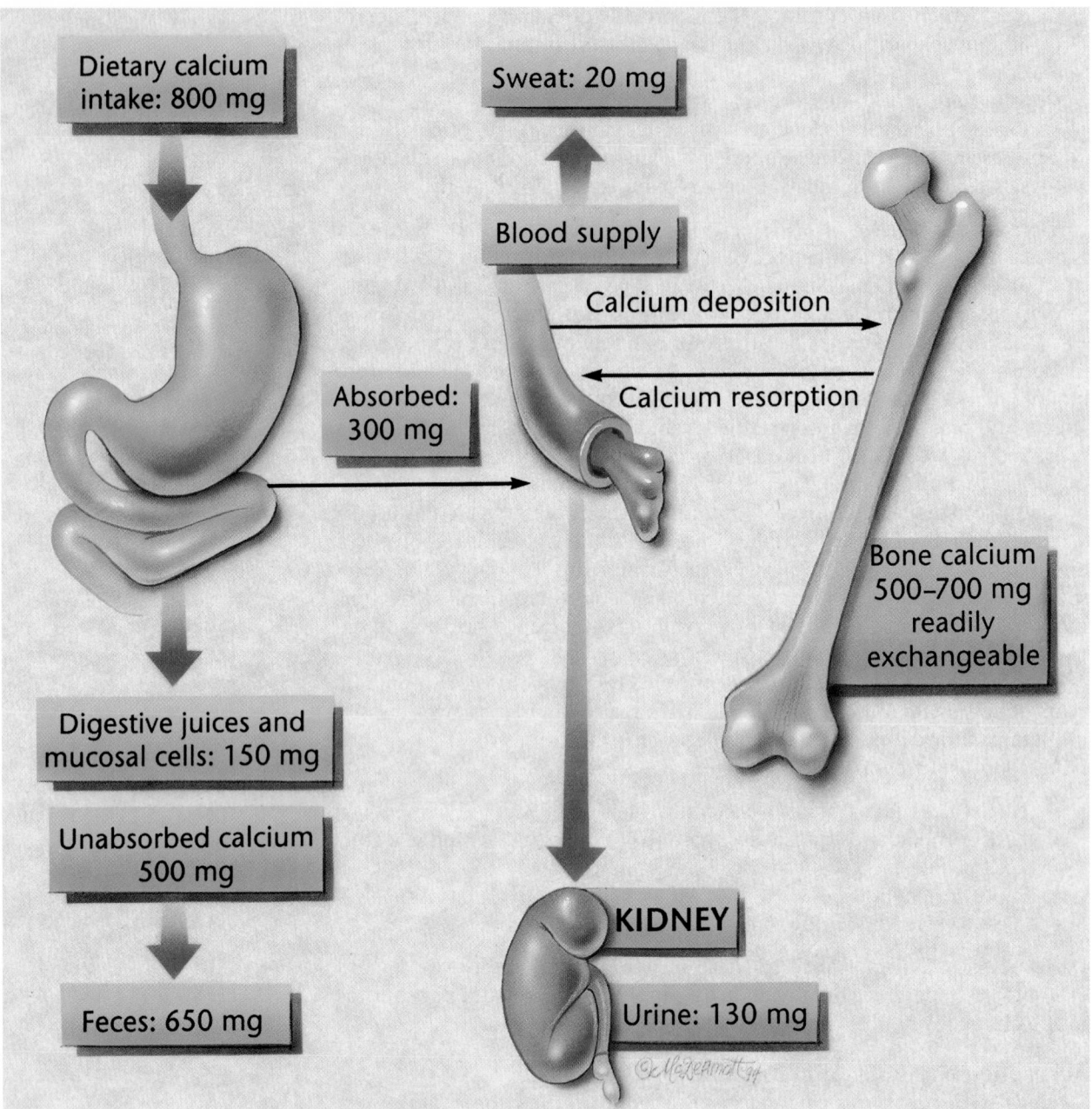

Figure 10-6. Digestion, absorption, utilization, and excretion of calcium. About 40% of the dietary calcium that a person consumes is absorbed into the blood. The rest is excreted through the feces, urine, and sweat. About 99% of the calcium retained in the body is located in the bones.

Calcium balance was once thought to be hindered by phosphate, which binds calcium in the GI tract, making it unavailable. However, recent evidence does not place as high an emphasis on phosphorus as a negative factor in calcium bioavailability. More work is needed before firm statements on the influence of phosphorus on calcium absorption can be made.

Fiber can bind calcium in the GI tract, making it unavailable for absorption. This calcium is excreted in the feces.

Oxalate and phytate may hinder absorption of calcium from the GI tract, but the significance of this on calcium balance in the body is debated by the experts.

Protein and amino acids at high levels of intake lead to increased loss of body calcium through the kidneys and urine.

Decreased gastric acidity decreases the absorption of calcium. This is common in the elderly and in patients taking antiulcer medications.[7]

Vitamin A in excessive amounts causes calcium loss from bone.

Sodium chloride (table salt) increases calcium loss through the kidneys.

Alcohol and caffeine in high amounts cause increased calcium loss from the body.

Medications including antacids and certain antibiotics decrease calcium absorption from the GI tract. Drugs such as the corticosteroids and thyroid extract increase calcium loss from the body. Athletes using steroids should be aware of this important negative effect on bone.

Disease states such as diabetes, kidney failure, and malabsorption syndromes (especially of fat) decrease calcium absorption.

Decreased physical activity causes bone loss. This is seen in bed-ridden patients and the elderly. Zero gravity causes calcium loss in astronauts. Increased physical activity slows the rate of bone loss, even in the elderly.

Osteoporosis is more common in women than in men

Everybody begins to lose bone mass by about 45 years of age. Osteoporosis ("porous bones") occurs when bone loss becomes so great that bone fractures occur after slight impact. Risk factors for osteoporosis include:

- Caucasian or Asian heritage
- Premature menopause or prolonged amenorrhea (absence or suppression of menstruation)
- Low calcium intake or absorption
- Positive family history of osteoporosis
- Short stature, low body weight
- Lack of exercise
- Not having given birth to children
- Cigarette smoking
- High alcohol consumption.

White, postmenopausal women are the population at greatest risk of osteoporosis. It is not as prevalent in men or in black women because of their higher bone mass. Lower-than-normal bone density is also found in people with anorexia nervosa. Most experts agree that the greatest protection against osteoporosis is a high bone mass in the early part of life.

The first sign of osteoporosis is back pain, caused by the collapse of one or more vertebrae. A "dowager's hump" can then result in older women (Figure 10-7).

Bones may be broken after slight impact, especially those in the spine, forearm, upper thigh, and hip.[4] Bone loss in the jaws, called alveolar bone

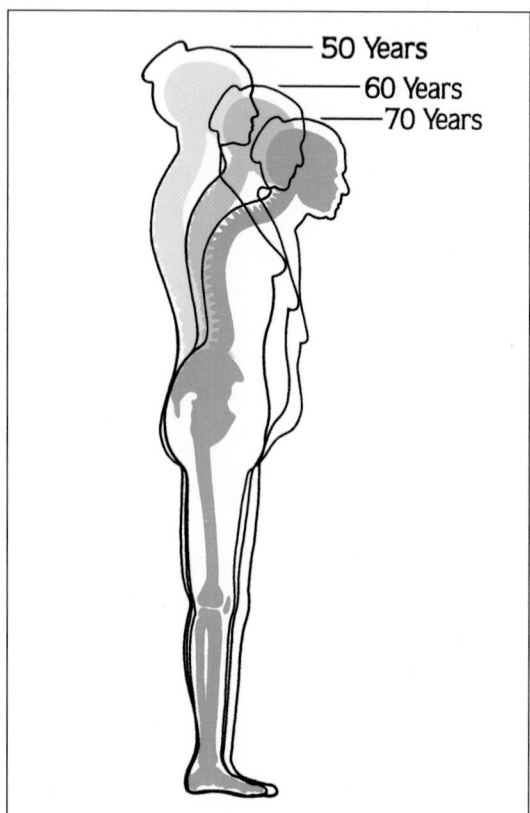

Figure 10-7. The dowager's hump, seen in some older women, is an indication of osteoporosis.

Estrogen: A female sex hormone responsible for development of secondary sexual characteristics; used to prevent osteoporosis.

loss, may be an early indicator of osteoporosis, and teeth can be lost as a result.

Osteoporosis is called "the silent disease" because it is difficult to diagnose until it has reached an advanced stage. If you are in your twenties, wouldn't it be nice to have a quick inexpensive checkup to tell you whether you will suffer from osteoporosis in later life? Unfortunately, the tests now available require sensitive equipment and are expensive. As one observer remarks, such tests are "premature, albeit profitable." Perhaps the best tactic is prevention of osteoporosis. For one expert, the method of choice is to fortify foods with calcium because

> pill taking doesn't get good compliance. We can't even get people who need medicines to take pills on a regular basis. Few individuals are going to maintain good nutrition by 40 years of pill taking.[8]

Why is osteoporosis more common in women than in men? Among the possible reasons are:

Women have lower calcium intake than men (see Table 10-2). Dr. Robert Heaney gives the following advice on calcium supplementation:

> . . . it seems prudent to increase the intake of calcium and vitamin D in most postmenopausal women–calcium to at least 1,000 mg and preferably to 1,500 mg per day, and vitamin D to 400 to 800 IU daily.[9]

Bone loss is greater after menopause. This suggests that hormonal factors are involved, especially the lack of *estrogen*.

Pregnancy and breast feeding increase calcium requirements (see the RDA table inside the back cover). This is especially important in teenage pregnancies. The higher RDA value for calcium (1,200 milligrams) is intended to meet calcium requirements for bone growth during the teenage years.

Weight-reducing diets are often low in calcium. Women are more likely to try them than are men.

Women live longer than men–and since osteoporosis is a disease of aging, it is seen more often in women.

Other factors suspected of contributing to osteoporosis are cigarette smoking, alcohol, and lack of exercise.

Rickets and osteomalacia are other calcium-related bone disorders. Rickets occurs in young children from a lack of vitamin D (see Chapter 9) and leads to poor absorption and deposition of calcium in bone. Osteomalacia occurs in adults and results from the combined deficiency of calcium and vitamin D. It is most common in women whose bones are depleted of calcium because of repeated pregnancies. The symptoms are the same in rickets and osteomalacia–distortion of bones and severe pain.

Sodium, Potassium, and Chloride: The Major Electrolytes

The major electrolytes–sodium, potassium, and chloride–are essential to health. Adults average about 100 grams of sodium and 95 grams of chloride in their bodies, which is equivalent to about 7 tablespoonfuls (half a cup) of salt, as well as 140 grams of potassium.

Sodium levels in the body regulate the amount of fluid inside and outside cells. The body is particularly sensitive to any increase in sodium within the cell; the excess is pumped back into the extracellular fluid. When the dietary intake of sodium is high, it is filtered from the blood by the kidneys and excreted in the urine. People with kidney disease require a diet low in sodium to spare the kidney this additional task.

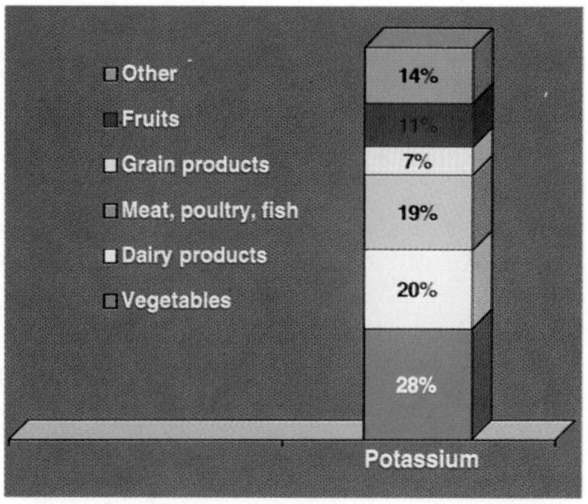

Sodium and potassium are required for muscle and nerve functioning. Both are important in carbohydrate nutrition–sodium for the absorption of glucose, potassium for the formation of glycogen–and potassium is involved also in protein synthesis. Chloride combines with hydrogen to form hydrochloric acid in the stomach, where it provides an acid medium that is important in the digestion of food. Potassium is depleted in severe diarrhea, which causes severe dehydration, paralysis, and death when prolonged.

☐ Other	14%
☐ Fruits	11%
☐ Grain products	7%
☐ Meat, poultry, fish	19%
☐ Dairy products	20%
☐ Vegetables	
	28%
Potassium	

Figure 10-8. Sources of potassium in the U.S. food supply.

Salt and sodium

Every day the average American consumes about 10 grams of salt, of which about 4 grams is sodium and the rest chloride. We are fortunate that these nutrients are freely available in most diets, but much of our sodium and chloride comes from table salt or from the salt added to processed foods. Potassium, which is closely related chemically to sodium, is found in many foods because it is an important ion inside the cells in animals and plants.

Salt has been added to foods since earliest of times to prevent food spoilage, to enhance flavor, and to influence the physical properties of

Table 10-3. Sources of Sodium in the U.S. Diet[a]

Sodium Source	Actual Intake (mg per day)	Contributed by
Nondiscretionary intake	3,340 by males 2,298 by females	Grain group, 24%
Naturally occurring in foods, 1/3		Combination foods (soups, gravies, mixed protein dishes) 20%
Added during commercial processing, 1/3		Meat group, 19% Fats, sweets, alcohol, 15% Milk group, 13% Fruits and vegetables, 11%
Discretionary intake, 1/3	1,300 by males 900 by females	Salt added by consumer

[a] Recommended intake from all sources: 1,100–3,300 milligrams per day for adults, equivalent to the sodium in 2.7–8.2 grams of salt (about ½ to 1¾ teaspoon) daily. Salt (NaCl) is 40% sodium.

some foods–strengthening bread dough and controlling cheese texture are two good examples. Salt is, in fact, the oldest food additive in the world. A new book with the title *Salt and Civilization*[10] makes the case that salt is among the most important natural commodities of all times, essential to human and animal life. But salt intake varies widely among different cultures. For example, high per capita use of salt has almost always been associated with meat preservation and flavoring. The intake of salt was sharply limited in India because of the vegetarianism required by the Hindu religion. Salt occurs in some obvious and some not so obvious foods:

- **Salted snacks**–saltine crackers, pretzels, salted potato chips, nuts, salted popcorn
- **Meat and fish that are salted or smoked**–frankfurters, ham, bacon, luncheon meat, sardines, anchovies, smoked salmon
- **Cheese**–especially processed cheese
- **Soups**–if canned or dehydrated
- **Sauces**–catsup, horseradish
- **Brine-soaked foods**–pickles, olives.

Sodium levels are high in:	
Steak sauce	Seasoned salt
Barbecue sauce	Celery salt
Worcestershire sauce	Onion salt
Chili sauce	Garlic salt
Catsup	Monosodium glutamate
Mustard	Meat tenderizer
Salad dressings	Baking powder
Pickles	Baking soda
Relish	Soy sauce

The U.S. Department of Agriculture issued the list of high-sodium commercially prepared condiments, sauces, and seasonings shown in the margin.

The list includes monosodium glutamate (MSG), which was investigated in an entire segment of a popular television news magazine program in November 1991. Since MSG has become a TV star (or villain), let's look at it more closely. MSG is the sodium salt of the amino acid glutamic acid. This acid is widespread in most foods, including tomatoes, peas, and mushrooms. MSG is a flavor enhancer important especially for the elderly, whose decreased taste sensitivity may have negative effects on their caloric and nutrient intake.[11] It is acknowledged that some persons report adverse reactions to MSG, including headaches and nausea, but these are the exception rather than the rule. It is now listed on many food labels and on the menu in many restaurants. If in doubt, people are encouraged to request the server to "hold the MSG."

Think about the list provided by the USDA. With sodium in so many places, it is difficult for some people to regulate sodium intake. There is good news–most herbs and spices are sodium free. But why are the government and the media fascinated with salt, MSG, sodium-containing condiments and sauces, and in general, the amount of sodium we consume? High sodium intake is associated with increased incidence of hypertension (high blood pressure). About one in five adult Americans suffers from hypertension, which is a risk factor in coronary heart disease and in stroke. The exact cause of hypertension is not known, but factors other than sodium intake are involved.[12] Weight loss is the most effective nonpharmacologic treatment for hypertension, followed by sodium restriction and stress management. More studies are needed to confirm suggestions that hypertension is controlled by the addition of either calcium, magnesium, potassium, or fish oil to the diet.

Evidence from anthropology, sociology, medicine, physiology, and epidemiology links sodium intake with hypertension in most parts of the world. The sodium level of the diet of most Americans, Canadians, and Europeans is far in excess of the amounts needed for functions performed by sodium in the body. So should we reduce this high sodium intake? Some experts who argue for reduction say there is no way to identify who may be among the approximately 20% of the population who are responsive to hypertension from high sodium intake. However, since adult hypertension may start in childhood, they argue that no one should go through life on a high sodium diet, just in case they are in the high-risk group. Most nutritionists make no argument against reducing very high intake of sodium. They do caution that wholesale elimination of sodium from foods may affect their microbiological safety.

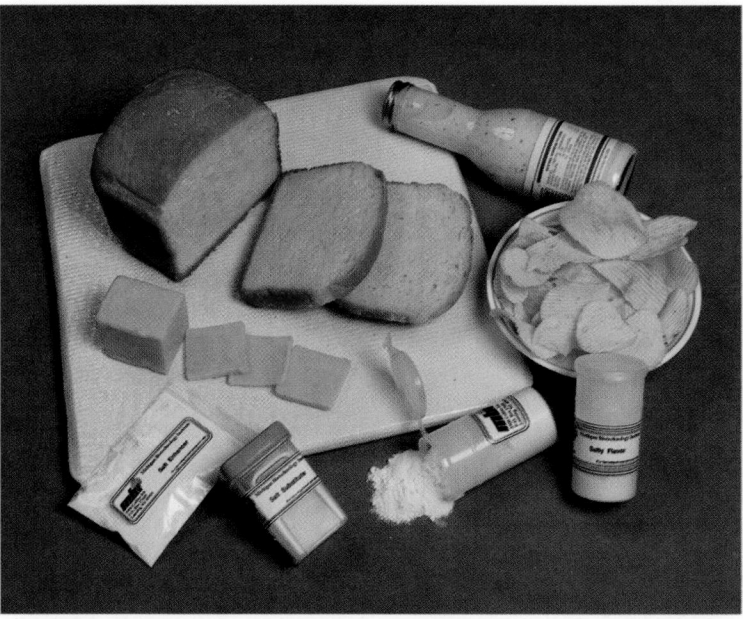

Figure 10-9. Foods containing salt substitutes. Salt substitutes give the taste of salt without containing sodium, which is a part of table salt. Sodium is a factor contributing to hypertension in some people.

Salt substitutes (Figure 10-9) can now be used instead of salt. They taste salty and leave a pleasant flavor and coolness as they dissolve on the tongue. Nutritionists are interested in them because of their low sodium content.

Recent evidence raises the question of whether chloride rather than sodium should be looked at in regard to hypertension. This evidence comes from some experiments showing that only sodium chloride is related to hypertension. Equal amounts of sodium in other sodium salts had little or no effect on hypertension. Much more must be learned about dietary and nondietary influences on this condition.

Magnesium

Magnesium is provided by many different food groups in the typical U.S. diet (Figure 10-10).

This wide variety of dietary sources of magnesium means that deficiencies are rare in the general population. Americans' average daily intake of magnesium is about 330 milligrams; the RDAs for adult men and women are 350 and 280 milligrams, respectively. Magnesium is an important part of chlorophyll, the green pigment in plants that is used in photosynthesis.

Adults have about 20–28 grams of magnesium in their bodies. About 40% of this is in muscle and soft tissue such as liver

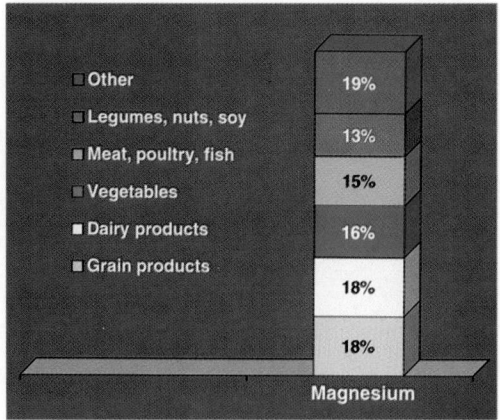

Figure 10-10. Sources of magnesium in the U.S. food supply.

and kidneys; 1% is in the extracellular fluid, and the remaining almost 60% is in bone. Magnesium assists over 300 enzymes involved in the synthesis and breakdown of carbohydrates, lipids, and proteins and in the synthesis of DNA and RNA within the cell.

It is needed for the functioning of nerves and muscles, including the heart. Deficiency symptoms include uncontrolled muscle twitching, leading to convulsions, heart failure, and death. They usually arise not from dietary deficiencies of magnesium but because of malabsorption from the GI tract or excessive fluid and electrolyte loss; malfunctioning of the kidneys, resulting in loss of magnesium in the urine; general malnutrition and alcoholism; or excessive use of certain medications that interfere with magnesium absorption and conservation within the body. Stress causes hormonal changes that lead to increased magnesium loss from the body. This stress can be either physical, including exhaustive exercise, surgery, and extremes of temperature, or psychological, including anger, fear, or overwork. In a study on U.S. Navy trainees, low blood magnesium levels were attributed to the stress of their hard physical training. Magnesium supplements are not needed in any of these stress situations.

Daily magnesium supplements improve glucose handling in elderly people, but these should be given only under medical supervision.[13] Hypermagnesemia does cause death. It is a major cause of death in northern India,[14] where the use of the chemical aluminum phosphide as a grain preservative can result in toxic accumulations of magnesium.

Sulfur

Sulfur has no RDA, and no sulfur deficiencies have been identified. Diets adequate in animal and plant protein are adequate in sulfur also. This is because three amino acids (methionine, cystine, and cysteine) contain sulfur. It is also found in the molecular structure of the vitamins thiamin and biotin.

Adjacent sulfur-containing amino acids can form rigid sulfur-sulfur bonds. These bonds are important in maintaining the three-dimensional structures of protein and are especially important for the functioning of enzymes. Increased numbers of sulfur-sulfur bridges in a protein molecule increase its rigidity. The best examples of this are the high-sulfur proteins in hair, nails, and skin.

■ Microminerals, or trace elements

Information on the microminerals has undergone rapid changes in the past 50 years. The importance of iron was established in the 17th century, but most discoveries on the essential nature of zinc, selenium, copper, and other trace elements are of recent vintage. The most important of the microminerals–iron, zinc, iodine, selenium, fluoride, copper, and a few others are examined in this section.

Iron–The Vital Carrier of Oxygen

We have already had the opportunity to examine the importance of iron in oxygen transport in the body in a number of places in this book. Now we are ready to take a closer look at this process. Muscles, in particular, need a lot of oxygen to quickly release the energy needed for physical work or athletic performance. To facilitate this, muscle has another iron-containing molecule called myoglobin, which picks up the oxygen from hemoglobin in the blood. Normal ranges in hemoglobin values in males and females over 14 years of age are 13–16 grams and 12–16 grams of hemoglobin per 100 milliliters of blood, respectively. Iron-deficiency anemia is diagnosed when hemoglobin values are less than 12 grams of hemoglobin per 100 milliliters of blood in females or males, or less than 11.0 grams in pregnant women.

Iron has other important functions in the body. It is part of some enzymes, and it helps maintain the immune system.[15] The negative effects of iron deficiency in early life have attracted considerable attention. Low hemoglobin levels in pregnant women result in lower oxygen-carrying capacity in the blood, which impairs fetal growth.[16] Iron deficiency decreases a child's learning capacity because of increased irritability, shortened attention spans, and fatigue.[17] These results must be interpreted carefully. Iron-poor diets are usually deficient in other nutrients also, and poor home and school environments may be complicating factors. However, investigators are confident that iron deficiency has a significant role to play in these learning problems. The encouraging fact is that they are correctable by iron therapy.

Iron is the only nutrient that has a higher RDA for women than for men. The RDA is 15 milligrams for premenopausal women and 10 milligrams for men. This difference is due to the loss of iron-containing hemoglobin during menstruation. About three quarters of the iron in the body is in the hemoglobin molecule in red blood cells. Iron-deficiency anemia in premenopausal women is usually the result of either heavy menstrual bleeding or of diets low in iron, or both. If an adult man is anemic, the first thing physicians suspect is a bleeding ulcer; men do not normally suffer from iron-deficiency anemia.

Sources of iron in the U.S. food supply are shown on the left in Figure 10-11, and the bioavailability of iron from different foods is shown on the right.

Grain products and meat are the most plentiful sources of dietary iron in the typical U.S. diet. Meats have the highest percent iron bioavailability of all foods. This means that people who don't eat meat must pay particular attention to having a variety of plant foods rich in iron in their diet. Vitamin C makes iron in plant foods more bioavailable. However, calcium supplements may inhibit the absorption of iron.[18] Taking regular calcium supplements with meals makes it more difficult for women to meet their daily iron requirement.

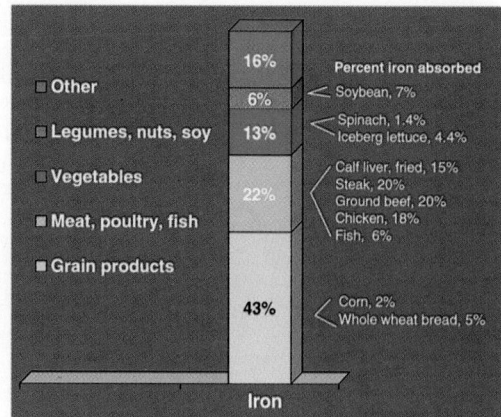

Figure 10-11. Sources of iron in the U.S. food supply (left) and the percentage of the iron in various foods that can be absorbed by the body (right). Notice that meat is the most bioavailable food source of iron.

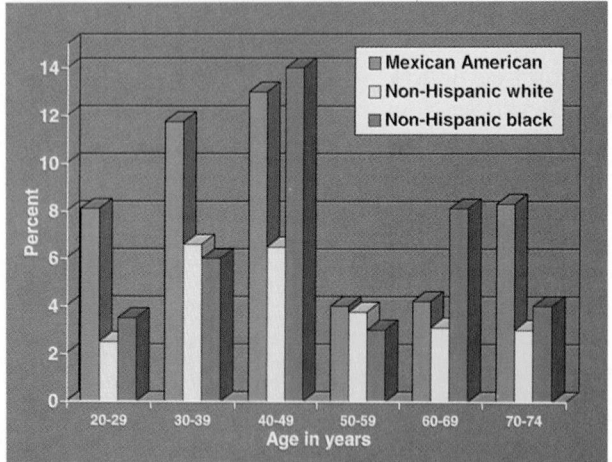

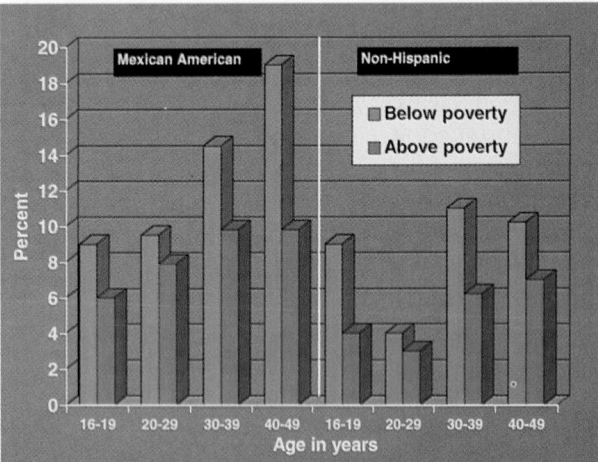

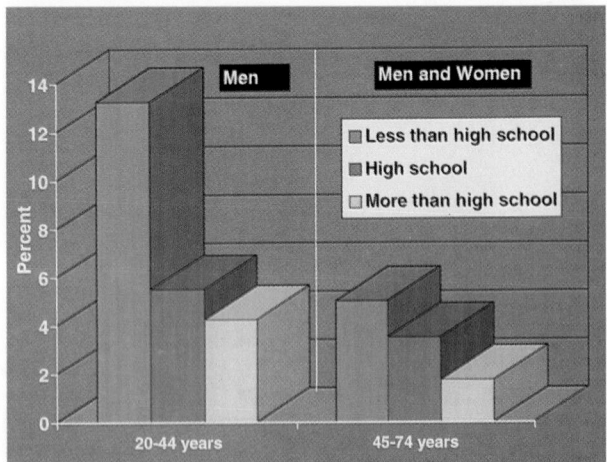

Figure 10-12. Iron deficiency in women of different ethnic and age groups (top), in women of different socioeconomic levels (middle), and in people with different education levels (bottom).

The information in Table 10-2 showed us that iron intake is a problem for 2-year-old children, teenage girls, and premenopausal women. This information is reflected in the incidence of iron deficiency among women, as seen in the Figure 10-12.

Certain trends are apparent from these graphs: 1) iron-deficiency is less prevalent after menopause; 2) it tends to be more common in African-American and Mexican-American women than in white women; 3) it is more prevalent in women living below the poverty level; and 4) it is more common among the less educated.

Most discussion about iron nutrition in the past concentrated on the effects of iron deficiency on health. Now there is also emphasis on the harmful health effects of iron overload.[19] *Hereditary hemochromatosis* is a form of iron overload with about a 5% frequency in the population of European descent in the United States, Australia, and Europe.[20] An abnormal gene is responsible for increased absorption of dietary iron, resulting in excess iron deposition in the liver, heart, and certain endocrine organs. Death may result from liver disease, cancer of the liver, or heart failure. Research and educational programs are being encouraged in order to alert health professionals and the public to the problem.

What happens here is an interesting combination of the effects of diet and the genetic composition of the individual. Some promising evidence pinpointing the genetic factor responsible for hemochromatosis in Africans may lead to a resolution of this problem, with significant nutritional implications for countries that permit addition of iron to foods, including the United States, Canada, and European countries.

Zinc–Food Sources a Problem for Many People

Information about zinc is very recent because only in 1963 was it shown to be essential in human nutrition. Since then we have learned that nearly half of our dietary zinc is provided by meats (Figure 10-13).

Zinc intake is a problem for many people, as was seen in Table 10-2. Part of the reason is that the best sources of zinc–meats and dairy products–are more expensive than other sources. Thus, economics may be at play here, as well as a lack of understanding of which foods are rich in zinc and of the important functions of zinc in the body. Another problem is that zinc absorption is reduced by plant substances such as phytate, by some types of fiber, and also by iron and calcium supplements. There is a fascinating chemical tug-of-war for absorption between different minerals after a meal.

Zinc is needed by over 70 enzymes in the body and for protein synthesis and is part of the insulin molecule. A deficiency of zinc produces delayed sexual development, growth failure, decreased immune function, loss of the sense of taste, skin changes, delayed wound healing, and reduced resistance to disease. A decreased ability of the eyes to adapt to darkness is a symptom of secondary vitamin A deficiency, which is caused by zinc deficiency. Dwarfism from zinc deficiency has been reported in a number of countries, including the United States, Egypt, China, Iran, and Morocco. Figures 10-14 and 10-15 show how deficiency appears in a zinc-deficient rat compared with a healthy animal of the same age.

Can the frightening consequences of zinc deficiency be prevented by zinc supplements? Yes, but be careful–low doses will correct most problems. A study in Canada showed that young boys short in stature increased their height after zinc supplementation. Improvements in severely malnourished children occur quickly after zinc supplements are given. But high doses of zinc cause a number of problems, including a negative effect on copper absorption and metabolism.[21]

Zinc RDAs for men and women are 15 and 12 milligrams, respectively. Increased amounts are recommended for pregnancy and lactation, in part for the increased protein synthesis required for growth and for the synthesis of milk proteins. Besides pregnant women, the people most likely to have low intake of zinc are premature infants, children, adolescents, and alcoholics. Many women taking oral contraceptive agents have low levels

Hereditary hemochromatosis: A genetic defect causing excess deposits of iron in the body, especially in the liver. Consequences include liver damage, heart failure, and diabetes; usually develops in middle age.

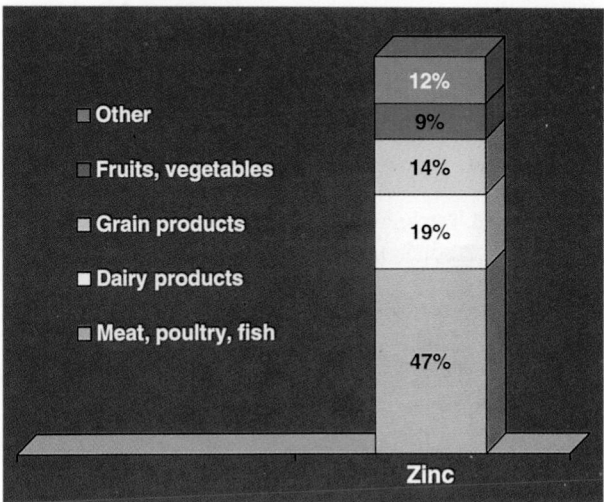

Figure 10-13. Sources of zinc in the U.S. food supply.

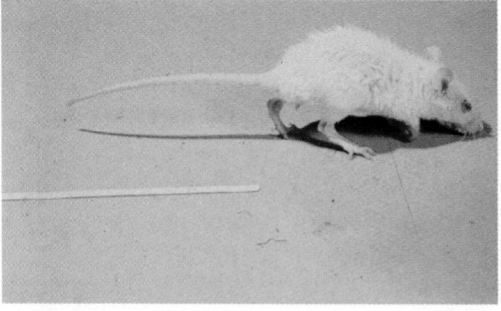 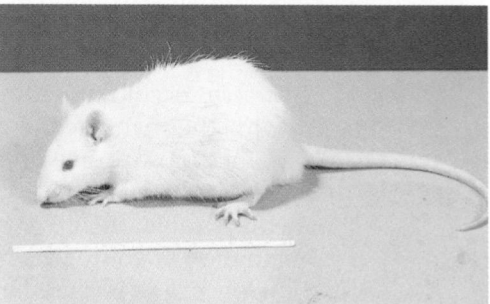

Figures 10-14 and 10-15. A zinc-deficient rat (left) and a rat of the same age that has consumed a diet adequate in zinc (right). The rat on the left did not grow as fast and has poor quality skin and coat. Experimental animals provide valuable information in human nutrition.

of zinc in the blood, but this is not a problem if the diet is adequate in zinc. Factors contributing to deficiency include poor diet, alcoholism, malabsorption of zinc, liver and kidney disease, and certain genetic disorders.

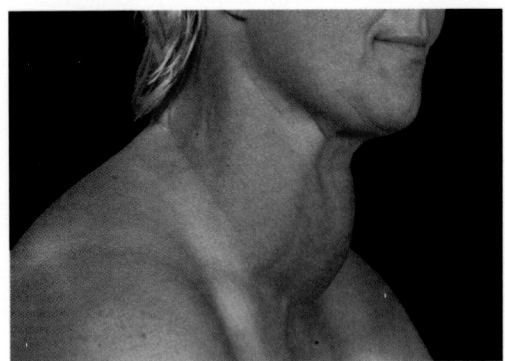

Figure 10-16. Person with goiter.

Goiter: An enlargement of the thyroid gland in the neck usually caused by dietary iodine deficiency.

Hypothyroidism: Deficiency of thyroid secretions, including the iodine-containing thyroid hormones, resulting in lower basal metabolism.

Iodine–A Major Deficiency Problem in the World

The man in Figure 10-16 suffers from iodine deficiency, which causes a swelling of the thyroid gland known as *goiter*. Goiter is more prevalent in women than in men. Since iodine is needed for thyroid hormone production, diets deficient in iodine cause *hypothyroidism*, resulting in mental retardation (cretinism), short stature, deaf-mutism, goiter, and an increased risk of death in childhood. If a woman is deficient in iodine during pregnancy, the child may be a cretin–permanently retarded in its mental and physical growth. This places an economic burden on the family and the society.

Unfortunately, these deficiency problems are not reversible when iodine intake is increased. About one-fifth of the earth's population, mostly in developing countries, is presently at risk of iodine deficiency. Yet a researcher over 60 years ago wrote,

> . . . simple goiter is the easiest of all known diseases to prevent . . . . It may be excluded from the list of human diseases as soon as society determines to make the effort.[22]

Some advances have been made, but mostly in developed countries. Since most foods rich in iodine are grown in or near the ocean, iodine deficiency used to be widespread in areas located far from the sea. In the early 1890s, many people in the upper Midwest and in central Canada were found to be suffering from goiter. This problem has been essentially eliminated by the availability of iodized salt, a process begun in Michigan in 1924. A second explanation of the elimination of goiter is the ease of distribution to all parts of the country of iodine-rich seafoods and other foods grown near the sea.

But not everybody is pleased with the addition of iodine to salt. Protesters in India point out that the government's proposal to add iodine to all salt will raise its price beyond the means of poor people. They also point out that environmental pollution and ecological imbalances created by new agricultural technologies are the real causes of the iodine depletion of the soil.[23]

Goitrogens: Substances that interfere with the normal functioning of the thyroid gland; found especially in cabbages, peanuts, and soybeans.

Thyroxin: One of the iodine-containing hormones produced by the thyroid gland.

Hyperthyroidism: Overactivity of the thyroid gland.

Goitrogens occur naturally in foods like cabbage and turnips. They interfere with the manufacture and synthesis of *thyroxin*, which contains iodine. Since most people do not eat large amounts of cabbage and turnips on a regular basis, this is not a problem. However, in parts of Africa where millet is a staple, there is a high incidence of goiter, probably caused by a combination of goitrogens in the millet and a low intake of iodine.

Hyperthyroidism is caused by an excess of iodine. Its symptoms include an increased basal metabolic rate, which causes an increased demand for food to support this metabolic activity. Concern that some people get too much iodine has been increasing since the 1970s. For a North American adult, a diet containing 2,850 calories per day will have about 700 micrograms of iodine, compared with an RDA value of 150 micrograms. Over half of this iodine is provided by dairy products, and grains and cereals provide a quarter. A typical fast-food meal of hamburger, french fries, and a milkshake provides three times the RDA of iodine. Much of this comes from iodine-containing chemicals used to kill bacteria and fungi on dairy equipment, and some comes from the iodine added as a dough conditioner in bread-making.

Selenium–Will It Prevent Cancer?

"Selenophilia," meaning "a love of selenium," is an interesting name coined for people with strong interests in selenium. Much of that interest is triggered by evidence that selenium may prevent cancer in experimental animals, but medical evidence of this occurring in humans is weak.[24] Scientists are still debating about the best form of selenium to take as supplements.[25] Be watchful for the following unproven promises of things that selenium supplements will prevent (these are *not* sanctioned by scientists): aging, cancer, cardiovascular disease, cataracts, sudden infant death syndrome, pollutant damage to cells, and others.

The minimum toxic dose for selenium is only five times in excess of the RDA. Clinical signs of selenium toxicity are difficult to detect. They include liver damage, numbness, nausea, vomiting, and rashes. Because of the added difficulties caused by toxicity, and because of fear of their abuse, nutritionists are slow to recommend selenium supplements.

Selenium is part of one enzyme that acts as an antioxidant. It interacts with vitamin E in its antioxidant capacity, thus preventing cell damage. Low levels of selenium in some parts of China produce Keshan disease in children, which leads to fatal heart damage. Poor diets coupled with acute alcoholism may cause selenium deficiency.

Plants low in protein (such as fruits and vegetables) are low in selenium. The best sources are meats and grains. The RDAs for selenium for men and women are 70 and 55 micrograms, respectively; intake levels in North America range from 60 to about 220 micrograms. Foods grown in different parts of the United States vary in their selenium content because of the variation in the concentration of this mineral in the soil. Low selenium levels are found in the soil in western Oregon and parts of the Midwest and in China, New Zealand, and Finland. In parts of the Great Plains in North America, plants can be grown that may produce selenium toxicity in animals.

Fluoride–Prevents Tooth Decay

Nutritional and medical information on fluoride may cause the general public to have a love-hate relationship with fluoride. Fluoridation of community water supplies was considered to be part of a Communist plot when first implemented in 1945, but this charge was quickly dropped. Fluoride added to water does prevent tooth decay.[26] Many studies have shown that increased levels of fluoride in water decrease the number of de-

Alzheimer's disease: An irreversible degenerative disease of the central nervous system characterized by loss of memory, mainly in 40–60 year olds.

cayed, missing, or filled teeth in children. In the 1970s, fluoride was suggested to be associated with cancer, but there is no strong evidence to support this relationship. The latest interest in fluoride stems from evidence of its possible beneficial effect in preventing *Alzheimer's disease*. That is because fluoride decreases the negative effects of aluminum, which has been suggested as a cause of this disease.[26] Original hopes that fluoride might be useful in preventing osteoporosis have not been borne out.[27] This is unfortunate because treatment of osteoporosis by estrogen causes unwanted side effects, and calcium supplements lead to interference with the absorption of other nutrients such as iron.

Good dietary advice is to consume an adequate diet and to use toothpaste with fluoride, which is shown to be effective against tooth decay. Water is the main source of fluoride for most people, but tea and seafood are also good sources. Adults consume about 1.0–2.3 milligrams of fluoride per day. A high intake of fluoride causes mottling or brown spots in teeth, but mottled teeth, although cosmetically unappealing, are strong and cavity-resistant. West Texas and parts of India are two places in the world with high fluoride intake. However, long-term intake of water containing up to eight times the recommended concentration of fluoride can eventually lead to severe bone and joint disorders. High use of aluminum-containing antacids causes significant losses of fluoride from the body.

Copper–Part of Many Enzymes

Take a close look at Figure 10-17.

These are the most important dietary sources of copper. How often do you eat lobster, shellfish, liver, nuts, and the other foods in this picture? It should not be a surprise that the copper intake is low for many people, as seen in Table 10-2. Many people may be marginally deficient in copper. Sources of copper in the North American food supply are equally distributed among foods of plant and animal origin (Figure 10-18).

Copper is a part of many enzymes, aids in iron absorption and metabolism, and is important for proper immune function and for blood clotting.

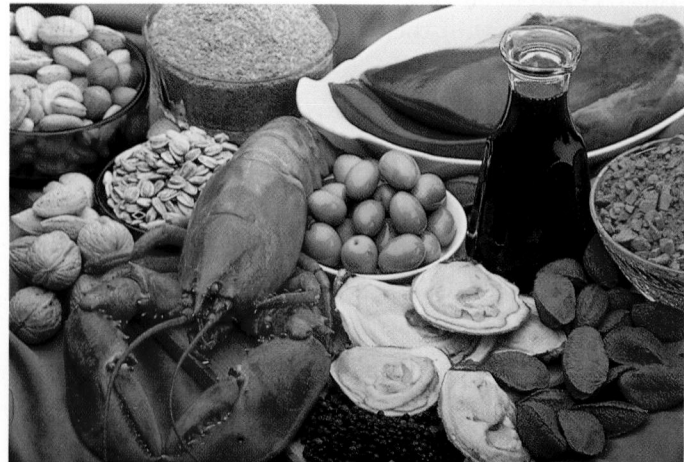

Figure 10-17. Copper-rich foods.

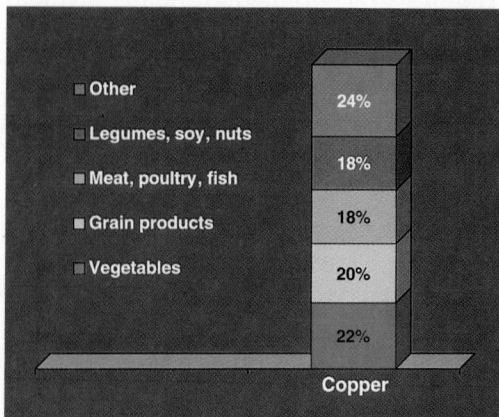

Figure 10-18. Sources of copper in the U.S. food supply.

Lower copper intake, in association with other dietary components, is thought to be a factor in coronary heart disease. The onset of heart abnormalities is rapid when experimental animals are given copper-poor diets.[28]

Trace Elements Recommended in Very Small Amounts

- **Manganese.** The absorption of manganese is not significantly affected by most dietary factors. It is needed for bone formation and for many enzyme reactions. Intake is low for teenage girls (see Table 10-2).

- **Silicon.** This is an essential element for plants and is probably an essential element for mammals.[29] Silicon is present in tiny amounts in most body tissues and fluids. The best dietary sources are unrefined grains of high fiber content, cereal products, and root vegetables. It may also be in drinking water, but that varies widely from one community to another. Foods of animal origin are low in silicon. Deficiency of silicon in experimental animals causes weakening of connective tissue.

- **Cobalt** is a part of vitamin B-12.

- **Molybdenum** is present in cereals and legumes. It is a part of some enzymes. No known deficiency symptoms occur in people.

- **Chromium** is present in liver, meat, seafood, and brewer's yeast. It is required for glucose metabolism, which is altered in the chromium-deficient state.

- **Nickel** is thought to be essential in human nutrition.

- **Boron.** Dr. Forrest Nielsen, a USDA scientist doing nutrition research on boron says,

  > Boron is of more nutritional importance than is generally recognized today, but is not a miracle nutrient, as suggested by some recent claims . . . it is clearly a biologically dynamic element that affects numerous metabolic processes in higher animals, including humans.[30]

It seems that each new nutrient attracts a long list of false claims on which fortunes are made. Boron seems to be no exception. Here is a sampling of *false* claims:[30]

"Miracle mineral (boron)–Substance could end bone disease in gals."
"Boron has a very positive effect on male libido."
"Boron is effective in suppressing postmenopausal hot flashes."
"Incredible strength gains using awesome boron."

■ People are different–Clay eating and lead contamination of food and drink

Clay eating and lead intoxication are two topics that may be a surprise in a chapter on mineral nutrition. Clay eating, also called *geophagy* or *pica*, is practiced by some people in various cultures in times of famine or economic deprivation.[31] It is sometimes considered an unusual behavior and a

---

Silicon in the water supply:

Chicago
0.68 milligrams per liter

Los Angeles
16.40 milligrams per liter

Geophagy or pica: Cravings for substances not fit for food, especially clay. Pregnant women are known to consume clay, starch, ashes, and plaster. Common throughout the world, especially in lower socioeconomic groups.

symptom of metabolic dysfunction, as is the consumption of laundry starch, paint, cigarette butts, and burnt matches. However, certain experts consider pica as a way to obtain minerals when intake in the diet is low. Some even consider that it has been important in the evolution of human dietary behavior since earliest times.[32] Some clay does provide calcium, copper, iron, magnesium, manganese, and zinc in amounts of nutritional significance. In the United States, pica is more common in pregnant women than in other people and more common than was originally thought. However, data on pica practices by pregnant women are limited.[33] Women at high risk of practicing pica are more likely to be African-American, to live in rural areas, and to have a childhood and family history of pica. Pica during pregnancy may cause anemia. (In the section on iron we saw how a number of other minerals interfere with iron absorption.) It has been associated with deaths of mothers and new babies. Researchers conclude that pica shows no sign of decline.

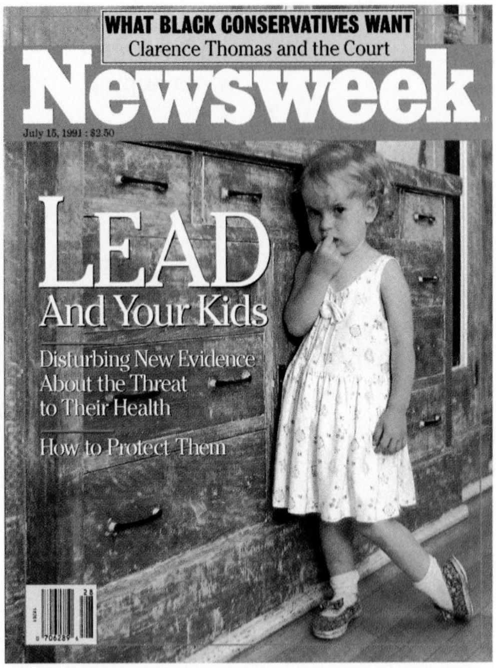

Think beyond the photograph in Figure 10-19. Why is lead a threat to children?

Lead gets into our bodies through lead in water, in contaminated food, in paint, and from car exhaust when leaded fuel is burned, as is still the case in many countries.

> Anyone can have lead poisoning . . . it occurs without regard for race, ethnic origin, income or social status

is how Dr. Sandra Andrews at Michigan State University describes the problem.

> No region is without a lead problem. Most people with lead poisoning do not know they have it.

We are fortunate that the amount of lead in our environment is much lower now than it was 30 years ago. Be assured that the level of lead in most food is now very low. It may occur in food under a variety of circumstances:

- If food is grown in lead-contaminated soil
- If water is high in lead
- If food (including infant formula) has been rehydrated with water high in lead
- If food has come from lead-soldered cans. These are now rare in North America.

Other sources of lead intake include:

- Lead paint on cribs and walls, eaten by small children
- Alcoholic drinks stored for long periods in lead crystal containers
- Ceramic wares that are usually high in lead (dishes, pottery)
- Bread wrappers imprinted with lead-based inks. A few years ago, wrappers were used that could transfer lead to food when the bags

WHAT BLACK CONSERVATIVES WANT
Clarence Thomas and the Court

Newsweek

July 15, 1991 : $2.50

LEAD
And Your Kids

Disturbing New Evidence
About the Threat
to Their Health

How to Protect Them

Figure 10-19. Lead poisoning causes slower mental development in children. It is a major environmental problem, as soil and water can be contaminated. One source of lead intake is water delivered through lead pipes.

were turned inside out. This finding forced bakers to switch to the use of new dyes with little or no lead.

Lead exposure has very damaging results, especially in young children. These include intelligence deficits and delayed behavioral and motor development.[34] Childhood exposure to lead is preventable, and there is a high intellectual cost for not preventing it among children. Improving nutrition is among the recommended ways to reduce or prevent further increases in blood-lead levels.[35]

■ Nutrition in action–Minerals and dairy products

It is time to examine the last of the major food commodities in our diet–dairy products. Information in Table 1-4 and in Chapter 4 showed how dairy products are important sources of calcium, phosphorus, protein, and vitamins, including riboflavin, other B-complex vitamins, and vitamins A and D. We also saw that some dairy products are high in fat. In this chapter we saw the nutritional importance of calcium and phosphorus and the possible problems with hypertension in some people when sodium intake is high.

Think about the numbers in Table 10-4.

Notice that the sodium content of dairy products varies considerably, but that the ones with the highest content are cheeses. Yogurt has the least sodium.

Let's examine how cheese and yogurt are manufactured. Cheese has been made since about 4000 B.C. by fermenting milk. Nowadays, the milk is pasteurized to kill harmful microorganisms and then cooled to about 20°C. This heat treatment is necessary because milk is an ideal medium for the growth of microorganisms. Bovine tuberculosis used to be a hazard in milk consumption, but the problem was eliminated by modern dairy hygiene practices. We saw in earlier chapters that not all microbes are harmful. Some harmless microbes are now put to work to make cheese. A *starter culture*, usually *Lactococcus lactis* in cheese manufacture, is added to the milk to convert lactose to lactic acid. That makes the medium so acidic that many harmful microbes are unable to grow. *Rennet* is added to the acid medium. It is an extract of calf stomach and contains the enzyme rennin, which clots the milk.

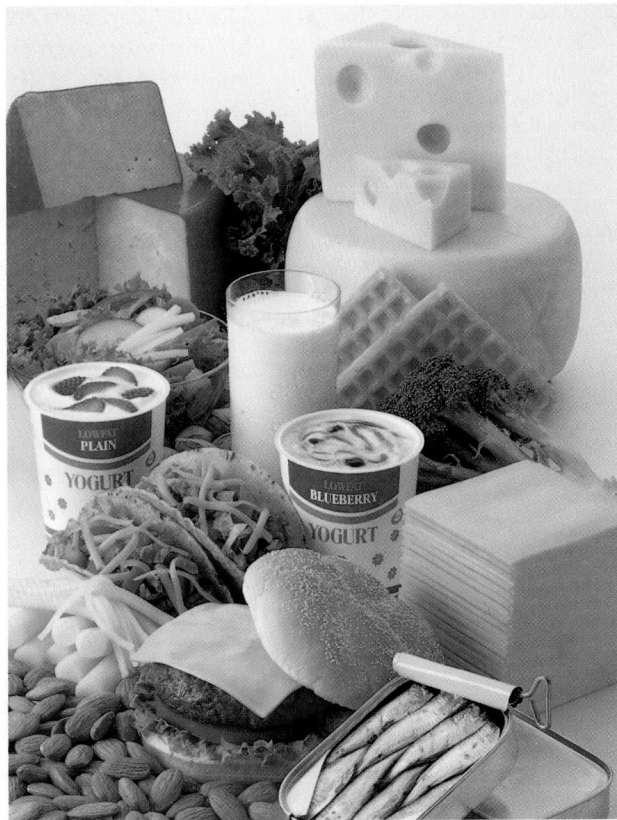

Figure 10-20. Calcium-rich foods.

Table 10-4. Calcium and Sodium in Dairy Products

Dairy Products	Calcium (milligrams)	Sodium (milligrams)
Cheese (per ounce)		
Blue	150	400
Brick	190	160
Brie	52	180
Cheddar	200	180
Cream	23	80
Gorgonzola	150	510
Swiss	270	70
Pasteurized (American)	170	400
Milk (per cup)	290	120
Ice cream (per cup)	150	110
Yogurt (per cup)	120	45

Starter culture: A culture of bacteria used to start bacterial growth in milk for cheese production, or in butter to develop the flavor, or in any fermentation.

Rennet: An extract of calf stomach containing the enzyme rennin, which clots milk; used in cheese-making.

Rennet can also be obtained from microorganisms, using techniques of biotechnology. A curd is now formed containing milk proteins, fat, fat-soluble vitamins, calcium, and most of the water-soluble vitamins. After the curd is hardened, it is cut into small pieces and the whey is drained off. (You probably first heard of these in the nursery rhyme in which Little Miss Muffet was eating her "curds and whey.")

Whey is a liquid containing proteins, lactose, and some minerals and water-soluble vitamins. Disposal of whey from cheese factories was formerly an environmental problem; because of its low economic value, it was dumped into rivers, causing much damage to fish and plants. Now it is incorporated into animal feeds or further processed for incorporation into human foods. The cheese curd is then pressed to give a firmer texture, and salt is added. This is where much of the sodium in cheese comes from. The salted cheese is then packed into molds and pressed. The typical flavors of individual cheeses develop during ripening and maturing, when microbes continue to grow in the cheese. With some cheeses (such as Camembert and Brie), these microorganisms grow as a mold on the outside of the cheese. The holes and "eyes" in Swiss cheeses such as Gruyere are formed when certain bacteria form carbon dioxide bubbles that burst into the cheese.

Cream cheese is made from cream rather than from milk and is simply the fresh curd; it will not last long at room temperature. Cottage cheese is typically low-fat because it is made from skim milk. Vegetarian cheeses are made from a rennet obtained not from calf stomach but from enzymes obtained from pineapples, figs, or fungi.

Yogurt has been made since about 2000 B.C. in the Middle East and countries of southeastern Europe, including Bulgaria and Romania. Within the past 20 years, it has become a popular item in the United States, where Americans consume over 4 pounds per year on average. Yogurt is nourishing, but many of the myths associated with it are just that–myths. Claims are made for slowing the aging process, reducing high cholesterol levels, and curing vaginal infections or even cancerous tumors in experimental animals.[36] Most of these health claims are based on mistaken beliefs about the beneficial effects of the bacteria *Lactobacillus bulgaricus* and *Streptococcus thermophilus,* which are used in yogurt manufacture.

Ice cream is both an emulsion and a foam. Fat globules are provided by milk fat in dairy ice cream and by vegetable fat in nondairy frozen desserts. Air cells along with the fat give ice cream its creaminess. Ice crystals formed from water should be small to avoid a gritty texture. And, finally, ice cream consists of dissolved sugar, milk proteins, stabilizers and emulsifiers, flavors, and colors. The stabilizers, which give ice cream its texture and prevent melting, come from carageenan (Irish moss), broad bean, or guar gum.

■ Now you know

- Minerals perform many important functions in the body, including transporting oxygen; assisting nerve-muscle function, enzyme activity, and energy metabolism; being part of the structure of some hormones;

regulating water balance and acid-base balance; and forming tissues, especially bones and teeth.

- Mineral intake in the diet is a problem for some parts of the population, especially teenage girls, premenopausal women, and the elderly.

- Deficiencies of some minerals have significant physical, psychological, and economic costs.

- The macrominerals are calcium, phosphorus, sodium, potassium, chloride, magnesium, and sulfur.

- Calcium is associated with bones and osteoporosis, and high sodium intake is associated with hypertension in some people.

- No problems are usually seen for the intake of phosphorus, potassium, chloride, magnesium, or sulfur.

- Important microminerals (trace minerals) include iron, zinc, iodine, selenium, fluoride, and copper. Less is known about manganese, silicon, cobalt, molybdenum, chromium, nickel, and boron.

- Getting adequate dietary intakes of iron, zinc, and copper are problems for some people. Iron is especially deficient in premenopausal women.

- The main function of iron is oxygen transport; zinc is needed for growth; iodine is a part of thyroid hormones, which are involved in energy regulation; selenium is part of antioxidant enzyme systems; and copper is a part of many enzymes.

- Clay eating (geophagy or pica) occurs in different parts of the world. Lead poisoning seriously retards learning in young children.

- Dairy products are important sources of calcium, phosphorus, and other nutrients.

Further Reading

1. Mertz, W. Chromium in human nutrition: A review. *Journal of Nutrition* 123:626, 1993.
2. Greger, J. L. Using animals to assess bioavailability of minerals: Implications for human nutrition. *Journal of Nutrition* 122:2047, 1992.
3. Scholl, T. O., and others. Anemia vs. iron deficiency: Increased risk of preterm delivery in a prospective study. *American Journal of Clinical Nutrition* 55:985, 1992.
4. Tolstoi, L. G., and Levin, R. M. Osteoporosis–The treatment controversy. *Nutrition Today* 27(4):6, 1992.
5. McCarron, D. A., and others. Dietary calcium and blood pressure: Modifying factors in specific populations. *American Journal of Clinical Nutrition* 54:215S, 1991.
6. Curhan, G. C., and others. A prospective study of dietary calcium and other nutrients and the risk of symptomatic kidney stones. *New England Journal of Medicine* 328:833, 1993.
7. Wood, R. J., and Serfaty-Lacrosniere, C. Gastric acidity, atrophic gastritis, and calcium absorption. *Nutrition Reviews* 50:33, 1992.

8. Randall, T. Longitudinal study pursues questions of calcium, hormones, and metabolism in life of skeleton. *Journal of the American Medical Association* 268:2357, 1992.

9. Heaney, R. P. Thinking straight about calcium. *New England Journal of Medicine* 328:503, 1993.

10. Adshead, S. A. M. *Salt and Civilization*. St. Martin's Press, London, 1992.

11. Institute of Food Technologists, Office of Scientific Public Affairs. Monosodium glutamate. *Food Technology* 46(2):34, 1992.

12. Pickering, T. G. Predicting the response to nonpharmacologic treatment in mild hypertension. *Journal of the American Medical Association* 267:1256, 1992.

13. Paolisso, G., and others. Daily magnesium supplements improve glucose handling in elderly subjects. *American Journal of Clinical Nutrition* 55:1161, 1992.

14. Singh, R. B., and others. Can aluminum phosphide poisoning cause hypermagnesemia? *Magnesium and Trace Elements* 9:212, 1990.

15. Hallquist, N. A., and others. Maternal-iron-deficiency effects on peritoneal macrophage and peritoneal natural-killer-cell cytotoxicity in rat pups. *American Journal of Clinical Nutrition* 55:741, 1992.

16. Mitchell, M. C., and Lerner, E. Maternal hematologic measures and pregnancy outcome. *Journal of the American Dietetic Association* 92:484, 1992.

17. Kanarek, R. B., and Marks-Kaufman, R. *Nutrition and Behavior*. Van Nostrand Reinhold, New York, page 63, 1991.

18. Cook, J. D., and others. Calcium supplementation: Effect on iron absorption. *American Journal of Clinical Nutrition* 53:106, 1991.

19. Bacon, B. R. Causes of iron overload. *New England Journal of Medicine* 326:126, 1992.

20. Gable, C. B. Hemochromatosis and dietary iron supplementation: Implications from US mortality, morbidity, and health survey data. *Journal of the American Dietetic Association* 92:208, 1992.

21. Boukaiba, N., and others. A physiological amount of zinc supplementation: Effects on nutritional, lipid, and thymic status in an elderly population. *American Journal of Clinical Nutrition* 57:566, 1993.

22. Dunn, J. T. Iodine deficiency–The next target for elimination? *New England Journal of Medicine* 326:267, 1992.

23. Balasubrahmanyan, V. India: Protests over salt iodization. *Lancet* 337:226, 1991.

24. Hunter, D. J., and others. Selenium and cancer. *Journal of the American Medical Association* 265:28, 1991.

25. Thomson, C. D., and others. Long-term supplementation with selenate and selenomethionine: Selenium and glutathione peroxidase in blood components of New Zealand women. *British Journal of Nutrition* 69:577, 1993.

26. Rifat, S. Fluoridation: A prophylaxis program for dental caries and dementia? *Canadian Journal of Public Health* 83:93, 1992.

27. Riggs, B. L. Treatment of osteoporosis with sodium fluoride or parathyroid hormone. *American Journal of Medicine* 91(suppl. 5B):37S, 1991.

28. Medeiros, D. M., and others. Electrocardiographic activity and cardiac function in copper-restricted rats. *Proceedings of the Society of Experimental Biology and Medicine* 200:78, 1992.

29. Randall, T. Implants aside, silicon is no stranger to the body. *Journal of the American Medical Association* 267:2442, 1992.

30. Nielsen, F. H. Facts and fallacies about boron. *Nutrition Today* 27(3):6, 1992.

31. Johns, T. Well-grounded diet. *The Sciences*, page 38, 1991.

32. Johns, T., and Duquette, M. Detoxification and mineral supplementation as functions of geophagy. *American Journal of Clinical Nutrition* 53:448, 1991.

33. Horner, R. D., and others. Pica practices of pregnant women. *Journal of the American Dietetic Association* 91:34, 1991.

34. Mahaffey, K. R. Exposure to lead in childhood. The importance of prevention. *New England Journal of Medicine* 327:1308, 1992.

35. Binder, S., and Matte, T. Childhood lead poisoning: The impact of prevention. *Journal of the American Medical Association* 269:1679, 1993.

36. Williams, R. D. Yogurt. The curds and whey of health? *FDA Consumer* 26(5):27, 1992.

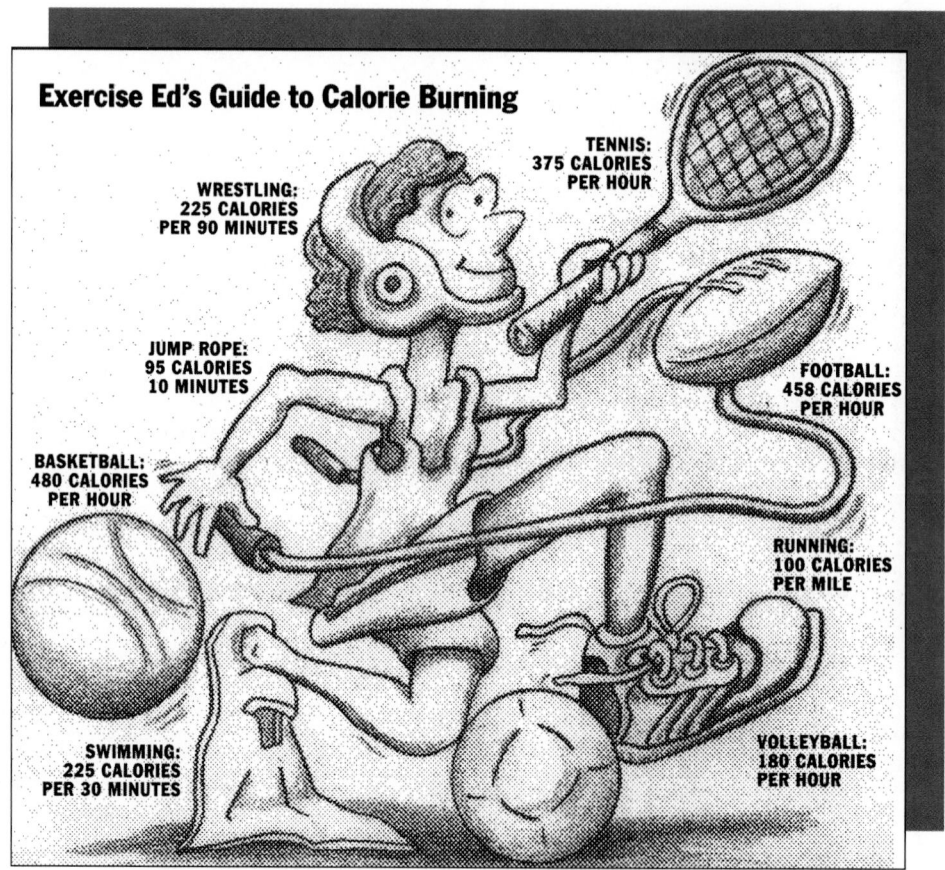

Figure 11-1. The amount of energy that a person expends varies among different sports and other activities.

Energy–Sources and Uses

■ Energy in our lives–More than just physical activity

Meet Exercise Ed (Edward or Edith), an athletic genius who is expending *energy* in a manner many of us may think of when the topic of energy expenditure is first introduced. It brings to our attention the caloric requirements of different activities for people who want to lose weight by increasing their physical activity. But there is more to the discussion of energy in this chapter than just admiring the athletic exploits of Exercise Ed. The information and concepts here lay the foundation for an understanding of many important issues in the world and in our lives. For example, to appreciate the causes and consequences of body weight loss in starvation, famine, AIDS, anorexia nervosa, or dieting, or of body weight gain in growth, pregnancy, or obesity, we need a knowledge of how we get and spend energy.

Let's think some more about the numbers Exercise Ed is generating. One pound of body fat tissue is lost when there is a deficit of about 3,500 calories. A slight digression is needed here to discuss this last sentence. First, one pound of body fat tissue is not all fat–it is 85% lipid, 11% water, and 4% protein. The lipid component obviously has almost all of the calories to contribute when body fat tissue is lost. Most experts on this topic consider that 3,500 calories are lost with the loss of one pound of body fat tissue during physical activity. A few nutrition texts and some nutritionists say it is 2,700 calories, especially during severe body weight loss due to extreme dieting or starvation. The reason for the lower number is that, in these situations, lean tissue is also lost, especially muscle. Lean tissue has a lower number of calories per kilogram than does body fat. We will stick with the majority of the experts and the conventional wisdom and use a value of 3,500 calories for the loss (or gain) of one pound of body fat tissue.

We can calculate how long it will take any one of us to lose one pound of body fat plus support tissue with each of the activities in Table 11-1. Divide the number of calories per hour into 3,500. The numbers are revealing.

Major Topics in This Chapter

You need energy for physical activity, for basal metabolic rate (to perform vital body processes such as breathing and maintaining body temperature), and for facultative thermogenesis (due to food intake and emotional stress).

■

Basal metabolic rate (or resting energy expenditure) is your greatest energy expenditure.

Exercise is a healthy way to lose body fat, but you must be patient.

Pregnancy, lactation, and growth require increased energy intake.

Fat added in the preparation and cooking of food increases energy intake significantly.

■

People Are Different– Cigarette smoking and body weight

Energy: The capacity of the body, a tissue, or a cell to do work. Measured in kilocalories ("calories" in popular terminology).

Losing one pound of body fat is a slow process, but we should not be discouraged. Having a regular exercise program that gives enjoyment is a recipe for success. Just as we emphasized moderation in eating, so we recommend moderation in exercise.

For some exercise-dependent people, workouts cease to be a means of improving life. They become an escape from it. Exercise makes them feel better about themselves when nothing else does anymore,

Table 11-1. Time Needed for an Average-Sized Person to Lose One Pound of Body Fat

Activity	Time (hours)
Tennis	9.3
Football	7.6
Volleyball	19.5
Swimming	7.8
Basketball	7.3
Jump rope	6.1
Wrestling	2.3
Running	35 miles

says Dr. Judith Rodin of Yale University.[1]

The benefits of good exercise programs are great, even beyond the loss of unwanted pounds of fat. They include improved muscle tone and body image and (usually) greater attention to a better diet. A person who exercises regularly is likely to pass over the high-fat foods at the tip of the Food Guide Pyramid in favor of the foods recommended in the other levels of the Pyramid (see Chapter 4) and in other dietary guidelines. For these reasons, nutritionists are interested in the relationship between exercise, energy intake, and *body composition*.

There are other reasons why nutritionists are interested in energy. These are summarized in Figure 11-2, which is your route map for the major topics in this chapter.

Body composition: Relative proportions of fat, bone, and lean tissue (muscle, kidneys, liver, brain, and other soft tissues) in the body.

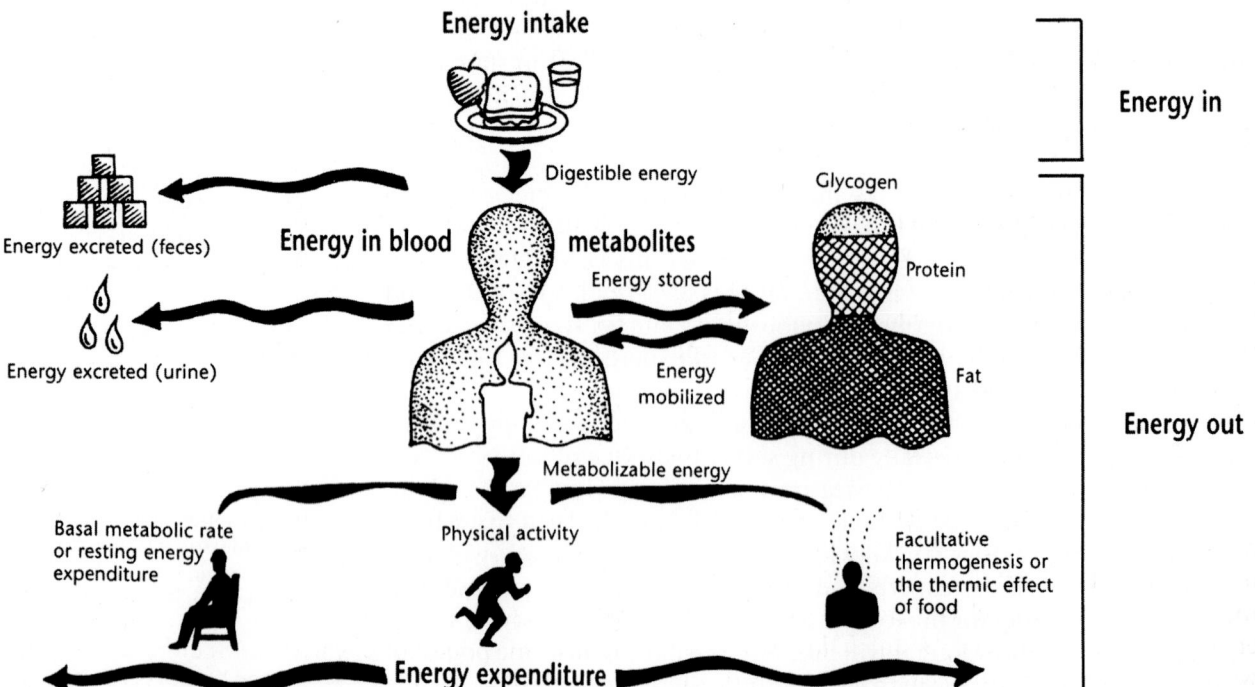

Figure 11-2. Summary of how you manage energy intake and energy expenditure.

If Exercise Edward/Edith in the cartoon never indulged in his/her many exercises, in fact if he/she never moved a muscle or blinked for 24 hours, energy expenditure would still occur. Think about what your body is doing within you right now to keep you alive:

- **Pumping** blood around the body
- **Inflating** the lungs in breathing
- **Secreting** substances from glands and cells
- **Firing** nerve impulses
- **Generating** heat to maintain normal body temperature
- **Maintaining** tension in muscles.

These actions require energy that is different from the energy expended by Exercise Ed in his/her multiple sporting activities in that we cannot voluntarily control the use of this energy. For example, you cannot at will lessen the tension in your muscles nor stop the functioning of heart and lungs. These metabolic processes needed to sustain life are collectively called *basal metabolism*, and the energy required for them is measured as *basal metabolic rate (BMR)*, or resting energy expenditure (REE).

One remaining energy requirement is the 8–10% of total daily energy expended in *facultative thermogenesis*. This is the energy expended due to changes in ambient temperature, food intake, emotional stress, and other factors. Energy is used for shivering when temperatures drop, for the digestion of food and absorption of nutrients, and to cope with emotional stresses such as changes in muscle tone when we feel stressed. Our total energy demands decrease as we grow older due to decreases in physical activity, in BMR, and in facultative thermogenesis.[2] The relative contributions of these three energy components also change as we age. The energy expenditure discussed thus far is summarized in Figure 11-3.

Notice that irrespective of age, a greater percentage of total energy goes to BMR and lower percentages to physical activity and facultative thermogenesis. Older people exercise less, and their facultative thermogenesis also decreases. The decrease in BMR for older people results from changes in body composition, a topic that we will examine shortly.

In summary, energy in our lives involves input from the food supply and output in physical activity, BMR, and facultative thermogenesis. Both input and output are measured in calories. When energy inputs and outputs are balanced, body weight is stable. When they are unbalanced, the following conditions result.

Basal metabolism: Metabolic processes needed to sustain life.

Basal metabolic rate (BMR): Energy needed to maintain vital body processes for a given period of time; measured in kilocalories.

Facultative thermogenesis: Energy expended in response to changes in ambient temperature, food intake, emotional stress, and other factors.

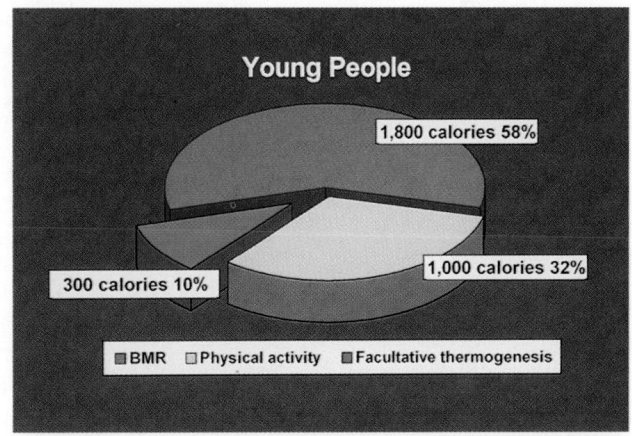

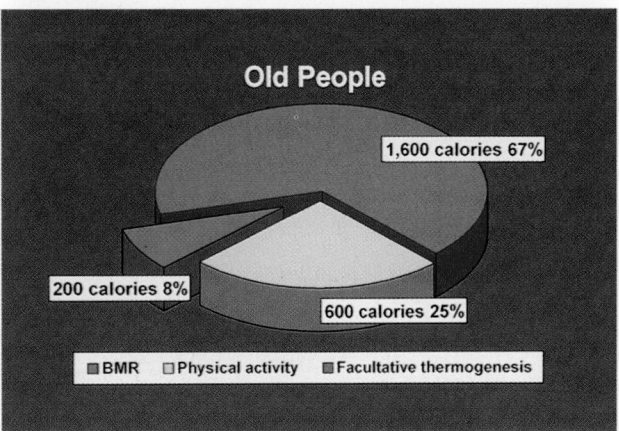

Figure 11-3. Energy expenditure by young people (top) and elderly people (bottom). Notice that the number of calories spent on each of the three forms of energy decreases with age, but the percentage of calories spent on basal metabolism rate (BMR) increases.

Weight gain results after:

- Overeating
- Decreased physical activity
- Decrease in BMR.

Weight loss results after:

- Starvation/weight-loss diets
- Increased physical activity
- Increase in BMR.

Changes in energy intake and energy expenditure affect body composition. Physiologists and nutritionists view the human body at five levels (Figure 11-4).[3]

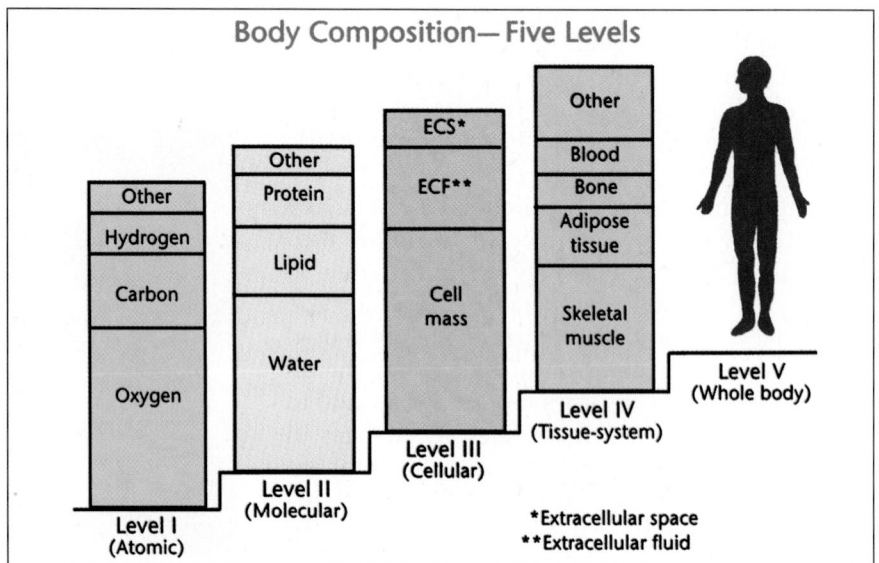

Figure 11-4. The composition of your body can be classified on five levels–atomic, molecular, cellular, tissue-system, and whole body. Measurements at each level may give useful information about how you store and use energy.

The first level is the atomic composition of the body–at your simplest chemical level, you are a collection of atoms of oxygen, carbon, hydrogen, and other elements. These are combined into water, lipids, protein, and "other," which includes minerals and vitamins and the small amount of carbohydrate stored as glycogen in the muscles and liver. All of these are distributed throughout the body in the cell mass, the extracellular fluid, and extracellular space. They are divided into various tissues, including skeletal muscle, adipose (fat) tissue, bone, and blood. All of these are combined to form your body. On issues of energy balance, nutritionists are most interested in the amount of adipose and muscle tissue (level IV in the figure). Adipose tissue increases in obese people and is greatly reduced in people who are starving. Skeletal muscle decreases also in starvation.

Let's begin the study of energy balance in our body by answering the questions: How much food do we need? What happens when food intake is too high or too low in relation to energy expenditure?

■ Food–The source of energy input to the body

The term "calorie" is used in many places in this book because reports in the popular literature on body weight loss, dieting, exercise, and the energy content of foods use that term. What "calorie" in these reports really refers to is the kilocalorie (kcal)–the amount of heat required to increase the temperature of 1 kilogram of water by 1 degree Celsius. Europeans count kilojoules instead of kilocalories (1 kilocalorie equals 4.18 kilojoules).

Food Is the Source of All Your Energy

All energy in your body comes from food and drink. This is seen most dramatically at both extremes of food intake. Starvation and famine cause severe wasting of body mass, whereas large food intake may results in obesity if the excess energy is not burned off in physical activity. Our attention here will focus on the energy nutrients–carbohydrates, lipids, and proteins–plus alcohol, if consumed. Vitamins and minerals provide no energy, even though B-complex vitamins are vital as coenzymes for energy metabolism, iron is needed for the delivery of oxygen to the cells, and some enzymes require certain minerals to function.

The number of calories you consume can be calculated if the amounts of carbohydrates, lipids, and proteins in the food are known. Try to monitor your energy intake by keeping a record of how much of each food and drink you consume in one day. You can then calculate total caloric intake by using one of the following methods.

Energy intake calculated from food labels

Note the number of calories listed on the food label. These are provided by the carbohydrates, fats, and proteins, described on the label. For example, the label on a rolled oats breakfast cereal on my kitchen shelf gives the following information for a serving:

Fat	2 g
Carbohydrate	18 g
Protein	5 g
Calories	110

If I want to know how many calories come from each of the three nutrients, I can multiply the fat grams by 9 and the carbohydrate and protein grams by 4.

Fat	18 calories
Carbohydrate	72 calories
Protein	20 calories
Total calories	110

The total of the three is the total that was given on the box. In order to find what percent of total calories is provided by one of the three nutrients (say, fat), I divide the calories for that nutrient by total calories (20/110 = 0.18, so 18% of the calories are from fat).

Bomb calorimeter: Instrument that measures energy (caloric content) present in a substance by burning it in oxygen and measuring the heat released.

Energy intake calculated from tables of food composition

Instead of checking the food label you can look at tables of food composition (see Appendix A). Nutrient data banks are also available on computer disks.

Nutrient information for the food label and the food table comes from chemical analyses by scientists in the laboratory. The total caloric content of a food can be obtained by burning it to an ash under carefully controlled conditions using an instrument called a *bomb calorimeter*. No, there are no explosions, just a measurement of the amount of heat liberated when the food is burned to an ash (or "bombed"). Caloric contents are thus measured by the amount of heat given off in this measurement. One correction must be made to the calculations if fiber is present in the food. Fiber is combustible, so it contributes to the total number of calories. However, we saw in Chapter 6 that fiber is not digested in the GI tract, and so the calories associated with fiber pass from the body in the feces. Therefore, the fiber content must be determined and the calories associated with fiber subtracted from the total number of calories.

Food preparation and cooking can influence energy content

We saw in Chapter 4 how the number of calories increase as a potato is turned into a French fry. Table 11-2 shows a greater refinement of this information.

Our desire for fatty foods has made the sources of calories in the modern American diet different from the sources in ancient diets. We now consume much more fat and much less protein than our ancient ancestors did (Table 11-3).

One reason for these changes is the huge difference in fat content between wild animals, which our ancient cousins depended on, and the domesticated, intensively reared animals of today. The bodies of wild animals contain 75% lean meat and only 4% storage fat, whereas domesticated animals today have 50% lean meat and 25% storage fat.

Table 11-2. Adding Fat to Potato Changes the Calorie Content

Method of Cooking	Kcalories per 100 grams
Baked, flesh only	93
Boiled, flesh only	86
Mashed, milk and butter added	106
In potato salad	143
French-fried	316
As potato chips	528

Table 11-3. Comparisons of Ancient Diet and Typical American Diet of the 1980s

Nutrient	Content of Diet (percent)		Recommended by Dietary Guidelines
	Ancient	Typical American	
Protein	34	12	12
Carbohydrate	45	46	58
Fat	21	42	30

■ Recommended energy intake

What is the recommended intake of calories per day to meet our total energy requirement? The Food and Nutrition Board of the National Research Council published its latest recommendations for energy intake in 1989. They were given in conjunction with median heights and weights. These values are for people with light to moderate activity.

Think about the numbers in Table 11-4. Which values apply to you?

RDAs for energy are listed in the extreme right-hand column in the table. They have been set to meet the needs for the three types of energy (physical activity, BMR, and facultative thermogenesis). Nutritionists have established RDAs for energy differently from the RDAs for other nutrients. *The energy RDAs represent the average of people in each age and gender group, whereas the RDAs for other nutrients represent the upper limits of variability for (almost) all people within the same age and gender group.* Setting the RDAs for energy at the upper limit might encourage obesity. Energy intake is recommended on the basis of an average desirable weight for men of 154 pounds or 70 kilograms and for women of 120 pounds or 55 kilograms. Additional

Table 11-4. Median Heights and Weights and Recommended Energy Intake

Category	Age (years) or Condition	Weight (kg)	Weight (lb)	Height (cm)	Height (in.)	BMR[a] (kcal per day)	Average Energy Allowance (kcal) Multiples of BMR	Average Energy Allowance (kcal) Per Kilogram	Average Energy Allowance (kcal) Per Day
Infants	0.0–0.5	6	13	60	24	320		108	650
	0.5–1.0	9	20	71	28	500		98	850
Children	1–3	13	29	90	35	740		102	1,300
	4–6	20	44	112	44	950		90	1,800
	7–10	28	62	132	52	1,130		70	2,000
Males	11–14	45	99	157	62	1,440	1.70	55	2,500
	15–18	66	145	176	69	1,760	1.67	45	3,000
	19–24	72	160	177	70	1,780	1.67	40	2,900
	25–50	79	174	176	70	1,800	1.60	37	2,900
	51+	77	170	173	68	1,530	1.50	30	2,300
Females	11–14	46	101	157	62	1,310	1.67	47	2,200
	15–18	55	120	163	64	1,370	1.60	40	2,200
	19–24	58	128	164	65	1,350	1.60	38	2,200
	25–50	63	138	163	64	1,380	1.55	36	2,200
	51+	65	143	160	63	1,280	1.50	30	1,900
Pregnant	1st trimester								+0
	2nd trimester								+300
	3rd trimester								+300
Lactating	1st 6 months								+500
	2nd 6 months								+500

[a] Basal metabolic rate, also known as resting energy expenditure (REE).

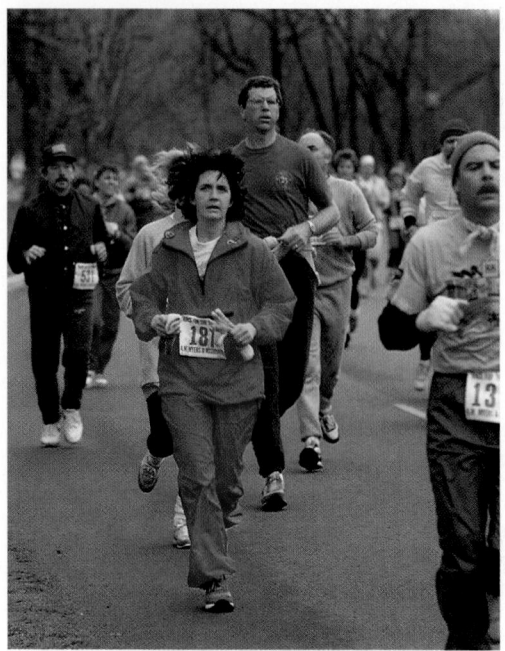

Figure 11-5. People who run races, or participate in other vigorous activity, are usually people who consume balanced, nutritious diets.

allowances must be made for people who are taller or who do intense physical activity.

RDA values for energy increase from birth to adulthood, as seen in the column on the extreme right of the table. The RDA for energy for adult men between the ages of 25 and 50 years is 2,900 calories and for adult women 2,200 calories. Pregnancy and lactation require increased energy, so pregnant women need higher energy intake to meet the demands of the growing fetus and the increased amount of maternal tissue such as the placenta. In a normal full-term pregnancy, a woman gains about 12.5 kilograms (28 pounds) and delivers a baby weighing on the average 3.3 kilograms (7 pounds). The total energy cost of the pregnancy is calculated to be about 80,000 calories. The energy allowance per day is figured by dividing the approximately 250 days following the first month of pregnancy into the total energy cost of 80,000 calories to give an increase of 300 calories per day for the entire pregnancy. Energy requirements for lactation are proportional to the amount of milk produced. Milk protein, fat, and lactose must be synthesized, and this requires energy input. Human milk from well-nourished mothers contains about 70 calories per 100 milliliters of milk. Some of the energy needed for milk production may come from the extra body fat stored by the woman during pregnancy. This fat is normally used during the first few months of breast feeding.

Much of the energy requirement of infants and children is for the growth of tissue. Under the age of 10, no distinction in energy requirement is made between boys and girls. After age 10, separate values are given because of differences in the age of onset of puberty and different physical activity patterns. Body composition changes for both girls and boys at puberty. This has an influence on energy requirements, as we will see shortly.

In the column second from the right in Table 11-4 under the heading "Average Energy Allowance per Kilogram," notice how values decrease as we get older. Infants have the highest RDA values per unit of body weight, and the elderly have the lowest values. This is because infants have the most rapid growth, while the elderly have decreased physical activity and lower BMR because of lower amounts of muscle and other lean tissue. The energy allowance beyond age 50 assumes continued light-to-moderate physical activity.

The information above is a foundation for our discussions on physical activity in the next chapter and on obesity and starvation in Chapter 13.

You can calculate your own energy needs

Think about your energy needs for today. You can calculate the number of calories you will need today by using Table 11-4. This is how it works. In the left-hand column, find the appropriate line for your age and gender. For example, if you are a 20-year-old female; locate the line for females 19–24 years of age. Move along that line to the right and see that the median weight for you is 58 kilograms (128 pounds) and median height is 164 centimeters (65 inches). The energy needed for your basal metabolic rate (BMR) is 1,350 calories. This means that you require about 1,350 calories to maintain the vital body processes discussed at the beginning of this chapter.

To determine what you need for average total energy expenditure (physical activity, plus BMR, plus facultative thermogenesis), the value for your BMR was multiplied by a factor of 1.60, giving 2,160 calories (this has been rounded up to 2,200 calories in the column on the right). Total energy expenditure can also be approximated by taking body weight in kilograms and multiplying it by a factor of 38 per kilogram. In this case, this would be 58 × 38 = 2,204 calories. This recommended energy intake should be adjusted upward to meet increased energy demands for increased physical activity and for larger body size. (Obviously, it should be decreased downward for decreased activity or smaller body size.)

In summary, energy intake from food is used by the body to supply energy for physical activity, BMR (or REE), and facultative thermogenesis. Let's move on to see how we spend energy on these activities.

■ Energy expenditure

Physical Activity

Physical activity is the only form of energy expenditure you can control. We saw that it is not the largest use of energy for most people. The actual number of calories burned is determined by your weight and by the type, intensity, and duration of the physical activity.

Body weight

Obese people use more energy than lean people to travel the same distance. We can confirm this easily by relating this observation to the automobile–heavy cars use more energy (gasoline) than do light or small cars. Look at the differences in calories expended by a 120-pound person and a 200-pound person when they engage in various activities for 60 minutes (Table 11-5).

We can tie information in this table to the caloric value for tennis shown in the cartoon at the beginning of the chapter. The table tells us that a 120-pound (54-kilogram) person will burn 360 calories during one hour of singles in tennis. Exercise Ed is shown to burn 375 calories, so he/she must have a body weight of about 120 pounds or 54 kilograms.

Table 11-5. Calories (kcal) Expended over a 60-Minute Period

Activity	Person Weighing 120 pounds (54 kg)	Person Weighing 200 pounds (91 kg)
Tennis		
Singles	360	600
Doubles	210	350
Volleyball	160	270
Dancing (fast)	550	920
Running or jogging (5 mph)	440	740

Type, intensity, and duration of activity

The figures above speak for themselves. The number of calories burned is highest when there is intense physical activity. Obviously, an hour of

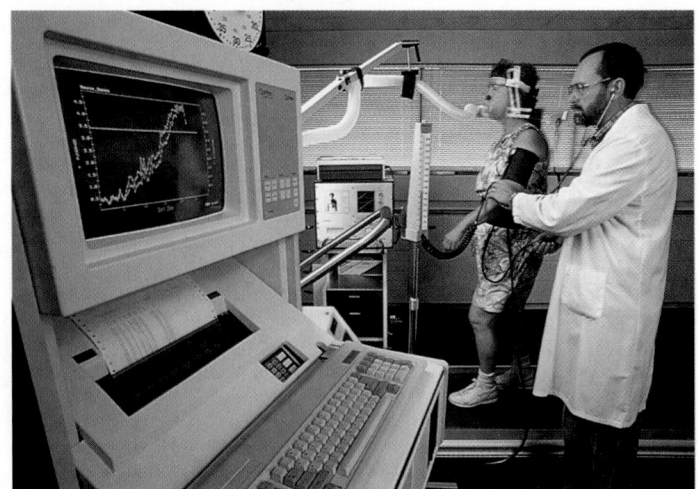

Figure 11-6. Measurement of energy expenditure under laboratory conditions.

leisurely tennis will require fewer calories than an hour in the finals at Wimbledon. Since duration is a factor, a two-hour finals match will require more calories than a one-hour match. If we want accurate measurements of energy expenditure, we must measure it in the laboratory. Figure 11-6 shows how that is done.

Basal Metabolic Rate

BMR, or REE, is the largest energy expenditure. All of the vital body processes to maintain life require energy–breathing, pumping blood around the body, maintaining normal body temperature, keeping muscles at a certain tension, firing of nerves, and secretion of substances from glands and cells. Measuring BMR accurately requires the elaborate procedures seen in Figure 11-7.

The person is placed in a supine or sitting position in a comfortable environment several hours after the last meal or significant physical activity. Then a number of different measures can be taken to obtain the amount of energy spent on basal activities. One way is to measure oxygen consumption, which is being done in this picture. Oxygen is needed to burn the body's energy stores of fat, carbohydrate, and, in emergencies, protein. So the amount of oxygen consumed by the person at rest over a given time is an indication of the resting metabolic activity. But you can do a quick calculation on yourself without being hooked up to the machine shown in the photograph.

For men: 1 calorie per kilogram of body weight per hour
For women: 0.9 calories per kilogram of body weight per hour

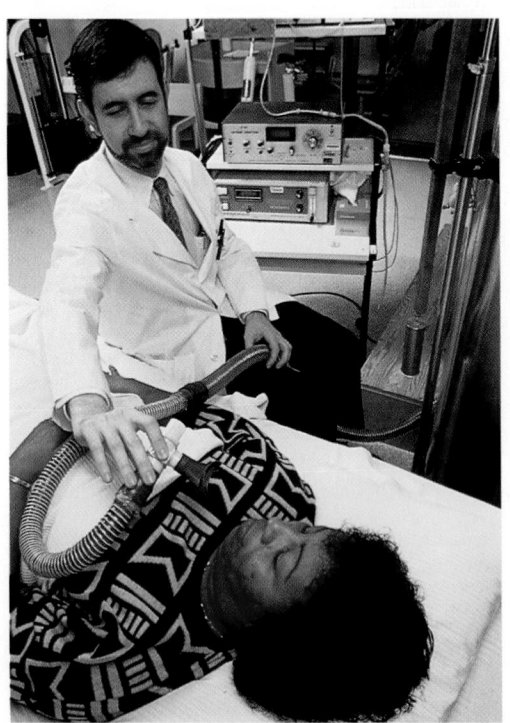

Figure 11-7. Measurement of basal metabolic rate (BMR) indicates how much energy is required for the vital body processes.

For example, if you are a young woman 20 years of age and weigh 128 pounds, your BMR is calculated as:

$0.9 \times 128 \times 24$ divided by $2.2 = 1,257$ calories

(The 2.2 converts from pounds to kilograms.) Notice that you multiply by 24 hours; you may work only an 8-hour day, but your vital body functions are working all 24 hours. The body weight of 128 pounds was chosen purposely because this is the recommended average body weight for a young woman of this age. Refer to Table 11-4 and note that the BMR is 1,350 calories for this person. The difference of about 100 calories is the result of rounding up the figures in the calculation we have just done.

Your BMR is a very useful number to know because it makes the application of weight control methods much more applicable to you. BMR is the number of calories you need each day just to keep yourself alive. Having a dietary intake below your BMR means that your body must draw on its own energy reserves to maintain vital body processes. This means it will use its greatest energy reserve–body fat. Therein lies the basis for weight reducing or slimming diets, to which we will return in Chapter 13.

Different tissues have different energy demands–muscle needs much more energy than fat or bone. Any changes in the proportion of fat to lean tissue changes BMR. A number of possible events in our lives will result in changes in BMR. This is what happens and why.

- **Body composition.** Muscular people have a greater proportion of lean tissue, resulting in higher BMR.

- **Exercise.** Any physical activity that increases muscle mass increases BMR. Weight lifting is a good example. Some evidence suggests that exercise may slow down the natural loss of muscle during aging.

- **Gender.** In general, men have a higher BMR than do women, as seen in Table 11-4. The main reason for this is that women have a higher proportion of body fat than men do, and men have more muscle, as seen in Table 11-6.

- **Age.** There is a dramatic decline in BMR as we grow older (Figure 11-8). Lean body mass decreases, mainly because of muscle loss. This decrease of BMR explains in part why some people suffer from "middle-aged spread." All people reaching their 40s and 50s have decreased BMR and therefore a lower energy requirement. But many are at a point in life where they have little time for physical activity, while business lunches and other eating opportunities add to the problem of controlling caloric intake.

Table 11-6. Proportion of Body Fat in Men and Women

	154-lb Man		125-lb Woman	
	Pounds	Percent	Pounds	Percent
Total fat	23	15	34	27
Essential fat	5	3	15	12
Storage fat	19	12	19	15
Muscle	69	45	45	36
Bone	23	15	15	12
Remainder	39	25	31	25
Lean body weight	136		107	

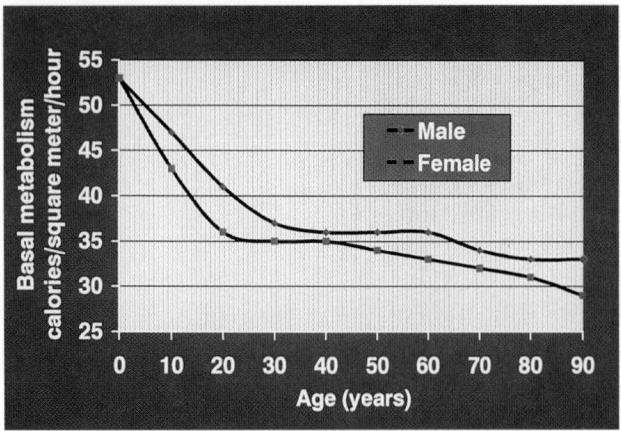

Figure 11-8. Basal metabolic rate decreases with age.

Thyroid gland: Gland in the neck that secretes thyroid hormones, which are involved in energy metabolism.

Dietary thermogenesis: Energy needed to digest, absorb, transport, and store nutrients in food; also known as specific dynamic action of food, or thermic effect of food.

Brown adipose tissue (BAT): Fat tissue with brown color given by a high concentration of mitochondria, which are energy-producing subcellular structures; found in high concentrations in hibernating animals such as bears and in newborn humans.

- **Pregnancy.** During pregnancy, the muscles in the uterus increase to the size needed for delivery. Muscle tissue increases in the fetus. These and other body changes in preparation for delivery and lactation result in increased BMR in pregnancy.

- **Health factors.** Ill health and trauma affect BMR. Lean body mass is lost in starvation, injury, after surgery, and in severe weight-loss diets. BMR is decreased in these cases; it is increased during a fever.

- **Thyroid hormone status.** An overactive *thyroid gland* produces excess thyroid hormone, resulting in elevated BMR.

Facultative Thermogenesis

Thermogenesis means the production of heat, and facultative thermogenesis is the third reason we need to consume energy. This category includes the effect of food, temperature, and stress. Let's take a brief look at how each of these affects energy balance.

Dietary thermogenesis

"Dietary thermogenesis," "specific dynamic action of food," and "thermic effect of food" are all terms that refer to the 5–10% of energy needed to digest, absorb, transport, and store nutrients in food. Digestion involves breaking large molecules into smaller ones, such as starch into glucose. Absorption sometimes requires pumping the nutrient against a gradient from the GI tract into the blood.

Transportation and storage of nutrients have their own energy costs. For example, surplus fat is synthesized from fatty acids and glycerol that are not needed for immediate energy. The synthesis of any chemicals in the body requires some energy input.

The importance of facultative thermogenesis in the overall energy balance of an individual is controversial. It is not clear yet whether dietary thermogenesis is different for obese and nonobese people. High energy intake in a meal does have an effect on dietary thermogenesis, but exercise seems to have no effect.

Brown adipose tissue

Brown adipose tissue (BAT) has attracted considerable attention recently as another factor in facultative thermogenesis. BAT was discovered not so long ago, and nutritionists became interested because it is thought to be important in maintaining body temperature. It is found in highest amounts in hibernating animals, such as bears, who have a high requirement to maintain body heat in cold climates. But what has this to do with people since, unlike bears, we do not hibernate? We know now that each one of us has BAT. It is in highest concentration at the back of the neck and shoulders. BAT is thought to be important in newborn infants to protect them from cold. Perhaps it is not much needed today for children born into centrally heated homes. But when we remember the less comfortable environments for many of our ancestors, we will understand why nature provided extra insulation for the newborn. BAT accounts for about 1% of body weight in adults. Its role in adults is not well understood, although some scientists have suggested that increased heat production in BAT may be one way that some people are able to burn off excess energy intake rather than gaining weight.

BAT is different from the white adipose tissue so many people struggle to control. Some researchers have found that it generates heat at a higher rate than the more common white adipose tissue. This high production of heat is achieved through the high concentration of mitochondria and an excellent blood supply, which together give BAT its brown color.

Why did the popular press write so many stories about BAT and weight control? Scientists found that obese people had smaller proportions of BAT. This means they had less opportunity to burn a lot of energy through BAT's heat-producing metabolism. Thus, the extra dietary calories taken in by an obese person are more likely to be stored as fat than burned for energy. The present state of information suggests that BAT has a minor but possibly meaningful role in energy balance.

■ People are different–Cigarette smoking and body weight

More than 1,000 years ago, Native Americans used tobacco, and they were probably aware of its appetite-suppressing and energy-instilling effects.[4] Scientific papers reporting that body weight gain was lowered by the use of tobacco began to appear more than 100 years ago. However, it was only about 10 years ago that the first detailed studies on the relationship between cigarette smoking and body weight were done. Much of the work was prompted by the fact that cigarette smoking is the single most important preventable cause of illness and death in the United States. More deaths are attributed to it than to alcohol, all other addictive drugs, accidents, and suicides *combined*. One concern of people who consider giving up cigarette smoking is the fear of gaining body weight.

Recent studies do confirm the general belief that cessation of cigarette smoking causes an increase in body weight.[4] Weight gains were, on average, 2.8 kilograms or just over 6 pounds for men and 3.8 kilograms or about 8¼ pounds for women. But about 10% of the men and women in the study gained over 13 kilograms or 28½ pounds. Some gender and race differences were observed that can be reported but not explained until further studies are done. For example, women who quit smoking gained more weight than men. African-Americans who quit smoking were more likely to gain weight than whites. People who smoked large numbers of cigarettes gained more weight after quitting than those who didn't smoke as often. Much more study is needed to explain these findings.

The negative health effects of cigarette smoking clearly outweigh the possible negative effects of weight gain after smoking cessation. The search is on for a mechanism to explain the weight gain so that preventive measures can be implemented for people who want to quit smoking. One thing we know is that when rats are infused with nicotine, body weight is always less than that of rats given no nicotine, but both groups have the same BMR.[5] When nicotine administration is stopped, food intake initially increases. The increase stops when the rats reach their stable body weight.

You don't have to gain weight when you quit smoking if you follow these recommendations from the National Institutes of Health.

- Lower the fat in your diet by cutting down on added fats (oils, margarine, sauces, and dressings), fatty cuts of meat, cheese, and whole-milk dairy products.
- Replace the high-fat foods in your diet with whole grains, breads, pasta, fruits, vegetables, and nonfat dairy products. These foods are filling and are naturally low in fat.
- Exercise by walking briskly for 20 minutes or more every day. This will help you to feel great and to keep your weight down.

■ Now you know

- Exercise in moderation is a healthy but slow way to lose body fat.
- Basal metabolic rate (BMR) or resting energy expenditure (REE) is the energy required to perform vital body processes such as inflating the lungs and pumping blood around the body.
- BMR is the largest energy expenditure by the body.
- BMR decreases as we get older because of the loss of lean tissue.
- In general, men have higher BMR than women because of their greater muscle mass and lower percentage of body fat.
- Facultative thermogenesis is the energy expended due to changes in ambient temperature, food intake, and emotional stress.
- Fat added in the preparation and cooking of food adds significantly to caloric intake.
- Pregnancy and lactation require increased energy intake.
- Body weight increases in many cigarette smokers who quit. This can be avoided by eating low-fat foods and increasing exercise.

Further Reading

1. Rodin, J. *Body Traps*. William Morrow and Company, Inc., New York, page 196, 1992.
2. Poehlman, E. T. Energy expenditure and requirements in aging humans. *Journal of Nutrition* 122:2057, 1992.

3. Heymsfield, S. B., and others. Body composition and aging: A study by in vivo neutron activation analysis. *Journal of Nutrition* 123:432, 1993.
4. Grunberg, N. E. Smoking cessation and weight gain. *New England Journal of Medicine* 324:768, 1991.
5. Schwid, S. R., and others. Nicotine effects on body weight: A regulatory perspective. *American Journal of Clinical Nutrition* 55:878, 1992.

Think beyond the power, elegance, and precision seen in these and other sporting activities. Think of the many chemical reactions needed to convert energy from food into the explosive burst of power of a sprinter, the precise timing of a hurdler, the grace of an ice skater, or the stamina of a world-class midfield soccer player, who may run up to 10 miles in a game.

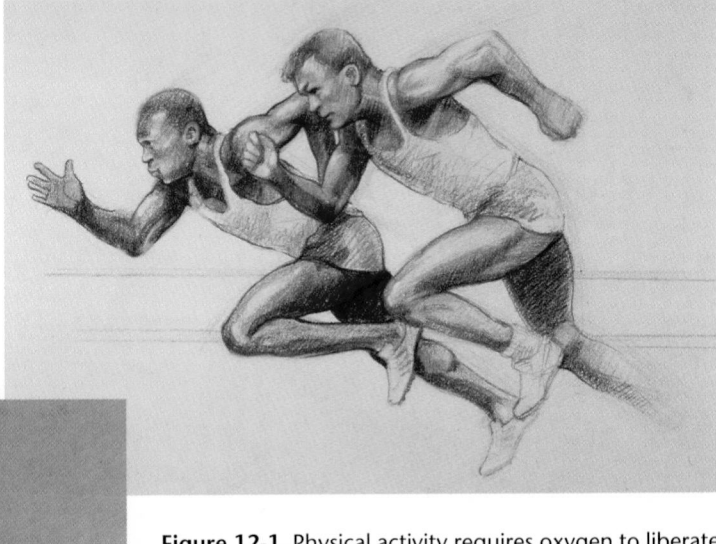

Figure 12-1. Physical activity requires oxygen to liberate the body's reserves of energy (carbohydrates, lipids, and proteins) with assistance from some vitamins and minerals and from water.

## CHAPTER 12

Nutrition and Physical Fitness

■ Nutrition and physical fitness in our lives

Food provides the calories for all of our energy needs, but some people have greater energy needs than others. Suppose you saw a shopping list containing, among other things, 2 dozen eggs, 8 loaves of bread, 10 pounds of ground meat, 5 gallons of fruit juice, 4 pounds of spaghetti, and 6 pounds of spaghetti sauce. Would you assume that it was this week's shopping list for a family of four? That would be a logical conclusion, but according to an article in *Sports Illustrated* (April 24, 1989), this is the amount of food purchased for *one* professional football player in one week. If most of us were to consume this amount of food, we would surely put on weight. Not so with the football player, who can eat this much and *not* gain weight. This incredible balancing act between caloric intake from food and caloric expenditure in physical activity shows that the key word in this relationship is *balance*.

The nutrition information in this chapter is important even if you are not on a varsity team, "into sports," or even a "weekend athlete." Physical activity has many biological and psychological benefits, some of which relate to nutrition.[1] Regular physical activity will give you the following benefits:

- The ability to eat more food while still maintaining body weight, because more calories will be burned for energy
- Improved functioning of the heart, lung, and blood system
- Improvement in the levels of two indicators of coronary heart disease–a reduction in low-density lipoprotein (LDL) cholesterol and an increase in high-density lipoprotein (HDL) cholesterol
- Reduced risk of stroke
- Increased lean body mass, which could lessen muscle loss during normal aging
- Stronger bones, which is important in protection against osteoporosis and consequent bone fractures

- Decreased stress, which could be important in reducing hypertension and improving appetite
- Decreased diabetic symptoms
- Better GI tract function with lower incidence of constipation.

Nutrient activities are coordinated brilliantly by the body to produce explosive energy for the 100-yard dash or sustained energy for walks or jogging. Energy requirements to support these and other activities in our modern lifestyle have been contrasted with those of our ancient ancestors by Dr. Boyd Eaton and colleagues at Emory University in Atlanta, Georgia. They say,

> There is little doubt that strenuous physical activity has been part of human and prehuman ancestral life for millions of years.

So why all the fuss about exercise? Dr. Eaton tells us that our ancient ancestors were

> strong, much stronger in fact than most people alive today. The earliest modern humans were much like current professional athletes, both men and women, whose strength generally greatly exceeds that of the average person.

We might add that they did not worry about vitamin and protein supplements and anabolic steroid use! They expended much energy in hunting for food and hauling it home, which may sound like endurance running and weight lifting in today's terms. They planted, gathered food, and carried water from rivers. How many of us exercise this much? Not very many, unfortunately–fewer than 10% of Americans older than 18 years meet the criteria for exercise proposed in the 1990 objectives for the nation. The next generation may not be much different; the physical activity levels of grade-school students are lower than levels called for in national health objectives.[2]

■ Oxygen–The spark to burn body energy

The air that we breathe is 21% oxygen, which is the spark to light the fire of life. Oxygen is required for the breakdown of carbohydrates, lipids, and proteins into energy, carbon dioxide, and water. Physical performance is reduced without an adequate supply of oxygen to cells, especially muscle cells. If the oxygen supply is inadequate, it is irrelevant to be concerned about identifying which nutrients are the best energy sources for the body and how the diet can provide them. Proof of this is seen in the difficulty of achieving maximum physical performance at high altitudes due to the lower oxygen concentrations there. At least several days of adjustment to lower oxygen concentrations are required by skiers, runners, climbers, and others involved in intense physical activity. This is the physiologists' area of study, so why should nutritionists be concerned? A person's nutritional status is critically important in understanding how oxygen gets from the air that we breathe to the cells that generate energy. Figure 12-2 shows what happens.

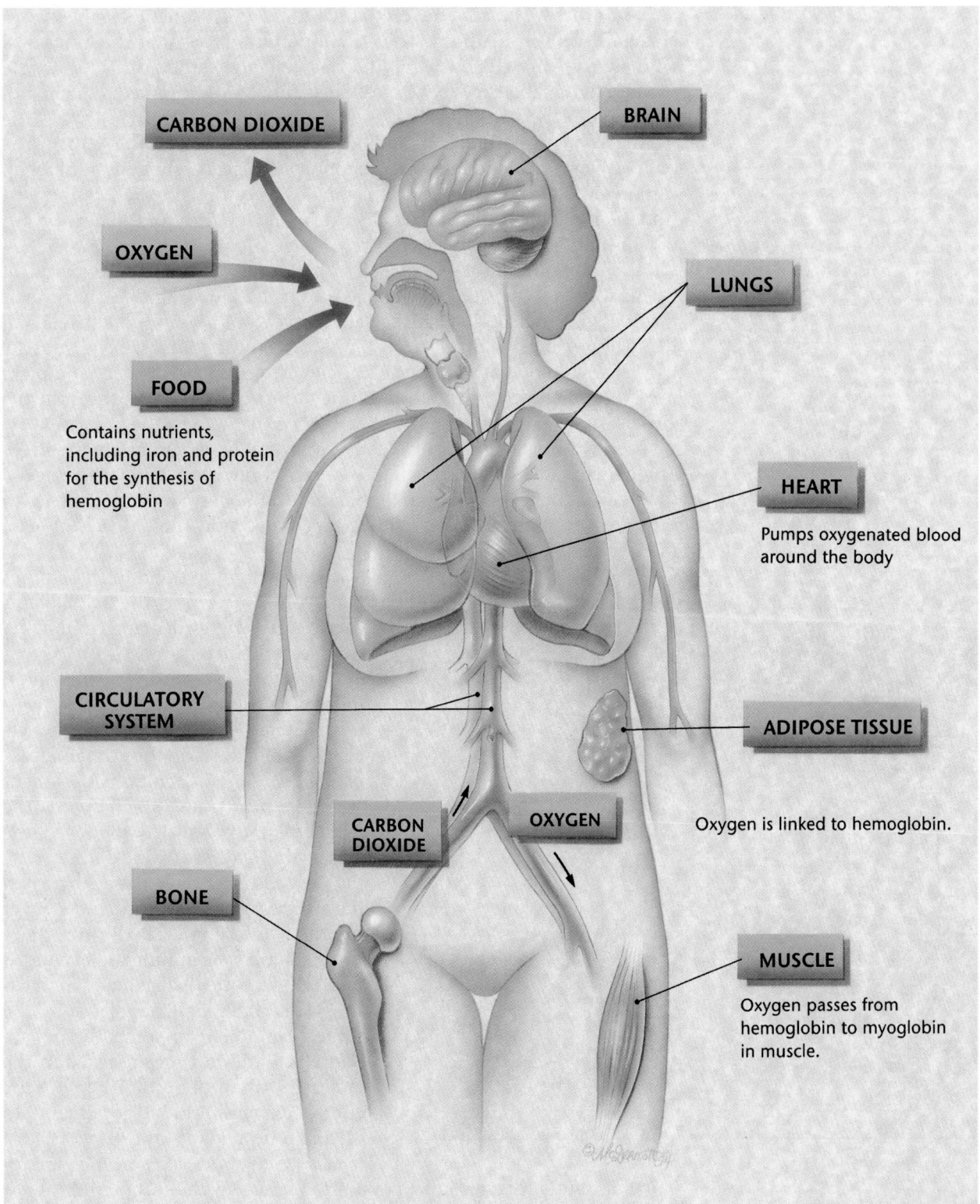

Figure 12-2. Delivery of oxygen to every cell in your body, and the removal of carbon dioxide from the cells, is essential to the cells' survival.

The air that we breathe travels to the lungs, which constitutes the gas exchange system in the body. The two important gasses that the lungs deal with are oxygen, which is vital for every cell, and carbon dioxide, a waste product of metabolism. Oxygen from the inhaled air is joined to hemoglobin in red blood cells as they pass through the lungs on their way to the heart. Oxygen-rich blood is pumped by the heart to all the cells in the body. When the blood releases its supply of oxygen to the cells, it picks up carbon dioxide and returns it to the lungs. The carbon dioxide is unhooked from hemoglobin, to be exhaled by the lungs in return for the next breath of "fresh air."

Muscles require a lot of oxygen to perform all the work we expect of them. To speed the supply of oxygen from the blood, muscles have their own oxygen transporter. This is called myoglobin, a molecule similar to hemoglobin but occurring only in cardiac (heart) and skeletal muscle. Oxygen-rich blood arrives at the muscles, drops off the oxygen, and picks up carbon dioxide for its return journey to the lungs. There, the cycle begins again.

When we engage in physical activity, several body tissues are involved. These include the lungs, the blood to transport oxygen from the lungs to the tissues, the heart to pump blood around the body, and the muscles to provide power for movement. Table 12-1 shows how these tissues interact in exercise.

Table 12-1. Metabolic Activity During Various Types of Exercise

Physical Effort	Oxygen Consumption (liters/min)	Heart Rate (beats/min)	Caloric Expenditure (calories/min)
Very light Sleeping, lying, sitting, driving, standing	<0.5	<80	<2.5
Light Walking (slow), golf, shopping, trade work	0.5–1.0	80–100	2.5–5.0
Moderate Walking (fast), cycling, tennis, dancing	1.0–1.5	100–120	5.0–7.5
Heavy Swimming, basketball, walking uphill with a load	1.5–2.0	120–140	7.5–10.0
Very heavy Running, climbing	2.0–2.5	140–160	10.0–12.5
Exhausting	>3.0	>180	>15.0

By following the trend in these numbers, you can see how the body adapts to increased energy demands in moving from very light physical effort to exercise capable of causing exhaustion. Oxygen consumption increases, ensuring that more oxygen gets to muscle cells, thereby allowing maximal release of energy. This is achieved by an increase in heart rate, which speeds the delivery of oxygen-rich blood to the cells. The increased work done by the muscle cells is reflected in the increased number of calories expended per minute. For example, about three times more calories per minute are expended in playing a basketball game than in sitting watching a game on television.

Take a moment to compare your favorite activities if they are listed in the table. This is an opportunity to see the energy expenditure categories and to calculate how many calories you burn over a given time. For example, a hard game of tennis requires an expenditure of 5.0–7.5 calories per minute or 300–450 calories per hour. Therefore, to burn off one pound of fat (3,500 calories), you need to play 7–12 hours of tennis. Ponder these numbers as confirmation that losing body fat is difficult (although your tennis game might improve!). It must be stressed that these are general estimates and do not account for variations in body size or in the degree of a person's physical fitness.

Returning to the job of getting oxygen to exercising cells, some environmental pollutants have negative effects on the delivery of oxygen to cells. Pollutants in the air may damage the lungs, and ozone, nitrous oxide, and lead hinder the uptake of oxygen by hemoglobin.

The adequacy of the diet to supply nutrients required for the synthesis of hemoglobin is a key factor in successful physical performance. Many nutrients are needed to synthesize hemoglobin. Let's start with iron, because hemoglobin cannot be synthesized without an adequate supply of iron from the diet.

Many factors affect the bioavailability of iron, as we saw in Chapter 10. An adequate dietary intake is critical, but not all athletes achieve this.[3] Another reason for insufficient amounts of iron for hemoglobin synthesis is the loss of iron from the body. There are contradictory opinions on the significance to athletic performance of iron loss through the skin, GI tract, and urine. Most marathon runners experience blood loss in the urine after a race. Loss of blood results in a loss of hemoglobin, and therefore a loss of oxygen-carrying capacity. However, the conventional wisdom seems to be that these losses do not greatly affect physical performance.

Dietary protein in adequate amounts is needed for the synthesis of globin, the protein part of hemoglobin. Other nutrients critical for the functioning of hemoglobin and the red blood cells containing it are vitamin E, vitamin B-6, and copper. Folacin and vitamin B-12 deficiencies result in red blood cells of irregular size and shape with decreased oxygen-carrying capacity.

Myoglobin in muscles is related chemically to hemoglobin. Also an iron-containing globin, it takes the oxygen from hemoglobin and transfers it to the muscle cells. Iron-deficient diets result in a reduction in myoglobin concentration and thus a reduction in muscle performance.

A not uncommon sight in football games is players leaving the field after a long run and placing masks over their noses to breathe oxygen. Oxygen is given in the belief that it helps in the removal of *lactic acid* from muscles because lactic acid requires oxygen for its breakdown to energy, carbon dioxide, and water. Some coaches and players think the extra oxygen quickens recovery and allows players to return to the game with renewed energy. In theory, this seems reasonable, given the importance of oxygen in liberating energy from muscles. But experiments show that breathing 100% oxygen during recovery from extensive exercise is of little value.[4] It seems that lower lactic acid concentrations are reached more rapidly if athletes walk during recovery rather than sit and breathe pure oxygen.

Lactic acid: An organic acid formed at the mid-point in the breakdown of glucose to energy, carbon dioxide, and water. It causes fatigue when it builds up in muscles during exercise.

■ Food–The fuel for physical activity

Athletes recognize that the amount and type of food eaten during training are important, as is the timing of a pre-event meal. In this section, we discuss the nutrient intake required for increased physical activity.

Energy and the Energy Nutrients

Energy requirements are determined by the type and duration of the sport or other activity and by the body weight and fitness of the individual. Figure 12-3 shows a wide range in the calories burned per hour by a preteenager; adults also burn different amounts of calories, depending upon their activities. A person's diet should reflect the level of energy he or she needs to expend–both the number of calories and the source of calories are important in meeting energy requirements.

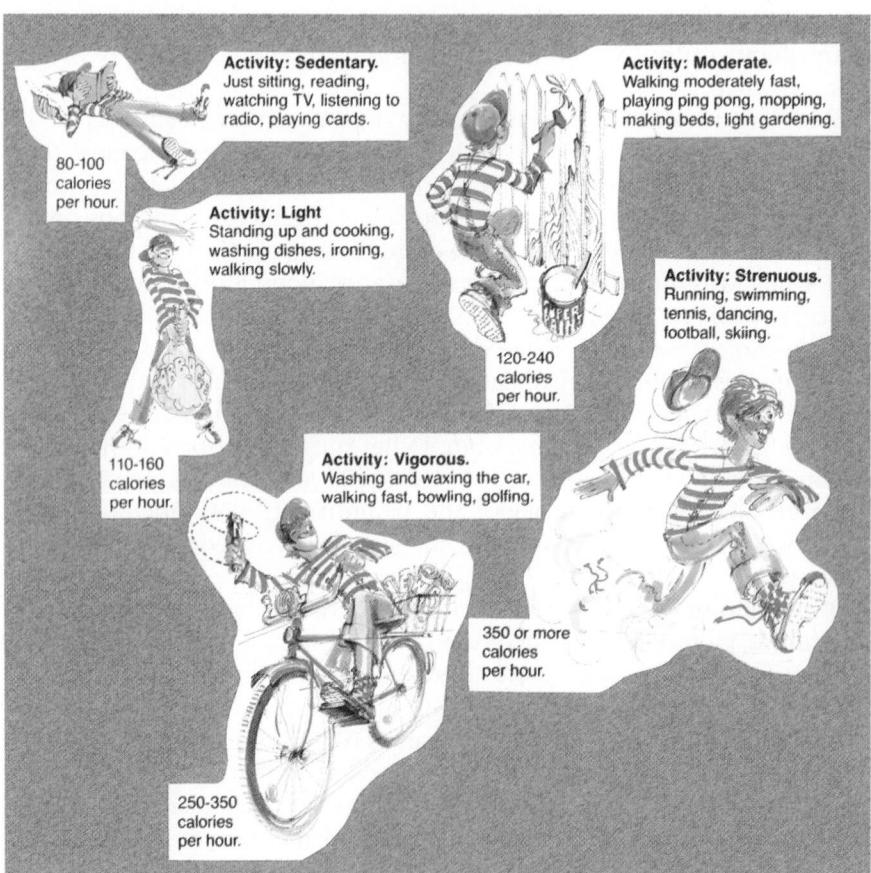

Figure 12-3. Energy expenditure varies for different activities. Remember that it takes an expenditure of 3,500 calories to lose one pound of fat.

Athletes should consume diets in which 55–60% of total calories come from carbohydrates, 30% from fat, and 15–20% from protein. These figures are similar to the recommended dietary intake for the general population.

Carbohydrates

An intake of carbohydrates providing 55–60% of total energy seems difficult to achieve for some athletes, including endurance runners. An example of such a diet, in which the starch content is high and sugar is low, is seen in Table 12-2, which lists the number of daily servings of each food group.

Dietary carbohydrates are now classified (by the glycemic index) according to the level to which they increase blood glucose.[5] This makes sense because glucose is the fuel of preference for the muscles, and so the need for speed in getting glucose to muscles is understandable. Foods such as bread and potatoes produce almost the same glycemic response as glucose ingestion. Carbohydrates with high glycemic index should therefore be selected for early recovery after exercise (see Table 6-5).

Protein

Protein requirements for athletes may be higher than previously thought.[6] However, this protein must come from a balanced diet, *not* from protein supplements, a subject we will deal with later. Protein intake up to 50% greater than the RDA for protein for adults is recommended, especially for athletes in endurance sports (marathons, cross-country skiing, and triathlons). Most experts suggest a protein intake of about 1.0 gram of protein per kilogram of body weight per day. This can usually be achieved because, when a diet is high in calories, it is usually high in protein. Exceptions to this situation occur only when carbohydrate intake is very high or when total energy intake is low. There is no need to rush to protein or amino acid supplements to achieve a high protein intake.

Higher protein intake is not as critical for intermittent-sport athletes such as soccer, softball, and basketball players or for golfers and weight-lifters. The reason for this difference is in the nature of the physical activity involved. Ultraendurance athletes train exclusively to maximize energy metabolism in skeletal and cardiac muscle. Although protein is not the preferred energy source (glucose and fatty acids are), the body turns to any energy source at the extremes of physical endurance. Therefore, amino acids are burned by these athletes. At the other end of the energy expenditure spectrum are weight-lifters and bodybuilders, who train mainly to increase muscle mass and strength. Their requirement for extra protein for increasing muscle mass is minimal.[6]

Table 12-2. Training Diet Consisting of 60% Carbohydrate, 15–20% Protein, and Less than 25% Fat, Showing Recommended Daily Servings

Food Group and Examples of Food in Group	Body Weight and Total Calories[a]	
	132 lb (60 kg) 3,000 kcal	176 lb (80 kg) 4,000 kcal
Milk group (90 kcal/serving)	4	4
Skim milk, 1 cup		
Plain, low-fat yogurt, 1 cup		
Meat group (55–75 kcal/serving)	5	6
Cooked lean meat, fish, poultry, 1 ounce		
Egg, 1		
Peanut butter, 1 tablespoon		
Low-fat cheese, 1 ounce		
Cottage cheese, ¼ cup		
Fruits (60 kcal/serving)	9	12
Fresh or juice, ½ cup		
Dried, ¼ cup		
Vegetables (25 kcal/serving)	5	7
Cooked or juice, ½ cup		
Raw, 1 cup		
Grain group (80 kcal/serving)	18	24
Bread, 1 slice		
Cereal, ½ cup (dry or cooked)		
Pasta, ½ cup (cooked)		
Dried beans, peas, lentils, ⅓ cup (cooked)		
Rice, ⅓ cup (cooked)		
Fat (45 kcal/serving)	6	10
Butter, margarine, oil, 1 teaspoon		
Nuts or seeds, 1 tablespoon		
Salad dressing, 1 tablespoon		

[a] An active athlete needs about 50 kcal of food per kilogram (23 kcal/lb) of body weight each day to provide enough calories for athletic performance. However, exact calorie needs are dependent on age, sex, and activity level.

Fat

Fat is consumed by many athletes at higher levels than the 30% of total calories recommended for the population in general.

Take a moment to examine the data in Table 12-3.

Table 12-3. Source of Dietary Energy for Athletes in Various Sports

Sport	Percent Energy Consumed as		
	Carbohydrate	Protein	Fat
Cycling	59	14	27
Basketball	48	17	34
Cross-country skiing	44	14	40
Football	44	16	38
Soccer	41	16	43
Bodybuilding	41	25	31

Notice that soccer players and bodybuilders have an almost identical percentage of total energy from carbohydrates. However, bodybuilders have a much higher percentage of calories from protein and a lower percentage from fat than do soccer players. This is a good example of how different sports require significant differences in the proportion of calories coming from the three energy nutrients. It also shows how difficult it is for athletes eating the North American or European diet to achieve a fat intake in which 30% of the total calories comes from fat.

Vitamins and Minerals

It makes biological sense that we examine the dietary intake of vitamins and minerals because of the involvement of some of them as coenzymes active in the breakdown and buildup of carbohydrate, fat, and protein in the human body. Many B-complex vitamins are vital in these processes, as we saw in Chapter 9. Dietary deficiencies of these vitamins can decrease physical performance, but there is no evidence that excessive intake by healthy people will improve physical performance. People who exercise but are marginally deficient in vitamin C and riboflavin may have increased requirements for these vitamins.

At the beginning of this chapter we saw the importance of iron in the delivery of oxygen to cells. A well-chosen, balanced diet should deliver the necessary amounts of vitamins and minerals without reliance on vitamin and mineral supplements, according to experts in this area of nutrition. However, women should pay particular attention to their intake of iron and calcium. Dietary intake of these nutrients is marginal for some women. Certain types of exercise–walking, running, and racket sports–promote an increase in bone size. This increases the dietary requirement for calcium. Also, some female athletes who have low caloric intake to keep their weight down have difficulty in meeting iron needs, especially when their intake of meat is low. This is further complicated by the loss of iron due to menstruation.

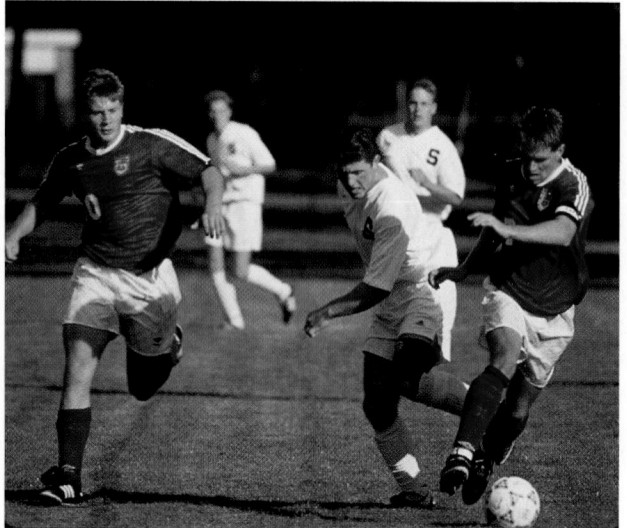

Figure 12-4. Soccer is a game that requires a high caloric expenditure.

Fluids and Electrolytes

Body fluid balance is critically important in achieving maximal physical performance. Figure 12-5 presents dramatic evidence of the drop in performance due to dehydration–about 12% dehydration causes death.

The figure shows how physical performance is decreased by increasing losses of body fluids. Sweating is an important regulator of body heat, and fluid losses are increased under conditions of heavy exercise, especially in warm environments. Special attention to fluid intake is necessary also because exercise seems to blunt the thirst mechanism. Cool water is the drink of preference for fluid replacement during moderate exercise; it can be drunk before, during, and after an event. After you exercise, it is wise to note the change in your body weight and drink two cups of water for every pound lost.

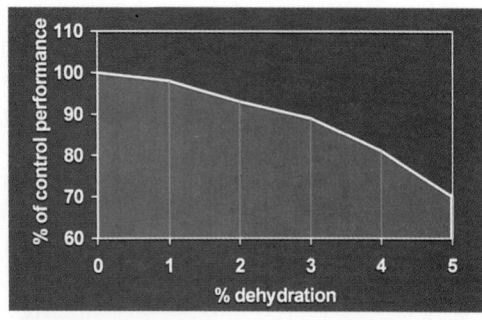

Figure 12-5. Dehydration of the body has dramatic negative effects on physical performance. Dehydration of 5% produces about a 30% reduction in performance. This is why adequate fluid intake is critical during athletic events.

■ Energy in the cell

Energy metabolism involves the storage and use of energy by the billions of cells in your body. *Catabolism* of the energy nutrients carbohydrate, fat, and protein involves many enzymatic reactions.

These chemical changes are taking place within you now as you read this information. If you were to go out and run to exhaustion, only slight shifts would occur in the contributions of amino acids and fatty acids to your energy needs, but the contribution from glucose would change greatly. *Glycolysis* is the means by which cells get most of their energy. A series of chemical reactions breaks each glucose molecule into two intermediate three-carbon units that are further broken down to carbon dioxide and water, generating energy in the process. The energy compound generated is called *adenosine triphosphate (ATP)*. High-energy bonds link the phosphate unit to the adenosine. The energy in ATP is available for your immediate use.

The breakdown of glycogen to glucose

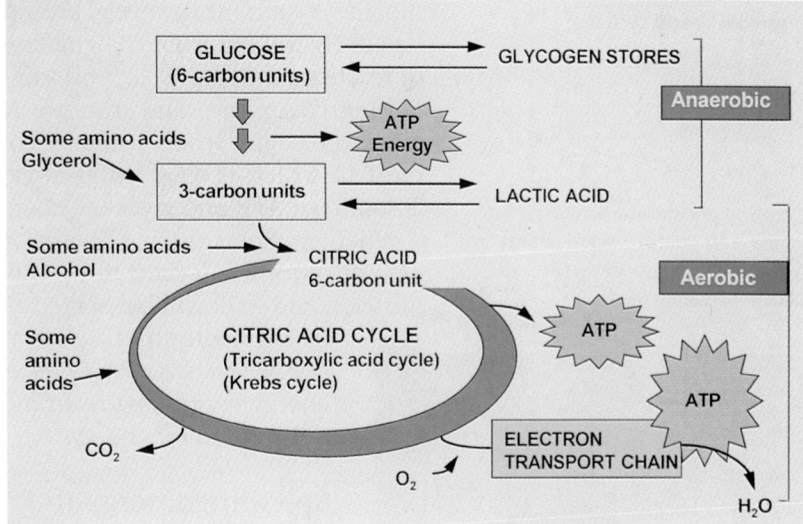

Figure 12-6. Metabolism of glucose. In the anaerobic stage, glucose is broken down into three-carbon units with the consequent production of adenosine triphosphate (ATP) and lactic acid. In the aerobic phase, the units enter the citric acid cycle, which results in the production of carbon dioxide, ATP, and water. Most of the energy (in the form of ATP) is released during the aerobic stage.

Catabolism: The breakdown of complex chemicals into their simpler units in living organisms. For example, glycogen is catabolized into its basic unit, glucose.

Glycolysis: The anaerobic series of reactions by which glucose is broken down to pyruvic acid, a three-carbon unit that is an intermediate chemical in the liberation of energy from glucose. For microbes, called "fermentation."

Adenosine triphosphate (ATP): The main energy reserve for enzyme activity, muscular contraction, pumping chemicals against a concentration gradient, and other work required of cells. Energy is released when one phosphate unit is removed from ATP, thus forming **adenosine diphosphate (ADP)**.

(a six-carbon unit, see Figure 6-5) and then to two three-carbon units, is an anaerobic process. This provides ATP quickly and is the preferred way to generate explosive energy in events lasting less than about 2 minutes. When you see a sprinter leap from the starting blocks, it is ATP that powers the muscles to the finish line by providing the energy for the repetitive muscle contractions and relaxations. Lactic acid is produced in strenuous anaerobic activity and can build up quickly in muscles, causing muscle fatigue. This is why anaerobic activity can be maintained for only about 2 minutes. The buildup of lactic acid lowers the pH of muscles, thereby reducing their ability to contract. However, lactic acid levels are reduced by the oxygen you breathe, which oxidizes the lactic acid back into the three-carbon units.

These units in turn pass through a cycle called any one of three names–the citric acid cycle, or the tricarboxylic acid cycle, or the *Krebs cycle* (named after the British biochemist, Sir Hans Krebs). Most of the ATP in the breakdown of glucose is generated in this cycle, which occurs in the presence of oxygen and is therefore called aerobic metabolism. Carbon dioxide is spun off the cycle, taken in the blood to the lungs, and then exhaled. Hydrogens from the glucose are taken through an important series of reactions called the electron transport chain. A number of vitamin-containing coenzymes and iron are involved in transferring the hydrogen along the chain, where it finally combines with oxygen to produce water, most of which is excreted as sweat. This aerobic process produces large amounts of ATP, and gives the energy for long-endurance events.

When energy is used, *adenosine diphosphate (ADP)* is formed. If you decide to go for a run right now, ATP will provide the energy to move your muscles, and ADP will be created. The ADP will later be built back to ATP by the addition of an extra phosphate unit. Extra ATP is stored as *creatine phosphate (CP)*, especially in muscles because of their high energy requirements for movement. CP is converted to ATP when it is needed for energy.

Krebs cycle: A series of biochemical reactions in the liberation of energy from the energy nutrients; also known as the citric acid cycle or the tricarboxylic acid cycle.

Creatine phosphate: A high-energy compound used to reform ATP from ADP; also known as phosphocreatine.

Spending Energy in Endurance Sporting Activities

The Tour de France is a bicycle race lasting 22 days with its start and finish in Paris. Dutch nutritionists monitored five competitors during the race and found that they expended about 6,100 calories every day.[7] This is about three times the energy requirement for a sedentary lifestyle. This energy demand must be met each day by the diet, or the cyclist will quickly become fatigued and drop out of the race. The researchers discovered that despite huge caloric expenditures, these cyclists maintained their body weight and body fat during the race. Therefore, their caloric intake must have balanced their energy expenditures, and this is indeed what happened. Their dietary caloric intake was measured at about 5,930 calories per day, with a top intake of 7,780 calories recorded on one day. The question then becomes: How did they consume enough food to achieve this caloric intake?

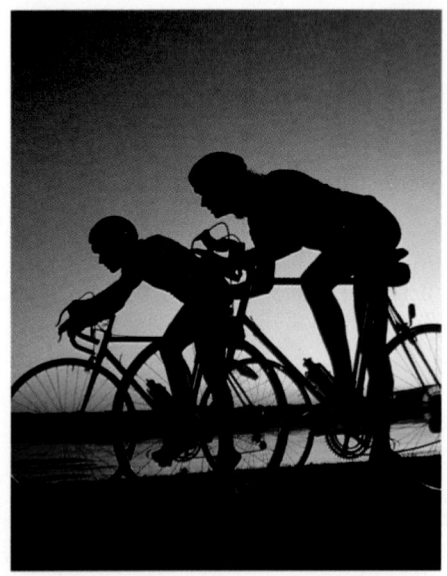

Figure 12-7. Long-distance cycle races, and similar endurance activities, involve high energy intake and expenditure.

Popular belief still maintains that high protein intake builds muscles and provides energy. However, this is *not* the case. As we saw previously, only about 12% of total dietary calories should come from protein. If athletes persist in the belief that high protein intake is helpful, they should be reminded that animal studies show that high protein intake leads to kidney damage. This is because of the large amounts of nitrogen produced as amino acids are metabolized. While there is no evidence of such damage in humans, neither is there any evidence that high levels of dietary protein benefit performance. Both the International Olympic Committee and the U.S. Olympic Committee stress that protein and amino acid supplements are unnecessary.

Having now dismissed protein as a major dietary source to meet the cyclists' enormous requirements for dietary energy, we can dismiss high fat intake as well. Fat moves slowly through the GI tract, making the athlete sluggish, and does not provide quick energy. This leaves carbohydrate as the main energy source.

High-carbohydrate diets are the best way to provide high dietary caloric intake to satisfy the energy demands of strenuous exercise.[8] The problem is that carbohydrate stores in the body are small. In the rested fed state, an adult male stores about 80–100 grams of carbohydrate as glycogen in the liver and about 350–400 grams of glycogen in muscles. (On the other hand, body fat stores are large–about 3 kilograms in the leanest male, and much more in others.) Hard exercise uses up about 3–4 grams of carbohydrate per minute. Therefore, the total supply of carbohydrate available for hard exercise is sufficient for less than 2 hours. When this is depleted, the athlete slows down or drops out of a race. In marathon runs, this is known as "hitting the wall" and usually occurs after about 18 miles. Consuming carbohydrates restores the glycogen that was burned.

Consuming up to 600 grams of carbohydrate per day is not easy. The Food Guide Pyramid and other dietary recommendations recommend a high intake of *complex carbohydrates* and a reduction in sugar intake. Complex carbohydrates are found in such foods as pasta, bread, rice, and potatoes. This presents a problem because all of these foods are bulky and have high fiber and water contents. Putting this in real terms, to get 100 grams of carbohydrate you must eat 350 grams of pasta or 500 grams of potatoes. A target carbohydrate intake of 800 grams per day would require the athlete to eat nearly 9 pounds of potatoes, which is about 25 medium-sized potatoes. Many serious athletes do achieve such a high intake of carbohydrates. One good aspect of high carbohydrate intake is that it is emptied from the stomach and digested faster than either fat or protein. However, this means a shorter wait before facing another plate of potatoes (or pasta, rice, or bread). Some athletes break this monotony by getting some carbohydrate from soft drinks and confectionery.

Carbohydrate loading (also known as glycogen loading, or glycogen supercompensation) is popular with athletes involved in endurance events such as the marathon, cross-country skiing, triathlon, or any high-intensity exercise lasting longer than 60–80 minutes. Carbohydrate loading allows maximum storage of glycogen in muscles; Figure 12-8 shows how it is done.

Complex carbohydrates: Polysaccharides, such as starch.

Carbohydrate loading: Consumption of carbohydrates (600 grams per day or 70% of total energy intake as carbohydrate, whichever is larger) for 6–7 days before certain athletic events to increase glycogen stores; also known as glycogen loading or glycogen supercompensation.

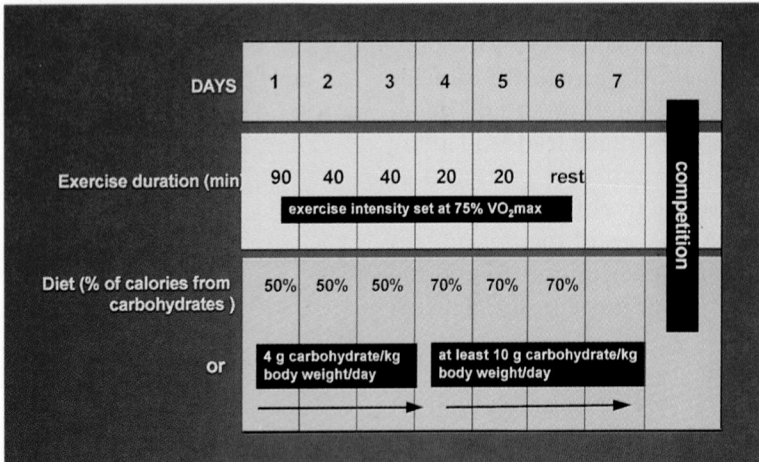

Figure 12-8. A modified regimen for glycogen loading. Carbohydrate, or glycogen, loading before an athletic event, such as a marathon run, requires attention to a number of factors. These include the amount and type of carbohydrate consumed, the amount of time before the event, and the duration, intensity, and timing of training before the event.

Table 12-4. Activities Appropriate and Inappropriate for Supercompensation (Carbohydrate Loading)

Appropriate	Inappropriate
Marathon	Football games
Long-distance swimming	10-km runs
Cross-country skiing	Downhill ski races
30-km runs	Walking and hiking
Soccer	Most swimming events
Cycling time trials	Basketball games
Long-distance canoe racing	Weight lifting
Triathlons	Most track and field events
Orienteering	Rowing events

T cell: (T lymphocyte) A type of white blood cell that fights infections within the body.

High carbohydrate intake is recommended not only immediately before the event, but also for hard training long before the endurance event. However, carbohydrate loading is not appropriate for all sports. Table 12-4 shows activities for which it is appropriate or inappropriate.

■ Can exercise damage your health?

This seems an odd question given the impressive list of benefits of physical activity we reviewed at the beginning of this chapter. This section will not correct or change all of those positives, but there are a few negatives, some of which have been researched intensively.

Exercise, Nutrition, and the Immune System

A puzzling negative about extensive physical activity by fit athletes is that they seem to have increased vulnerability to certain infections. This is how a recent scientific article introduced the problem:

> Regular exercise is a good thing: conventional wisdom says so, and the experts . . . agree. But what about infectious diseases? Does exercise help us to ward them off, or does it make us succumb more readily by impairing the immune system?[9]

There is evidence that exercise has marked effects on the body's immune system. Have a look under the microscope (Figure 12-9) at some of our defenders, the killer *T cells*. These cells, also called T lymphocytes, are a type of white blood cell. Such cells are your body's scavengers, which help it fight infections. T cells are an important part of the body's protective mechanism against foreign substances, including viruses such as HIV, the causative agent of AIDS.

World-class athletes train for up to 35 hours per week. Swimmers, rowers, canoeists, cyclists, and runners spend at least four hours each day on the water, road, or track. Some coaches and sports doctors suspect that this type of heavy exercise can impair immunity to infections. But there is no scientific evidence to confirm this impression. There are observations that when infections such as respiratory diseases, GI tract infections, skin complaints, and polio break out in a community, it is usually the very fit who are most affected. However, we cannot immediately jump to the conclusion that a faulty immune system is involved with very fit athletes. An alternate reason is that athletes train and travel together, with plenty of opportunities to spread a virus. Experts are also uncertain how each component of the immune system, especially the B cells and T cells, responds to different types of exercise. However, there is no shortage of theories.

One theory is that depleted nutrition for immune cells may suppress the immune system. This theory involves nutrition because immune cells seem to have high demands for the amino acid glutamine and to rely on high levels of it in the blood. When levels of glutamine decrease, there is a decrease in some immune functions. Glutamine is found in plants and is a chemical relative of glutamic acid, a nonessential amino acid. The immune cells use glut-

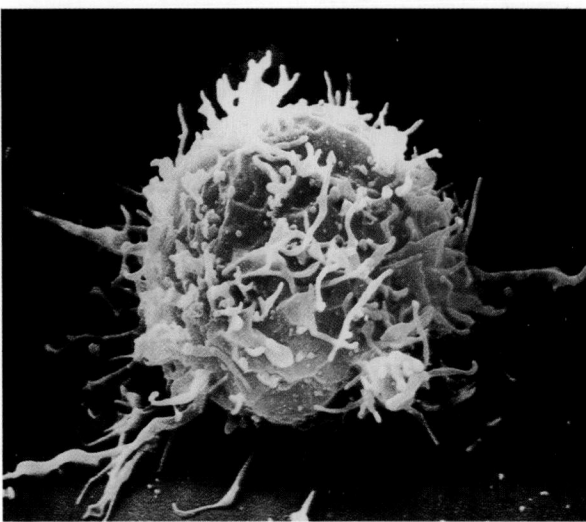

Figure 12-9. T cells, also called T lymphocytes, help fight infection in the body. Recent evidence suggests that intense physical activity decreases the level of T cells, thus increasing the possibility of infections in highly trained athletes.

amine to provide energy and as a source of nitrogen to synthesize DNA and RNA. It may also have a role in controlling the metabolism of immune cells. Marathon runners may have a 25% decrease in blood levels of glutamine after a race. Athletes suffering from the overtraining syndrome also have low glutamine blood levels. Feeding glutamine to patients suffering from immune suppression increases glutamine levels in the blood, and a significant improvement in resistance has been noted. Much more will be heard in the future about the immune system, the role of glutamine, and the work of nutritionists in this important area.

Exercise and Menstrual Disorders

Strenuous exercise may produce abnormal menstrual cycles. These are likely to occur if, for instance, a woman runs 4 miles per day, progresses to 10 miles per day by the fifth week, and engages daily in 3½ hours of moderate-intensity sports. Menstrual abnormalities arise with vigorous exercise, especially if compounded by body weight loss. Normal menstruation usually resumes when the strenuous exercise stops. Bone injuries are more common when women have menstrual disorders. We need to learn more about the long-term effects of a lack of estrogen on bone loss and on osteoporosis.[10] These effects are particularly important in young, growing athletes.

Sports Anemia or Runners' Anemia

Some athletes have low hemoglobin concentrations compared to those of the general public. This could be caused by low dietary intake of iron and other nutrients assisting iron absorption and metabolism or to a condition called "sports anemia" or "runners' anemia." The most common cause of runners' anemia is an increase in plasma volume. This allows blood to move faster to muscles during exercise, but the increased amount of plasma dilutes the concentration of red blood cells in a given volume of blood. Hemoglobin is in red blood cells, so a decrease is apparent in the concentration of hemoglobin. This causes no harm to the person, prompting one researcher to entitle a paper in a medical journal "Runners' anemia: A paper tiger." Runners' anemia may be caused also by the breaking of red blood cells, resulting in a loss of hemoglobin. This breakage is probably caused by the constant pounding of the feet in long-distance running. The resulting small drop in hemoglobin level can cause a problem if the person has a barely adequate iron status at the start of the race.

Anabolic Steroids

Abuse of anabolic steroids is also a concern. The steroid most associated with the term "anabolic steroids" is testosterone, or a steroid hormone resembling it. Testosterone is the principal sex hormone produced by males. Anabolism means the building up of body tissues such as muscles. Among the nutrition-related problems produced by steroid abuses are liver damage and an increase in the blood lipids that are thought to increase the risk of coronary heart disease.

Some Similarities to Anorexia

Eating disorders, including anorexia nervosa, are examined in Chapter 13. However, it is appropriate to examine some similarities and dissimilarities between the athlete who is obsessive about exercise and body fitness and the young person obsessed about food intake and body weight. Dr. Judith Rodin of Yale University reserves a section in her book *Body Traps* for what she describes as "exercise addicts."[11] The two groups share some common features relating to food and nutrition.

Dietitians' Advice for Athletes and Exercisers

The following advice is an appropriate summary of our discussion on diet and physical performance. It comes from SCAN, the American Dietetic Association's Sports and Cardiovascular Nutritionists group.[12]

- Drink plenty of water; dehydration can really hurt your performance.

- Eat more carbohydrates and less fat before an event and during training.

- Use carbohydrate and fluid replacement drinks during long events (competitions and training) to maintain a normal blood sugar level. (Before a long training run, you might have to "plant" a sports drink at water stops along the way.) Without these carbohydrates, your thinking will become fuzzy and you'll lose your competitive edge.

- Recovery carbohydrates and fluids are important, so pay attention to postevent meals! Rapid carbohydrate replacement 15–30 minutes after

Table 12-5. Shared and Distinguishing Features of Athletic and Anorectic Women

Athletic Woman	Anorectic Woman
Shared features	
Dietary faddism	
Controlled calorie consumption	
Specific carbohydrate avoidance	
Low body weight	
Slow heart rate and low blood pressure	
Increased physical activity	
No or few menstrual periods	
Anemia (may or may not be present)	
Distinguishing features	
Purposeful training	Aimless physical activity
Good muscular development	Poor or decreasing exercise performance
Accurate body image	Poor muscular development
Body fat level within defined normal range	Flawed body image (believes herself to be overweight)
Increased plasma volume	Body fat level below normal range
Increased O_2 extraction from blood	Electrolyte abnormalities if abusing laxatives and/or diuretics
Efficient energy metabolism	
Increased HDL_2 (high-density lipoprotein)	Cold intolerance
	Dry skin
	Irregular heartbeat
	Downy hair covering the body
	White blood cell dysfunction

exercise can make a big difference; e.g., don't skip breakfast after a morning workout.

- Eat a small meal 2 hours before an event; don't try to exercise "on fumes."

- Be sure to get adequate iron; lean meats can help cut fatigue.

- Don't try to lose weight quickly while training and competing. With inadequate glycogen replacement, you'll feel chronically tired and perform poorly.

- Have a very positive attitude and always think successful thoughts.

We have been through a lot of information, so it may be refreshing to learn that even knowledgeable sports nutritionists sometimes make food mistakes that interfere with top performance.[12] The most common mistakes were eating too much fat, too much food, or too soon before exercising. Some had food rituals or superstitions such as avoiding peanuts, nuts, popcorn, and protein-rich foods.

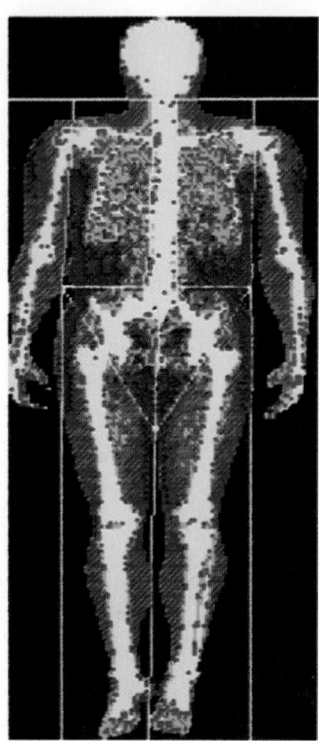

Figure 12-10. X-ray absorptiometric view of the human body, showing bones (white), muscles (green), and fat tissue (purple).

■ People are different–Variable responses to the effects of exercise on lean body mass

Figure 12-10 shows how the body of a young man appears using dual-energy X-ray absorptiometry. What is important for our purposes is that this technique shows bones, muscles, and body fat in white, green, and purple, respectively. If we differ in body composition, different proportions of these colors will show up for each of us.

The amount and type of muscles in your body are the products of many factors. Certainly, nutrition is important because dietary protein synthesizes muscle proteins, some dietary carbohydrates are stored as glycogen, and some fats and fatty acids are also energy sources available to your muscles. We have different amounts of muscle in our bodies because of differences in our genes, the amount of exercise we exert on muscles, and our degree of mobility. Muscle loss is a serious problem for people who are bedridden or confined to wheelchairs. Astronauts living in zero gravity in space also experience muscle loss. Irrespective of dietary quality, muscles that cannot contract and relax can lose up to 40% of their mass within a few weeks.[13]

A question this raises is: How do the muscles of embryos grow? They do very little mechanical work and thus may not be much different in that respect from the bedridden person. Yet by birth an explosive amount of muscle growth has occurred. We still await an answer.

The foregoing information puts some of the relationships between nutrition and athletic performance into perspective. We inherit muscles that are biologically programmed for sprinting or for endurance competition. No amount of nutritional manipulation will alter that fact. The search is on to trace the biochemical steps leading to the switching on and off of muscle genes. When that is understood, we will have a better understanding of the role of specific nutrients. It is not unreasonable to assume that a way will be discovered to artificially stimulate muscle fibers to grow. However, before we get too excited about the prospects of programming specific muscles for specific events, we should remember that athletic potential depends as much on the brain and the cardiovascular system as it does on having the right types of muscle fibers in the right place.[13] And it also takes the right combination of nutrients to maintain and fuel all of these tissues.

Another area of interest to nutritionists is why successful athletes have larger lean body mass (LBM) than sedentary people. Lean body mass is the weight of the body excluding the weight of body fat, and this has a significant influence on a person's body weight. The debate continues as to whether the increased LBM in athletes is due to training and exercise or to genetic factors. Recent evidence suggests that exercise programs cannot prevent a decrease in lean weight when body weight is being lost also.[14] We also know that exercise can induce a modest increase in LBM and a decrease in body fat, but to do this you must maintain your body weight at its preexercise level. Accordingly, exercisers wishing to increase, or even maintain, their lean weight (mainly skeletal muscle) must consume a sufficient number of calories to compensate for the increase in energy expenditure produced by exercise. Obese people have an advantage over thin people in this regard because they lose proportionately less lean weight during weight loss.[14]

Advances in molecular biology, exercise physiology, and genetic engineering will open up many new aspects of physical activity that will be of interest to nutritionists.

■ Nutrition in action–Do supplements help physical performance?

Many consumers use food supplements for their pharmaceutical properties but may not consider such food supplements to be drugs, and physicians may not take a history of their use from their patients. This is why there are major gaps in our understanding of the use and effectiveness of various dietary supplements. A recent study of popular health and bodybuilding magazines (Table 12-6) showed that amino acids were the most frequently advertised nutritional supplement; the most frequently promoted health benefit was muscle growth.[15] Here are some details of this study, which will help us understand why some of these are popular and why many are useless and may be dangerous to our health.

Researchers in the survey identified some general characteristics of nutrient supplements and their users.[15] They found that: 1) food and nutrient supplements are readily available to the public; 2) supplements are consumed by a large number of people; 3) many ingredients are not readily identifiable, and potential side effects are not known; 4) supplement users may combine two or more products and usually set their own dosage; and 5) unanticipated side effects may occur, as was the case with tryptophan supplements (see Chapter 8).

Is a great athlete born or made? The answer is: "both, it appears."[16] Experts agree that the keys to success include training, genetic attributes, and proper nutrition, especially adequate carbohydrate and fluid intake before and during a competition. Yet many athletes continue to believe that some special food or nutrient supplement can bring instant success. If one exists, no one has found it yet.[9] That does not stop enterprising individuals and con artists from hyping "performance enhancers" and other aids.

Ergogenic aids are products supposed to enhance physical performance, to improve energy utilization, and to prevent fatigue.[16] They are classified into five

Ergogenic aids: Products supposed to increase physical performance.

Table 12-6. Categories and Principal Effects Attributed to Advertised Products in Study of Food Supplement Advertisements

Category of Ingredient	Percent of Mentions[a]
Amino acids	21.7
Miscellaneous	19.1
Herbs	14.2
Vitamins	11.5
Trace minerals	7.5
Minerals	5.1
Steroids	4.3
Protein	3.9
Fats	3.9
Enzymes	2.5
Glands	2.5
Carbohydrates	2.3
Over-the-counter medication	0.8
Bacteria	0.4
Prescription medication	0.1

Attributed Effects	Percent of Products Claiming the Effect[b]
Muscle growth	19.0
Increased testosterone levels	8.7
Nutritional supplement	6.8
Energy enhancer	5.5
Fat reduction	4.8
Increased strength	3.8
Growth hormone releaser	2.6
No effect listed	28.9
Other effects	19.9

[a] Out of 914 mentions.
[b] Out of 311 products claiming effects.

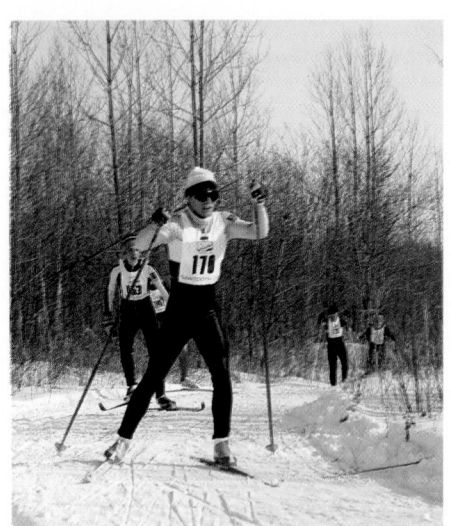

Figure 12-11. To improve their physical performance, athletes should understand the scientific principles underlying diets and nutrient supplements.

groups: mechanical (e.g., lightweight racing shoes), psychological (e.g., hypnosis), physiological (e.g., soda doping), nutritional (e.g., carbohydrate loading), and pharmacological (e.g., recombinant erythropoietin, a hormone that regulates red blood cell production on the theory that having more red blood cells increases hemoglobin and, therefore, the oxygen-carrying capacity of the blood).

Some interesting facts emerge from this list. For example, by using lightweight shoes, a runner improves energy efficiency by 1.2% or more. This means that an athlete running a marathon in 2 hours and 10 minutes can shave at least 90 seconds off that time by using these shoes. But better nutrition can do more–a 160-pound runner who loses 5% of body weight as *fat* (about 8 pounds) can save 5.6 minutes in the same marathon run. Amino acids are included among the psychological aids because their biological and nutritional advantages remain to be determined.

Sodium bicarbonate is listed as a physiological aid because it helps neutralize metabolic acids, especially the lactic acid that accumulates in muscle and induces fatigue. Ingestion of sodium bicarbonate is known as soda doping. Studies show that an intake of 300 milligrams of sodium bicarbonate per kilogram of body weight improves performance in high-intensity exercise lasting 1–5 minutes. The effects on long-distance events are unknown. The use of sodium bicarbonate is safe and legal, but it is not recommended because of gastrointestinal disturbances such as diarrhea and abdominal distention.

Pharmacological aids include two food drugs that are partially banned–alcohol and caffeine. Alcohol use is outlawed only in certain sports (shooting), and caffeine can be used in moderate amounts by all athletes. Alcohol is thought to increase energy, but there is no scientific evidence that it does. It may actually depress energy efficiency by decreasing glucose release from the liver, resulting in fatigue. Caffeine's supposed ability to increase energy has been of interest for over 100 years. It is thought to increase the release of fatty acids, thereby sparing muscle glycogen. This could be important in endurance events because it is glycogen concentration that often separates winners from dropouts. Small amounts of caffeine are usually allowed before an event, but intake of about 800 milligrams, the equivalent of 6–8 cups of coffee, results in a caffeine level in the urine that can cause disqualification.

Nutritional ergogenic aids are *not* substitutes for a balanced diet. Research data are limited, but experts' opinions are that they are of little value and may even be harmful. Vitamin E supplements are supposed to increase aerobic endurance, but there is no evidence that they do. Phosphate salts are sold on the basis that phosphorus is part of both the ATP molecule and some coenzymes and has buffering abilities in cells. Results of scientific studies are mixed, and it may be concluded that the jury is still out on the effectiveness of phosphate salts as an ergogenic aid.

We cannot continue with details on specific ergogenic substances supposed to improve athletic performance because there are too many of them. The list in Table 12-7 is a summary. Care must be exercised with all

Table 12-7. Unproven Ergogenic Aids for Athletes

Ergogenic Aid	Description	Claim
Bee pollen	Mixture of bee saliva, plant nectar, and pollen	Increased energy levels, enhanced physical fitness
Brewer's yeast	By-product of beer brewing	Increased energy levels
Carnitine	Compound synthesized in the body from glutamate and methionine	Improved cardiovascular function and muscle strength, delayed fatigue, decreased muscle pain
Choline	Precursor of the neurotransmitter acetylcholine	Improved performance
DNA, RNA	Deoxyribonucleic acid, ribonucleic acid	Tissue regeneration
Gelatin	Obtained from collagen	Improved muscle contraction
Ginseng	Extract of ginseng root	Protection against tissue damage
Glycine	An amino acid that is a phosphocreatine precursor	Improved muscle contraction
Inosine	Purine	Enhanced physical strength
Kelp	Seaweed	Vitamin/mineral source
Lecithin	Phosphatidylcholine	Prevention of fat gain
Octacosanol	Alcohol isolate extracted from wheat germ oil	Improved energy and performance
Pangamic acid	Also referred to as vitamin B-15; varied composition, depending on supplier	Increased delivery of oxygen
Royal jelly	Substance produced by worker bees and fed to the queen bee	Increased strength
Spirulina	Microscopic blue-green algae	Protein source
Superoxide dismutase	Enzyme	Protection of body against oxidative cell damage incurred from aerobic metabolism

of the substances discussed in this section because most can produce some undesirable side effects.[16]

■ Now you know

- Physical activity gives many health benefits, but many people, including the young, are not meeting national fitness objectives.

- Oxygen is carried by hemoglobin to cells to help in the release of energy; the oxygen-carrying capacity of the blood may be reduced by certain nutritional and environmental factors.

- Athletes should get 55–60% of calories from carbohydrate, 30% from fat, and 15–20% from protein.

- Athletes in different sports consume different amounts of calories and in different proportions of carbohydrate, fat, and protein.

- Adequate fluid intake is essential for maximum physical performance.

- Cells get their energy from the breakdown of carbohydrate, fat, and protein to produce adenosine triphosphate (ATP) and creatine phosphate (CP) both anaerobically and aerobically. Carbohydrate is the dietary fuel of preference, especially for endurance activities. Some athletes get additional glycogen into muscles by carbohydrate loading.

- Intense and prolonged exercise seems to damage the immune system, resulting in higher rates of infections among athletes. The amino acid glutamine may be an effective preventive.

- Intense exercise causes menstrual changes.

- Female athletes and patients with anorexia nervosa have some shared and some distinguishing features regarding food habits and health indicators.

- Exercise has different effects on lean body tissues in athletic people and nonathletic people.

- Supplements to a balanced diet do not improve physical performance. Ergogenic supplements have no known benefits and may have negative side effects.

Further Reading

1. Gloag, D. Exercise, fitness, and health. *British Medical Journal* 305:377, 1992.
2. Simons-Morton, B. G., and others. The physical activity of fifth-grade students during physical education classes. *American Journal of Public Health* 83:262, 1993.
3. Weight, L. M., and others. Dietary iron deficiency and sports anaemia. *British Journal of Nutrition* 68:253, 1992.
4. Cooper, K. H., and others. Oxygen and athletes. *Journal of the American Medical Association* 262:264, 1989.
5. Simopoulos, A. P. Nutrition and fitness: A conference report. *Nutrition Today* 27(6):24, 1992.
6. Houston, M. E. Protein and amino acid needs of athletes. *Nutrition Today* 27(5):36, 1992.
7. Maughan, R. Success on a plate. *New Scientist* 135(1831):36, 1992.
8. Jensen, C. D., and others. Dietary intakes of male endurance cyclists during training and racing. *Journal of the American Dietetic Association* 92:986, 1992.
9. Sharp, C., and Parry-Billings, M. Can exercise damage your health? *New Scientist* 135(1834):33, 1992.
10. Shangold, M., and others. Evaluation and management of menstrual dysfunction in athletes. *Journal of the American Medical Association* 263:1665, 1990.
11. Rodin, J. *Body Traps*. William Morrow and Company, New York, page 217, 1992.
12. Clark, N. Sports nutritionists practice what they preach. *Journal of the American Dietetic Association* 92:419, 1992.

13. Goldspink, G. The brains behind the brawn. *New Scientist* 135(1832):28, 1992.
14. Forbes, G. B. Exercise and lean weight: The influence of body weight. *Nutrition Reviews* 50:157, 1992.
15. Philen, R. M., and others. Survey of advertising for nutritional supplements in health and bodybuilding magazines. *Journal of the American Medical Association* 268:1008, 1992.
16. Williams, M. H. Nutritional ergogenics: Help or hype? *Journal of the American Dietetic Association* 92:1213, 1992.

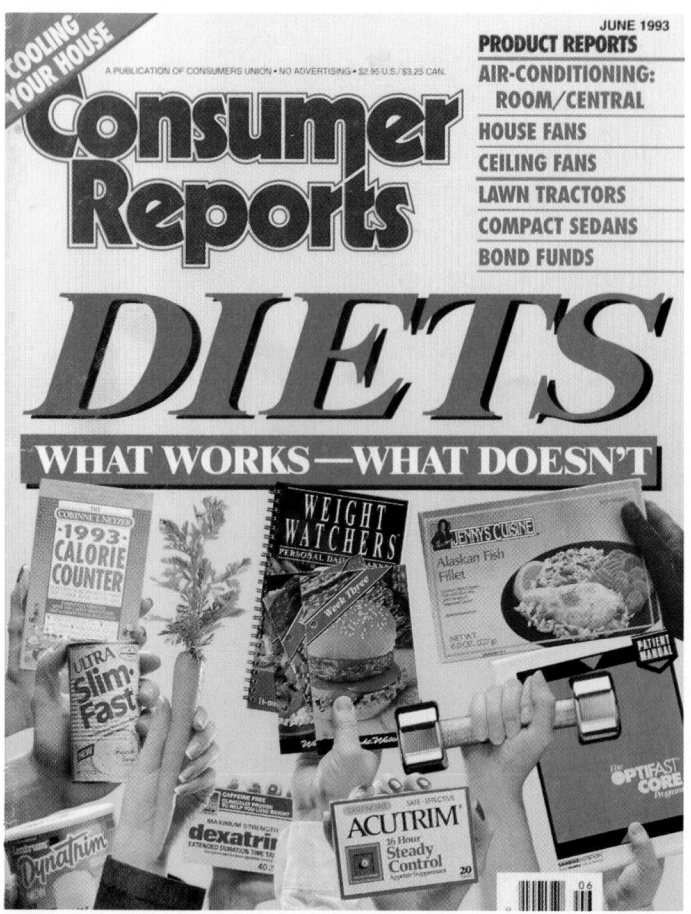

"Eating disorders" is a group term that includes anorexia nervosa and bulimia. In the United States, about 11,000 cases of anorexia and 10,000 of bulimia are diagnosed each year. It is estimated that by the first year of college, 4.5–18% of women and 0.4% of men have a history of bulimia and that as many as 1 in 100 females aged 12–18 have anorexia. Eating disorders are apparently more prevalent in females, with males accounting for a total of only 5–10% of all cases.[1]

Percent Obese Individuals

Country	Males	Females
United States	12	12
Canada	9	12
Great Britain	6	8
Netherlands	4	6
Australia	7	7

Figures 13-1 and 13-2. The two ends of a nutrition spectrum–overweight and underweight–are common all over the world. Left, about 34 million adults in the United States are overweight.[2] Right, over 500 million children in the world suffer from protein-energy malnutrition, according to the World Health Organization. Millions of people are also underweight because of eating disorders.

Obesity, Starvation, and Eating Disorders

■ Nutrition in our lives–The pain and problems of dietary excesses and deficiencies

The photographs and information on the preceding page indicate that obesity is a concern for men and women in developed countries and that eating disorders exist in some teenagers, especially girls, while, at the same time, many people in developing countries, especially the children, suffer famine and starvation.

Figure 13-1 reflects a developed society that seems greatly interested in weight loss. The numbers show that obesity occurs more frequently in North America than in Europe or Australia. It occurs when energy intake is greater than energy expenditure. Figure 13-2 is the outcome of famine resulting from crop failures, war, poor food distribution, or political oppression. Too little food also can result when people consume very low-calorie diets or have too little money for food or when teenagers have eating disorders. All of these problems may result in death. In this chapter, we will discuss the effects of inadequate or excess food consumption.

A starting point for an understanding of obesity, starvation, and eating disorders is to examine what influences body weight. As we work through this list, think of how many of these factors are under your direct control–the answer may surprise you. Examples are given for most of the factors affecting body weight, but you are encouraged to think about each category and come up with your own examples.

■ Obesity

Factors Affecting Body Fat

The following factors are *not* listed in order of importance.

- **Age.** The amount of body fat increases with age.

- **Gender.** Women have more fat than men per unit of body weight. We saw in Chapter 7 one reason why nature gave women more body fat than men–to maintain reproduction in times of food shortages.

- **Genetics.** Heredity plays an important part in whether we fight a weight problem or not. Studies with twins raised by biological parents and twins raised by adopted parents show that genetic background rather than family environment determines whether a person becomes obese. In general, if both of your parents were obese, there is about a 75% probability that you will be also. If one parent is obese, the probability drops to about 40%, and if neither parent is, it drops to 10%. Even though genetics plays a strong role in determining the extent of obesity in the next generation of a family, the eating habits of parents also have a role. Consider the two mice in Figure 13-3–genetics is the reason why the one on the right is obese and the one on the left is lean.

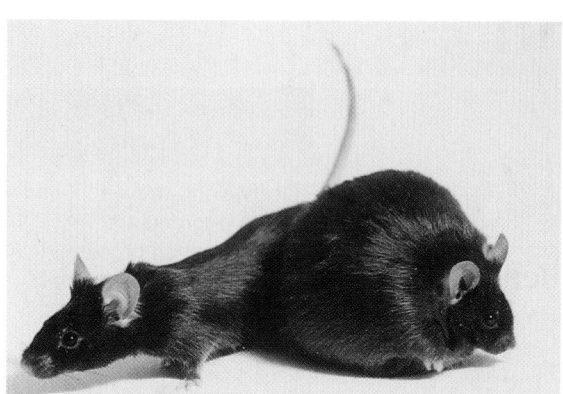

Figure 13-3. Genetics is an important factor in determining obesity in both people and animals. These two mice are similar in all respects (age, gender, diet) except for their heredity and their weight.

Thyroid hormone: Iodine-containing hormone secreted by the thyroid gland, located in the neck.

Adrenal gland: Gland that influences the metabolism of carbohydrates, body water, muscle, bone, the nervous system, the GI tract, and the cardiovascular system. Located near the kidney. Produces epinephrine (adrenaline).

Pituitary gland: A small gland located at the base of the brain. Secretes hormones that regulate growth, reproduction, and many metabolic activities. Often referred to as the "master gland."

Hypothalamus: Part of the brain that influences body-water balance, carbohydrate and fat metabolism, and the regulation of body temperature.

- **Basal energy requirement.** Basal metabolic rate (BMR) decreases during aging because of the normal loss of lean tissue (see Chapter 11). Body weight increases if there is no decrease in energy intake from food. This is a partial explanation for "middle-age spread."

- **Physical activity.** You will lose weight if you burn more calories in exercise *and* hold caloric intake constant. See Table 11-5 to refresh your memory about activities that burn up extra calories.

- **Pregnancy.** Body fat increases during pregnancy but is usually lost during lactation. However, if the mother gives infant formula instead of her own breast milk, she may retain much of the body fat accumulated in pregnancy.

- **Hormone levels.** Low production of *thyroid hormone* and abnormal activity of the *adrenal* or *pituitary glands* can cause obesity. However, the popular belief that all obesity is caused by "glandular problems" is not borne out by clinical evidence.

- **Brain/nerve signals.** Obesity may be produced by brain tumors or by physical injury affecting the *hypothalamus*, the feeding center of the brain.

- **Disease.** Loss of appetite, resulting in loss of body weight, occurs in cancer, AIDS, and other diseases.

- **Emotions.** Most of us have probably experienced changes in food intake due to anger, boredom, frustration, or depression. Over a long period of time, these changes in food intake can produce weight gain or loss. Stress produces various results in people–a difficult divorce or a death in the family could cause one person to eat more food and another to eat less.

- **Attractiveness of food.** People tend to eat more when several foods with different tastes, textures, and appearance are offered. They will eat less when just one food is offered, even if that food is a favorite. Does this mean that if you eat a monotonous diet you will lose weight? Not necessarily; many people quit commercial weight-reducing diets because they are monotonous. Two factors may be at work here. One is that we are naturally attracted to a variety of foods, thus ensuring a sufficient intake of nutrients. Many times in this book the advice is given to eat a varied diet. The second reason is that the sensory aspects of food are among the great pleasures of life for most people.

- **Type of food.** Obese people seem to prefer foods high in fat rather than in carbohydrates.[3] They consume carbohydrate foods less frequently, and only if the foods are sweet or are also major sources of fat (doughnuts, cookies, cakes). A low incidence of obesity exists among Native Americans and South Pacific islanders who consume their traditional diets, which are low in fat and sugar. The incidence of obesity increases when they eat a Western-type diet high in fat. Surveys show that the incidence of obesity among Native Americans developed over the past 40 years.

- **Meal patterns.** Meal patterns may play a role in obesity. Nibblers are less likely to put on weight than large meal eaters when caloric intake is the same. These observations have implications for the 12 million Americans who skip breakfast and possibly for the 68 million who use low-calorie foods, two behaviors that are often followed by the eating of large meals.

- **Temperature.** Food temperature can determine the amount of food eaten and therefore the amount of energy intake. Children find lukewarm food more appealing than the same food either hot or cold.

- **Socioeconomic status and cultural factors.** Obesity is prevalent in the following groups (although certainly not in everybody in these groups):
  - Lower income groups–especially women. This group may consume more energy-dense foods, especially foods high in fat.
  - Certain ethnic groups. In the United States, high incidences of obesity are found in people of Hungarian and Czech origin.
  - Succeeding generations. First-generation immigrants have less obesity than later generations of immigrants in the United States.

- **Drugs.** The following drug treatments for obesity are *not* clinically effective even though they are sold to dieters: 1) drugs designed to inhibit absorption of nutrients from the GI tract and 2) those designed to increase energy expenditure. Also available are appetite suppressant, or anorectic, drugs designed to reduce hunger, thus making dieting more acceptable. But a British expert on obesity states: "I do not believe that benefits derived from the use of anorectic drugs outweigh the disadvantages."[4]

  However, others think that drugs affecting the nervous centers that control eating and appetite are effective and safe. Barriers do exist to their proper and effective use, including expectations of medical doctors that anorectic drugs should decrease obesity, hindrance by state licensing agencies, regulatory rigidity over some drugs that may be effective, and limited research funding to discover safe drugs.[5] This is another good example of the interactions of medical science, economics, politics, and the law in a nutrition issue.

It is worth reviewing the list again to see which factors influencing body weight you can control. Changes from ideal body weight occur in obesity, overweight, starvation, anorexia nervosa, and bulimia. But what is your ideal body weight?

Ideal Body Weight May Be Obtained from Height and Weight Tables

One of the most frequently asked questions in nutrition is: What is my ideal body weight? It is also one of the most difficult questions to answer. Here's why–ideal body weights are obtained from insurance companies, who correlate body weight with age at death. On the average, obese people die at an earlier age than nonobese people.

If you weigh considerably more or less than ideal body weight, you should get medical advice about the health implications. Not everyone who is obese is unhealthy, and a weight-reducing program might do more harm than good. We will see shortly that there are plenty of harmful weight-reducing diets available. We have seen already that body weight is very much influenced by our genetic makeup. As a result, we may be programmed genetically for a particular body weight.

You should also be aware of precautions in the interpretation of your recommended weight from the height and weight tables. The first problem is that weight scales tell total body weight, *not* the weight of body fat. Two people can have the same body weight but different amounts of muscle and body fat. A second problem with the tables is that they reflect the average body weight of Americans in their twenties. These weights may be neither ideal nor desirable for people aged 30 and older. Body composition does change during aging, including an increase in the amount of body fat. Finally, the tables are based on people who buy life insurance, a fairly homogeneous socioeconomic and ethnic group. This means that biases due to economic status, age, race, health, personal habits (quality of diet, exercise, smoking), and stress levels may be involved.

All of this information is given not to disillusion or frustrate you but to again illustrate that standardizing measurements of interest in nutrition, even body weight, is difficult because of the number of variables each of us contributes to the measurement.

Now you can compare your body weight with those of average Americans in Table 13-1, which is from the National Institutes of Health.

Body Mass Index Defines Overweight

Body mass index (BMI): A measure for ideal weight and for obesity used by some nutritionists. Determined as body weight (in kilograms) divided by height (in meters) squared.

Body mass index (BMI) is widely used to define overweight.[6]

BMI = body weight (in kilograms) divided by height (in meters) squared

You can get your BMI easily from Table 13-2 (next page), using the instructions in the footnote. Government and scientific groups have suggested slightly different desirable ranges for BMI, extending from 20 to 27 for adults through middle age. There is general agreement that people with BMIs over 29 are obese. Obesity is defined as weight more than 20% in excess of ideal body weight.

Overweight is defined by experts in obesity research as 0–20% in excess of the ideal body weight. About one-quarter to one-third of the adults in the United States are classified as overweight, with the prevalence increasing during the last 20 years.[6]

Is the Ideal Body Weight the Same for Health and for Beauty?

Think about the information in Table 13-3 (next page). Are North Americans and Europeans different from the rest of the world in relating body weight to beauty?

The information from different cultures certainly suggests that "beauty is in the eye of the beholder." If you visit the great art galleries of Europe, you will see that Rubens, Goya, Frans Hals, and others painted their beautiful women with full, rounded figures. In the United States and England at the turn of this century, fat babies were welcomed because they were considered to have better protection against tuberculosis and other diseases. People in parts of Africa and the Pacific islands see bountiful bodies as beautiful. Contrast this with a report in the *New York Times* (November 22, 1992):

> In a recent study of formerly fat people who had lost weight after intestinal bypass surgery, researchers at the University of Florida reported that virtually all said they would rather be blind or deaf or have a leg amputated than be fat again.

Measuring Body Fat

Fat floats on water–you can see that oil separates on the top of salad dressings and cream floats on milk. This principle is used to measure the amount of fat in people. Fat people should have better floatation on water, and this is measured by weighing a person under water. This measurement

Table 13-1. Average Weights of Americans (in pounds)

Height (inches)	Age					
	20–24	25–34	35–44	45–54	55–64	65–74
Men						
62	133	141	145	144	144	140
63	137	146	149	148	148	145
64	142	150	154	153	153	150
65	146	155	159	158	158	154
66	151	160	164	168	163	159
67	155	165	169	168	168	164
68	160	170	174	173	173	169
69	165	175	179	178	178	174
70	170	180	184	183	183	179
71	174	185	190	189	189	184
72	179	191	195	194	194	189
73	184	196	201	199	199	195
74	189	210	206	205	205	200
Women						
57	114	120	127	129	132	130
58	117	123	131	133	135	133
59	120	126	134	136	139	137
60	123	129	137	140	142	140
61	126	133	141	143	146	144
62	129	136	144	147	150	147
63	132	139	148	150	153	151
64	135	142	151	154	157	154
65	138	146	155	157	161	158
66	142	149	158	161	164	162
67	145	153	162	165	168	165
68	158	156	166	169	172	169

Table 13-2. Body Weights in Pounds According to Height and Body Mass Index[a]

	Body Mass Index (kilogram per square meter)													
	19	20	21	22	23	24	25	26	27	28	29	30	35	40
Height (inches)	Body Weight													
58	91	96	100	105	110	115	119	124	129	134	138	143	167	191
59	94	99	104	109	114	119	124	128	133	138	143	148	173	198
60	97	102	107	112	118	123	128	133	138	143	148	153	179	204
61	100	106	111	116	122	127	132	137	143	148	153	158	185	211
62	104	109	115	120	126	131	136	142	147	153	158	164	191	218
63	107	113	118	124	130	135	144	146	152	158	163	169	197	225
64	110	116	122	128	134	140	145	151	157	163	169	174	204	232
65	114	120	126	132	138	144	150	156	162	168	174	180	210	240
66	118	124	130	136	142	148	155	161	167	173	179	186	216	247
67	121	127	134	140	146	153	159	166	172	178	184	191	223	254
68	125	135	138	144	151	158	164	171	177	184	190	197	230	262
69	128	135	142	149	155	162	169	176	182	189	196	203	236	270
70	132	139	146	153	160	167	174	181	188	195	202	207	243	278
71	136	143	150	157	165	172	179	186	193	200	208	215	250	286
72	140	147	154	162	169	176	183	191	199	206	213	221	258	294
73	144	151	159	166	174	182	189	197	204	212	219	227	265	302
74	148	155	163	171	178	186	194	202	210	218	225	233	272	311
75	152	160	168	176	184	192	200	208	216	224	232	240	280	319
76	156	164	172	180	189	197	205	213	221	230	238	246	287	328

[a] Find the appropriate height in the left-hand column. Move across the row to the appropriate weight. The number at the top of the column is the body mass index for that height and weight. Pounds have been rounded off.

Table 13-3. Cross-Cultural Standards of Female Beauty

	Percent of Societies That Consider This Beautiful
Overall body	
Extreme obesity	0
Plumpness/moderate fat	81
Thin/abhorrence of fat	19
Hips and legs	
Large and fat	90
Slender	10

is done in clinics and is accurate but expensive. On the other hand, to measure the extent of obesity in a community setting, the only method available is the skinfold thickness measurement (Figure 13-4).

Greater accuracy is achieved when measurements are made in a number of different regions of the body and the results compared with a standard. Because body fat is distributed differently in men than in women, the skinfold thickness measurements should be measured in men in the chest near the armpit, the abdomen, and the thigh. In women, the measurements should be made at the triceps muscle (at the back of the upper arm), suprailium (top of the hip), and thigh. Clearly these measurements cannot be easily made in full view of everybody at a local mall. In such circumstances, the thickness at the triceps is measured, although this limits the accuracy of the measurements.

How Is Obesity Classified?

The following is an abbreviated classification of obesity, based on its causes.[7]

- **Simple obesity**, caused by energy intake greater than energy expenditure.

- **Symptomatic obesity**
  - **Endocrine**–caused by hormonal imbalance
  - **Hereditary**–genetic transfer of obesity from one generation to the next
  - **Hypothalamic**–defect in the hypothalamus in the brain
  - **Frontal**–defect in the frontal lobe of the brain
  - **Metabolic**–usually a defect in the storage of lipids.

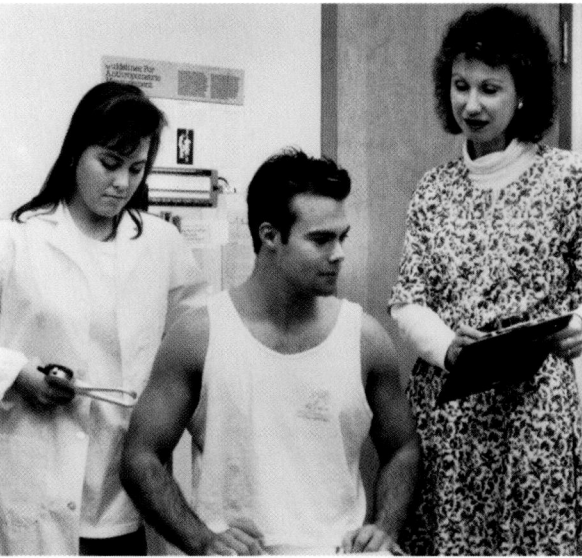

Figure 13-4. Measurement of skinfold thickness. Fat accumulation under the skin is measured with calipers in several parts of the body (the abdomen, the thigh, and behind the shoulder and upper arm).

Experts also classify obesity by the number and size of fat cells and by the distribution of fat in different parts of the body. Perhaps the classification that has best captured public interest in recent years is the grouping of people into pear types and apple types (Figure 13-5).[7]

Metabolic disorders are more likely with the apple type of obesity than with the pear type. It seems that pot-bellied men and women (apple type) have greater risks of diabetes, hypertension, and elevated blood lipids than do pear types, who have the fat deposited on the hips. The suspected reason is the higher metabolic activity associated with abdominal fat, which causes a higher level of fat in the blood. Another reason could be that pot bellies result from lack of exercise, with accompanying hypertension and high blood cholesterol. More research is obviously needed on this important aspect of obesity.

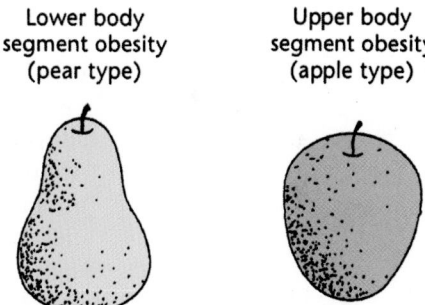

Figure 13-5. Apple and pear body shapes. Apple-shaped people are pot-bellied, and pear-shaped people have more fat on thighs and buttocks. Apple-shaped people have a higher risk of coronary heart disease, diabetes, and hypertension.

Risks of Obesity

Obesity is a health hazard, especially in developed countries, for the reasons implied by Figure 13-6. Obesity increases the risk of potentially fatal diseases–certain cancers, cardiovascular disease, respiratory disease, and non-insulin-dependent diabetes. It may also cause disability because inactivity due to extreme obesity can lead to osteoarthritis and back pain. Other related problems include gall stones, infertility, and hypertension.

Obese people also must contend with economic and social risks. A *New York Times* article (November 22, 1992) gives us a sense of the risks.

> Studies have found that fat people are less likely to be admitted to elite colleges, are less likely to be hired for a job, make less money when they are hired, and are less likely to be promoted. One study found that businessmen sacrifice $1,000 in salary for every pound they are overweight.

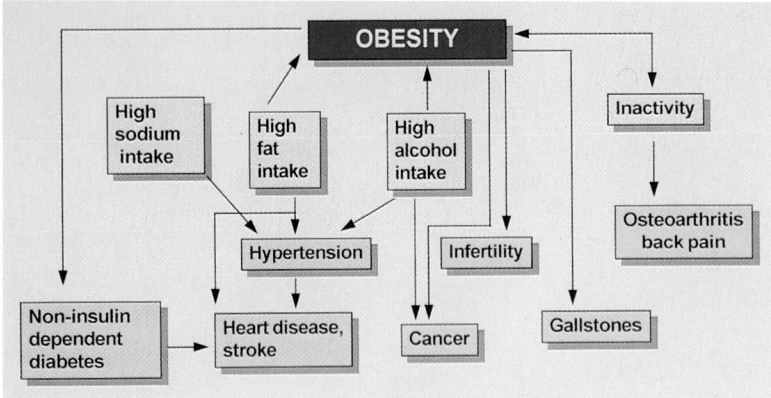

Figure 13-6. Relationship of obesity to various diseases. The effects of obesity and the activities leading to obesity are factors in many illnesses.

But there are more costs–obese people buy special clothing and foods, and they may buy weight-reducing "cures." They may not be able to get life insurance and may have higher transportation costs (flying first class only because of the wider seats, for example).

Social costs for obese people often include loneliness and negative feelings about themselves. This may lead to less participation in sports, dancing, and other types of social activities. Add to all of this the economic cost and personal disappointment of failed weight-loss diets.

■ Losing weight–Many problems, many costs, and many failures

Why do people want to lose weight?

The reasons are many–for better health, to improve fitness, to improve self-image, to avoid the discrimination shown to the obese, or to lose the weight gained after quitting smoking or after pregnancy.[6]

Who is trying to lose weight?

Government surveys in the United States show that over one-third of adult women and about one-quarter of adult men are trying to lose weight. Attempts at weight loss are more prevalent in middle age and increase with income and education. People with high BMI are most likely to be on a diet, but surprisingly, weight-loss efforts are not restricted to people with high BMI (check your BMI value again). This suggests that some people may be trying to lose weight more to conform to cosmetic and societal demands than for real health reasons. The percentage of women trying to lose weight does not differ by race, although a higher proportion of African-American and Hispanic women than white women are overweight.

People stay on their weight-loss diets for an average of 6–7 months. Within a two-year period, women and men averaged two and a half and two attempts, respectively, to lose weight.[6] These observations are meaningful statistics, confirming that people move from one weight-loss program to another or make several attempts to lose weight with the same diet. Thus, new diets appear each year. We will not deal here with specific diets because their popularity changes from year to year. What we will do is concentrate on why some diets are healthy and others are unhealthy or may even be fatal. You will then be equipped with the correct questions to ask regarding weight-loss diets as well as the ability to interpret the effectiveness of new diets. (Rest assured that by this time next year more "revolutionary" or "new" diets will be on the market.)

What weight-loss methods are people using?

Eating fewer calories was the most popular method, followed by increased physical activity. Much lower among the methods cited were vitamins, meal replacements, over-the-counter products including appetite suppressants, participation in a weight-loss program, and dietary supplements.

A survey of college students showed that exercise and skipping meals are the most popular ways to lose weight (Table 13-4).

Table 13-4. Students' Methods of Losing Weight

	Percent of Students	
	Female	Male
Exercise	51	30
Skipping meals	49	18
Using diet pills	4	2
Self-induced vomiting	3	1

Right Ways to Lose Body Weight

The weight-loss and diet-control market is enormous. In a recent year, some 48 million Americans spent over $32 billion on weight-loss products and programs, averaging about $670 per person.

Think about the numbers in Table 13-5.

Table 13-5. The Weight-Loss and Diet-Control Market

	Sales (1989 estimate, in $ millions)	Growth Rate (% forecast through 1995)
Diet soft drinks	11,380	9.0
Health spas/exercise clubs (nonresidential)	8,480	6.5
Hospital weight-loss programs	5,490	15.4
Commercial weight-loss centers	1,782	18.0
Low-calorie prepared foods	1,750	12.8
Residential spa weight-loss programs	1,662	20.0
Artificial sweeteners	1,090	9.0
Diet books and cassettes	418	9.5
Over-the-counter appetite suppressants[a]	370	13.9
Total market	32,400	10.6

[a] Includes diet pills, tablets, gums, skin patches, candy, liquid protein, and powders and mixes.

And now think about the three effective ways to lose body fat:

• Increased physical activity
• Decreased energy intake
• A combination of both.

Increased physical activity

Physical activity increases energy output and uses up stored body energy. We saw in Chapters 11 and 12 that loss of body weight by expending energy in increased physical activity is a slow process. For example, about 5–6 hours of high-intensity racquetball is needed to lose 1 pound of body fat. But exercise brings other advantages, including increased muscle tone and

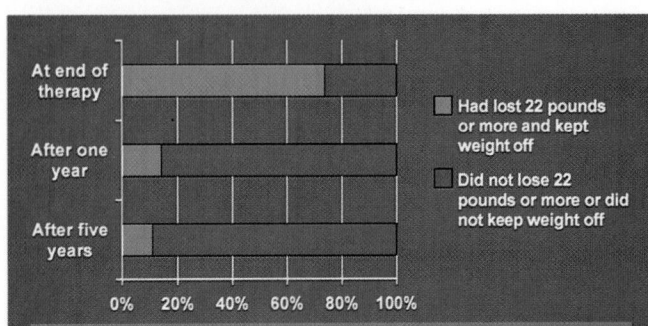

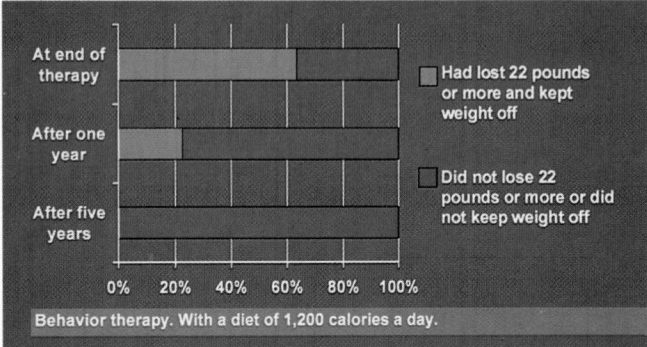

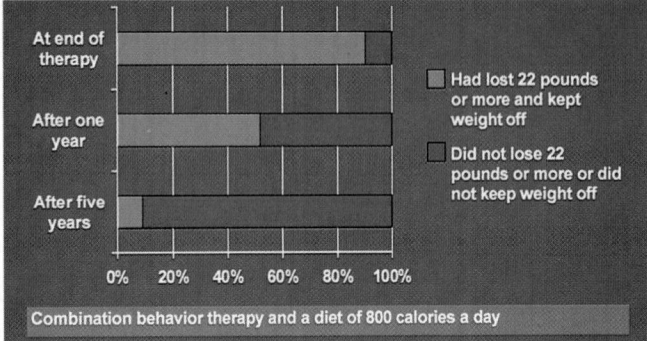

Figure 13-7. Successfulness of diets. Percentage of women who lost 22 pounds (10 kilograms) or more and kept off the weight for one or five years, showing type of weight-loss program used.

bone strength, and there is some evidence of a short-term decrease in appetite.

Decreased energy intake

This can be achieved by:

- Decreasing food intake. Many people do this through commercial diets, of which only some are effective.
- Varying the composition of the diet. Diets high in fat are more likely to cause obesity than are diets high in carbohydrate.
- Using pharmacologic agents as appetite suppressants. This method is not recommended.
- Surgical treatment to the GI tract to reduce the absorption of energy. This is not recommended and is performed only in extreme obesity that does not respond to any other treatment.
- Behavior modification. This includes changing eating behavior and attitudes toward food.

The choices are rather limited, and commercial diets seem to many people to be the easy way out. Before embarking on any program, it is useful to know your chances of success.

Think about the numbers in Figure 13-7 in terms of your chances of long-term successful weight loss.

Even dieting plans that provided initial success could not guarantee success after several years. In fact, studies shows that none of the current popular commercial methods of losing weight can deliver long-term success. But overweight people using these diets paid a price for their failure. Some weight-loss diets have a health price because of their imbalance in nutrients, and some have even been known to cause death. Diets also carry an economic price, as shown in Table 13-6.

Successful Dieters Use Input from Many Sources

One expert likens the difficulty and the probability of success of eliminating severe obesity to trying to master a foreign language–it can be done by almost anybody who has reasonably competent guidance and who is prepared to invest sufficient effort, but it always takes a considerable amount of time and trouble.[8] This seems a good analogy because "reasonably competent guidance" is frequently in short supply. Many of the popular diet books are written by people with little or no training in nutrition. The reference to "considerable time and trouble" is also appropriate; there are no quick fixes in correcting overweight problems.

A recent study gives us an insight into people who maintained weight loss and had successful strategies for handling food cravings.[9] These people had kept their weight down for over four years. Their success was attributed to (in decreasing order of frequency of mention) cognitive/psychological factors such as "determination" ("I was really sick of being fat"); changed eating habits; improved appearance; social support; and exercise, especially for men. Strategies they used for handling food cravings included (in decreasing order) wait it out; eat small amounts; substitute another food; drink fluids; satisfy the craving; and finally, call a friend.[9] In summary, successful weight loss takes determination and know-how.

Table 13-6. Cost of Losing Weight[a]

Cost (Range)	Type of Weight-Loss Program
$8.96 ($6.35–11.56)	Medically supervised, very low calorie diets
$6.21 ($1.10–10.43)	Balanced low-calorie diets run by dietitians or nonmedical personnel
$0.02 ($0.00–0.03)	Volunteer-staffed or self-help support groups

[a] Average cost per pound of weight loss during various 12- week diet programs. Women were an average of 37% above their ideal body weight at the program's start; men were 27% above.

What Makes a Healthy Weight-Loss Diet?

Low in calories

Safe weight-loss diets must be low in total calories but adequate in all other nutrients. Nutritional adequacy cannot be achieved on diets less than 1,000–1,200 calories per day–more in the case of active college students. Refer to the Food Guide Pyramid to plan a diet to achieve this reduced caloric intake (see Chapter 4). Many commercial diets are as low as 600–800 calories per day. Some commercial diets have caused serious nutrient deficiencies and even death because of nutrient imbalances. Vitamin and mineral supplements are only a partial solution.

Palatable food

This is a difficult problem because presumably the diet that made the person overweight was preferred. This is where behavior modification and training in proper food selection are important. Food in the weight loss diet must be palatable, familiar, easily available, and economical. Lack of one or more of these factors is sufficient to make people stop the diet. Many of the commercial diets fail in one or more of these counts. As an exercise, go to your local store, look at the ingredients in some diet foods, and guess at the palatability. Also, are they easy to prepare, especially for busy people? Do some cost comparisons.

Reasonable body weight loss per week

Dealing with what is a reasonable weight loss is also difficult for many people to understand. Advertisements seduce people into believing that they can lose 8–10 pounds or more per week, can eat all they want of any food, and need no exercise program. Another case of too good to be true? Unfortunately, yes. The 8–10 pounds of lost weight are frequently just a loss of body water. Some weight-loss programs use diuretics to increase fluid loss from the body. This produces a loss in body weight but little loss in body fat. Diuretics are dangerous because they cause dehydration and the loss of electrolytes. Other diets contain bulking agents that absorb fluid in the stomach, thereby giving a full feeling. Methylcellulose and glucomannan are substances of this type. They are widely used but are not effective in the long term.

A safe rate of weight loss on a medically approved diet must not exceed 2 pounds of body weight per week, as recommended by the American Medical Association. The Dietary Guidelines recommend the loss of ½ to 1 pound of body weight per week. This weight loss is not as popular as the more drastic loss promised by other programs, but it does assure more chance of success. Consider what happens when rapid body weight loss occurs. The individual is pleased, and the weighing scales continue to display the desired decreasing weight for the first few weeks of the diet. But such rapid weight loss causes a type of shock to the body. It suddenly recognizes a crisis and begins to take corrective action as a survival mechanism. The outcome is the same whether the weight loss is due to famine or to a severe weight-loss diet because the body makes no distinction between them. It responds to severe restrictions in caloric intake by reducing caloric expenditure to match its caloric intake. It does this by reducing the major energy expenditure in the body–basal energy. Therefore, extreme cases of weight loss cause a loss of lean tissue and decreases in heart rate, body heat, muscle tone, breathing, and the thermic effect of food. In general, there is a slowing of vital body processes so that energy can be saved. A possible conflict of interest results. The body is pleased with its adjustment because it has saved energy and slowed the slide to death from starvation. However, the individual is frustrated because this very survival mechanism has slowed down the weight loss.

Composition of the diet after the weight is lost

This is a factor frequently not considered by much of the public wishing to lose weight. Unfortunately, many people return to their original eating habits once they arrive at their desired body weight. But this is the very diet that made them overweight. In many cases, they end up heavier than when they began to lose weight. Weight cycling happens when a person's body weight yo-yos up and down from different unsuccessful diets. These people are more likely to have heart attacks and face premature death than people who maintain a relatively constant weight.[8] The answer is to find a combination of exercise and diet that will take weight off and keep it off permanently.

Behavior modification has not lived up to some of its earlier promise. This method concentrates on the food consumed and the environment in which it is consumed. People are asked to notice when and how they eat and to begin eating deliberately only in certain ways and in certain times and places. Behavioral approaches to obesity are usually employed in short-term treatments of 10–20 weeks. They produce weight losses averaging 10 kg (22 pounds) at the end of the program and about 7 kg at 1-year follow-up.[10] Food diaries seem to be a useful and inexpensive way of making people aware of the amount and type of food they eat.[8] We can postpone further discussion of this topic to the end of this chapter, where we examine how little all of us know about the food we eat.

Various Surgical Treatments May Reduce Obesity

About 30 surgical techniques can be used to treat obesity.[11] They are classified into three groups:

- **Physical or mechanical**, including the removal of adipose tissue by *liposuction*. This is considered inappropriate by many surgeons, and deaths have occurred in the past when this surgery was performed under inadequate conditions. Other surgical procedures include restricting food intake by stapling a portion of the stomach or by placing an inflated balloon in the stomach. In both cases, the stomach space is smaller, and thus a "full feeling" occurs with a smaller amount of food.
- **Malabsorptive**, a bypass of the portion of the GI tract where energy is absorbed
- **Regulatory**, directly affecting hunger or thirst.

Any form of surgery is drastic treatment with risks to the person. That is why surgery to control extreme obesity is usually done when all other methods to reduce body weight have failed. Experts agree that the ineffectiveness of many weight-loss methods makes it likely that surgical techniques will still be available in the foreseeable future.[11]

Liposuction: Surgical removal of fat deposits; not considered a safe way to lose weight.

Unfortunately, You Cannot Melt Away Fat

Advertisements claim that you can "melt away" body fat–these are false and are contrary to all of the scientific principles of body weight loss. Body fat is supposed to melt after you buy special wraps, sweat suits, mechanical or electrical stimulators, or various creams or use certain chemicals from food (such as grapefruit). There are good reasons why the FDA bans most of these treatments.

Think about the logic of these claims.

If these treatments really do melt fat, it must be removed from the body to achieve weight loss. Liquid, oily fat supposedly floating around in you will keep you at the same body weight. So this "melted" fat must be removed from the body. Fat is insoluble in water, and it is not excreted through the urine or sweat. So how does it get out of the body? The only way to deplete body fat is to burn it off as energy through physical activity or to reduce caloric intake in the diet. The case of the grapefruit fraud was interesting because it was based on the false proposition that the acidity in grapefruits "melted" body fat after you ate grapefruit pills, which were sold at a high price. If you looked at the very small print in the commercials singing the praises of this "weight loss breakthrough," you would see that you were advised also to have a caloric intake of less than 800 calories per day. As we noted earlier, safe weight-reducing diets should not be less than 1,000–1,200 calories per day.

Table 13-7. Recommendations for Adult Weight-Loss Programs

Program Feature	Recommendation
Screening	The client should be screened to verify that there are no medical or psychological conditions that would make weight loss inappropriate. The client's level of health risk should be identified: low, moderate, or high.
Individualized treatment plan	Factors contributing to the client's weight status should be identified. These factors should serve as the bases for nutrition, exercise, behavioral change, medical monitoring or supervision, and health supervision.
Staffing	Weight-loss service providers should be trained and supervised adequately for the level of health risk of clients receiving care.
Full disclosure	The client should give informed consent, having been informed of potential physical and psychological risks from weight loss and regain, likely long-term success of the program, full cost of the program, and credentials of the weight-loss service.
Reasonable weight goal	The weight goal for the client should be based on personal and family history, not exclusively on height and weight charts.
Rate of weight loss	The advertised and actual rate of weight loss, after the first two weeks, should not exceed an average of 2 pounds per week.
Calories per day	The daily calorie level should be adjusted so that each client can achieve but not exceed the recommended rate of weight loss. The daily caloric intake should not be lower than 1,000 kilocalories without medical supervision. If the daily caloric level is below 800 kilocalories, additional safeguards should be in place. Even with medical supervision, 800 kilocalories was the lowest recommended intake.
Diet composition	• Protein: between 0.8 and 1.5 grams per kilogram of goal body weight, but no more than 100 grams per day. • Fat: 10–30% of energy as fat. • Carbohydrate: at least 100 grams per day without medical supervision; at least 50 grams per day even with medical supervision. • Fluid: at least 1 quart of water daily.
Nutritional adequacy	The food plan should allow the client to obtain 100% of the client's recommended dietary allowances (RDAs). If nutrition supplements are used, nutrient levels should not greatly exceed 100% of the RDA.
Nutrition education	Nutrition education encouraging permanent healthful eating patterns should be incorporated into the weight-loss program.
Formula products	The food plan should consist of a variety of foods available from the conventional food supply. Formula products are not recommended for the treatment of moderate obesity and should not be used at low-calorie formulations without specialized medical supervision.
Exercise component	The weight-loss program should include an exercise component that is safe and appropriate for the individual client. • The client should be screened for conditions that would make medical clearance before exercise appropriate. • The client should be instructed to recognize and deal with potentially dangerous physical responses to exercise. • The client should work toward 30–60 minutes of continuous exercise five to seven times per week, with gradual increases in intensity and duration.
Psychological component	Behavior modification techniques appropriate for the specific client should be taught.
Appetite suppressants	Appetite suppressant drugs are not recommended and should not take the place of changes in diet, exercise, and behavior.
Weight maintenance	A maintenance phase should be included in the treatment program. Programs should place as high a priority on helping clients maintain weight loss as on achieving initial weight loss.

This should be a warning that there is no shortage of useless and sometimes dangerous diets. A few years ago, a scientist at Johns Hopkins University in Baltimore documented the existence of 29,000 claims, theories, and treatments for losing body weight. Unfortunately, the list has grown since then, and we still wait for a safe, effective, and economical way to lose weight. In the meantime, some responsible recommendations for adult weight-loss programs are available. These provide the summary for our examination of obesity.

Some Do's for Dieters

- Do include exercise as part of your weight-loss program.
- Do be patient with the time taken to lose those extra pounds of body fat.
- Do be aware of portion sizes of food.
- Do include foods with no hidden fat, and avoid those foods with hidden fat, such as muffins, pastries, and casseroles.
- Do pick your weight-loss program carefully.
- Do have the correct motivation to lose weight.

All of this is stated more specifically in Table 13-7.

■ Starvation and hunger in the world

We started this chapter with the photograph of a starving child. Let's start the discussion of starvation and hunger with hope, as seen in Figures 13-8 and 13-9.

Francis is 13 months old and is from Uganda, a country in East Africa. His skin problems and some facial edema in Figure 13-8 are symptoms of

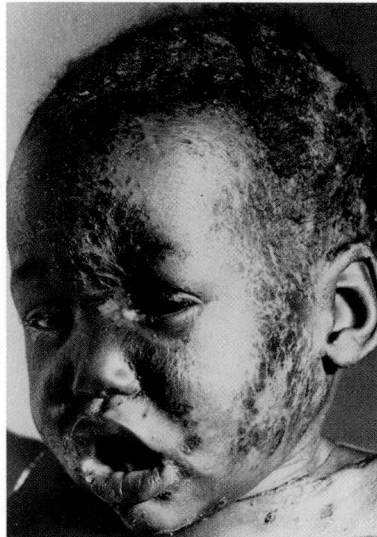 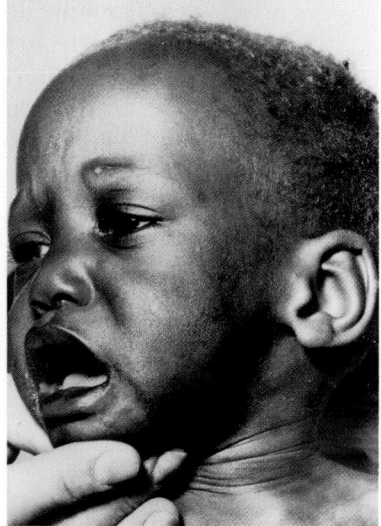

Figures 13-8 and 13-9. A 13-month-old child showing effects of severe malnutrition (left) and the same child after 15 days on an adequate diet (right).

protein-energy malnutrition. The remarkable change in Francis's appearance shown in Figure 13-9 took only 15 days to achieve on an adequate diet. But why do so many people in the world starve? Here are some of the reasons.

- **Inadequate food distribution.** Enough food is produced in the world to feed everybody adequately. That this food does not get to all people equally has multiple causes–economic, political, historical, and personal.

- **War.** Somalia and the Sudan were in the news in 1993 because of famines caused mainly by wars. Some of the worst famines in history were caused by wars. The sieges of Paris in 1871 and of Leningrad (now St. Petersburg) in Russia in 1942, and the starvation of the Jews in Poland's Warsaw Ghetto during World War II are but a few examples.

- **Drought.** Chronic drought is a problem in some African countries.

- **Floods.** Although these are less of a problem than droughts, they nevertheless have caused problems in India and China.

- **Plant and animal disease.** The failure of the potato crop caused the Irish potato famine in the 1840s. Development of disease-resistant breeds of plants and animals by techniques in genetic engineering should lessen this cause of famine in the future.

- **Loss of food to rodents, insects, and other creatures.** This is a major problem in all countries. Figure 13-10 may seem, at first glance, to be out of place in a nutrition book. But consider the important work these USDA scientists are doing in developing a package to better protect food from insects and rodents.

- **Income inequality.** The very poor cannot buy adequate food, housing, sanitation, education, or health services. Combinations of some or all of these factors lead to undernourished babies, adults with limited potential for earning money, poor food choices, inadequate food preparation and storage facilities, diarrhea and food poisoning from unsafe food and water, and high mortality rates from infectious diseases such as measles.

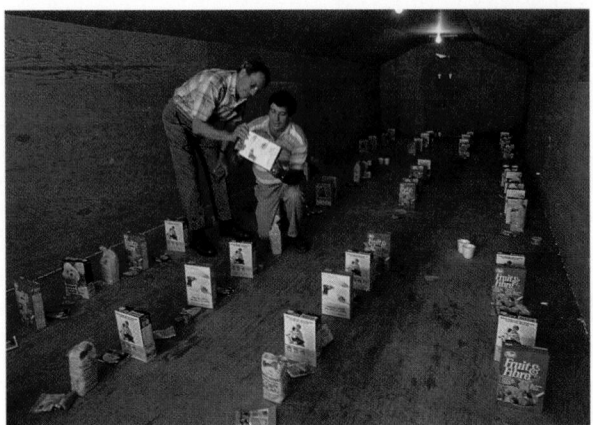

Figure 13-10. Testing to develop insect-resistant packages. Food losses to insects and rodents are major problems in some communities and may be factors contributing to undernutrition.

- **Land tenure systems.** Where land is owned by many people, food production and nutritional status are usually good. However, in many developing countries, only a small number of wealthy families control the land. Renters have little ability or incentive to improve the land, and food shortages occur often.

- **Industrialization and urbanization.** These have increased mechanization, which has drawn workers from the land with little compensation. Food production has actually decreased in some developing countries.

Much of the food that is produced is exported to developed countries rather than being consumed within the country.

- **Failed economic policies.** In the 1930s, the government of Ukraine, in the former Soviet Union, tried to collectivize its farms. The policy disrupted food production to such an extent that famine resulted.

- **Other factors.** This category includes corrupt politicians who use food as a political weapon; black markets that make food too expensive for poor people; and high population density relative to available food.

The Chinese proverb "Give a man a fish and you feed him for a day; teach him how to fish and you feed him for life" is appropriate in the context of the long list of causes of hunger and starvation. Even the delivery and distribution of food by relief agencies is still far from satisfactory.[12] Usually there is failure to supply an adequate balance of food. Most feeding programs are designed to provide about 1,900 calories per day and usually contain cereal, a legume, and an oil. Particularly vulnerable groups such as children under 5 years of age and the elderly get a little extra food. However, deficiencies of some vitamins and minerals are common in children receiving international food aid. Scurvy due to vitamin C deficiency was common in Somalia in 1992. A diet of cereal, legume, and oil for any length of time produces deficiencies in vitamins A and C, niacin, and iron. In addition to cases of severe deficiency, the incidence of marginal deficiency of these and other nutrients must be high in areas where food is very scarce. Some governments have been known to withhold vegetable oil and legumes and to supply only cereals to starving people, but starving children need energy-dense foods such as oil in addition to cereal to satisfy their needs.[12]

The role of women is critical in times of starvation. Even in nonfamine times, they expend large amounts of energy to obtain food, fuel, and water for the family. In times of famine, women must forage for wild foods, and petty trading in the village becomes essential for survival. Mothers must also find time to accompany malnourished children to a relief feeding center, which can take a whole day. Because of this, mothers may stop attending the relief center, resulting in a lack of relief food for the children. Thus, the malnutrition gets worse. Relief feeding centers are criticized because of this, yet they continue to be a central part of famine relief. One reason given for their continuation, despite the reservations of some nutritionists, is their high profile for media coverage.[12]

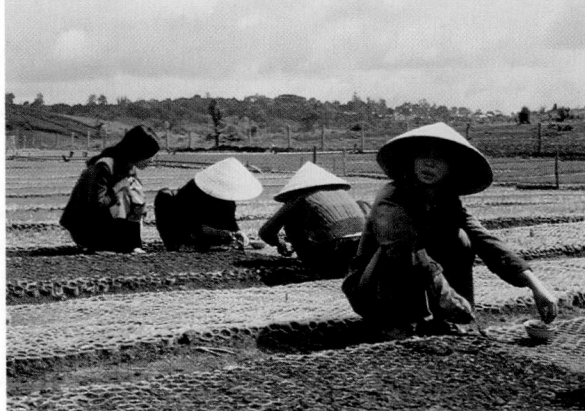

Figure 13-11. The role of women in providing food for the family is important at all times and critical in times of famine.

The extent of the starvation problem is enormous. Worldwide, 15–30 million people each year are at risk of death by famine. About 450 million people live in rural households where economic deprivation, environmental destruction, or restriction of the people to marginal land has made it impossible for them to grow or buy sufficient food.

Women of reproductive age and young children are the most vulnerable to malnutrition. Major nutrition problems include wasting and stunting in the children. The child in Figure 13-2 is wasted; much of his muscle has been broken down by his body to provide him enough energy just to survive. Women of child-bearing age and infants suffer from iron-deficiency anemia. About 280 million children in the world are at risk of vitamin A deficiency, and more than 180 million cases of goiter occur because of iodine deficiency. In summary, malnutrition is widespread in communities suffering from a lack of adequate food.

It is informative to go through the checklist used by relief workers in determining the extent of risk for protein-energy malnutrition among young children in a community.[13] The following is an abbreviated form.

- **Demographic/biologic factors:** Includes data on family size, birth order, number of children, birth weight, and marital status
- **Socioeconomic factors:** Includes parents' education and occupation, size and type of house, family income and debt, land ownership and use, amount of food (rice, wheat) stored, religion, and household possessions
- **Morbidity:** Includes history of diarrhea episodes, hospital admissions, attendance at health clinics, respiratory infections, and illnesses of the mother and father
- **Dietary factors:** Includes breast-feeding status, use of bottle or formula foods, age at introduction of solid foods, and food consumption in the previous 24 hours
- **Environmental factors:** Includes household water sources/distance, water quality/use, latrine presence and use, refuse disposal, and hand-washing materials used.

This list emphasizes again that many environmental, family, and socioeconomic factors as well as food are involved in malnutrition.

Education Is Important in Preventing Malnutrition

The decision whether to breast-feed or bottle-feed is relatively easy to make in developed countries. The nutritional advantages of breast-feeding are examined in Chapter 15. In many developing countries, this decision may be a matter of life or death for the baby. Bottle-feeding requires education, nutritious breast-milk substitutes, clean water, and a sanitary environment. These are frequently missing in many countries.

There are two forms of protein-energy malnutrition. One form is *marasmus*, which involves the total wasting of muscle and other soft tissue, as seen in Figure 13-2. This is due to dietary deficiencies of protein, calories, and other nutrients, resulting from too little food. The other form, called kwashiorkor, is due to a severe lack of protein coupled with a less than adequate intake of calories.

The word "kwashiorkor" comes from the Ga tribe in Ghana in western Africa.[14] It means "the disease of the displaced child," and it usually occurs in this way. The mother breast-feeds her first child. This child grows normally and is healthy until the mother becomes pregnant with her second

Marasmus: Starvation symptoms of no body fat and muscle wasting, due to little or no intake of dietary protein and energy.

child. She can no longer breast-feed, so she looks for an alternative to her breast milk. In western Africa she finds it in a watery extract from the cassava plant, a root plant with low protein and a high carbohydrate content in the form of starch. It is white, and when it is mixed with water it looks like milk. However, its nutritional value is much lower than that of milk, and that is the first cause of the kwashiorkor. This situation is made worse by the fact that the water is usually unsafe because of high bacterial counts, which results in diarrhea. The mother forces the baby to drink this unpalatable, unsafe, non-nutritious drink because she thinks it is a suitable alternative to her milk. But the child does not grow well and has all of the symptoms of kwashiorkor by the time the second child is born. These symptoms include:

- Failure to grow
- Diarrhea, which can cause death within 4–5 days if uncorrected with oral rehydration therapy (see Chapter 5)
- Infections, because protein deficiency impairs the immune system
- Skin changes, resulting mainly from deficiencies of B-vitamins, vitamin A, and essential fatty acids. The undernourished child in Morocco shown in Figure 13-12 has skin rashes in the lower trunk and limbs.
- *Anorexia*, which is common in kwashiorkor
- Edema due to decreased levels of the blood protein albumin
- Hair changes, including changes in texture, strength (when pulled, it comes away easily in the hand), and color (black hair sometimes turns red)
- Swelling of the liver due to excessive accumulation of fat, giving the child a pot-bellied appearance
- Mental changes–the child is listless, irritable, and unsmiling.

Protein-energy malnutrition has two different effects on body dimensions. The body may be wasted, with great loss of muscle, or it may be stunted, so that the child will never reach its genetically determined height. Some experts are puzzled as to why some children are wasted and others are stunted.[15] Stunting is considered less damaging than wasting. In summary, protein-energy malnutrition is a major nutrition problem for millions of children and is caused in most cases by poverty, poor education, lack of food, and poor food choices.

■ Eating disorders

The term "eating disorders" includes *anorexia nervosa* and bulimia. People with anorexia nervosa have extreme body weight loss, distorted images of their bodies, and a great fear that they will become fat. Because their body images are distorted, they mistakenly see themselves as being very fat, so they voluntarily starve themselves. Anorexia has devastating effects on the amount of bone and other tissues in the anorectic person's body.

Bulimia, sometimes called bulimia nervosa, is different from anorexia

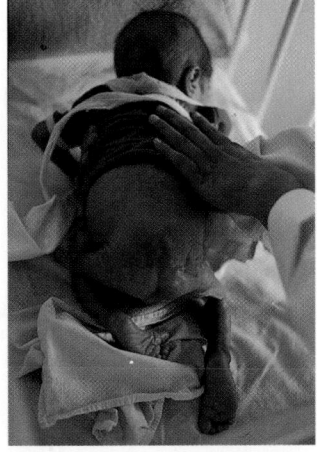

Figure 13-12. An undernourished child with typical thin legs and arms and a skin rash.

Anorexia: Loss of appetite.

Anorexia nervosa: An eating disorder usually associated with puberty. Involves a psychological loss of appetite and self-starvation. May be produced by a distorted body image and by social pressures, especially those associated with body weight.

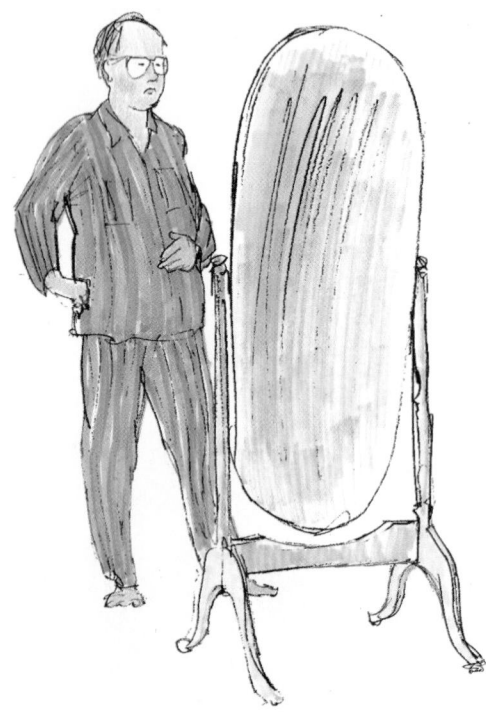

Figure 13-13. Some people see themselves as fat even though their body weight may be normal. This distorted body image may lead to eating disorders.

nervosa. It involves secretive binge eating episodes, followed by self-induced purging by means of vomiting; the abuse of laxatives (50–100 tablets at a time), diuretics, or diet pills; or the taking of saunas. Between binges, the individual may fast or exercise excessively.

The American Psychiatric Association states that a person diagnosed as bulimic or anorectic must have all of that disorder's specific symptoms:

Bulimia nervosa
- recurrent episodes of binge eating (minimum average of two binge-eating episodes a week for at least three months)
- a feeling of lack of control over eating during the binges
- regular use of one or more of the following to prevent weight gain: self-induced vomiting, use of laxatives or diuretics, strict dieting or fasting, or vigorous exercise
- persistent over-concern with body shape and weight.

Anorexia nervosa
- refusal to maintain weight that is over the lowest weight considered normal for age and height
- intense fear of gaining weight or becoming fat, even though underweight
- distorted body image
- in women, three consecutive missed menstrual periods without pregnancy.

Bulimia develops during the teens and 20s. Persons with bulimia may binge and purge up to 20 times per day.[2] They may consume up to 3,400 calories in 1¼ hours compared to a total daily intake of 2,000–3,000 for nonbulimic people. Some bulimic people have been known to consume up to 20,000 calories in an 8-hour period. This amount of food costs over $50 per day. Recent evidence shows that bulimic people eat more high-energy food than do anorectic people. In so doing, they still respond to the sensory characteristics of the food–they are not eating food just for the sake of eating.[16] They usually appear healthy and successful, but in reality they have electrolyte imbalance and erosion of enamel on their teeth, both due to the extensive vomiting. They usually have low self-esteem, suffer from depression, and may indulge in compulsive behaviors, including shoplifting and alcohol abuse.

Anorexia usually develops in the teens and has been reported in people aged 5 to 60. The incidence of anorexia in preteens is said to be increasing.[2] Anorexia may be present for a few months or for many years. Adult women may lose weight rapidly until they are 80–90 pounds. In such extreme starvation, the body behaves as it would in starvation from famine. Basal energy expenditure decreases, menstruation ceases or never begins in the case of girls in their early teens, growth rate slows, the skin becomes dry, and hair and nails are brittle. Swelling of joints and loss of bone and muscle are other characteristics of anorexia. A person with thinner bones has a higher possibility of bone fractures.

Causes and Treatment of Eating Disorders Are Complex

A look through journals publishing research on eating disorders reveals that the search continues for an understanding of the problem. Here is a sampling of some recent research to suggest where you can expect further developments.

Eating disorders involve distorted images of body weight, but women with eating disorders are neither more nor less accurate in reporting their body weight than are normal women.[17] Childhood sexual abuse as a risk factor for bulimia has been reported in the scientific literature for the past several years, but a recent study failed to find any evidence to support this hypothesis.[18] Puberty may be a risk factor for the development of eating disorders.[19] The hormonal changes at puberty have long been suspected to be a trigger for the problem. It is suggested that prevention efforts might best be directed at prepubertal adolescents. A seasonal pattern seems to be emerging in the identification of bulimia nervosa; it seems to be practiced more often in winter than in summer.[20]

Over 90% of people with eating disorders share these characteristics:

- Are teenage girls, usually white
- Have parents who are usually middle- or upper-income and family members who all are high achievers
- Usually have siblings.

Most therapies for people with eating disorders involve other members of the family. The American Anorexia/Bulimia Association has put together a list of tips for parents.

- Do not urge your child to eat, or watch her eat, or discuss food intake or weight with her. Your involvement with her eating is her tool for manipulating you.
- Do not allow yourself to feel guilty. Once you have checked out his physical condition with a physician and made it possible for him to begin counseling, getting well is his responsibility.
- Do not neglect your spouse or other children. Focusing on the sick child can perpetuate her illness and destroy the family.
- Do not be afraid to have the child separated from you, either in school or in separate housing, if it becomes obvious that his continued presence is undermining the emotional health of the family. Don't allow him to intimidate the family with threats of suicide. (But don't ignore the threats either.)
- Do not put the child down by comparing her to her more "successful" siblings or friends. Do not ask questions such as "How are you feeling?" or "How is your social life?"
- Love your child as you should love yourself.
- Trust your child to find his own values, ideals, and standards rather than insisting on yours.

- Do everything to encourage her initiative, independence, and autonomy.
- Be aware of the long-term nature of the illness. Families must face months and sometimes years of treatment and anxiety.

■ People are different–Do you know your eating pattern?

We have seen many examples in this book of the difficulty of measuring our food intake. The following study shows that, for many of us, "eating very little" may not be as little as we think when our food intake is measured accurately.

> Dietitians all across the country encounter patients who say they eat very little but can't lose weight. Many are convinced they have a metabolic problem, and there may be some grain of truth to it,

says principal investigator Dr. Steven Heymsfield, deputy director of the Obesity Research Center and associate professor of medicine at Columbia College of Physicians and Surgeons, New York.

> We decided to set up an experimental protocol to test whether the culprit was an abnormal metabolism or a misreporting of food intake.[21]

Ten "diet-resistant" patients were chosen for the study. These were people who reportedly ate fewer than 1,200 calories per day yet maintained stable weight. Some had unsuccessfully attempted as many as 20 diets. The 10 "diet-resistant" patients and 80 overweight people in a control group were given a series of physiological and psychological tests. Individuals in the two groups had similar metabolic rates at rest, after meals, and while exercising. Extensive psychological testing showed no major abnormalities, and both groups were able to accurately estimate the size of food portions.

However, when the diet-resistant patients were asked to report foods eaten in a hospital lunch the previous day, they remembered eating only 80% of their actual intake, whereas the control group, while also underreporting, did not misjudge the amounts by as much. Studies show that most individuals, when asked to keep a food log, underreport the amounts they have eaten by 20–25%. The researchers believed that the "diet-resistant" individuals did not intentionally lie about their activities; they had participated in very time-consuming experiments and seemed genuinely upset when told the results of the study. It seems that they misperceive the amounts of food they eat, or convince themselves that they're eating less than they actually are. One reason for this may be social desirability; it is socially desirable to have a normal weight and to have tight control over food intake. By not admitting to overeating, these people can say, "It's not my fault, it's my genes. Don't blame me."

It is estimated that as many as 5% of obese people believe that they are diet-resistant, and some of them may be right. The only way to find out is to monitor the patient in the manner outlined above.

Table 13-8. Types of Eating Styles[a]

Type	Eating Style or Attitude Toward Food	Other Characteristics
Night eaters	Wake in the middle of the night and raid the refrigerator Or eat just before going to bed–as a kind of sleeping pill Usually don't eat three balanced meals a day; often skip breakfast and/or lunch	10% of obese are night eaters Have stressful lives Many are also heavy smokers and big coffee drinkers
Compulsive eaters/eating addicts	Use food either to block out fears and anxieties or as a substitute for love Eat constantly–often until they are sick. Some are closet eaters But rarely sit down to an entire meal	Children who are obese during development are often compulsive eaters
Liquid drinkers	Drink quarts of coffee, soft drinks, and/or alcohol a day Get most of their calories from fluids Diet often low in essential nutrients and fiber because they tend to fill themselves with non-nourishing fluids	Often workaholics who rarely relax Under stress, they can become addicted to some fluids
Binge eaters	Have sudden, uncontrolled eating binges often triggered by stress, frustration, hostility, anger, or depression But do not purge themselves after a binge Average three binges a month May eat sensibly for weeks or months between binges	5% of obese are binge eaters Three-quarters of all binge eaters are women
Traditional overeaters	Trained by their families to eat three substantial meals a day with several snacks Food represents security, family love, and a link to the past Many encounter opposition from their families when they try to change their eating habits	15% of obese are traditional overeaters
Environmental eaters	Ads, parties, luncheons, friends, and the sight and smell of food all trigger an eating response Eat because food is accessible Although impulse eaters, they usually have regular meals	Tend to be executives, shift workers, or working women Have active social, civic, and business schedules
Gastronomic overeaters	Love to cook More concerned with food quality and preparation than with calories Eat because food gives them pleasure Seldom eat large amounts of food or have between-meal snacks	High percentage are male Often professionals with middle to high incomes who are single or divorced
Snackers	Become overweight out of ignorance or indifference to nutrition Never eat real meals Prefer to snack on foods they enjoy Likely to try fad diets and diet pill–looking for a way to lose weight fast and still eat whatever they want	Prevalent among students and young working women with hectic schedules
Sedentary gainers	Are physically inactive and don't compensate enough for this in their eating habits Live in a vicious cycle–gain weight from reduced activity, which makes future exercise more difficult and embarrassing	Can be anyone with a sedentary lifestyle Some athletes are in this category once their athletic careers end
Convalescent overeaters	Sudden lack of accustomed exercise and no cut in calories result in weight gain Often use food to relieve the boredom, depression, and frustration felt during convalescence One-third continue to overeat after recuperation	Affects almost two-thirds of those recovering from an accident, surgery, or illness
Chronic dieters	Know everything about dieting but still cannot lose weight Often have visited doctors, joined weight-loss groups, used diet pills, and even tried bizarre weight-reducing gadgets Try several fad diets a year Usually are looking for instant results	Usually women in their late 30s and early 40s

[a] Although there are objective characteristics associated with individuals who are obese, these characteristics are not meant to categorize people. Rather, they are meant as guidelines to identify those characteristics that could influence a person's weight. Individuals may exhibit behaviors from more than one of these types.

We end as we began this chapter, with some comparisons. Table 13-8 applies to the well-fed peoples of this world. It is meant as a guide to characteristics that might influence weight gain and is not meant to describe individuals.

■ Now you know

- Obesity and starvation are at opposite ends of a long spectrum of amounts of food eaten.

- Many factors influence our body weight, including age, gender, genetics, basal energy requirements, physical activity, pregnancy and lactation, hormone levels, brain/nerve signals, disease, emotions, attractiveness and type of food, meal patterns, temperature, socioeconomic status, cultural factors, and drugs.

- Ideal body weight can be obtained from insurance tables.

- Different cultures have different interpretations of body weight and beauty.

- Obesity is caused by many factors–hormonal, hereditary, brain dysfunction (hypothalamic and frontal), and metabolic.

- Obesity increases the risk of coronary heart disease, stroke, cancer, non-insulin-dependent diabetes, gallstones, infertility, respiratory disease, and osteoarthritis.

- Body weight can be lost by increasing energy expenditure through increased exercise, by decreasing energy intake through reducing food intake, or by a combination of these.

- Failure is more common than success in most weight-loss programs. Successful weight-loss diets must not be too low in calories and must be adequate in all nutrients, be palatable, give a reasonable body weight loss per week, and train the dieter for an appropriate eating pattern after the weight is lost.

- Surgical procedures to reduce obesity are performed only after all other methods to lose weight have failed.

- Starvation and famine are caused by one or more of the following: inadequate food distribution, war, drought, floods, plant and animal diseases, income inequality, land tenure systems, industrialization and urbanization, failed economic policies.

- The role of women is critical in times of starvation–for getting food and water and for small amounts of trading in villages.

- Protein-calorie malnutrition involves a number of causative factors, including family size, the child's birth weight and birth order, the parents' education and occupation, illnesses, and sanitation conditions.

- Education is important in preventing malnutrition.

- Eating disorders include anorexia nervosa and bulimia.

- Anorexia nervosa is self-induced starvation, and bulimia involves bingeing and purging.

- Most treatments for eating disorders usually involve the entire family.

- Many people have poor knowledge of how much food they consume.

- There are many different eating styles ranging from "night eaters" to "chronic dieters."

Further Reading

1. Farley, D. *Eating Disorders Require Medical Attention.* Department of Health and Human Services Publication No. (FDA) 92-1194, March 1992.
2. Kuczmarski, R. J. Prevalence of overweight and weight gain in the United States. *American Journal of Clinical Nutrition* 55:495S, 1992.
3. Drewnowski, A., and others. Food preferences in human obesity: Carbohydrates versus fats. *Appetite* 18:207, 1992.
4. Garrow, J. S. Importance of obesity. *British Medical Journal* 303:704, 1991.
5. Bray, G. A. Drug treatment of obesity. *American Journal of Clinical Nutrition* 55:538S, 1992.
6. National Institutes of Health. Methods for voluntary weight loss and control. *Nutrition Today* 27(4):27, 1992.
7. Matsuzawa, Y., and others. Classification of obesity with respect to morbidity. *Proceedings of the Society for Experimental Biology and Medicine* 200:197, 1992.
8. Garrow, J. S. Treatment of obesity. *Lancet* 340:409, 1992.
9. Ferguson, K. J., and others. Characteristics of successful dieters as measured by guided interview responses and restraint scale scores. *Journal of the American Dietetic Association* 92:1119, 1992.
10. Wing, R. R. Behavioral treatment of severe obesity. *American Journal of Clinical Nutrition* 55:545S, 1992.
11. Kral, J. G. Overview of surgical techniques for treating obesity. *American Journal of Clinical Nutrition* 55:552S, 1992.
12. Shoham, J. Emergency feeding programmes. Still not delivering the goods. *British Medical Journal* 305:596, 1992.
13. Henry, F. J., and others. The risk approach to intervention in severe malnutrition in rural Bangladesh. *American Journal of Epidemiology* 136:460, 1992.
14. Konotey-Ahulu, F. I. D. Kwashiorkor. *British Medical Journal* 302:180, 1991.
15. Victoria, C. G. The association between wasting and stunting: An international perspective. *Journal of Nutrition* 122:1105, 1992.
16. Rolls, B. J., and others. Food intake, hunger, and satiety after preloads in women with eating disorders. *American Journal of Clinical Nutrition* 55:1093, 1992.
17. Smith, G. T., and others. Accuracy of self-reported weight: Covariation with binger or restrainer status and eating disorder symptomatology. *Addictive Behavior* 17:1, 1992.
18. Pope, H. G., Jr., and Hudson, J. I. Is childhood sexual abuse a risk factor for bulimia nervosa? *American Journal of Psychiatry* 149:455, 1992.
19. Killen, J. D., and others. Is puberty a risk factor for eating disorders? *American Journal of Diseases of Children* 146: 323, 1992.
20. Blouin, A., and others. Seasonal patterns of bulimia nervosa. *American Journal of Psychiatry* 149:73, 1992.
21. Anonymous. Dieters' Truth or Consequences. *NCRR Reporter* 17(3):8, 1993.

Think about this life-threatening
cancer cell and these numbers.
Does your family have a history
of diet-related diseases?

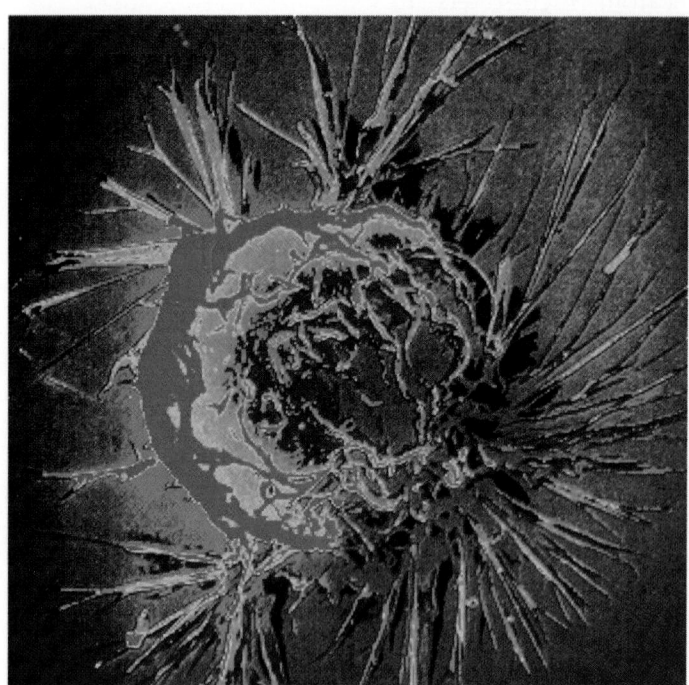

Figure 14-1. Digitized scanning electron micrograph of a single breast cancer cell. Breast cancer is the most common cancer type in women. Diet is suspected as a factor in this cancer.

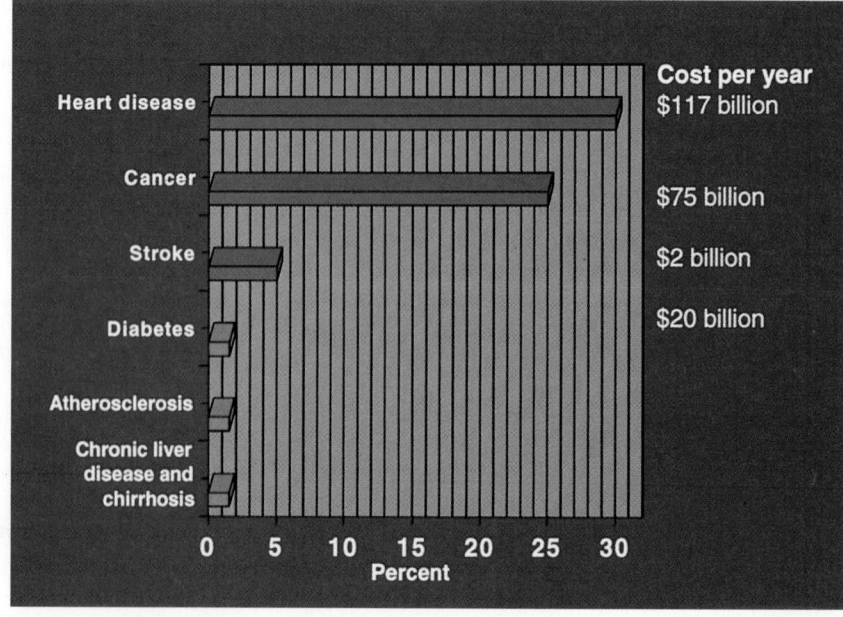

Figure 14-2. Proportion of U.S. deaths due to major diet-related causes (1989 data) and the cost per year for four of them.

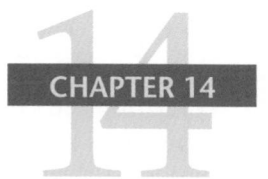

## CHAPTER 14

Nutrition and Disease

■ Nutrition in our lives–The economic costs of nutrition-related diseases

Nutrition plays a role in all of the diseases listed, but other factors such as genetics, environment, and lifestyle are also important. An entire chapter is devoted to these nutrition-related diseases because of how much there is yet to learn about the relationship of nutrition and other risk factors to various diseases. The dollar values above are enormous and add to the rapid increases in health care costs. Since good nutrition is important in decreasing the incidence of these diseases, it makes economic sense to learn more about how nutrition is related to health and disease.

Let's begin by making a couple of connections with previous chapters. You will notice as we go along that obesity is a factor in some diseases. Annual health care costs of nearly 40 billion dollars are attributed to the excess weight associated with coronary heart disease, hypertension, breast and colon cancer, diabetes, and gallbladder disease.[1] Also, many of the nutrition-related symptoms in acquired immunodeficiency syndrome (AIDS) are similar to those in protein-energy malnutrition. AIDS is the first disease we will examine.

■ Acquired immunodeficiency syndrome (AIDS)

"Poor man's plague" is how an article on AIDS was introduced in *The Economist* (September 21, 1991). It might be appropriate to add "poor women's and children's plague" because of the information in the following figure. AIDS has been rapidly increasing in the developing countries of Africa, Asia, and Latin America (Figure 14-3).

As of early 1992, about 10–12 million people worldwide were suspected of being infected with the human immunodeficiency virus (HIV), which causes AIDS. About 90% of these were in sub-Saharan Africa, and about half of the remaining individuals were in North America and Europe.[2] The number of people infected with HIV is increasing rapidly in Latin America

Major Topics in This Chapter

AIDS has many symptoms similar to those of protein-energy malnutrition.

Side effects from drugs used to treat AIDS have negative nutritional implications.

Diet-related factors are associated with certain cancers.

■

Hypertension (high blood pressure) is related to high sodium intake in some people.

Diabetes is most likely to develop in the overweight, the elderly, certain ethnic groups, and women.

Diet is one of several risk factors in coronary heart disease.

■

People Are Different– Low-calorie alternatives for the health-conscious

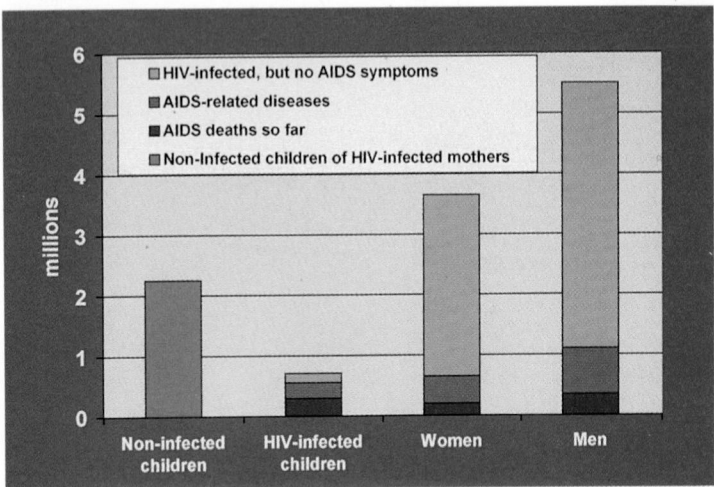

Figure 14-3. Number of cases of AIDS/HIV in the world (1991 estimates).

and in parts of Asia. The World Health Organization (WHO) predicts that during the 1990s as many as 10 million children under 10 years of age will lose their mothers to AIDS. Projected infant and child deaths from AIDS may increase child mortality rates by as much as 50% in parts of sub-Saharan Africa. In many countries this will wipe out the gains in child survival achieved over the past two decades. WHO projects that by the year 2000 there will be a cumulative total of 30–40 million HIV infections in men, women, and children, more than 90% of whom will live in developing countries. In the United States and other developed countries, AIDS has primarily affected homosexual men and intravenous drug users, but health experts warn that the incidence is already spreading to other parts of the population. It is therefore important that we look at the role of nutrition in AIDS.

People with AIDS have significant decreases in nutritional status, as shown in Table 14-1.[3]

Table 14-1. Trends of Changes in People with AIDS

Characteristic	Direction of Change
Body weight	↓
Proteins in blood	↓
Amino acids (most) in blood	↓
Lipids in blood	
Triglycerides	↑
Fatty acids	↓
Cholesterol	↓
Folate (in nerves and blood)	↓
Vitamin B-12 in blood	↓
Zinc	
In blood	↓
By zinc taste test	↓
Selenium	↓
Iron (hemoglobin and serum iron)	↓

Since the amount of these nutrients in the blood is a good indicator of the amount in the tissues, we know that many nutrients are at low levels in people with AIDS. They experience many difficulties in consuming and digesting food and absorbing nutrients. These include nausea and vomiting, diarrhea, loss of appetite, and difficulties in eating and swallowing, all of which make eating a difficult experience. As a result, major changes must be made in the type and amount of food eaten, as seen in Table 14-2.

Further nutritional complications usually arise for the AIDS patient because of side effects from a wide range of drugs. Some of these drugs are given to control various infections (viral, parasitic, fungal, and bacterial), and some are to correct the immune system and to control cancer. The side effects of many of the drugs include nausea, loss of appetite, vomiting, diarrhea, sore throat, and poor wound healing, all of which clearly have a negative impact on nutritional status.

Similar immune system changes occur in AIDS and in protein-energy malnutrition. These negative changes are caused by deficiencies of specific nutrients–protein, amino acids, lipids, zinc, iron, selenium, magnesium, copper, folacin, thiamin, riboflavin, pantothenic acid, biotin, or vitamins A, E, C, B-6, and B-12. Single nutrient deficiencies are relatively rare; people with AIDS usually have multiple deficiencies of nutrients. It is clear that optimal nutritional status must be maintained in the

Table 14-2. Nutrition-Related Problems and Dietary Intervention Strategies for AIDS

Problem	Symptoms	Dietary Intervention	Practical Food Tips
Oral lesions	Difficulty in chewing and swallowing	Mechanically modified diet (bland, soft semiliquid foods)	Mashed, pureed, or blended fruits and vegetables
		High-calorie/high-protein supplements	Prepare baked and steamed foods like fish, ground beef, custard, pudding
		Mild flavored foods at room or cold temperature	Canned fruits (skin and seeds removed)
		Avoid acidic or tart foods	Use a straw for drinking vitamin C fortified apple or grape juice
Esophageal lesions	Feeling of obstruction in chest and difficulty in swallowing	Mechanically modified diet (see above)	Drink liquids like milk shakes (milk and ice cream), egg cream (chocolate syrup and carbonated water), diluted or undiluted fruit nectars (apricot, pear, or peach)
GI infections	Nausea and vomiting	Eat carbohydrate foods in the morning	Dry toast or crackers first thing in the morning
		Small frequent meals and snacks	Chew food slowly and eat small portions frequently
		Frequent intake of liquids, slowly between meals	Drink fruit juices and eat smooth soups (creamed, pureed)
		Avoid fried foods	Bake, broil, boil, and steam foods
			Open windows while cooking
	Diarrhea	Frequent fluids and electrolyte supplements (including high-potassium juices)	Fruit ices, fruited gelatin and high potassium juices (cranberry, orange if tolerated)
		Low-fiber, low-lactose foods	Diluted or undiluted fruit nectars (apricot, pear, peach)
		Small, frequent feedings	Pureed banana and canned peaches
		If diarrhea is severe and persistent, use enteral nutrition formulas or parenteral nutrition only, under the direction of a physician	
	Loss of appetite, anorexia	Small, frequent feedings	Eat a number of small meals and snacks throughout the day
		Calorically dense foods	Add nonfat dry milk to potatoes, casseroles, and soups
		Drink fluids after meals	Foods should be served attractively
		Rearrange the time of large meals/snacks to coincide with the time the appetite is best	If appetite is good in the morning, eat a large morning meal
		Calorically dense enteral formulas to supplement diet as directed by a physician	
		If significant weight loss occurs, tube feeding may be indicated as directed by a physician	

AIDS patient, just as in the individual with marasmus or kwashiorkor, who also has depressed immune activity. These people are more vulnerable to life-threatening infections because of reduced resistance.

AIDS patients typically have suboptimal intakes of nutrients. In one study, hospitalized patients consumed only 70% of what they needed for basal energy and 65% of the protein they needed.[4] This nutrient level does not allow for the increased energy needed for the elevated metabolism associated with acute infection; nor does it permit any physical activity.

"Wasting syndrome" is a term applied to the weight loss in AIDS patients. They lose lean body mass, total body water, and body fat.[5] This weight loss results from decreased food intake due to nausea, vomiting, and loss of appetite. Other factors are also involved; among them are nutrients malabsorbed from the GI tract and nutrients lost through diarrhea. Energy metabolism is inefficient because of an increased basal metabolic rate, thought to be caused by increases in serum thyroid hormones.

AIDS patients must be fed in special ways to correct the multiple nutrient deficiencies.[5] Patients with more than 10% weight loss should be fed by either *enteral* or *parenteral feeding*. The word *enteral* means "within the intestine"; the feeding involves passing liquid diets down a tube through the nose and into the GI tract or directly into the stomach or intestine. *Parenteral* means "situated or occurring outside of the intestines" and involves the delivery of total caloric and nutrient needs through the veins. Parenteral feeding is also referred to as total parenteral nutrition (TPN), or hyperalimentation. TPN may be used in cases of severe diarrhea or malabsorption.

Think beyond the picture in Figure 14-4. How are these things related?

Enteral feeding: Feeding a liquid diet down a tube through the nose into the GI tract, or directly into the stomach or intestine ("within the intestine").

Parenteral feeding: Feeding nutrients into veins ("outside the intestines"). Also referred to as total parenteral nutrition (TPN) or hyperalimentation.

Advances in modern nutrition allow the nutrient equivalent of all of the foods in the photograph (and others not shown) to be delivered directly into the digestive system. This system is used for people with AIDS and other medical problems hindering the normal digestion of food.

Dietary counseling has been found to be better than nutrient supplements in improving the nutritional status of people with HIV infection complicated by weight loss.[6] AIDS patients are advised to seek medical advice regarding supplements because nutritional problems in HIV-related diseases vary from patient to patient.

Some people turn to unproven nutritional therapies and unconventional diets because of the desire to control their own treatment, and the irreversible, incurable nature of AIDS.[3] Many of these so-called therapies may cause either toxicity or deficiencies in certain nutrients. Food safety can be a significant problem for AIDS patients because food can be a vehicle for various infectious agents. It may bring pathogenic bacteria and viruses to the digestive system. One study in San Francisco showed that the incidence of food poisoning

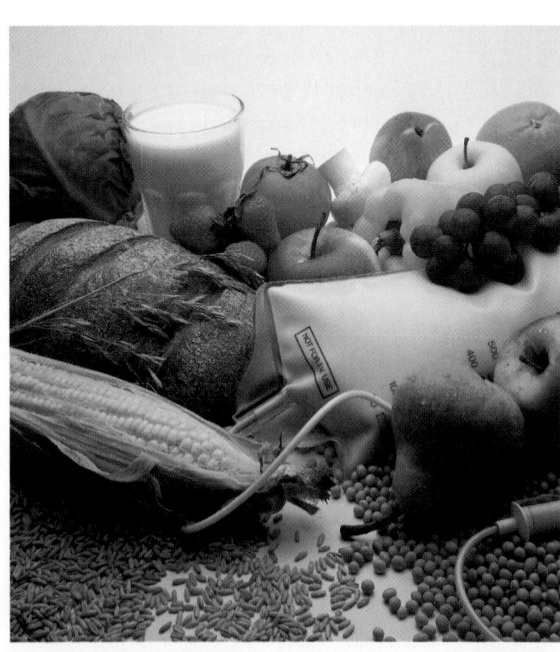

Figure 14-4. Major advances in medicine allow nutrients to be supplied to a patient by tube.

from *Salmonella* in men with AIDS increased nearly 20-fold over that in comparable normal subjects. Increased incidence of infections from *Listeria monocytogenes* and *Campylobacter jejuni* also have been reported for AIDS patients.[3]

HIV-infected children are frequently born to infected mothers with incomes below the poverty level.[7] Poverty and poor prenatal care add to the nutritional problems of the HIV-infected child. HIV does not affect birth weight, but subsequent body weight gain is less than in uninfected infants. An explanation for the poorer growth of HIV-infected children is the higher incidence of vomiting and diarrhea; also, their energy utilization may be adversely affected. Researchers recommend early supplementation with high-energy diets to decrease the adverse effects and to prolong the life of the child.

Feeding infants and children with AIDS requires certain precautions because their immune systems are weakened, thus making them more open to infections. No shortcuts must be taken in the usual safety precautions for preparing infant food. All utensils and dishes should be washed in a dishwasher or in hot soapy water and air dried. Food in opened jars should be refrigerated and used within 24 hours. Fruits and vegetables should be peeled or cooked, and meats should be well cooked. Unpasteurized milk and products from unpasteurized milk should never be given to these or any infants and children because they may contain *Salmonella* species or other organisms that can cause intestinal infections. Proper hygiene procedures in formula preparation are needed for bottle-fed infants. Children with AIDS who live in poverty may have additional nutrition problems because of poor education, improper housing conditions, and inadequate facilities for the storage and preparation of food.

■ Cancer

It is estimated that about 20 million people throughout the world suffer from cancer, and over 5 million people die from the disease in any one year.[2] Cancer is primarily a disease of the elderly, who will form an increasing proportion of the population in all countries and particularly in developing countries in the future. In the United States, the incidence of most cancers since the 1950s has gone up for men and fallen slightly for women.[8] Nutritionists are concerned about how various cancers affect food intake as well as about possible linkages between diet and cancer. People with low incomes and education are the least likely to be aware of or able to apply preventive dietary measures. They should be especially targeted for education about cancer risk reduction.[9]

Food Intake of the Cancer Patient

It goes without saying that the majority of patients with cancer will eventually lose weight and a proportion become *emaciated* to the extent that they appear to die of starvation.[10]

Emaciated: Excessively thin.

This statement from an article in the *Proceedings of the Nutrition Society* acknowledges that cancer patients frequently experience extreme weight

Chemotherapy: In the treatment of disease, the application of chemicals that have a specific and toxic effect on the disease-causing agent.

loss. The importance of weight loss in cancer has been recognized since the early 1900s.[11] Why do cancer patients decrease their food intake? The reasons may include one or more of the following medical, nutritional, or psychological factors:

- Ulcers or infections in the mouth
- Atrophy (wasting away) of the GI tract
- Tumor obstructions in the GI tract
- Nausea and/or vomiting caused by *chemotherapy*
- Altered taste sensitivity, which could be due to the treatment or to zinc deficiency
- Depression, stress, and anxiety
- General weakness
- Tumor products that depress food intake.

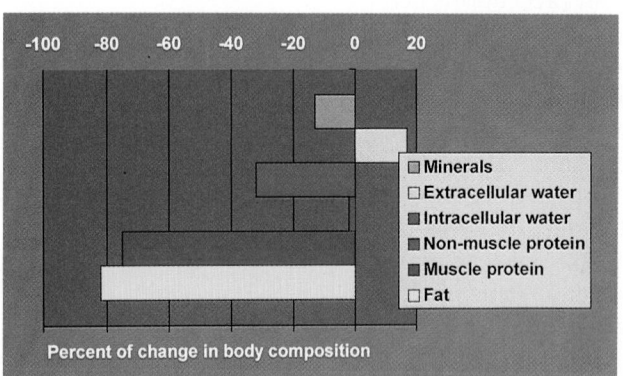

Figure 14-5. Percent change in body composition of cancer patients compared to that of persons without cancer.

The reduction in food intake brings about major changes in body composition, as shown in Figure 14-5 for cancer patients who have lost 30% of their precancer body weight.

The body composition changes caused by some cancers have some similarity to the changes seen in starvation. For example, a person with cancer loses much storage fat, as well as muscle protein. You would see this person as skinny with very little muscle. The person's nonmuscle protein is maintained, however, whereas a starving person without cancer would lose nonmuscle protein.[10] All the loss of tissue significantly decreases the amount of intracellular water in the cancer patient, but the total mineral content of the body is not changed.

Cancer treatments such as surgery, radiation therapy, and chemotherapy can change the patient's nutritional needs, as well as his or her ability to consume nutrients, as outlined in Table 14-3.

Diet and Cancer

Think about the numbers in Figure 14-6. Are they affected by personal choices?

The figure shows that 65% of cancer deaths can be attributed to tobacco and diet. According to the American Institute for Cancer Research, more than 80% of all cancers are within our control. For example, a modest reduction in energy intake is a simple and inexpensive approach to reducing your risk of cancer.[11] The other risk factors, including pollution and other environmental risks, are small.

The pamphlet from the American Cancer Society (Figure 14-7) lists seven nutritional things (in addition to some nonnutritional things such as not smoking) that

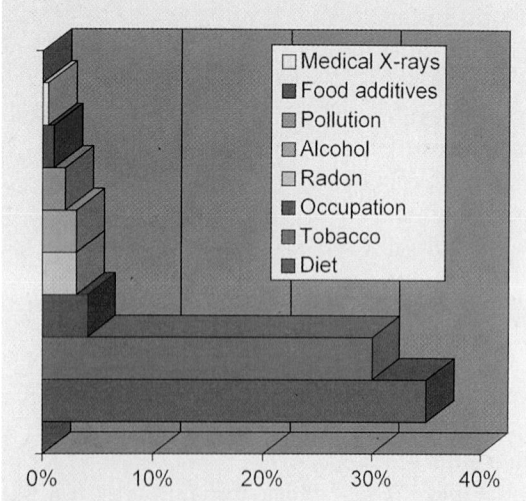

Figure 14-6. Percentage of cancer deaths attributed to various factors. The highest percentages are from diet and tobacco, two factors that we can control.

Table 14-3. How Cancer Treatments Can Affect Eating

Treatment	Why It Can Affect Eating	Possible Side Effects
Surgery	Increases the need for good nutrition by putting stress on the body. May stop parts of the body that are needed for eating, such as the stomach, from working properly. May also make them sore.	Before surgery, a high-protein, high-calorie diet may be prescribed if a patient is underweight or weak. After surgery, some patients may not resume normal eating at first. They may receive nutrients: – Through a needle in their vein (intravenous or IV feeding) – Through a tube in their nose or stomach – By drinking clear liquids – By following a special diet
Radiation therapy	May harm parts of the body as it damages cancer cells	Treatment of head, neck, or chest may cause: – Dry mouth – Sore mouth – Sore throat – Change in the taste of food – Dental problems Treatment in the area of the stomach may cause: – Nausea – Vomiting – Diarrhea
Chemotherapy	May harm parts of the body needed for eating as it destroys cancer cells	– Nausea and vomiting – Loss of appetite – Diarrhea – Constipation – Sore mouth or throat – Weight gain – Change in the taste of food

you can do to help reduce your cancer risk and most likely make you feel better, too.

- **Watch your weight.** Get some exercise like walking every day to help keep your weight down. Obesity is linked to cancers of the uterus, gallbladder, breast, and colon. Check with your doctor before you begin an exercise routine or go on a strict diet.

- **Eat a varied diet.** A varied diet, eaten sensibly, offers the best hope for lowering the risk of cancer.

- **Eat a lot of vegetables and fruits every day.** Choose foods rich in vitamins A and C. They may help protect you against cancers of the throat, stomach, or lungs. Choose vegetables such as sweet potatoes, carrots, broccoli, cabbage, and green peppers, and fruits such as oranges, strawberries, peaches, tomatoes, and watermelon.

Figure 14-7. The American Cancer Society's pamphlet shows how each of us can take control of our diet to reduce the risk of cancers.

- **Add more high-fiber foods such as whole-grain cereals, vegetables, and fruits.** A high-fiber diet may protect you against colon cancer. Fiber is found in peaches, strawberries, potatoes, and popcorn; whole-wheat breads, cereals, and pastas; and tortillas, rice, and beans.

- **Trim fat from your diet.** A high-fat diet increases your risk of breast, colon, and prostate cancers. Eat lean meats, skinned chicken or turkey, and fish. Cut down on butter, margarine, fried foods, and rich desserts. Drink low-fat milk; eat low-fat cheese.

- **Cut down on foods like ham, bacon, bologna, and hot dogs.** These smoked or cured meats have a chemical in them that keeps them from spoiling–but it will add to your risk of cancer.

- **Greatly restrict the use of alcohol.** If you drink a lot, your risk of liver cancer increases. Smoking and drinking alcohol greatly increase your risk for cancer of the mouth, throat, and stomach, and, possibly, the breast.

Most doctors consider this to be useful advice, even though we do not yet know the exact relationship between diet and cancer. But a small minority in the medical profession doubt that a relationship exists at all. "Diet and Cancer: Causal Relation or Just Wishful Thinking?" is the title of a paper in a leading international medical journal.[12] We take a brief look at this viewpoint here as an illustration of how experts can differ on some nutrition issues. The author examines some evidence linking diet and cancer and concludes:

> Most of these theories are in the twilight zone, yet dietary prevention has become a multimillion-dollar industry, with low-fat/low-cholesterol labels on a multitude of commercial products including club soda.

He gives some reasons for what he terms "this exploitation." One is that diet seems to be one risk factor that can be treated without stopping the wheels of industry. Second, diet is commonly regarded as controllable by almost anybody. Third, most countries do not regulate health claims about food as rigorously as they do claims for drugs. In these arguments we see again that nutrition and health are usually bound up with economics, risk/benefit analysis, environmental issues, and consumer protection.

Unproven Nutrition Treatments and Cancer

Many people try unproven nutritional treatments because of the medical, emotional, and psychological impact of cancer. Better-educated people seem to be the ones most often seeking these ineffective nutritional remedies.[13] Among the unproven dietary treatments for cancer are:

- Vegan-type diets, including macrobiotic diets, which are extremely restricted diets (such as one consisting mainly of whole grains) that may be deficient in some essential nutrients.
- Drugs and formulations, such as hydrogen peroxide or laetrile, that are meant to work as nutrients once they enter the body.

- Food supplements consisting of vitamins, minerals, or various extracts of herbs, animal glands, or other foods.
- Specific diets, including wheatgrass supplements and enemas, and the "Gerson therapy," which is a vegetarian-type diet with liver extracts and coffee enemas. This latter treatment is high in bulk and low in vitamins D and B-12, iron, and calcium; it is relatively low in calories.

Each decade seems to bring its share of unproven treatments for cancer. In the 1970s it was vitamin B-17, or laetrile, which is not a legitimate vitamin; in the 1980s it was megadoses of vitamins A and C and selenium. Perhaps we will know more about this kind of treatment in the future; the National Institutes of Health (NIH) has created an office to examine some alternative medical practices, including diet, in the treatment of cancer and other diseases. In the meantime, beware of promises from unusual dietary treatments for cancer, and seek reliable dietary advice from dietitians and physicians.

■ Hypertension and diet

Hypertension (high blood pressure) is one of the most prevalent vascular diseases in the world. It increases the risk of coronary heart disease and stroke. In the United States, about 500,000 strokes and 1.25 million coronary attacks occur each year.[14] The World Health Organization identifies hypertension as having a strong relationship with obesity and high alcohol intake.[15] Sodium intake has a weaker, but significant, effect on the rise in blood pressure with age. Blood pressures of populations with low salt intakes show no increase as the people age. Epidemiological studies consistently suggest that blood pressures are lower among vegetarians than nonvegetarians.

Older women have a higher risk of hypertension than younger women. It is more common in African-American women than in white women. Use of birth control pills can contribute to high blood pressure in some women.

Diet therapy for hypertension includes these recommendations:

Type of Blood Pressure	Range (millimeters of mercury)	Category
Diastolic	<85	Normal
	90–104	Mild hypertension
	>115	Severe hypertension
Systolic, when diastolic blood pressure is <90		
	<140	Normal
	>160	Hypertension

- If obese, reduce weight.
- Restrict dietary sodium to 2 grams per day.
- Consume more fiber and less saturated fat.
- Limit alcohol intake to 1 ounce per day.
- If a deficiency of potassium, magnesium, or calcium exists, take supplements under medical supervision.

Canadian research shows promising indications that families can adapt to dietary intervention for hypertension.[16] Young children accepted healthy alternatives to foods low in nutrients and high in fat. The snacks that were recommended included low-fat yogurt, yogurt dips, frozen yogurt, fruit bars, pasta with low-fat vegetable sauce, toast with fruit spreads, fresh fruits and vegetables, and vegetable juice cocktail. These are worthwhile recommendations for all children.

Stress is a contributor to hypertension and coronary heart disease and should be considered when dietary changes are made. One study reports that low promotion prospects, competitiveness at work, and feelings of sustained anger contribute as much to hypertension as do overweight and smoking.[17] These researchers found that hypertension and elevated blood lipids are more likely to exist in blue-collar men than white-collar men, when both groups are working under stress and also smoke and are overweight.

If certain diets, smoking, obesity, and stress are contributing factors to hypertension, and if these factors are shared by many Americans, why do African-Americans have, on the average, a higher incidence of hypertension than other American population groups? Present-day West Africans do not have a high incidence of hypertension, so genetics cannot be the reason. One hypothesis suggests that present-day hypertension results from the malnutrition experienced by their African ancestors on slave ships, but an article in a health journal refutes that idea, saying,

> No evidence has been advanced that a dietary trauma experienced by 80% of one's ancestors over a period of less than 1 year, 220 years ago, could bring about a genetic change lasting to the present.[18]

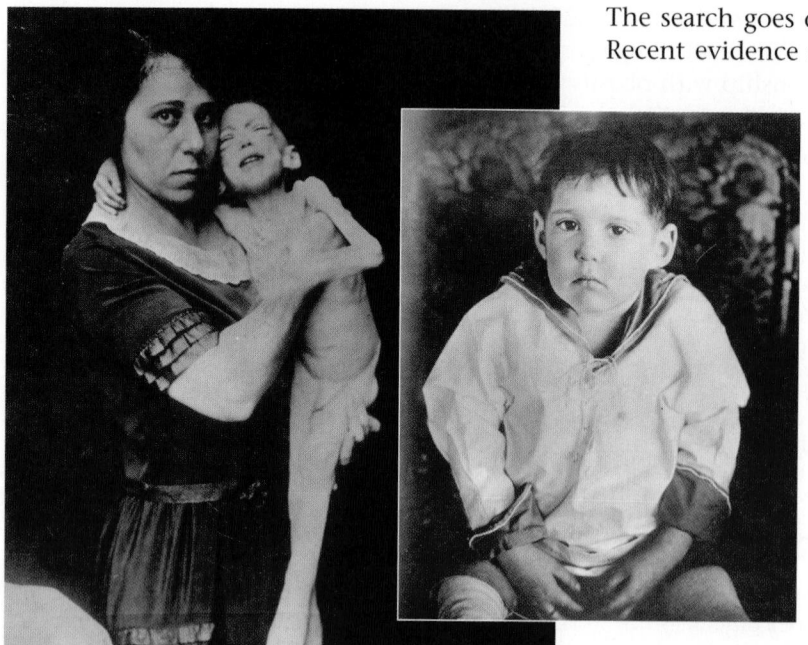

The search goes on for an explanation and a solution. Recent evidence suggests that moderate restrictions in potassium rather than excesses in sodium might be the cause of hypertension in salt-sensitive African-Americans but not in Caucasians. Higher levels of dietary potassium within the normal range of intake might decrease the hypertension that is sensitive to salt.[19] Potassium is widely distributed in many foods.

■ Diabetes

About 11 million Americans suffer from diabetes, a disease in which the body isn't able to handle food properly. This is due to a lack of the hormone insulin or to the body's inability to use it properly. Insulin removes glucose from the blood and takes it to cells to be used for energy. The effects of insulin deficiency and subsequent administration of the hormone are dramatic. Figure 14-8 shows a mother with her diabetic child and the same child after he received insulin treatment.

Figure 14-8. Photographs taken in 1922 to introduce the positive effects of insulin to the medical profession. A mother holds her diabetic son, who is 3 years old and weighs 15 pounds. The same boy is shown in the inset after treatment with insulin for two months; he weighs 29 pounds.

The diagram in Figure 14-9 shows how insulin helps glucose get into fat and muscle cells.

If glucose cannot enter cells, it is filtered from the blood by the kidneys and is excreted in the urine. High blood-glucose levels can result in damage to eyes, kidneys, nerves, blood vessels, and other parts of the body, as well as causing complications in pregnancy and increased infections.

Diabetes was described over 3,000 years ago, but we are still refining its definition. There are two main types of diabetes: insulin-dependent (or Type I, formerly called juvenile) diabetes mellitus and non-insulin-dependent diabetes mellitus (NIDDM or Type II, formerly called adult-onset). These two types of diabetes are different in several ways, as shown in Table 14-4.

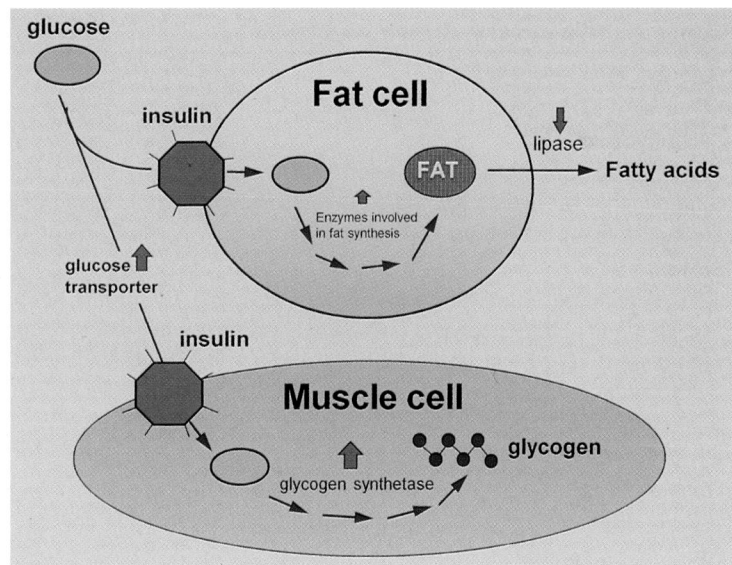

Figure 14-9. The metabolic effects of insulin. The actions of insulin in the body include assisting glucose to enter cells for storage. Glucose is stored as glycogen in muscles or as fat in fat cells.

Table 14-4. Types of Diabetes

	Insulin-Dependent (ID) or Type I (Juvenile)	Non-Insulin-Dependent (NID) or Type II (Adult-Onset)
Percent of diabetic population	<20%	>80%
Age at onset	Young (under 30)	Older (over 50)
Body weight	Normal	80% are overweight
Blood insulin level	Low or zero	Normal or raised
Treatment	Requires insulin	Diet, may need oral agents and/or insulin

Who is likely to develop NIDDM?

- **People who are overweight.** About 80% of people with NIDDM are overweight. Weight loss decreases the incidence of NIDDM.
- **Women.** Diabetes is twice as common in women as in men. Family history of diabetes is important in identifying women who may be susceptible to the disease.[20]
- **African-Americans.** This diabetes is twice as common as in whites.[21]
- **Hispanic-Americans.** The disease is five times more common than in other population groups in the United States.[21]
- **Native Americans.** The incidence of NIDDM in this group is higher than for whites.
- **The elderly.** The risk of diabetes increases with each decade of life. In addition, many elderly people have difficulty in following dietary recommendations for diabetes.[22]

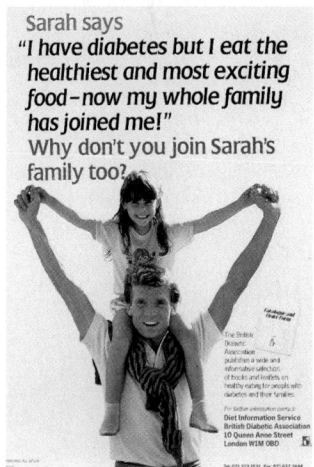

Sarah says
"I have diabetes but I eat the healthiest and most exciting food – now my whole family has joined me!"
Why don't you join Sarah's family too?

Figure 14-10. In this poster from the British Diabetic Association, Sarah has good advice for all of us. Diseases such as diabetes should not prevent people from eating healthy and exciting foods.

Target Nutrition Goals for People with Diabetes[a]

Calories
Sufficient to achieve and maintain reasonable weight.

Carbohydrate
May be up to 55–60% of total calories. Liberalized; individualized; emphasis on unrefined carbohydrate with fiber; modest amounts of sucrose and other refined sugars may be acceptable contingent on metabolic control.

Protein
Usual intake of protein in most Americans is double the amount needed; exact percentage of total calories is unknown. Usual recommendation for people with diabetes is 12–20% of total calories. Recommended daily allowance is 0.8 gram per kilogram of body weight for adults; intake is modified for children, pregnant and lactating women, the aged, and individuals with special medical conditions, e.g., renal complications.

Fiber
Up to 40 grams per day; 25 grams per 1,000 kilocalories for low-calorie intakes.

Fat
Ideally <30% of total calories. However, this needs to be individualized because 30% may be unachievable for some individuals.
- Polyunsaturated fats, up to 10%
- Saturated fats, <10%
- Monounsaturated fats, remaining percentage (10–15%)

Cholesterol
<300 milligrams per day.

Alternative sweeteners
Use is acceptable.

Sodium
Not to exceed 3,000 milligrams per day; modified for special medical conditions.

Alcohol
Occasional use; limit to 1–2 alcohol equivalents one to two times a week.

Vitamins/minerals
No evidence that diabetes caused increased need.

[a]Each goal needs to be individualized. The above goals should serve as a guide for establishing short- and long-term goals.

- **People with a family history of the disease.** Having a family history of NIDDM increases the likelihood of getting it.

Diet is important in the control of diabetes. Refer to the Exchange Lists for diabetics, which we discussed in Chapter 6. The recommendations on this page are made by the American Diabetes Association and The American Dietetic Association.

■ Coronary heart disease

Cardiovascular diseases account for half of all deaths in industrialized countries.[2] The encouraging news is that mortality from coronary heart disease (CHD) fell by 40% in the last 20 years in the United States.[23] We have discussed certain aspects of this disease in different parts of this book because of the confirmed or suspected involvement of a number of dietary components, especially the amount and type of lipids (Chapter 7). We can now look at all risk factors in CHD.

Risk Factors for Coronary Heart Disease

One expert warns us that everybody is at risk of CHD, but some are much more than others.[23] Family history is important if relatives developed the disease before age 60. Even those in the lowest risk group are more likely to die of CHD than of any other single cause, but it will happen later in their lives. Therefore, it is appropriate that we all pay attention to the risk factors involved. Some factors are within your control–smoking, obesity, hypertension, exercise, coffee consumption, diabetes, diet. Other risk factors are outside your control–age, gender, genetics. Let's deal with the risks outside our control first.

- **Age.** CHD increases in incidence after 35–40 years of age in men and after menopause in women.

- **Gender.** The incidence of coronary heart disease is greater in men than in women but is increasing at a greater rate in women. Some of this is attributed to a decrease in cigarette smoking by men and an increase by women. Gender differences are much reduced after menopause in women.

- **Genetics.** Family history of the disease is an indicator of the risk of developing CHD.

Here are some CHD risk factors you *can* control.

- **Smoking**–especially cigarettes, but probably also pipes and cigars if the smoke is inhaled. Smoking doubles the risk of heart disease. The number of cigarettes smoked seems less important than the mere fact of smoking, and for the heart there is no "safe cigarette." Stopping smoking brings quick benefits.[23] Smoking lowers HDL cholesterol, the beneficial cholesterol.

- **Being overweight.** If you lose weight, you reduce serum cholesterol and therefore reduce the risk of CHD.

- **High blood pressure.** Even slightly high levels double the risk of CHD. High blood pressure combined with smoking and high blood-cholesterol levels gives the highest risk of coronary heart disease.

- **Sedentary lifestyle.** Exercise reduces blood cholesterol. Exercise alone is no absolute guarantee of escaping heart disease in middle age, but people who exercise are more likely to monitor their body weight and diet, and they rarely smoke.

- **Coffee.** Heavy coffee drinkers (who thus have high caffeine intake) have higher incidences of heart disease than do people who don't drink coffee. Some of this may be due to cigarette smoking because smokers are often heavy coffee drinkers.

- **Diabetes.** Nondiabetics have lower incidences of CHD. (Some cases of diabetes can be controlled.)

- **Diet.** Reduced intake of fat, saturated fat, cholesterol, and sodium; no alcohol in excess; and increased intake of fiber and complex carbohydrates are thought to decrease the risk of CHD. Studies on animal protein, coffee, and sugar have shown them to have variable associations with increased blood-lipid levels. Much current research on heart disease is directed toward antioxidants.[24] Increased risk of heart disease exists when the dietary intake of the antioxidant nutrients beta-carotene and vitamins A, C, and E is low. There is no strong evidence for increasing vitamin or mineral intake above the normally recommended levels.

"Is Baldness Bad for the Heart?" is not a title you would expect to see in a scientific paper in the *Journal of the American Medical Association*.[25] However, it is not a joke; it refers to a serious scientific study showing that baldness in men under the age of 55 years is associated with coronary artery disease. Baldness is an indicator of changes in male hormone metabolism that increase the risk of heart disease. What has this to do with nutrition? Directly, very little, because the hormones have no known relationship with nutrient deficiencies or excesses. Indirectly, this information is relevant to nutrition in that it shows the multitude of factors apart from diet that may be risk factors in CHD.

■ Other diseases

Gallstones

Gallstones are composed mainly of cholesterol, along with other bile salts, calcium salts, and protein. They form when the level of cholesterol in bile becomes high. Women have higher incidences of gallstones than men.[26] Obesity is an established risk factor for gallstones.[27]

Cystic fibrosis

This is a genetic disease affecting mainly whites from infancy to young adulthood. Symptoms include malfunctioning of the pancreas. This tissue normally secretes enzymes essential for the digestion of food in the GI tract. When the enzymes are reduced or absent, some nutrients, including fat and the fat-soluble vitamins, are maldigested and malabsorbed. Individuals with cystic fibrosis should restrict their intake of dietary fat and should be monitored for essential fatty acid deficiencies, as well as for deficiencies of vitamins E and K (because of the fat malabsorption), electrolytes, zinc, and iron. Another symptom with nutritional implications is the excessive loss of electrolytes, including sodium, potassium, and chloride, via sweat.

Children with cystic fibrosis can surmount some of these difficulties and maintain normal growth and energy stores. This is done with a diet relatively high in calories and moderate in fat, as well as with an aggressive pancreatic enzyme supplement program.[28]

■ People are different–Low-calorie alternatives for the health-conscious

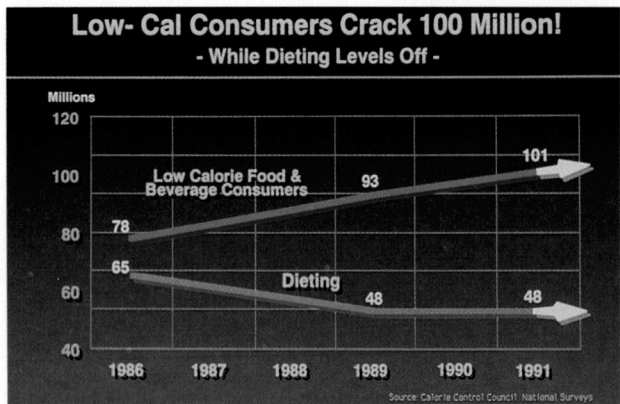

Figure 14-11. Some people are switching from dieting to consuming low-calorie foods as a means of losing excess body fat.

The number of people consuming low-calorie foods has increased since the mid-1980s (Figure 14-11). Many of these people switched to low-calorie products as an alternative to dieting to lose weight. Reduction in fat intake (and caloric intake) has beneficial effects on coronary heart disease, diabetes, and hypertension. Reducing the intake of saturated fatty acids reduces blood cholesterol.[29] Low-calorie, low-fat, and light foods and beverages were once called dietetic or "diet" food.[30] They were originally designed for diabetics and others with diet-related medical problems. Low-calorie products first appeared in health food stores or in dietetic sections of supermarkets, but they are now located throughout the store. In Chapter 7 we saw what goes into low-fat products. Now, let's see why they are consumed.

People consume low-calorie products for a variety of reasons (Table 14-5). Notice that refreshment or taste value is near the bottom of the list. Health, weight, and appearance are the main reasons. Three out of every four Americans (141 million) consume low-fat or low-calorie foods and beverages, with women consuming more than men.

Table 14-5. Reasons for Using Low-Calorie Products

Reason	Percent of Consumers of Low-Calorie Products
Stay in better overall health	67
Maintain current weight	60
Maintain attractive physical appearance	53
Reduce weight	48
Refreshment of taste	43
Prevent or control dental cavities	38
Help with a medical condition	33

Table 14-6. The Most Popular Reduced-Fat Products

	Percent of Total Population	Percent of Consumers of Low-Fat Products
Cheese/dairy products	49	74
Beverages	43	64
Ice cream/frozen desserts	34	51
Chips/snack foods	31	46
Cakes/baked goods	25	37
Dinner entrees	23	34

Diet beverages were introduced in the late 1950s. Saccharin and cyclamate were the early sweeteners, but saccharin had the problem of a bitter aftertaste. It is now used to sweeten some dietetic canned fruits. Cyclamate was widely used as a sweetener in canned fruits in the 1960s but was banned by the FDA as a result of the publication of research results (since discredited) suggesting that it was a carcinogen. These problems were overcome by the introduction of aspartame in the early 1980s. "Sugar-free" gum containing xylitol and other low-calorie sweeteners are also available.

Fat-reduced dairy products are popular (Table 14-6). Sales of skim milk keep increasing while those of whole milk decrease. Skim milk is now used extensively as an ingredient in many reduced-fat foods. Low-fat/low-calorie cheeses continue to increase in popularity, as do reduced-fat sour cream, yogurt, ice milk, and frozen desserts.

Think beyond the picture in Figure 14-12. Do you consume reduced-calorie foods? Do you know how they are made?

Many low-calorie or low-fat breads, cookies, frostings, and desserts are available. Low-calorie frozen entrees and dinners are popular because of their reduced caloric content and their convenience. "Healthy" and "lean" are two terms frequently used in the titles of these products.

Meat is more than 25% leaner than it was in the mid-1980s, thanks to the efforts of animal geneti-

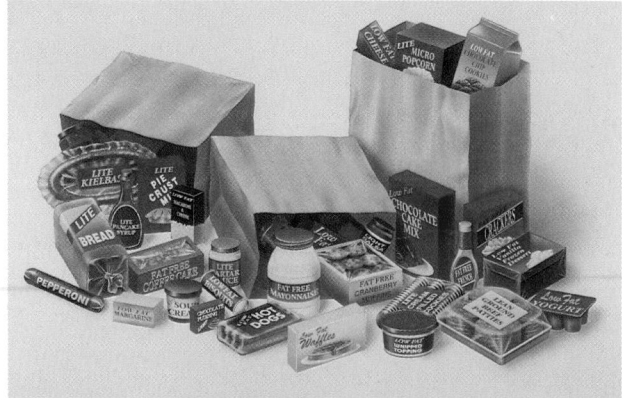

Figure 14-12. Reduced-calorie foods present both opportunities and challenges for the food industry.

cists, farmers, and retailers. The geneticists identified breeds of animals with less body fat and more muscle (meat). Farmers are more aware that consumers want lean and not fat, and retailers trim fat from meat. The fat content of frankfurters has been reduced from about 30 to 20%. Most of this was done by the addition of water, which diluted the fat. Lean ground beef products are now commonplace in supermarkets and fast food restaurants.

Low-fat and no-fat salad dressings have become a big market as marketing of these and other products moved from an emphasis on consumers with special diet-related medical needs to an emphasis on consumers who pay attention to fat and calorie intake. Low-fat, no-cholesterol dressings are available now. Many of these products owe their existence to the work of food scientists, who made innovative use of gums to help reduce the fat content while retaining the physical characteristics of fat. Low-calorie versions of potato chips, popcorn, and other snacks have been marketed.

In summary, the food industry has provided attractive low-fat, low-cholesterol, and low-calorie alternatives to conventional foods.

■ Now you know

- AIDS has many of the symptoms of protein-energy malnutrition–wasting of the body; decreases in blood proteins, fatty acids, folate, vitamin B-12, zinc, selenium, and iron; and immune system changes.

- AIDS patients have many changes in the mouth, esophagus, and GI tract that make eating, swallowing, and digesting food difficult.

- AIDS patients have side effects from treatment drugs that have negative nutritional implications.

- Feeding of severe AIDS cases must be done by tube either into the GI tract or through a vein.

- AIDS patients frequently adopt unproven nutritional therapies.

- Food safety is an important factor for the AIDS patient–foodborne illnesses must be avoided.

- Cancer causes nutritional problems as a result of loss of appetite or difficulties in consuming or digesting food. The seriousness of the difficulties may depend on the location of the tumor.

- Body composition changes similar to those seen in protein-energy malnutrition occur in the cancer patient.

- Nutrition problems may arise for the cancer patient following surgery, radiation, or chemotherapy.

- Diet is one important factor in the development of cancer, and changes in diet may provide protection against some types of cancer.

- Many unproven nutrition treatments for cancer exist that should not even be tried.

- Hypertension is related to obesity, high alcohol intake, and sodium intake. Diet therapy includes losing weight and restricting sodium.

- The reasons why African-Americans have higher incidences of hypertension are not fully known. Low dietary potassium is a possibility being investigated further.

- Diabetes exists as insulin-dependent or juvenile diabetes mellitus (Type I) and non-insulin-dependent diabetes mellitus (NIDDM or Type II, formerly called adult-onset).

- People most likely to develop diabetes include the overweight, women, African-Americans, Hispanic-Americans, Native Americans, and the elderly.

- Diet is important in the control of diabetes; intake of low-fat and high-carbohydrate foods is recommended.

- Risk factors for coronary heart disease that are not under your control include age, gender (higher in males), and genetics. Risk factors under your control include smoking, hypertension, lack of exercise, coffee drinking, and elevated blood cholesterol. In some cases, obesity and diabetes are risk factors that can be controlled.

- Low-fat, low-calorie, low-cholesterol products are increasing in popularity with health-conscious consumers.

Further Reading

1. Colditz, G. A. Economic costs of obesity. *American Journal of Clinical Nutrition* 55:503S, 1992.
2. Anonymous. *Global Health Situations and Projections. Estimates.* World Health Organization, Geneva, Switzerland, 1992.
3. Raiten, D. J. Nutrition and HIV infection. A review and evaluation of the extant knowledge of the relationship between nutrition and HIV infection. *Nutrition in Clinical Practice* 6:1S, 1991.
4. Trujillo, E. B., and others. Assessment of nutritional status, nutrient intake, and nutrition support in AIDS patients. *Journal of the American Dietetic Association* 92:477, 1992.
5. Singer, P., and others. Nutritional aspects of the acquired immunodeficiency syndrome. *American Journal of Gastroenterology* 87:265, 1992.
6. Murphy, J., and others. Dietary counselling and nutritional supplementation in HIV infection. *Journal of the Canadian Dietetic Association* 53:205, 1992.
7. Miller, T. L., and others. Growth and body composition in children infected with the human immunodeficiency virus-1. *American Journal of Clinical Nutrition* 57:588, 1993.
8. Anonymous. The cancer epidemic: Fact or misinterpretation? *Lancet* 340:399, 1992.
9. Cotugna, N., and others. Nutrition and cancer prevention knowledge, beliefs, attitudes, and practices: The 1987 National Health Interview Survey. *Journal of the American Dietetic Association* 92:963, 1992.
10. Fearon, K. C. H. The mechanisms and treatment of weight loss in cancer. *Proceedings of the Nutrition Society* 51:251, 1992.

11. Kritchevsky, D. Undernutrition and chronic disease: Cancer. *Proceedings of the Nutrition Society* 52:39, 1993.

12. Modan, B. Diet and cancer: Causal relation or just wishful thinking? *Lancet* 340:162, 1992.

13. Dwyer, J. T. Unproven nutritional remedies and cancer. *Nutrition Reviews* 50:106, 1992.

14. Kannel, W. B., and Wolf, P. A. Inferences from secular trend analysis of hypertension control. *American Journal of Public Health* 82:1583, 1992.

15. WHO Commission on Health and Environment. *Report of the Panel on Food and Agriculture.* World Health Organization, Geneva, Switzerland, page 150, 1992.

16. McNicol, J., and Kaplan, B. J. Long-term adherence to dietary restrictions for hyperactivity. *Journal of the Canadian Dietetic Association* 53:287, 1992.

17. Siegrist, J., and others. Psychological and biobehavioral characteristics of hypertensive men with elevated atherogenic lipids. *Atherosclerosis* 86:211, 1991.

18. Curtin, P. D. The slavery hypothesis for hypertension among African Americans: The historical evidence. *American Journal of Public Health* 82:1681, 1992.

19. NIH Nutrition Coordinating Committee. *15th Annual Report, National Institutes of Health Program in Biomedical and Behavioral Nutrition Research and Training.* NIH Publication No. 92-2092, page 75, 1992.

20. Wing, R. R., and others. Environmental and familial contributions to insulin levels and change in insulin levels in middle-aged women. *Journal of the American Medical Association* 268:1890, 1992.

21. The American Dietetic Association. Testimony of The American Dietetic Association: Non-insulin-dependent diabetes mellitus–An unrelenting but undeserved threat to the health of minorities. *Journal of the American Dietetic Association* 92:671, 1992.

22. Horwath, C. C., and Worsley, A. Dietary habits of elderly persons with diabetes. *Journal of the American Dietetic Association* 91:553, 1991.

23. Rose, G. Epidemiology of atherosclerosis. *British Medical Journal* 303:1537, 1991.

24. Gey, K. F., and others. Increased risk of cardiovascular disease at suboptimal plasma concentrations of essential antioxidants: An epidemiological update with special attention to carotene and vitamin C. *American Journal of Clinical Nutrition* 57(suppl):787S, 1993.

25. Wilson, P. W. F., and Kannel, W. B. Is baldness bad for your heart? *Journal of the American Medical Association* 269:1035, 1993.

26. Johnston, D. E., and Kaplan, M. M. Pathogenesis and treatment of gallstones. *New England Journal of Medicine* 328:412, 1993.

27. Thijs, C., and others. Is gallstone disease caused by obesity or by dieting? *American Journal of Epidemiology* 135:274, 1992.

28. Tomezsko, J. L., and others. Dietary intake of healthy children with cystic fibrosis compared with normal control children. *Pediatrics* 90:547, 1992.

29. Hegsted, D. M., and others. Dietary fat and serum lipids: An evaluation of the experimental data. *American Journal of Clinical Nutrition* 57:874, 1993.

30. Nabors, L. O., and Lemieux, R. History of the commercial development of low-calorie foods. In: *Low-Calorie Foods Handbook.* A. M. Altschul, editor, Marcel Dekker, Inc., New York, page 91, 1993.

Think beyond these pictures.
When does our need for
nutrients begin?

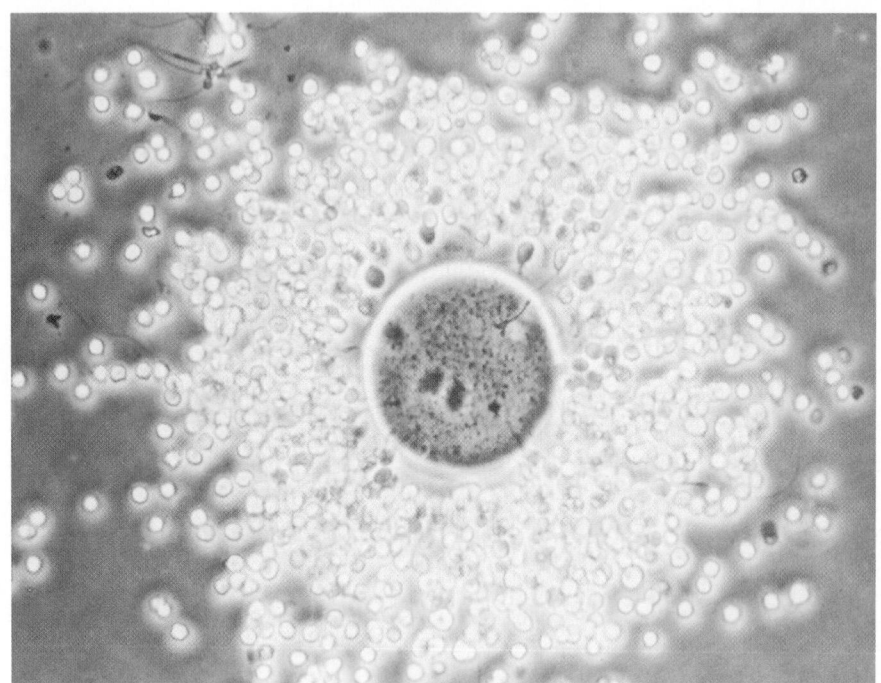

Figure 15-1. A fertilized egg. The nutritional status of the mother is important even in early pregnancy.

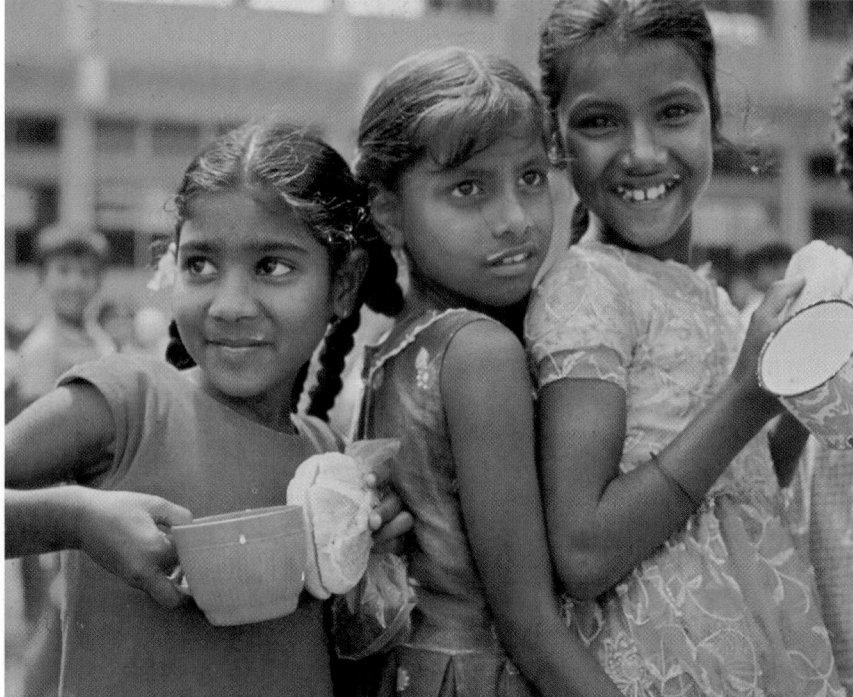

Figure 15-2. Adequate nutrient intake and a safe environment are major factors in a healthy start to life.

Nutrition and the Early Years

■ Nutrition in our lives–Food and nutrient needs begin with the fertilized cell

In this part of the book we take the information for each nutrient and apply it to the changing needs for nutrients from conception to death. This chapter covers the early part of that process.

Nutrient needs begin at conception and change continuously during infancy and throughout the preteen years. The unborn child's nutritional needs are met from the mother's nutrient reserves and from increased nutrient intake. This is why RDA values are higher for pregnant women.

The utilization of these nutrients is influenced by some nondietary factors. Think of the consequences to the growing fetus of certain behaviors of the pregnant mother–going on a weight-loss diet; consuming drugs, caffeine, or alcohol; or smoking cigarettes. We discussed one of these consequences, fetal alcohol syndrome, in Chapter 5. Think also of the stresses beyond the mother's control, such as famine or the transfer of environmental toxicants through the mother to the fetus. Now pause for a moment and consider how many of these influences are of recent origin. Excessive concern with body weight, even in pregnancy, and the widespread use of tobacco, alcohol, and drugs are of recent vintage. Environmental toxicants are mainly products of the industrial revolution of the past 200 years. Only famines have been with us since the earliest of times. It is remarkable that the species survives such stresses.

One other practice during pregnancy is worth mentioning because of its obvious nutritional implications. Since the earliest times, people have manipulated diet during pregnancy in the hope of influencing the gender of the baby.[1] If you wanted a boy, some cultures suggested eating a lot of lettuce or cowpeas or drinking lion's blood and wine. For a girl, they suggested oysters boiled in salted water or a diet high in sweets. Of course, all of these approaches are without scientific basis, but interest in them remains. Some popular books on this topic can be found in your local bookstore.

Think of the implications of the decision either to breast feed or to bottle feed. In the past, breast feeding was the rule, because nutrition knowledge and the science of food were not developed sufficiently to assure a nutritionally balanced substitute for human milk. Bottle feeding has added convenience to people's lives, but there are risks. We saw in Chapter 13 how kwashiorkor is caused mainly by a combination of poverty, lack of education, and poor sanitation in providing a substitute for human milk. Famine and starvation cause a reduction in the quantity of human milk produced by the mother, but there is no reduction in its nutritional value.

Think beyond the photograph in Figure 15-2. Consider the magnificent combinations of nutrients necessary to form the next generation as it grows to adulthood.

Now think of the impact that pregnancy has on the nutrient needs of a 10- to 15-year-old child and her developing fetus. "Children giving birth to children" is how teenage pregnancy is sometimes described. Great care must be exercised to ensure that the growing fetus and the growing mother both meet all of their nutrient needs. This may be difficult in low-income families.

■ Nutritional status before and during pregnancy is important

Pregnancy imposes increased energy and nutrient demands on the woman. Part of the extra nutrient intake is needed for the growth of the fetus–the most rapid growth of a child's life takes place between conception and birth. Part of the extra intake is for tissues in the mother to support pregnancy and lactation, as seen in Figure 15-3.

Figure 15-3.
The recommended dietary allowance (RDA) of nutrients for a woman during pregnancy is higher than for other women (left) in order to meet the additional nutrient demands of the mother and the developing fetus (right).

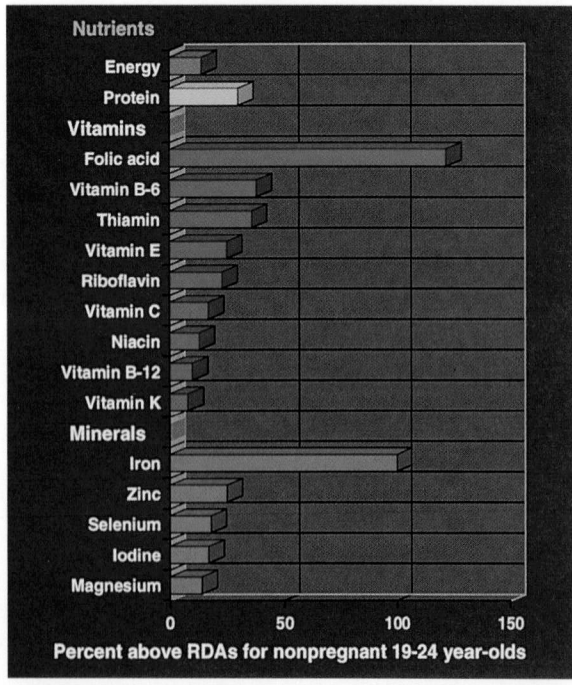

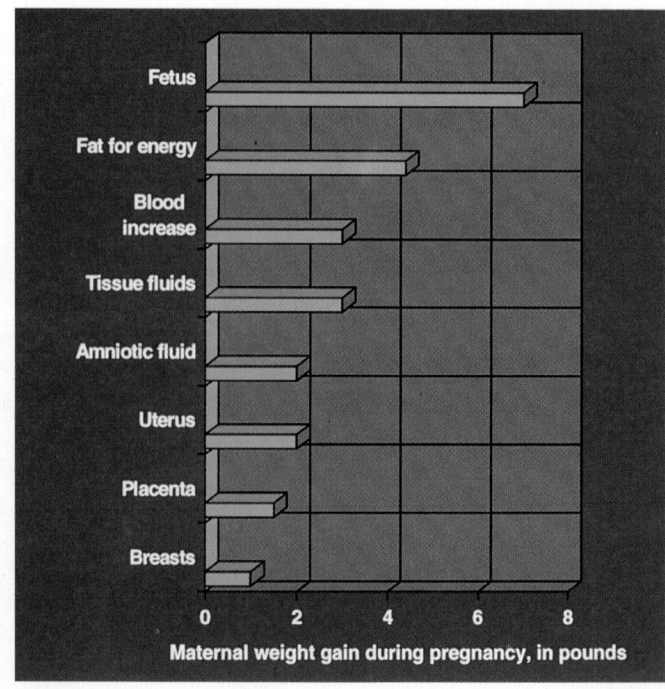

Weight gain in early pregnancy goes mainly toward the mother's tissues (*uterus*, *placenta*, amniotic fluid, increased blood and tissue fluid volume, fat as an energy reserve, and breasts). Weight gain later in pregnancy goes mainly to the growth of the fetus. Certain factors necessitate an even higher weight gain during pregnancy, including low prepregnancy body weight, being a young teenager (less than 2 years after *menarche*), or carrying more than one fetus. Nutrient supplementation for women with poor nutritional status before and during pregnancy improves their nutritional status and prevents the child from having a low birth weight.[2] This is important because babies with low birth weight have lower reserves of nutrients for the rapid growth period after birth and are also more vulnerable to disease. Appropriate nutrient intake is critical for a successful pregnancy, so dietetic and medical advice should be sought as soon as possible.

The following conditions should be monitored before and during pregnancy.[3]

- **Weight and height.** Either obesity or a rapid and substantial weight loss may decrease a woman's ability to conceive.[3] Eating disorders may be suspected if she has a preoccupation with weight, has rapidly changing weight, or has excesses in exercise or diet. Obesity is also associated with many health complications in pregnancy. Women with low weight-to-height ratios are more likely to deliver a low-birth-weight baby with a higher probability of mortality. If weight must be gained or lost, it must be done gradually–no more than 1–2 pounds per week.

Uterus: The organ that contains and nourishes the embryo and fetus from time of conception until time of birth.

Placenta: The organ linking the uterus to the fetus. Nutrients are transferred to the fetus through it.

Menarche: The onset of menstruation.

Think about Figures 15-4 and 15-5. How do they each contribute to "a good start"?

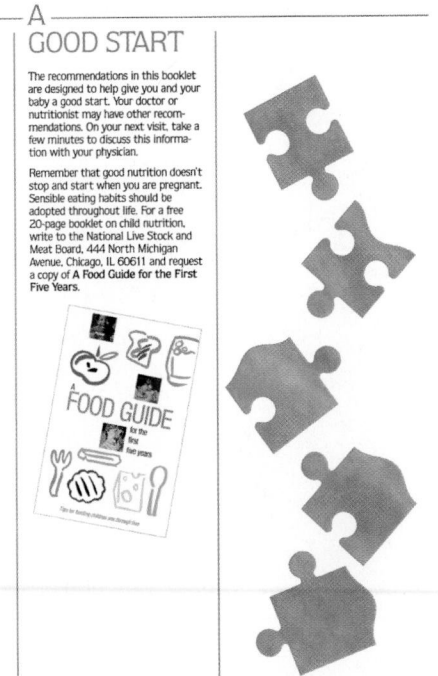

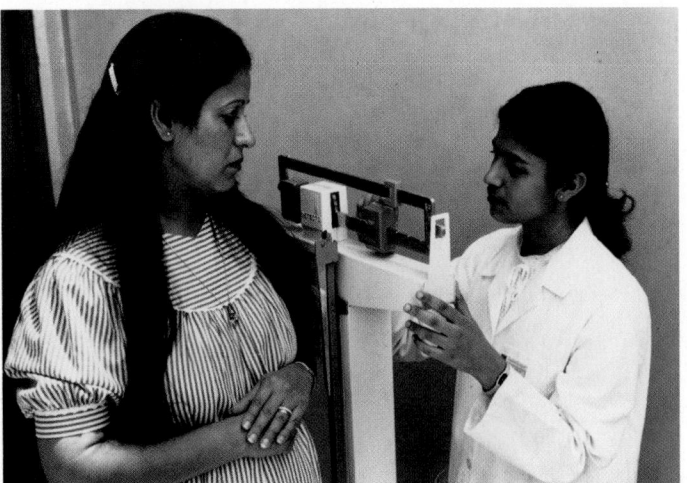

Figure 15-4. Nutrition education allows an expectant mother to successfully fit together the pieces of the dietary puzzle during pregnancy.

Figure 15-5. Monitoring body weight during pregnancy helps to ensure that mothers give birth to children of appropriate body weight.

Teratogen: Anything that causes the development of a severely deformed fetus.

Neural tube defect: A defect in the tube formed where the brain and spinal chord develop, causing brain and motor injury.

- **Use of vitamin and mineral supplements.** Excessive use should be avoided. For example, vitamin A at high levels is a *teratogen*; dosages exceeding 800 RE (4,000 IU) are discouraged. However, not all high intakes of vitamins may be harmful. For example, folacin in larger than normal amounts seems to prevent *neural tube defects*. The Centers for Disease Control in Atlanta recommends that if a woman has a child with a neural tube defect she should consult a physician as soon as she plans another pregnancy. A supplement of 4 milligrams of folacin may be recommended and taken under medical supervision. Folacin supplements after the third month of pregnancy don't protect against neural tube defects; adequate folic acid intake is required *before* conception. This is why there is a growing demand for fortification of foods with folic acid.

Iron supplementation is recommended by the National Academy of Sciences[3] (Table 15-1) because, as we saw in Chapter 10, consuming sufficient iron to meet the demands of menstruation, pregnancy, and lactation may be difficult for women of childbearing years.

Table 15-1. Indications for Nutrient Supplementation

Reproductive Period and Condition	Iron		Low-Dose Multi-Vitamin/Mineral Preparation	Calcium, 600 mg
	30 mg[a,b]	60–120 mg [b,c]		
Preconception, interconception				
Iron deficiency anemia		x	x	
Pregnancy				
Normal	x			
Complete vegetarian			x	
Multiple gestation			x	
Poor-quality diet and resistant to change			x	
Heavy cigarette smoking			x	
Alcohol abuse			x	
Under 25, consuming no protein-rich milk products, and resistant to change			x[d]	x
Iron-deficiency anemia		x	x	
Lactation				
Low energy intake			x	
Low intake of milk products			x[d]	x
Iron deficiency anemia		x	x	

[a] Begin routine iron supplementation for all pregnant women by the 12th week of gestation.
[b] Iron should be taken with juice or water, apart from meals.
[c] Therapeutic doses of iron should be taken apart from other supplements.
[d] The vitamin supplement is indicated to supply vitamin D. Regular exposure to sunshine reduces the need for a supplement.

- **Eating habits.** Habits such as poor appetite, skipping meals, dieting, or omitting a major food group should be corrected. Unfortunately, eating disorders, dietary cravings, and aversions are not uncommon during pregnancy.[4] Women on special diets for medical reasons should consult a dietitian. All other women should follow the Dietary Guidelines to ensure that they get satisfactory nutrient intakes. Table 15-2 contains some suggested measures for improving the nutrient intake of women who restrict what they eat in various ways.

Think about the reasons why nutrient supplementation may be needed in the circumstances shown in the table.

Table 15-2. Suggested Measures for Improving Nutrient Intake of Pregnant Women with Restrictive Eating Patterns

Type of Restrictive Eating Pattern	Corrective Measures
Excessive restriction of food intake, i.e., ingestion of <1,800 kcal of energy per day, which ordinarily leads to unsatisfactory intake of nutrients compared with the amounts needed by lactating women	Encourage increased intake of nutrient-rich foods to achieve an energy intake of at least 1,800 kcal per day. If the mother insists on curbing food intake sharply, promote substitution of foods rich in vitamins, minerals, and protein for those lower in nutritive value. In individual cases, it may be advisable to recommend a balanced multivitamin-mineral supplement. Discourage use of liquid weight-loss diets and appetite suppressants.
Complete vegetarianism, i.e., avoidance of all animal foods, including meat, fish, dairy products, and eggs	Advise intake of a regular source of vitamin B-12, such as special vitamin B-12-containing plant food products or a 2.6-microgram vitamin B-12 supplement daily.
Avoidance of milk, cheese, or other calcium-rich dairy products	Encourage increased intake of other culturally appropriate dietary calcium sources, such as collard greens for people from the southeastern United States. Provide information on the appropriate use of low-lactose dairy products if milk is being avoided because of lactose intolerance. If correction by diet cannot be achieved, it may be advisable to recommend 600 milligrams of elemental calcium per day taken with meals.
Avoidance of vitamin D-fortified foods, such as fortified milk or cereal, combined with limited exposure to ultraviolet light	Recommend 10 micrograms of supplemental vitamin D per day.

- **Use of cigarettes, smokeless tobacco, alcohol, and drugs.** This use should be significantly reduced and preferably eliminated. Here are the reasons why.[3]

  - Impaired fetal growth. Babies born to smokers have lower birth weights, partly because of the negative effect of tobacco and partly because smokers have lower nutrient intake than nonsmokers.[5]
  - Low food intake by the mother. This may be due to decreased appetite (cocaine and amphetamines are appetite suppressants), substitution of alcohol for food, lack of money to spend on food, or any combination of these. Some women who quit smoking or who quit using other harmful substances may be anxious about gaining too much weight. Appropriate diet counseling should help avoid this problem.
  - Increased nutrient requirements. Cigarette smoking increases the metabolism of vitamin C and therefore more of it is required. Alcohol restricts the absorption and utilization of several nutrients and may inhibit the transfer of some nutrients across the placenta.

- **Mental and physical well-being.** The National Academy of Sciences report *Nutrition During Pregnancy and Lactation* emphasizes that signs of depression, battering and other abuse, and poor hygiene usually suggest a less than adequate nutritional intake.[3]

Dietitians and health professionals who are trying to improve a pregnant woman's diet should be aware of cultural differences. Nutrition education for pregnant women in a culturally friendly environment is important.[6] For instance, the foods used in some supplemental feeding programs may be culturally biased and even unfamiliar to people in some cultures. The needs of vegetarians and people who do not absorb lactose (who must obtain calcium from nondairy sources) may not be addressed in some recommendations. Even within the United States, regional differences exist in beliefs about nutrition during pregnancy.[7] Many people harbor unscientific beliefs about food cravings and weight during pregnancy. Examples include:

- If you crave a food, your baby will like that food
- Give in to your cravings or you will give the baby a birthmark
- When you are pregnant, you will crave pickles and ice cream
- Pregnancy is a good time to lose weight
- Obese women don't need to gain weight during pregnancy.

These beliefs are *not* supported by scientific information.

An unscientific practice that is common in some areas during pregnancy is clay eating (pica, see chapter 10). Pica should be discouraged because it may limit nutrient intake, have adverse effects on blood levels of nutrients and on the normal functioning of the GI tract, and introduce toxic substances to the fetus.

So far, we have discussed what a pregnant woman should *not* do. What are the *right* things for her to eat? Here are specific dietary recommendations for pregnant women.

- Eat enough food to gain weight at the rate recommended by your health care provider, as shown on your weight gain chart. Include fruits, vegetables, grains, meat or meat alternates, and milk products in your meals and snacks every day.

- Eat small to moderate-sized meals at regular intervals, and eat nutritious snacks. This will help you to be comfortable and to have the best chance of getting all the nutrients you and your baby need.

- Take three or more servings of milk products daily, either with or between meals. One cup (½ pint) of milk is an example of one serving. Choose low-fat or skim milk products often.

- To absorb more iron, include some meat, poultry, fish, or vitamin-C-rich foods (such as orange juice, broccoli, or strawberries) in your meals.

- Salt your food to taste unless your physician advises you to curb your salt intake because of a medical problem. Your need for salt increases somewhat during pregnancy.

- If you drink coffee or other caffeinated beverages such as cola, do so in moderation (two to three servings or less daily).

- While you are pregnant, the only sure way to avoid the possible harmful effects of alcohol on the fetus is to avoid drinking alcoholic beverages entirely.

■ Lactation: Is breast feeding better than bottle feeding?

Nutritional, economical, and psychological advantages suggest that breast feeding is better for the infant and the mother. The advantages to the infant of breast feeding include the following.

- **Breast milk is the most nutritious first food of life.** Nutrients in breast milk are better balanced and more bioavailable than nutrients in a formula. Human milk has hormones and other bioactive compounds that help in the growth and development of young infants.[8] In developing countries, breast feeding is associated with a substantial reduction of the risk of vitamin A deficiency, extending to the third year of life.[9] This is important because, as we saw in Chapter 9, vitamin A deficiency causes blindness in young children in many countries.

- **Breast milk is less likely to be contaminated by harmful microorganisms.** Contamination is a major problem when formula is prepared

---

Treating Dietary Discomforts During Pregnancy

Nausea and vomiting
Eat crackers, dry cereal, or melba toast.
Eat frequent small meals.
Consume adequate liquids, especially fruit juices.
Avoid tea and coffee or citrus fruit drinks (orange or grapefruit juices) early in the morning. Drink liquids mainly between meals.
Avoid or limit the intake of high-fat or spicy foods.

Heartburn
Eat small, low-fat, and nonspicy meals, slowly.
Eat low-fat snacks–fruit or dry toast.
Drink fluids mainly between meals.
Do not lie down for 1–2 hours after eating or drinking, especially before going to bed.
Wear loose-fitting clothes.

Avoiding constipation
Drink 2–3 quarts of fluids daily (water, milk, juice, soup).
Eat a high-fiber diet–cereals, whole-grains, legumes, fruits, and vegetables.
Increase physical activity, including walking.

Heartburn: A burning sensation caused by acid liquid from the stomach being forced into the esophagus.

under unhygienic conditions and/or with unclean water, resulting in diarrhea.

- **Antibodies in breast milk help prevent infections.** The immunologic properties of breast milk help reduce infant illnesses and deaths during the breast-feeding period.

- **Breast milk is unlikely to cause allergic reactions.** Some proteins in cow's milk may cause allergic reactions in some babies.

- *Colostrum,* **the first milk, protects against infections,** especially in the GI tract during the critical first few days after birth. It also contains growth-promoting substances that are not in cow's milk or formula.

- **Breast feeding provides psychological benefits for the infant** resulting from its intimate relationship with the mother.

- **Breast feeding is considered beneficial in reducing the incidence of infantile obesity.** The infant is not force-fed a bottle formula.

Breast feeding also benefits the mother in several ways.

- **Breast feeding gives the mother feelings of well-being** because of hormonal changes during lactation.

Colostrum: The milk secreted within the first two or three days of lactation; so-called "first milk."

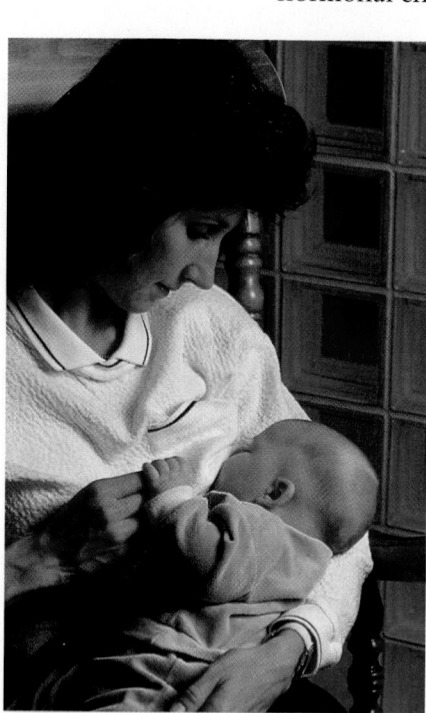

Figure 15-6. Breast feeding is recommended by many doctors because breast milk provides most of the nutrients in amounts required by the infant, provides protection from infections, and is less likely than formula to cause allergic reactions.

- **Loss of fat tissue.** Some of the body fat accumulated during pregnancy is lost during lactation, especially the fat that accumulated on the hips.[10] However, breast feeding does not eliminate all of the fat accumulated during pregnancy, and the amount varies with different women.

- **Breast feeding can be a type of birth control.** Most women who have a complete and uninterrupted breast feeding schedule do not ovulate or menstruate for at least 10 weeks after delivery. However, experts differ on the reliability of breast feeding as a form of birth control.[11] Most say don't count on it.

- **Breast feeding increases the bonding between mother and infant.**

- **Many mothers like the convenience of breast feeding.** There is no preparation, no waste, and little cleanup for breast feeding. It is also becoming acceptable in public places in many countries. If a mother cannot breast feed her child at work or while traveling, she can pump the milk from her breast and leave it in a refrigerator for later use, which allows another person to feed the baby during the mother's absence. The volume of milk secreted is variable among mothers. However, exclusive breast feeding by well-nourished mothers can be adequate for 2–15 months.

- **Breast feeding is economical.** Infant formulas may be costly for low-income families and families in developing countries.

Some suggestions for successful lactation

The following dietary recommendations should be followed for successful lactation.[3]

- **Avoid diets and medications promising rapid weight loss.** Weight loss is usually gradual; it may take several months to reduce to prepregnancy weight.
- **Eat a wide variety of food each day**–breads and cereal grains, fruits, vegetables, dairy products, and meats or meat alternates (for example, beans).
- **Take three or more servings of dairy products each day.**
- **Eat vitamin A-rich fruits and vegetables often.** See Table 4 in Chapter 1 for good sources of vitamin A.
- **Drink fluids often to avoid thirst.**
- **Have only a moderate intake of coffee and other caffeinated drinks such as cola and tea.** Two servings daily are unlikely to harm the infant. Higher intakes result in caffeine passing into breast milk.
- **If environmental contaminants such as mercury or pesticides are problems in the area where certain foods are grown, these foods should be avoided.**

Exercise is encouraged for the lactating mother to reduce some of the body fat accumulated during pregnancy. But some lactating women have difficulty nursing their infants after exercise. When they exercise, some lactic acid is produced in the breakdown of glucose for energy (Chapter 11) and is transferred into the milk. This negatively alters the taste of the mother's milk to the baby.[12]

Smoking and drug use during lactation

No smoking should take place during the months that the baby is being nursed.

If prescription drugs or legal mood-altering drugs are to be used, medical approval should be sought on a case-by-case basis.[3]

Special concerns of some low-income women during pregnancy and lactation

Sometimes women face problems that affect their ability to feed themselves and their children. These may be crisis situations that are short-lived and unanticipated and for which short-term solutions are needed. Here are suggestions for handling some possible problems.

If the local water tastes bad, water containers can be taken to the woman's clinic and filled with water there. Bottled water may be a temporary solution. If there is no refrigeration, ice can be put into a cooler. Many

Special Supplemental Food Program for Women, Infants, and Children (WIC): A government-funded program in the United States that provides food, as well as nutritional and medical support, for low-income women during pregnancy and the first few years of the child's life.

nutritious foods such as peanut butter, bread, fruit, vegetables, and canned foods do not require refrigeration.

For times when there is no money or food stamps to buy food, food pantries and shelters may be available. Pregnant women and women with young children should be sure to sign up for the *Special Supplemental Food Program for Women, Infants, and Children (WIC)*, a U.S. government program that provides extra food for this important period of their lives. This program is discussed in the People Are Different section of this chapter.

If the family has no cooking facilities, a hot plate may sometimes be used in place of a stove. Charcoal grills should never be used indoors. People on the WIC program should ask about the special food package for women without cooking facilities.

Factors influencing the prevalence of breast feeding

Breast feeding is currently "in" in most developed countries, whereas it is declining in popularity in many developing countries. Where it is increasing in popularity, some of the reasons include the following:

- Mothers are educated about the advantages of breast feeding.
- "Natural foods" have been popular since the 1970s, so it became popular to use the most natural food to feed babies.
- Better facilities are now available in hospitals and workplaces.
- Organizations such as the La Leche League offer advice and support on breast feeding.

A number of factors are involved in determining which mothers are most likely to breast feed their infants. In the United States, breast feeding is performed by over half of all white women and nearly half of all Hispanic women, but by only a quarter of all African-American women. It is more popular among older women in all racial groups and among high-income and college-educated women. Women living in the Pacific and Mountain regions of the United States are most likely to breast feed their infants. Many fathers harbor myths and misconceptions about breast feeding. To provide greater family support for nursing mothers, fathers should be included in breast-feeding education programs.[13]

We return to the topic of breast feeding at the end of this chapter, where we consider some connections between breast milk and the environment.

■ Undernutrition in pregnancy and lactation

Think beyond Figures 15-7 and 15-8. How might undernutrition be related to bottle feeding or to food contamination?

Undernutrition results from lack of food or lack of nutritious food. During a child's early life, it may be caused by unsanitary environments, especially in the preparation of substitutes for breast milk. One or more of the many sources of contamination may affect the baby's food and have negative effects on its nutritional status. However, the hygienic quality of the food, including the water in formula, can be controlled by appropriate food safety measures, as shown in the diagram.

Undernutrition during pregnancy and lactation usually is found where many nutrition problems begin–with a lack of money. The babies in Figure 15-7 have been born into a situation characterized by poverty, lack of education, too many young children, poor hygienic conditions, and lowered resistance to infection–the result of a series of interacting factors at the local and national level.

The poorest countries in the world have the highest prevalence of undernutrition. Lack of capital for industrialization or for farm improvements leads to insufficient renewal of agricultural investments and practices. Food production drops, and there is less variety in available foods. Family income decreases, resulting in less food being available for the family. Malnutrition results, which decreases the working capacity of the parents, resulting in low productivity. This in turn reduces family income further, causing a progressive worsening in living conditions, including sanitation. Diarrhea and infectious diseases result, which in turn worsen the malnutrition.

Economics and the ability to grow or purchase food are at the center of this discussion. The effect of undernutrition on brain development is of great concern because undernutrition influences the child's motor and intellectual development, hindering the child's physical and mental abilities to function satisfactorily in modern society. Hence, it affects the nation's ability to compete globally. The latest research suggests that poor diet has relatively more negative effects on motor development than on mental development in young children.[14]

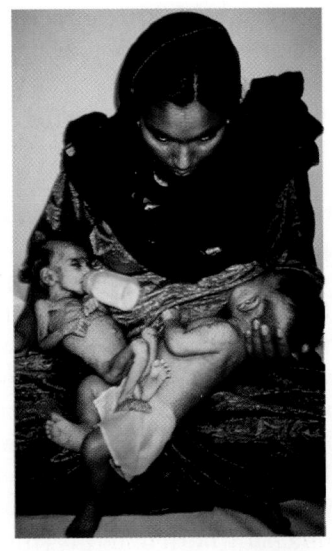

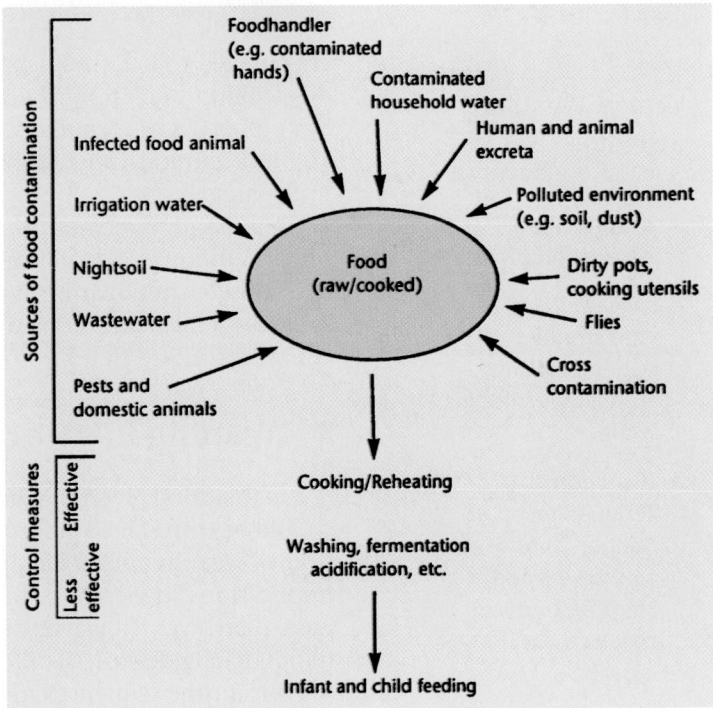

Figures 15-7 and 15-8. Bottle feeding (left), although necessary or desirable in some situations, may introduce harmful bacteria and toxins into the infant's food unless precautions are taken. The sources of contamination (below) are numerous but can be controlled by proper handling of food.

In some cultures, the father is given the largest amount of scarce food, with the smallest amount going to the mother and young children. Some Dutch and Indonesian researchers remind us that the health of undernourished mothers is frequently forgotten.

> Maternal nutrition has been studied in relation to fetal growth, lactation, and infant growth but the effect of reproduction on woman's nutritional status has received limited attention.[15]

They conclude that undernutrition among women of reproductive age is primarily a result of low energy intakes.

Premature Babies and Nutrient Intake

Human milk banks: Expressed human milk saved for future use; found in many countries, including the United Kingdom.

Until recently, the mortality rate among premature babies was high, mostly because of respiratory problems. Advances in technology have helped manage these problems, but the remaining problems associated with premature births can involve nutrition. A large flow of nutrients from the mother to the fetus occurs in the last three months of pregnancy. The infant's fat is increased sevenfold, and there are increases in the amount of calcium, iron, phosphorus, potassium, nitrogen, and other nutrients in its body. When the infant is born 3 months premature, these nutrients must be provided by the diet. Some studies suggest that fat content is higher in the mother's milk when the baby is born preterm but that the concentrations of most minerals and vitamins are similar to those in milk produced for a baby born at term. This amount may not be sufficient for the premature baby, in which case medical advice is necessary. Moreover, preterm babies may be too weak or immature to suck effectively. Mothers should be encouraged to help the baby overcome this difficulty because of the better digestibility and immunological properties of their milk compared with the properties of formulas or of term milk drawn from a *human milk bank*. Medical opinion is mixed on the effectiveness, cost, and need for human milk banks.[16]

There is no agreement on the amount of supplementation needed for preterm infants' diets. Formulas designed for preterm infants are preferred over pooled milk-bank samples if the premature infant's own mother's milk is not available. Pooled milk-bank samples have nutrient contents adequate for full-term infants only.

■ Weaning foods are important

The first food given to a baby teaches it to eat rather than to suck. Foods should be introduced gradually, beginning at about 4–6 months. The exact time of weaning has social, psychological, environmental, and nutritional implications. If weaning starts too early, the infant may become sick and have diarrhea.[17] However, the baby's GI tract and kidneys are capable of handling a wide variety of foods by its first birthday.

Typical time sequences for the introduction of various foods in a regular feeding pattern are shown in the margin.

The choice of foods given at weaning varies throughout the world. They should be chosen carefully because body weight increases about 150% during the first year of life. Changes in body weight should be measured against reference standards (Figure 15-9).

Energy intake during the first year of life is critical for the synthesis of tissues. The liberation of energy needs thiamin, riboflavin, and niacin as coenzymes; protein and amino acid metabolism requires vitamin B-6. Infants born to mothers who took megadoses of vitamin C during preg-

Typical Weaning Schedule

4–6 months
Iron-fortified cereals for infants.

6–8 months
Add strained vegetables and fruits. Give juice in a cup.

7–10 months
Strained meats, "finger" foods such as crackers and small amounts of ready-to-eat cereals.

9–12 months
Gradually change from strained foods to chopped, well-cooked foods or canned foods prepared without added salt or sugar.

nancy may have higher requirements for vitamin C. These infants should probably be given 25–50 milligrams of vitamin C per day. Breast milk may not contain sufficient vitamin D. Extra vitamin D may be necessary for infants born in the northern United States and Canada because of the lack of sufficient sunshine. If the child is fed a vegan diet, it is critically important that a wide variety of plant foods be offered.

Education is sometimes needed to ensure that food is safe for the baby when it is prepared in the home. These precautions include:

- Clean hands and utensils thoroughly before starting.
- Use fresh, high-quality fruits, vegetables, and meats.
- Use as little water as possible to prepare the food to prevent loss of water-soluble nutrients.
- Do not overcook because heat-sensitive nutrients such as some vitamins and amino acids may be lost.
- Do not use salt, and use sugar sparingly. Do not give honey to babies under 1 year of age because of the risk of botulism.
- Do not allow food to stand at room temperature for long periods for microbiological safety reasons.
- Strain or puree the food.
- To make extra servings, pour the puree into an ice cube tray and freeze it.
- Thaw and heat in a serving container the amount of food needed for a single feeding. Heat in a microwave oven or a water bath. Be careful to handle the food in such a way that foodborne microbes are not introduced.

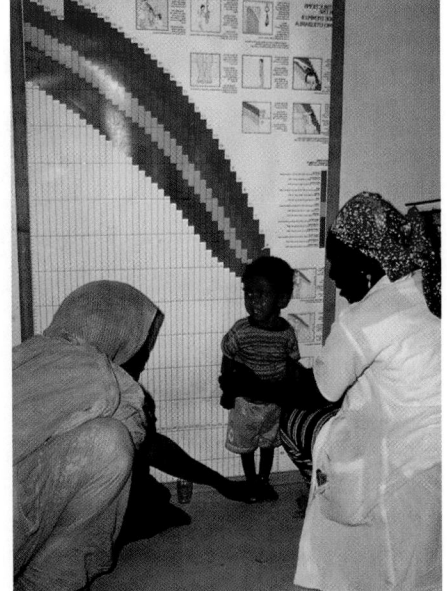

Figure 15-9. Changes in body weight and height are useful measures of dietary quality during the growing years.

Some nutrition habits should be avoided during weaning. Don't force the baby to empty its bowl, plate, or cup. Balance the baby's food intake with its activity. Never use food or drink as a reward. Don't cultivate a liking for sweet or salty foods. Infants can appreciate the natural flavors of fruits and vegetables just as they are; it is adults who feel that food needs more sugar or salt for it to taste "right." Babies develop a liking for salt at about 4 months of age. We are still learning about their taste buds and their short-lived dislikes for particular foods.

Adults can help prevent tooth decay at an early age. Don't check the temperature or taste of the baby's food by putting the spoon in your mouth and then placing it in the baby's mouth. The baby's teeth are just erupting, and they are sensitive to a bacterium called *Streptococcus mutans*, which causes dental caries. Saliva from adults is the usual transmitter of the bacterium to the infant. If you must test the temperature of a baby's food, it's best to just touch it to your wrist so that it will not come into contact with your saliva.

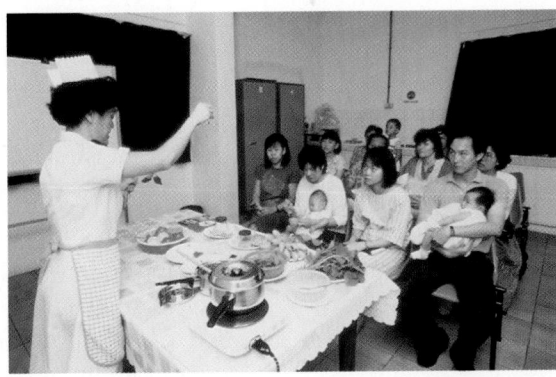

Figure 15-10. Parents in a nutrition class. Information about the nutritional value of different foods and how to increase food safety can help parents improve their children's diets.

■ Toddler to teen: A period of changing eating patterns

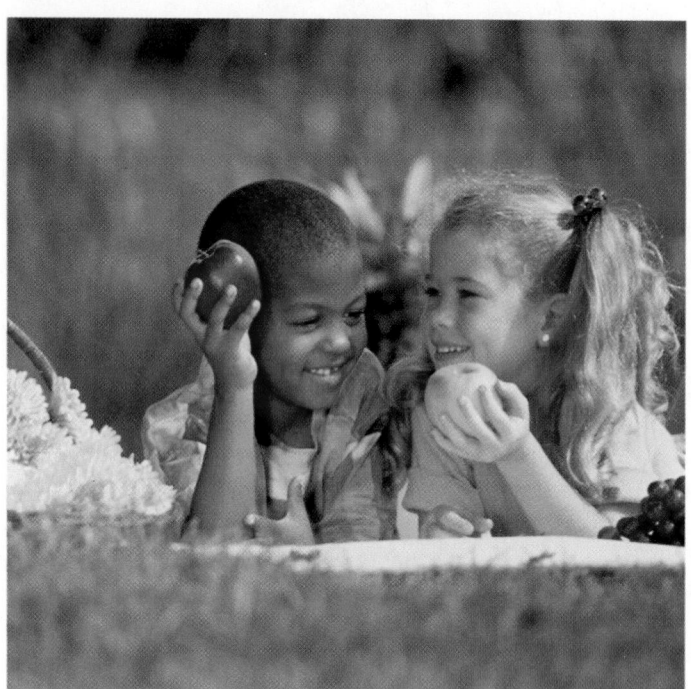

Figure 15-11. Having fun while eating nutritious foods is part of developing a healthy attitude toward eating.

Morbidity: The state of being diseased.

The Preschool Years

These children are at a period of life where food choice is an expression of independence from parents; it helps them express their individuality. If the children in this picture had been born with low birth weights due to nutritional and other problems during pregnancy, they probably would not be the healthy children you see here. Children born with low birth weight have increased *morbidity* at early school age.[18] Proper nutrition for children is critical during this period of rapid growth.

Healthy preschoolers have a variety of emotional, eating, and feeding behaviors of which people looking after young children should be aware, according to Dr. Madeleine Sigman-Grant of Pennsylvania State University. Some of these are listed in Table 15-3.

Food is fun during the preschool age, although children at this age have dislikes as well as likes. For example:

- **Flavors.** Mild flavors are liked; strong or tart flavors are disliked.
- **Colors.** Best liked are orange, green, and yellow.
- **Textures.** Dry foods are difficult to eat. It is best to serve a variety of textures at each meal–one soft food, one crisp, one chewy.
- **Familiarity.** Children like familiar foods. New foods should be introduced gradually in small amounts.

Preschoolers should be allowed to play with their food. Watch a child have fun making a "gravy lake" using meat as "boulders," mashed potatoes as "concrete," and peas to plug any holes in the dam. The child is using food for fun and to attract attention–and the food is eventually eaten.

Parents should not be alarmed if appetite and interest in food vary from time to time. The preschool stage is a time of great change, including the type of food eaten. Many children at this age are not ready biologically or psychologically to be regulated into an adult pattern of three meals per day.

If eating patterns are sometimes irregular, how can balanced nutrient intake be assured? Here are a few suggestions:

- Choose from the suggested foods in the Food Guide Pyramid.
- Use variety within each food group.

Table 15-3. Observed Emotional, Eating, and Feeding Behaviors of Preschoolers

Age (yr)	Emotional Behaviors	Eating Behaviors	Feeding Behaviors
1–2	*Neophobia* Sharing is difficult Requires constant supervision Enjoys helping but can't be left alone Curious Often defiant Eager for attention	"Finicky" eater Food jags Holds food in mouth without swallowing	*One-year-old* Uses spoon with some skill (especially if hungry) Has good control of cup-lifts, drinks, sets it down, holds with one hand Helps self-feed *Two-year-old* Masters big arm muscle movements
3	The "me too" age—wants to be included in everything Responds well to options rather than demands Sharing is still difficult Somewhat rigid about the "right" way to do things	Eats most foods except for certain vegetables Dawdles over food when not hungry Comments on how foods are served	Uses spoon in semiadult fashion; may spear with fork Medium hand muscle development Feeds self independently, especially if hungry
4	Shares well Needs adult approval and attention—shows off Understands; needs limits Follows rules most of the time Still rigid about the "right" way to do things	Eating and talking get in the way—prefers to talk Strong food likes and dislikes Refuses to eat to the point of tears	Uses all eating utensils Small finger muscle development
5	Helpful and cooperative with family chores and routines Still somewhat rigid about the "right" way to do things Very attached to mother, home, and family	Likes familiar foods, prefers most vegetables raw Latches onto food dislikes of family members and declares these as own	Fine coordination in fingers and hands

- Restrict the intake of low-nutrient foods such as sweets, fats, oils, and sugar.
- Fiber intake should be adequate but not so high as to cause GI tract disturbances.
- Supplements are not necessary if the diet is adequate and varied. Iron is the one nutrient for which supplementation may be necessary. Children from families with inadequate food may need supplementation of a number of nutrients.

Neophobia: Dread of or aversion to novelty.

Parents who are vegans can successfully rear their children on a vegan diet provided sufficient care is taken to avoid foods that are too bulky or

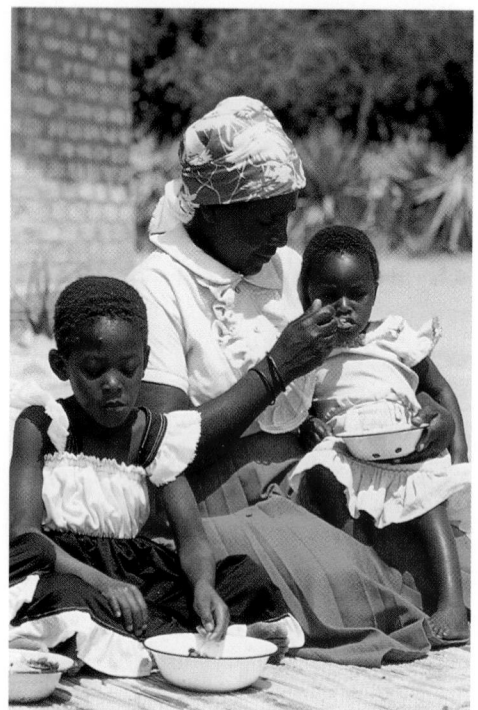

Figure 15-12. Food is an integral part of social interaction for all age groups in all parts of the world.

diets that are deficient in vitamin B-12. Diets exclusively from plant foods tend to be bulky, which is a problem because the stomachs of infants and preschoolers cannot deal with large volumes of food. Children on vegan diets may also have deficiencies in vitamin D, riboflavin, iron, zinc, calcium, and protein because these nutrients are found in highest amounts in foods of animal origin. In addition, limited food choices are offered by some vegan diets, and appropriate meals and snacks may be harder to find for vegan children than for nonvegan children. Diet counseling may improve their nutrient intake.

Parents who consume macrobiotic diets with almost no foods of animal origin or fat are usually highly educated, yet their dietary practices can cause their children to have energy and calcium intakes that are up to 60% less than the intake by children of similar age on conventional diets.[19]

The Preteen Years

The years from 6 to 12 are peaceful relative to those of infancy and adolescence. Appetite and growth show no wide fluctuations, and there is greater interest in food. Energy is expended in sports, and most children do not yet have the preoccupation with body size that comes with adolescence.

Surveys show that intakes of magnesium, copper, and vitamin B-6 may be low in North American children. Although some children may have low intakes of vitamins A and C and calcium, clinical signs of deficiency are not usually evident. This is a period of ready acceptance of food. Plate waste is less than in adolescence, even for school lunch programs. Still, there is some waste–girls seem to do more of it than boys–and some food is refused. Usually the lowest refusal rate is for desserts, fruits, and milk, and the highest is for vegetables and mixed casseroles.

The Cost of Feeding a Family

Food is an investment in future growth and health, and it comes at considerable cost to most families. The USDA gives detailed estimates of food costs for families and for family members at various ages. Table 15-4 gives some of the latest figures.

Table 15-4. Cost of Food at Home

	Cost for 1 Week			
	Thrifty Plan	Low-Cost Plan	Moderate-Cost Plan	Liberal Plan
Family of four	$72.30	90.50	110.40	135.60
Each additional child (9–11 years)	$20.50	26.20	33.60	38.80

This means that a family of four on the thrifty plan will pay $3,760 a year and one on the liberal plan will pay $7,050. Do your own quick calculation to see the amount of money spent on food to bring you from a toddler to a teen.

Do these numbers seem high to you? Feeding a family is expensive. Yet, the cost of providing nutritious food is less than the cost that results when children are poorly fed. The amounts above do not include the extra costs brought about by nutrition problems, such as medical costs for the treatment of diarrhea, infections, or protein malnutrition. They do not count the economic costs and nutritional impact of the drug and alcohol abuse that are growing problems among preteens[20] or of eating disorders. Nor do they include the costs that will result later from faulty nutrition. These range from reduced earning power resulting from slow brain development due to malnutrition, to the high medical costs of treating coronary heart disease and other diseases of affluence or money wasted on worthless weight-loss programs. Since food is an important component of many costs, we should better understand the factors that are important in making nutritious food choices.

Food Selection

Many factors determine the quantity and quality of food consumed. Family resources important in food choices include income, the number of children and their ages, the education and occupations of the parents, and the type of housing and kitchen facilities. When housing is poor and kitchens have inadequate refrigeration, food choice may be limited and food safety may be a problem.

The way a family operates and communicates is important to a child's nutritional status. For example, the ability of the parents to prepare nutritious meals and the amount of permissiveness they show in allowing their children to consume any kind of food irrespective of its nutritional value have direct influences on the nutrient intake of the child's diet. Their ability to understand that a child's pattern of food intake changes as the child develops affects the kinds and amounts of foods they offer. Parents may also influence their child's attitude about food and thus indirectly affect what the child eats. For instance, if they use food as a weapon in disciplining the child or transfer fears, phobias, and tensions about food to the child, they may cause the child to avoid all or some types of food. Researchers at the University of Nebraska, Omaha, tell us that more than one-quarter of American children have eating problems that began before adolescence. Table 15-5 shows some behaviors they found.

Think beyond the information in Table 15-5. Which of these behaviors will probably have a positive impact on the child's long-range nutritional status?

According to the authors of an article that considers the important topic of nutritional messages,

Table 15-5. Food-Related Behaviors of Parents: Some of the Most and Least Used Behaviors

Behavior	Percent Reported Using
Allow the child enough time to eat	87
Ask child to help prepare food or set table	85
Allow child to make decisions about the type of food eaten	81
Give small portions when introducing a new food	81
Promise a special food, such as dessert, for eating a meal	56
Withhold food as a punishment	55
Threaten punishment for not eating	11
Make child clean the plate	10
Give food to calm the child	10
Praise child for eating healthy foods	8

Sibling: One of two or more children of the same parents.

The ultimate intervention to combat fear of obesity and restrictive eating among growing children must be at the societal level. Parents, significant others, and the media must alter their expectations for children's body sizes and shapes and help children feel that they are loved and respected regardless of physical appearance.[21]

Some characteristics of the child also influence the important process of food selection. Age and birth order are important, especially in poor families. There may not be much food left for the youngest child in some large families. Gender bias in some parts of the world, Latin America for example, favors boys with respect to the amount of food available.[22] Due to gender bias in energy intake, boys typically have higher rates of weight gain than girls at 1–2 years of age.

Benefits of School Lunch and Breakfast Programs

The National School Lunch Program began in 1946 as a consequence of the U.S. military's dissatisfaction with the nutritional status of recruits for World War II. Today the program provides subsidized lunches either free or reduced in price for needy children. Full-priced lunches are provided for nonneedy children. The School Breakfast Program was started in 1966 for low-income children and by 1972 was available to all children in school districts having the program. School districts encourage parents to cooperate with the program. Of concern to nutritionists is the fact that many eligible children do not participate. Reasons given include negative or indifferent attitudes of parents and children and the structure of the family. This includes the age of *siblings*, family schedules, walking distance to school, and the appeal of ethnically appropriate menus at school. Factors within schools that may discourage participation in the programs include a lack of atmosphere and support in terms of busing schedules, cafeteria facilities, meal preparation, content and variety, time allowed for breakfast, supervision, and ineffective promotion of the program.[23] Recently, many school lunch programs have worked to provide tasty food choices that are low in fat and sodium and acceptable to the students.[24]

Correction of Children's Diets Is Attracting the Attention of Nutritionists

Nutrition research is finding increasing evidence that some adult nutrition problems begin in childhood. For example, obesity in childhood is related to increased mortality in middle age, with coronary heart disease being the greatest cause of death.[25] Restricting calories in the diet, as a means of inducing weight loss, has seldom been used as a treatment of obesity in infancy for fear that permanent stunting of growth may occur. However, new evidence suggests that caloric restriction and weight reduction may be achieved safely in selected obese infants when the weight loss clearly will bring nutritional and clinical advantages.[26] Changes in weight, growth in height, head circumference, and the amount of fat-free mass in the body must be carefully monitored.

Think about the numbers in the margin. Children can put on unwanted pounds as easily as adults can.

Some attention to weight loss in childhood is important because predictions of overweight in middle age are related to body mass index (BMI) in early life. These predictions are more reliable for males than for females.[27] Several explanations are given for this gender difference. One is that the growth spurt at puberty is associated with a greater increase in adipose tissue in females than in males. Another reason is that adult women are far more likely than adult men to consciously alter their weight by dieting, and thus their BMI later in life may be lowered.

We have seen several times that obesity is a high risk factor in coronary heart disease. Another risk factor is high levels of cholesterol in the blood. Screening of blood cholesterol is done for adults and can also be done for children. However, the American Academy of Pediatrics is concerned that cholesterol screening of children may lead to overly restrictive diets at a time of maximum growth. One study found that about one-third of the children screened had cholesterol levels above the recommended cutoff point of 175 milligrams per 100 milliliters.[28] Adults would have been rechecked. But hints of a lack of enthusiasm for further testing of the children came from statements such as "not sure test machine was accurate," or "child too traumatized by finger stick," or "will try low-cholesterol diet before recheck." Many parents thought that concentrating on the elevated cholesterol level "would make the child worry too much." Also, pediatricians and parents are interested in immediate health rather than in a problem that may or may not develop until 30–50 years later. In summary, many children may benefit from cholesterol screening, but the medical community is divided on its advantages.[29] Some argue that children with high blood cholesterol levels do not necessarily become adults with high cholesterol levels. A counterargument is that potential public health benefits support childhood screening of cholesterol

> Only 50 extra calories per day will put on 5 pounds of body fat in 1 year. Children can get these extra 50 calories from a variety of foods, including any one of the following:
>
> 1/3 of a small ice cream cone
>
> 1/4 of a serving of french fries at a fast-food outlet
>
> 1/3 of an ounce of plain chocolate
>
> 1/2 of an ounce of hard candy
>
> 1/3 of a can of regular cola beverage.

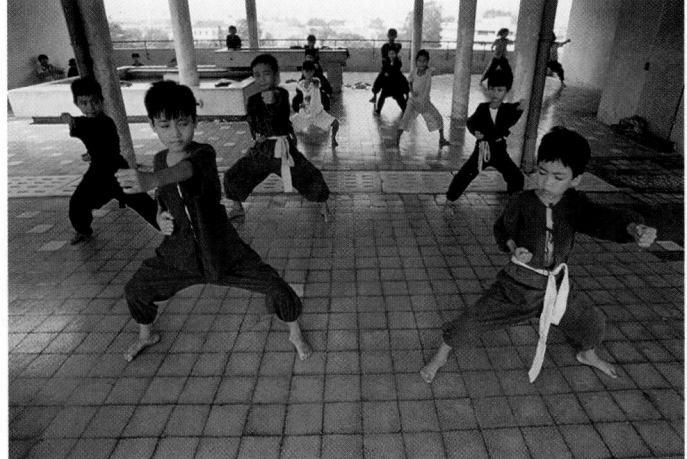

Figure 15-13. Exercise is important for children as well as for adults.

levels. The argument as to whether the medical and economic gains outweigh the risks of screening has yet to be settled, although the evidence tends to suggest that they do.

Behavioral Problems Do Not Seem to Have a Connection with Diet

Hyperactivity, also called hyperkinesis, attention deficit hyperactivity disorder (ADHD), or minimal brain dysfunction, occurs in some children. It has many ill-defined symptoms including overactivity, short attention span, and impulsive behavior. The child has an inability to stick to activities, including play. Measurement of these symptoms is often done subjectively, and thus a child's behavior may appear different to parents than to teachers. We are even unsure as to the exact number of children who may suffer from hyperactivity. The American Psychiatric Association estimates that about 3% of preadolescent children suffer from ADHD, with the disorder about six to nine times more common in boys than in girls. Other estimates place the incidence in the United States at levels up to 20%. Hyperactive children are of normal or above-average intelligence.

Here is why nutritionists are interested in hyperactivity in children. In the 1970s, Dr. Benjamin Feingold, a pediatrician and allergist, proposed a connection between hyperactivity and a range of food additives, including salicylates. His ideas appealed to many parents of children with discipline problems. This was at a time when people were finding links between natural foods and the environment, having concerns about the safety of food, and feeling alarm about the overuse of medications.

Dr. Feingold suggested that foods containing natural salicylates should be removed from the diets of hyperactive children. These foods include apples, all berries, oranges, raisins, tomatoes, green peppers, and cucumbers. Removal of salicylate-rich foods and foods containing additives was supposed to decrease hyperactive behavior. Even though experiments were conducted, they were not conclusive; it was difficult to avoid subjective input into the conclusions and the involvement of other components in the diet. Most scientists now conclude that claims about diet and hyperactivity were overstated and that only a small percentage of hyperactive children react negatively to food additives.[30] Preschool children may be more sensitive to them than older children. Most experts agree that further research is needed with better methodology to determine whether there are any relationships between diet and hyperactivity.

Does sugar intake cause hyperactivity in children? Many educators, parents, and some physicians think that it has a negative effect on classroom behavior.[30] However, to date, no well-designed experiment has shown a relationship between sugar intake and ADHD.

■ People are different–Supplemental feeding programs during pregnancy and lactation

Think about the importance of the following recommendation from the American Dietetic Association, published in March 1993.

To protect the nutritional health of children and to promote their optimal health and nutritional status, The American Dietetic Association recommends that the following basic child nutrition services be available to all children, regardless of economic status, race, special needs, or national origin:

- Access for all children to optimal amounts of health-promoting foods.
- Food programs that provide nutritious, appealing, wholesome foods that reflect the U.S. Dietary Guidelines for Americans, served in an environment that encourages its acceptance.
- Meals that serve as a laboratory to apply critical thinking skills to food selection.
- Nutrition education for parents and their children, and professional education and in-service training for teachers and others involved in the nutrition care of children.
- Nutrition screening to identify children at risk.
- Dietary assessment and counseling to meet special health needs.
- Referral to food assistance programs and services.

This statement recognizes that some children have inadequate nutrient intake and discourages discrimination because of economic status, race, special need, or national origin. Children at risk of nutrient deficiencies live in all countries throughout the world. In the United States, the Special Supplemental Food Program for Women, Infants, and Children (WIC), which serves women and children during pregnancy and early childhood, is associated with reduced *Medicaid* costs and increased infant birth weight. For every $1.00 spent on WIC services, the Medicaid saving in costs for newborn medical care was estimated to be $2.91.[31]

Medicaid: A U.S. government program covering medical expenses of low-income individuals.

WIC meets the nutritional needs of eligible pregnant women and preschool children by providing nutritional screening, food assistance, nutrition education, and health and social service referrals. Among the requirements for participation in WIC are having an income of 185% of the poverty level or less and being at nutritional risk as determined by a medical or nutritional assessment. Risk factors include anemia, extreme thinness or obesity, the mother being young, a poor pregnancy history, and dietary risks resulting from unsatisfactory food intake. Women must be pregnant or breast feeding or have an eligible child less than 5 years old. Supplemental food is provided through vouchers or checks that are exchanged for certain foods in stores. Included are iron-fortified infant formula, eggs, fruit and vegetable juices rich in vitamin C, milk and cheese, dried peas or beans, iron-fortified adult and infant cereals, and peanut

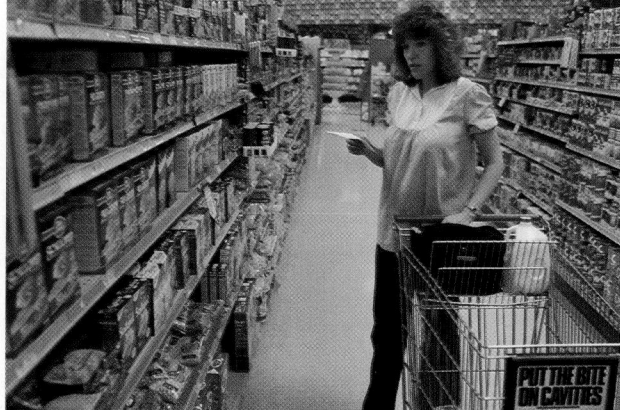

Figure 15-14. Good food choices are necessary before and during pregnancy. The Special Supplemental Food Program for Women, Infants, and Children (WIC) provides food assistance, nutrition education, nutritional screening, and health and social service referrals.

butter. These foods are chosen to prevent the deficiencies of protein, vitamins A and C, iron, and calcium that are often found in low-income families. A portion of the WIC funds that go to local agencies must be spent on nutrition education and counseling.

The WIC program now serves over 5 million people at a cost of over $2.3 billion and has had considerable success in combating malnutrition. Its successes include improvements in average birth weight, reductions in the incidence of low birth weight, decreased incidence of fetal mortality, and reduced Medicaid costs after birth. An additional advantage is that it gets mothers from low-income families to use health-care facilities more often.[32] In summary, WIC is seen by most nutritionists, medical practitioners, social workers, politicians, and participants to be a success in meeting the nutrient needs of low-income women and their young children.

■ Nutrition in action–Environmental factors and foods eaten by the young

How best to feed infants is an area of nutrition with plenty of incomplete scientific observations, folklore, emotion, and commercial manipulation. It is understandable that people want the first food of life to be as nutritious, pure, and healthful as possible. Experts contend that breast feeding is the best way to ensure that the baby gets the most appropriate food. This point has been emphasized in editorials and commentaries in medical journals in recent years. For example, the *British Medical Journal*[33] has pointed out that the European Community may ban advertising of infant formulas (substitutes for breast milk) and follow-on milks (formulas for babies over 4 months) to encourage breast feeding. Laws of this kind were passed in Australia[34] and in India.[35]

Although there is little argument that breast feeding is the best way to feed infants, there is growing concern that problems caused by society are affecting some breast milk. We have mentioned that the HIV virus may be transmitted in breast milk to the infant (see the Preface). Pesticides such as DDT and some drugs have been found in human milk since the 1950s and 1960s. In fact, testing human milk has been proposed as an effective way to determine whether the general population is exposed to environmental chemicals.[36] Many environmental toxicants that come through in the food supply are fat-soluble and therefore soluble in the fat in breast milk. It is much easier and less painful to test milk fat than to take a biopsy sample from a body fat deposit. Some studies show that children fed milk containing fat-soluble environmental contaminants have reduced body weight, slower psychomotor development, and a vitamin K deficiency that causes hemorrhages. Human milk samples were used also to measure the impact on the food supply of a major disaster that occurred at a nuclear power station in Chernobyl in the former Soviet Union in the mid-1980s.

All of this is of great concern, but the British Medical Association puts the problem in perspective with respect to the presence of one type of contaminant, pesticides, in human milk.

> Although the presence of pesticide residues in breast milk is an area of genuine concern, both because of the risk to infants and as an indicator of levels of pollution in the environment, it is important that women should not be led to believe that breast feeding is in some way less healthy than using formula feeds.[37]

Breast milk still remains the most effective way to feed infants for the reasons explained earlier in this chapter. Bottle feeding often presents problems because of inadequate sanitation and unsafe water supplies. Even where the water is safe, large amounts of lead are sometimes found in infant formula when domestic water supplies are used.[38] This problem arises as a result of the popularity of powdered and concentrated formulas, which are economical and convenient, requiring the addition of water only.

An additional environmental hazard that may exist in infant feeding is infant botulism, which can occur in either bottle feeding or breast feeding. Many cases of infant botulism were traced to the consumption of honey, corn syrup, or other nonsterilized foods and nonfood items that contained *Clostridium botulinum* spores. It is recommended that food not essential for nutrition, such as honey or corn syrup, not be given to infants. Some cases of infant botulism are fatal, and others cause nerve problems for the infant.[39]

We have looked at a few documented and scientifically confirmed environmental hazards in infant foods. Of even greater concern is the manipulation of the media and the public to create an unnecessary scare about the safety of food fed to infants.

Think beyond the picture in Figure 15-15. How could apples cause a nutritional uproar?

There is little argument about the positive nutritive value of apples. Take a moment to check the table of food composition in the Appendix to find the significant amounts of minerals, vitamins, and other nutrients that apples contribute to our diet. Apple sauce and apple juice have been a staple in infants' diets for decades. Yet, apples, like some other foods, have been the subject of some consumer concern in recent years. Not all of this concern has been based on sound scientific facts–the Alar scare with apples is a good example.

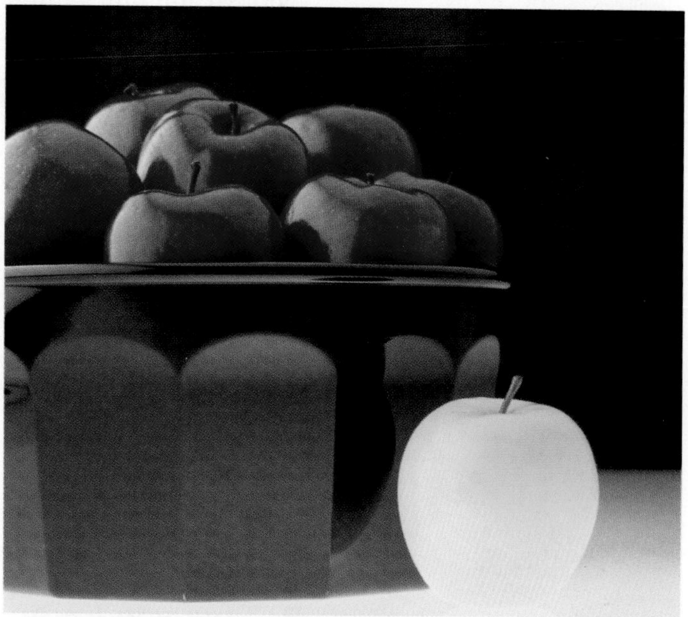

The controversy over Alar and apples was a classic case of a false scare that damaged the apple industry, unnecessarily scared parents, and damaged the credibility of sections of the media. Here is how one observer introduces the topic:[40]

Figure 15-15. Apples make nutritious snacks for both children and adults. The safety of this familiar food was questioned for a short time during the Alar scare.

The Great Apple Scare of 1989 [was] the result of one of the slickest, most cynical fear campaigns in recent American history. The immediate target was Alar . . . a growth regulator used to promote uniform ripening of red apples and to improve the fruit's appearance. That chemical, which had been used for twenty-one years with no observable ill effects and which had been knowingly allowed to remain on the market by the Environmental Protection Agency (EPA), was suddenly tried, convicted, and sentenced to death by the media.

Here is some background showing why some people were concerned about the use of Alar in foods for infants and young children. When Alar is heated, it is transformed into another chemical called UDMH (unsymmetrical dimethylhydrazine), which causes tumors in mice. Apple juice and apple sauce are popular foods fed to babies. They are heated in their manufacture, resulting in the conversion of Alar into UDMH.

In 1989, the Natural Resources Defense Council (NRDC), an environmental pressure group in the United States, published a report alleging that children under 6 years of age are especially vulnerable to cancer-causing pesticides because of the likelihood of their consuming more fruits and vegetables than adults relative to body size. The news media, especially television, picked up on the report, resulting in much public attention. Schools removed apples, apple juice, and apple sauce from lunch menus. Organic food stores reported increased demand for pesticide-free food. Some Hollywood personalities joined the campaign against Alar. Regulatory agencies at the federal and state level issued conflicting opinions on the safety of Alar. In this atmosphere of confusion, the manufacturer of Alar withdrew it from the market. Next to appear was an independent report on behalf of the North American Chemicals Association, which described the NRDC report that originated the problem as emotive and unscientific. Among the problems listed were mathematical errors that led to overestimation of the degree of risk from Alar use. Nevertheless, a statement from the manufacturer stated that the removal of Alar was based on commercial grounds because

> even if further tests were successful, growers and the food industry would be very unlikely to come back to the product in any meaningful way.[37]

What are we to learn from this information? First, the science of risk assessment is a new discipline and open to different conclusions from the same databases. For the record, Alar was regarded as safe for use by the EPA in the United States, the Advisory Committee on Pesticides in the United Kingdom, and the World Health Organization. Second, misuse of science, especially by the media, can produce unnecessary public anxiety about the food supply.[37] And here is a question worth thinking about:

> The withdrawal of Alar may increase the use of other pesticides. . . . Has the removal of this pesticide made the situation safer, or have we cast out one demon and left a place for seven to rush in?[39]

■ Now you know

- The most rapid growth in our lives occurs between conception and birth.

- Famine and hunger have always been problems in pregnancy. Environmental contaminants and the widespread use of alcohol, drugs, tobacco, and caffeine are of recent origin.

- "Children giving birth to children" places additional nutritional stresses on the young mother and on the fetus.

- RDA values for many nutrients increase during pregnancy and lactation. Things to avoid during pregnancy are rapid body weight change, excessive use of nutrient supplements, faulty dietary practices, and the use of alcohol, drugs, and tobacco.

- Cultural preferences for food, vegetarianism, and the problems of lactose malabsorbers should receive consideration from health providers. Pica should be discouraged.

- Changes in diet while maintaining nutrient intake can alleviate nausea, vomiting, constipation, and heartburn during pregnancy.

- Breast milk is the most nutritious and safest first food of life. Its use also has psychological, allergic, and economic benefits.

- Adequate intakes of fluid and food are important during lactation.

- Severe undernutrition decreases the quantity but not the quality of breast milk.

- Premature babies require special dietary attention. Formula diets designed for premature infants should be used only if the mother's milk is not available.

- Weaning foods and the time at which they are introduced to the infant are influenced by social, psychological, environmental, and nutritional factors.

- Food choices by preschool children are highly influenced by color, flavor, texture, and familiarity.

- North American children 6–12 years of age may have low intakes of magnesium, copper, and vitamin B-6.

- Feeding young children is costly, but the costs of poor nutrition are also high.

- Whether a child receives a nutritious diet depends, in part, on the family structure, attitudes of the family, and, in some parts of the world, on the child's characteristics, including gender.

- School lunch and breakfast programs can correct low nutrient intake for some low-income children.

- Nutritionists are starting to look at childhood as a time to correct obesity and higher than normal cholesterol levels. Not all medical professionals or parents are in agreement with these interventions.

- No proven relationship exists between hyperactivity in children and the consumption of food additives or sugar.

- The Special Supplemental Food Program for Women, Infants, and Children (WIC) in the United States provides food for low-income mothers and their young children. Birth weight and growth of the children and the health of the mothers are improved by this program.

- Environmental contaminants can come through to the child from human milk, but breast feeding is still much safer than the use of bottle formulas. Health scares, involving claims not based on reliable, scientific evidence, such as that involving Alar, are damaging to everybody.

Further Reading

1. Palmer, C. A., and Dwyer, J. T. Boys or girls by the flick of the fork??? The questionable basis of the preconception gender diet. *Nutrition Today* 27(3):32, 1992.
2. Wharton, B. Food and biological clocks. *Proceedings of the Nutrition Society* 51:145, 1992.
3. National Academy of Sciences, Institute of Medicine. *Nutrition During Pregnancy and Lactation. An Implementation Guide.* National Academy Press, Washington, DC, 1992.
4. Fairburn, C. G., and others. Eating habits and eating disorders during pregnancy. *Psychosomatic Medicine* 54:665, 1992.
5. Haste, F. M., and others. The effect of nutritional intake on outcome of pregnancy in smokers and non-smokers. *British Journal of Nutrition* 65:347, 1991.
6. Stowers, S. L. Development of a culturally appropriate food guide for pregnant Caribbean immigrants in the United States. *Journal of The American Dietetic Association* 92:331, 1992.
7. Carruth, B. R., and Skinner, J. D. Practitioners beware: Regional differences in beliefs about nutrition during pregnancy. *Journal of the American Dietetic Association* 91:435, 1991.
8. Ellis, L. A., and Picciano, M. F. Milk-borne hormones: Regulators of development in neonates. *Nutrition Today* 27(5):6, 1992.
9. Mahalanabis, D. Breast feeding and vitamin A deficiency among children attending a diarrhoea treatment center in Bangladesh: A case-control study. *British Medical Journal* 303:493, 1991.
10. Kramer, F. M., and others. Breast-feeding reduces maternal lower-body fat. *Journal of The American Dietetic Association* 93:429, 1993.
11. Kennedy, K. I., and Visness, C. M. Contraceptive efficacy of lactational amenorrhoea. *Lancet* 339:227, 1992.
12. Wallace, J. P., and others. Infant acceptance of postexercise breast milk. *Pediatrics* 89:1245, 1992.
13. Freed, G. L., and others. Attitudes of expectant fathers regarding breast-feeding. *Pediatrics* 90:224, 1992.
14. Smart, J. L. 'Malnutrition, learning and behavior': 25 years on from the MIT Symposium. *Proceedings of the Nutrition Society* 52:189, 1993.
15. Kusin, J. A., and others. Chronic undernutrition in pregnancy and lactation. *Proceedings of the Nutrition Society* 52:19, 1993.
16. Davies, D. P. Future of human milk banks. *British Medical Journal* 305:433, 1992.
17. Hendricks, K. M., and Badruddin, S. H. Weaning recommendations: The scientific basis. *Nutrition Reviews* 50:125, 1992.
18. McCormick, M. C., and others. The health and developmental status of very low-birth-weight children at school age. *Journal of the American Medical Association* 267:2204, 1992.

19. Herens, M. C., and others. Nutrition and mental development of 4–5-year-old children on macrobiotic diets. *Journal of Human Nutrition and Dietetics* 5:1, 1992.

20. Bush, P. J., and Iannotti, R. J. Alcohol, cigarette, and marijuana use among fourth-grade urban schoolchildren in 1988/89 and 1990/91. *American Journal of Public Health* 83:111, 1993.

21. Gustafson-Larson, A. M., and Terry, R. D. Weight-related behaviors and concerns of fourth-grade children. *Journal of The American Dietetic Association* 92:818, 1992.

22. Frongillo, E. A., Jr., and Begin, F. Gender bias in food intake favors male preschool Guatemalan children. *Journal of Nutrition* 123:189, 1993.

23. Sampson, A. E., and others. School breakfast program participation and parental attitudes. *Journal of Nutrition Education* 23:110, 1991.

24. Snyder, M. P., and others. Reducing fat and sodium in school lunch programs: The LUNCHPOWER! Intervention Study. *Journal of the American Dietetic Association* 92:1087, 1992.

25. Nieto, F. J., and others. Childhood weight and growth rate as predictors of adult mortality. *American Journal of Epidemiology* 136:201, 1992.

26. Peipert, J. M., and others. Infant obesity, weight reduction with normal increase in linear growth and fat-free body mass. *Pediatrics* 89:143, 1992.

27. Casey, V. A., and others. Body mass index from childhood to middle age: A 50-y follow-up. *American Journal of Clinical Nutrition* 56:14, 1992.

28. Lannon, C. M., and Earp, J. Parents' behavior and attitudes toward screening children for high serum cholesterol levels. *Pediatrics* 89:1159, 1992.

29. Resnicow, K., and others. The case against 'the case against childhood cholesterol screening.' *Journal of the American Medical Association* 265:3003, 1991.

30. Kanarek, R. B., and Marks-Kaufman, R. *Nutrition and Behavior.* Van Nostrand Reinhold, New York, page 137, 1991.

31. Buescher, P. A., and others. Prenatal WIC participation can reduce low birth weight and newborn medical costs: A cost-benefit analysis of WIC participation in North Carolina. *Journal of The American Dietetic Association* 93:163, 1993.

32. Gielen, A. C., and others. Determinants of breastfeeding in a rural WIC population. *Journal of Human Lactation* 8:11, 1992.

33. Robinson, R. Baby milk advertising in Europe. *British Medical Journal* 302:744, 1991.

34. Ragg, M. Australia: Infant milk formulae. *Lancet* 340:661, 1992.

35. Prakash, P. India: Advertising of infant foods to be restricted. *Lancet* 340:962, 1992.

36. Sim, M. R., and McNeil, J. J. Monitoring chemical exposure using breast milk: A methodological review. *American Journal of Epidemiology* 136:1, 1992.

37. British Medical Association. *The BMA Guide to Pesticides, Chemicals and Health.* Edward Arnold, London, page 126, 1992.

38. Shannon, M., and Graef, J. Hazard of lead in infant formula. *New England Journal of Medicine* 326:137, 1992.

39. Jones, J. M. *Food Safety.* Eagan Press, St. Paul, Minnesota, 1992.

40. Fumento, M. *Science Under Siege: Balancing Technology and the Environment.* William Morrow and Company, Inc., New York, page 19, 1993.

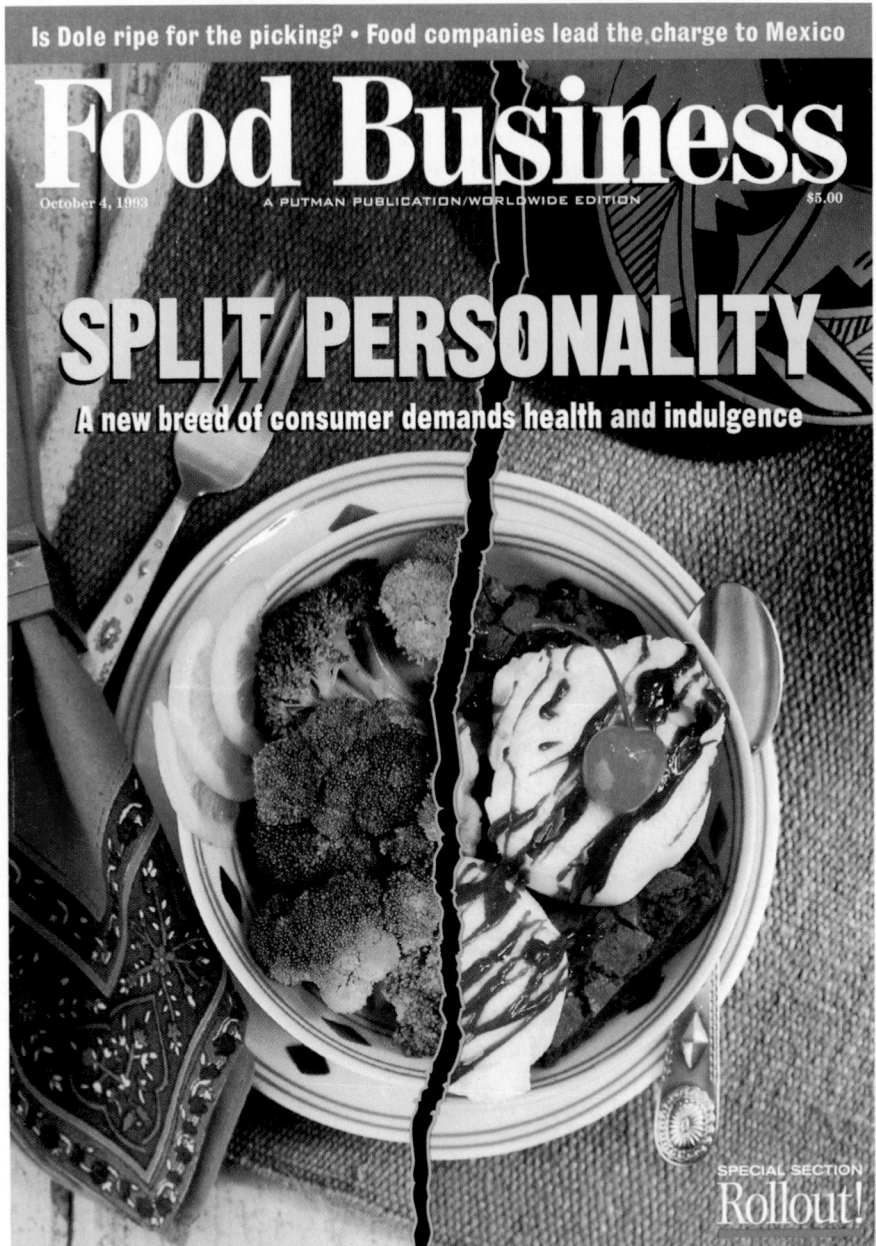

Think beyond this picture.
Does your eating pattern have a split
personality?

Is Dole ripe for the picking? • Food companies lead the charge to Mexico

Food Business

October 4, 1993   A PUTMAN PUBLICATION/WORLDWIDE EDITION $5.00

SPLIT PERSONALITY
A new breed of consumer demands health and indulgence

SPECIAL SECTION
Rollout!

Figure 16-1. As the cover of this magazine suggests, many people pay attention to the nutritional value of only a portion of their total diet.

## CHAPTER 16

Nutrition and Food for Adults

■ Nutrition for the middle and later years

One food industry executive defined the attempt to balance health and indulgence by saying, "consumers will sacrifice and eat something healthy for the main course, and then have their indulgent desserts." Are you in this category? Should adults make major dietary changes to correct potential problems resulting from diet? People's nutrition concerns change as they age. Body image and body weight are important to the teenager. Middle-aged adults worry about "middle-age spread," hypertension, blood cholesterol levels, and other diet-related medical problems. For most people, the greatest physiological and physical changes occur in old age, and they usually result in dietary adjustments. For example, the number of calories required per unit of body weight decreases as we age. This happens to all of us as we get older, due to the changes in growth patterns, body composition, and exercise that accompany aging.

■ Adolescence–Nutrient needs and food acceptability

A recent study of health-risk behaviors and health concerns among young adolescents ended with the researchers suggesting to adults

> [that] we stop viewing young adolescents as naive children and begin to view them as observers of and participants in a changing social environment that has important implications for their current and future health status.[1]

Parents as well as researchers are aware of adolescent health issues, including nutrition, and many want to have more involvement with their physicians and schools in these issues.[2]

Adolescents do observe and participate in an environment that contains

Table 16-1. Dieting Practices of Adolescents

	Females (%)[a]	Males (%)[a]
Eat less food	57	23
Exercise more (than usual)	57	26
Avoid sweets	53	22
Eat low-calorie foods/beverages	50	18
Skip a meal	45	19
Eat only salads	41	16
Eat only fruits	39	18
Hardly eat, fast	33	12
Eat only high-protein foods	30	16
Drink only liquids	27	13
Use diet pills or diet candies	11	3
Vomit after eating	8	3
Take laxatives	4	3

[a] Percentage of total

nutritional messages, and they have opinions about them. Table 16-1 shows some adolescents' views on one nutrition-related issue–dieting.

Notice that adolescent girls are more concerned than boys about the amount and type of food they eat. The reasons for these concerns are mainly social, but they are in response to biological changes in body composition at puberty. At the start of puberty, boys and girls both have about one-sixth of their weight as body fat. After puberty, the boys put on more muscle, which drops their body fat content to one-tenth of their weight, while girls increase their body fat to about one-quarter of body weight.[3] In most developed countries, social approval is given to slender female body types. Girls consider extra fat to be threatening, and so some are attracted to dangerous slimming methods or eating disorders as the solution.

Eating habits developed by adolescents may last throughout life, which may lead to problems because this is an age when the intake of many nutrients is often marginal. For example, 14- to 16-year-old girls in the United States have low intakes of calcium, magnesium, iron, zinc, copper, and manganese (see Table 10-2).

Diet and Nutrition Concerns of Teenagers Now and 100 Years Ago

Nutritional and dietary problems, concerns, knowledge, and responses may change over the decades. One useful way to observe the extent of change is to examine how nutritional and dietary issues for teenagers today differ from those of a century ago.

Body size
Today's teenagers weigh more and are taller at any given age than teenagers 100 years ago. Average height continues to increase with each generation.

Puberty onset
Puberty begins at an earlier age now than it did in the 1890s. Menarche occurs at about age 12 or 13 today, compared to about age 17 then. Among the nutritional implications of this change is the fact that more iron is required at an earlier age to replace the iron lost in menstruation. Pregnancy can now occur even before age 12, resulting in considerable stress for the still-growing mother and the growing fetus. Body compositional changes resulting in higher proportions of body fat in girls after puberty now occur at an earlier age. As a result, some girls become preoccupied with body weight and body image at an earlier age, leading to early dieting and eating disorders.

Weight-loss diets and eating disorders

"Each epoch has had different tolerances for weight and for fatness," writes Hillel Schwartz in his book *Never Satisfied: A Cultural History of Diets, Fantasies and Fat.*

> Since the 1880s, those tolerances have grown especially narrow, especially demanding. We take for granted now a constant personal vigil against overweight and obesity.

There was some interest in weight loss in the 1890s but not to the extent of the billions of dollars collected by the weight-loss industry of today. This was because female beauty was seen in heavier women than is the case today. Clothes covered more of the body then; today, fashions show much of the body, especially in advertisements, and thinness is considered an asset.

Were eating disorders a problem in the 1890s? Scientists don't know because medical records give no indication, but we might guess that they were not so troublesome then. We do know that many individuals never lived to the teenage years because of the much higher rates of infant and child mortality.

Skipping meals and consuming snacks, fast foods, and unconventional meals

Teenagers often skip meals, especially breakfast. In the 1890s, more people lived on farms, where they usually started the day with a large breakfast from the products of the farm.

Snacks are now a significant part of the eating pattern of teenagers,[4] as they are of people of all ages. Snack foods are growing in popularity all over the world. Nations with the highest spending per person on snack foods (according to statistics in the *Economist*, June 11, 1994) are, in decreasing order: the United States, Norway, Japan, Britain, Spain, Holland, Australia, and Canada. The Snack Food Association of America tells us that Americans consume $8 billion worth of

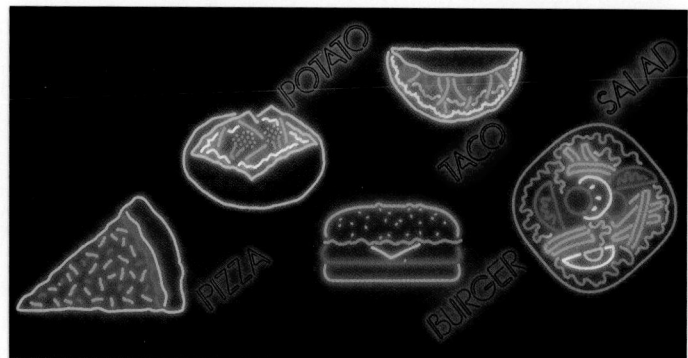

Figure 16-2. Fast foods are a relatively new type of product in the marketplace. This style of eating has developed in the last 30 years or so.

snacks each year. From 60 to 70% of American children and teenagers eat snack food at least once a day, and snacks contribute 12–17% of the RDA energy intake of teenagers. Snacking has even been referred to as the "art of grazing."[5] Snacks can range from very nutritious to a nutritional zero. Some are high in fat, sugar, cholesterol, or salt and/or are low in fiber, vitamins, and minerals. An extensive list of good and not-so-good snacks is given in *The Real Life Nutrition Book: Making the Right Choices Without Changing Your Life-style.*[5] The authors say that fast foods and carryout foods will continue to undergo changes, with even more changes by the 21st century.

Under the constant pressure of the clock, we embrace anything that promises greater speed and efficiency. In the twenty-first century, we define fast food as something that can be prepared in minutes or even seconds.

Snacks preferred by teenagers include those shown in Figure 16-3.

Teenagers 100 years ago had no concept of the fast foods we have today. Their meals usually followed the food traditions of the family and consisted of food that was available in the neighborhood. The teen of today can have nutritious food from most corners of the globe by visiting the restaurants on Main Street. The fast-food industry has responded to government dietary recommendations by improving the nutritive value of some of their food items and by providing salads and low-fat options. Still, many teens prefer fast foods high in fat, sodium, and sugar, including potato chips, cheeseburgers, and french fries. Figure 16-4 presents one way of looking at a french fry–the high magnification shows many droplets of fat.

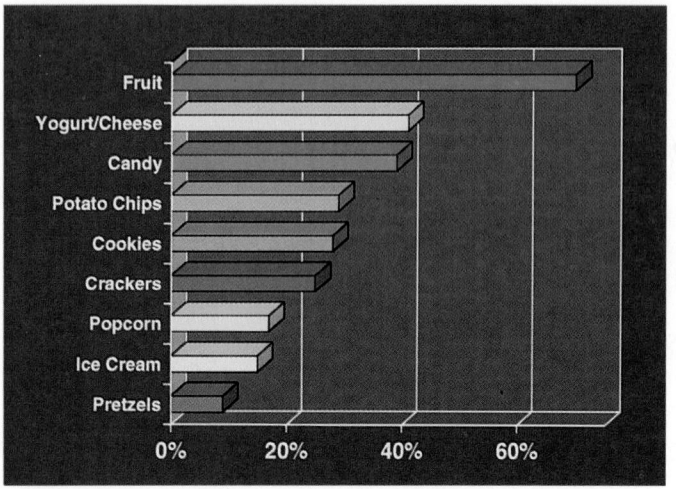

Figure 16-3. Snack food choices of teenagers, showing percentages of snacks chosen.

Some teens may switch to a vegetarian diet or to unconventional ways of eating. Nutritionists must be aware of the psychological and social issues involved in any dietary change during the adolescent years. For example, psychologists have identified a range of internal and external environmental cues that stimulate eating even when a person has no physiological need for food.[6] Emotional eating, restrained eating, and eating in response to external cues, all eating patterns frequently exhibited by teenagers, are considered to be factors in obesity. Restrained eating is sometimes associated with negative attitudes to foods other than those associated with slimming. Instances of emotionally cued eating, negative emotional responses to episodes of overeating, and extreme steps taken to compensate for overeating are frequently noted. Psychologists stress that the resulting emotional conflict can lead to serious difficulties in eating control.[6]

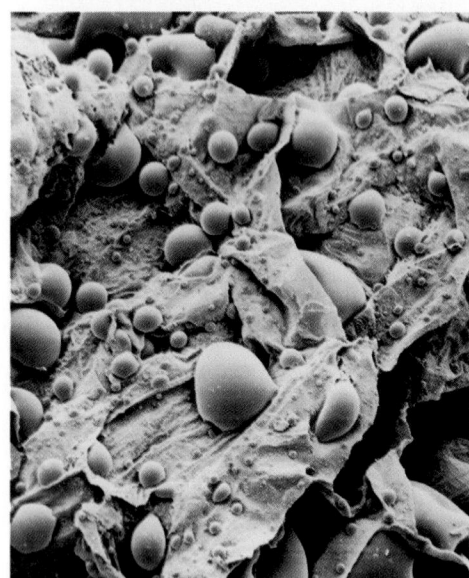

Figure 16-4. Fat droplets on a french fry, seen under a microscope, give visual proof that french fries are high in fat.

Different tastes

Likes and dislikes in foods among teenagers can vary between males and females, among cultures, and between those interested in sports or in artistic performances. In addition, the actual sources of taste in food have changed over the past 100 years. We can now experience the sweet taste of sugar without the sugar and the taste and mouthfeel of fat from food that is fat-free. Food scientists have provided us with these options.

Alcohol, drugs, and tobacco use

Think beyond the picture in Figure 16-5. Do you think young people in this era had as much access to alcohol as they do now?

The abuse of alcohol and drugs is certainly more common among teenagers now than it was 100 years ago. The book *Drinking in America*[7] refers to "the dry offensive" in the 1870s and 1880s, when many people campaigned against the use of liquor. Alcohol was not nearly as readily available to teenagers then as it is today.

Cigarette smoking has been tried by 70% of students in grades 9–12, according to the Centers for Disease Control,[8] and similar numbers are reported for other countries. Smoking is a major risk factor in coronary heart disease and may depress food intake to levels where nutrient intake is low. For teenage girls who smoke, the risks are even greater if they take oral contraceptives, since this increases the chance of having a stroke. Smokers have an increased requirement for vitamin C, and the diet of teenage smokers may be already low in vitamin C.

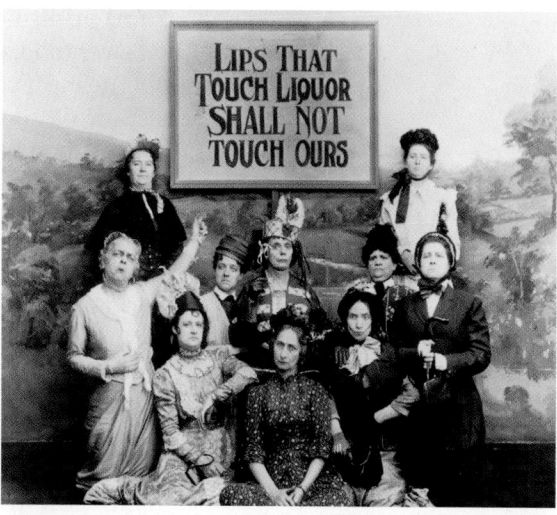

Figure 16-5. Attitudes toward alcohol vary with time and with location in the world. Facts about alcohol show that excessive use consistently creates nutritional problems.

Soft drinks

Both regular soft drinks containing sugar and those not containing sugar and marketed as low-calorie are clearly products of the 20th century. Did our ancestors miss anything in not having these drinks? Clearly, soft drinks provide only calories and no other nutrients. Soft drinks may replace milk in the diet, thereby reducing the intake of calcium, a particularly important nutrient for teenage girls. A higher percentage of 12- to 29-year-olds drink regular soda than any other age group.[9]

Level of nutrient intake and dietary supplements

We have no idea whether teenagers 100 years ago had an adequate intake of nutrients; dietary surveys were not conducted and accurate food intake records were not usually kept. We do know that there was no knowledge of vitamins and that the nutritional role of some minerals remained to be discovered. Vitamin and mineral supplements were not available.

When girls reach approximately age 12 and boys reach age 14, they may suddenly need high energy intakes, reaching as much as 4,000 calories per day. Some teenagers today may not attain that level of intake for a number of reasons, including lack of money or fear of becoming fat. Teenagers typically have a low intake of many nutrients, especially iron, zinc, copper, calcium, and vitamin B-6. Folacin intake is sometimes low because green leafy vegetables are not at the top of the favorite food list for many teens. The social dimension of food must be taken into consideration here. Nutritionists can stress the importance of nutrient intake, but this is also a time of experimentation with eating styles, when food is used to send personal and social messages.

Food additives

Fewer food additives were used a century ago. Sugar and salt were probably the most common because chemists had not yet invented the great collection of additives we have today. As a result, food waste usually was greater then because food spoiled more quickly. We saw in Chapter 15 that some relationship between food additives and hyperactivity and other behavioral disorders is suspected, although not proven. Such concerns did not exist until recently.

Food advertising and television viewing

The teens of the 1890s were not exposed to the high-pressure advertising we have today, especially the mixed messages from television.[4] Coupled with advertisements for nutritionally adequate foods are those for foods high in fat, cholesterol, sodium, and sugar. Viewers also see the very slim bodies of successful models and hear the constant babble on talk shows about how to lose weight. Studies show that as television viewing increases, so also does the tendency to consume calorically dense food, producing the classic "couch potato." In addition, television viewing is one of the reasons that teenagers today are less physically active than teens a century ago.

Teen pregnancy and birth control

The United States has a higher rate of teenage pregnancy than any other developed country. It is more common today than 100 years ago, and the incidence continues to increase. Besides change in societal attitudes toward pregnancy and birth control, one reason for this difference may be the earlier age of menarche today. From a nutrition standpoint, a nutritionally marginal diet for the teenage mother may present problems for the fetus and child. Teenagers are more likely to have low-birth-weight babies.

Work

More teenagers have jobs outside the home today than did teenagers in the 1890s. Working teens are more likely to eat sandwich-type food and to skip the evening meal. They have a lower intake of calcium and riboflavin than nonworking adolescents.

Athletics and nutrition

Today there are more athletic events than in the 1890s and higher standards that require control of body weight. Gymnastics is one example. There is also much more emphasis on special foods and dietary supplements. A balanced diet does not require the taking of additional supplements, yet that is common practice among athletes. This can be seen in the multitude of advertisements for nutritional supplements in health and body-building magazines.[10]

Nutrition and illness

Modern medicine makes nutritional support available during illness in ways that could not be imagined in the 1890s. Hospitals and clinics employ dietitians, and nutritional therapy is an important part of the recovery programs for many diseases.

A particular problem for adolescents is acne–about 85% of teenagers have acne at some point. There are nondietary reasons for acne, such as hormonal imbalances, but popular belief (although little medical evidence) blames chocolate, fatty foods, soft drinks, and alcohol (especially beer). Since teenagers consume many of these, it is difficult to isolate dietary causes. It is good nutritional advice for adolescents to reduce the intake of these foods anyway.

■ Nutrition in young and middle-aged adults

For the purposes of this discussion, we will consider young adults to be those in the 21–40 age range, and middle-aged adults those 40–60. The elderly (those over 60 years) are discussed later in this chapter.

Eating patterns for young and middle-aged adults should follow the recommendations in the Food Guide Pyramid (Chapter 4) for maximum health. It is rare that people in middle age die from undernutrition even in developing countries, provided they do not experience famine. Contrast this with the high death rates from undernutrition among infants and children. One reason is that adults have lower nutrient requirements because nutrients are needed for maintenance only, not for growth. Another reason is that adults have a higher resistance to infection.

Even in developed countries some adults experience low intake of some nutrients, especially vitamin B-6, magnesium, calcium, zinc, folacin, and in premenopausal women, iron.

Nutrient intake is lowest among the poor in this age group. There is increasing evidence that nutrition education, such as the recommendations in the Food Guide Pyramid, has a positive effect on the eating practices of many adults. Various surveys have noted increases in the intake of low-fat and skim milk, poultry, fish, grain products (especially pasta and mixes with grains), and nonalcoholic beverages, as well as decreases in the intake of whole milk, beef, pork, and eggs.

We live in a time of increasing economic pressures for employment and for excellent job performance. The American Dietetic Association offers the following helpful and healthful advice for beating "brain drain" on the job.

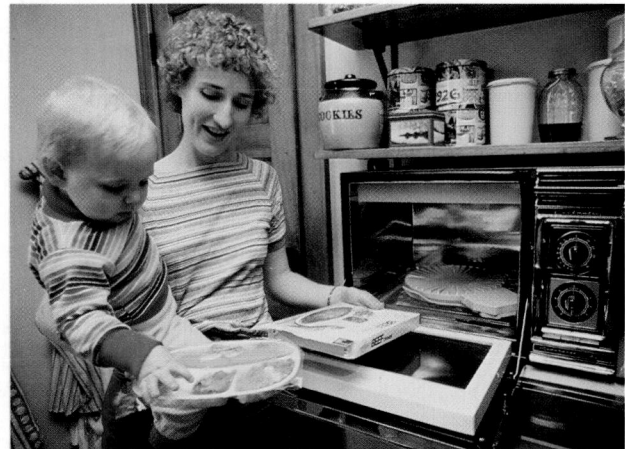

Figure 16-6. Today, many adults, especially working people with families, rely on quickly prepared foods. The food industry has developed many new products to meet their needs.

- Don't leave home without it–breakfast.
- Space your meals throughout the day. Go no longer than five hours without eating.
- Snack on low-fat foods when there's no time for lunch.
- Pack your desk and briefcase with snacks such as low-fat crackers, pretzels, or juice boxes.
- Drink lots of water. Also, contribute to your daily water needs (a minimum of eight cups) by drinking herbal teas or hot water with a twist of lemon.

- Limit coffee to two cups a day. Too much coffee can drain vital fluids. Caffeine is a diuretic, which causes the body to lose water.
- Pass on the doughnuts, except as a special treat. Try bagels and fresh fruit for a breakfast on the run.
- Keep power lunches light. Overeating during midday can cause drowsiness.
- Take five–a five-minute walk or stress break beats eating to ease stress.
- Keep the office kitchen stocked with energizing snacks such as nonfat yogurt, snack-size cereals, low-fat cheese, and single servings of water-packed tuna.

Nutrition and the College Student

Any or all of the following can negatively affect a college student's nutritional intake–missed meals because of busy schedules; low-nutrient food bought because of limited budgets; the easy availability of junk food; pressure to alter one's diet for athletic reasons, to lose weight, or to conform to a religious or cultural creed; or perhaps even varying nutritive value in dining hall food.

What does all of this produce in some college students? Potential nutrition-related problems include dental caries, obesity, anemia (in women), acne, and the multiple nutrition problems created by abuse of alcohol and drugs. Eating disorders seem to be as prevalent among female college students as among females in the general population. Students who view themselves as being more maladjusted than their peers may have a higher risk of bulimia. Some studies conclude that many college students don't eat correctly because they don't eat the right proportions of the most nutritious foods. A recent study showed that college students need information about making nutrient-dense choices, especially for iron and calcium, and about ways of reducing fat intake.[11]

Look at the great diversity in off-campus eating locations reported by college students (Table 16-2). Where do you fit in this pattern of eating?

The nutritive value of food is what is important, not the location where it is served, but location may give a good clue to nutritive value. An acceptable nutrition education program can improve nutrient intake, as shown by a study on some British university students.[12]

Gender Differences in Nutrition-Related Diseases

Many of the gender differences in nutrition-related diseases begin to emerge in middle age. We have looked at some nutrition-related diseases in Chapter 14, but it is worth making a quick review and adding a discussion of diseases that tend to be gender-specific.

Table 16-2. Eating Out Practices of College Students

Location of Meal or Snack	Seldom or Never (%)
Delivery (mostly pizza)	9
Fast-food restaurant	10
Family-style restaurant	14
Ice cream/yogurt shop	23
Ethnic food shop	27
Vending machine	28
Bar	39
Better restaurant	40
Bookstore, movie, drugstore	40
Bake shop/doughnut shop	47
Conventional cafeteria	69

Nutrition-related problems that are more prevalent in women

Women experience some nutrition problems that are gender-related. Food choices made by women are frequently influenced by weight-control problems, money, time pressure, and nutrition-related concerns. The following nutrition-related problems are either specific to or more common in women than in men.

Obesity is related closely to hypertension, high blood cholesterol levels, diabetes (Type II), certain cancers, arthritis, varicose veins in the legs, gallstones, and blood clots, as well as a decrease in life span. Many of these problems are complicated further during pregnancy.

Why there is a higher incidence of obesity among poor adult women in the United States is an unsolved puzzle. This is a particular problem among African-American and Native-American women but not among the men and children of these ethnic groups. The switch from thin to fat begins at about age 15. By age 50, a low-income woman averages 17 pounds more than her high-income counterpart even though the poorer woman is generally shorter in height. A researcher at the University of Michigan concluded that none of the accepted theories on obesity seems to explain this type of obesity. One theory is that the low-income men may be doing harder physical work than the women, with corresponding higher energy expenditures.

Some cancers with possible association with diet are more prevalent in women; breast cancer is an example.

Osteoporosis and **anemia** are often seen in women but are uncommon in men.

Premenstrual syndrome (PMS) is a collection of symptoms experienced by some women before and during menstruation. The symptoms include both physical and emotional pain. PMS is going through a redefinition.

> To the dismay of some feminists, the American Psychiatric Association has created a new class of depression based on hormonal changes in women,

writes Marilyn Chase in the *Wall Street Journal* (May 28, 1993). She continues,

> . . . the association voted . . . to list a severe form of premenstrual syndrome, or PMS, as a 'depressive disorder' in its new diagnostic manual of mental illness.

What upset some people is that this definition will give PMS the stigma of a mental disorder, with serious social and economic penalties for women. Currently, there is no accepted treatment for monthly depression associated with the menstrual cycle.

Where does nutrition enter into a discussion on PMS? Nutritionists cannot add much at the moment, but that does not prevent commercial exploitation of the problem. Although claims have been made that vitamin B-6, vitamin E, and magnesium decrease PMS, there is no strong evidence for this.

Goiter due to iodine deficiency is more common in women than in men. It is also more prevalent in countries where the diet is low in iodine and salt is not iodized.

Premenstrual syndrome (PMS): Physical and emotional symptoms experienced before and during menstruation by some women; includes water retention.

Nutrition-related problems that are more prevalent in men

Men have a high incidence of **colon cancer. Prostate cancer** also occurs at a high frequency, especially in older men.

Men may have **shorter life expectancy**, but they don't seem to have as many problems as women do in obtaining enough nutrients.

Coronary heart disease (CHD) is more prevalent in men, but the gap in the incidence between men and women is narrowing in many countries. The increasing number of women who smoke cigarettes is among the reasons given for the increased CHD in women.

Nutrition-related problems common to both women and men

Growing older means getting better in a number of ways but not in terms of the following nutrition-related problems that are equally common in women and men.

Hypertension. High blood pressure was discussed in Chapter 14.

Periodontal disease: Degeneration of bone and gum tissue around teeth.

Dental and gum disorders. The loss of teeth before age 35 is mainly the result of dental caries, whereas after 35 it is caused mainly by *periodontal disease*. This disease affects the gums and causes loss of bone surrounding the teeth. It is thought to be increased when diets are low in calcium, protein, vitamin C, and/or zinc, nutrients needed for the production of collagen and dentin, which are both important in the structure of teeth. Dietary deficiencies of protein and vitamin C are not problems for most Americans.

Diabetes. We discussed this disease in Chapters 6 and 14. As we have seen throughout this book, there is still much to learn in nutrition, and the treatment of some nutrition-related diseases is still at the trial-and-error stage. It is understandable that this frustrates people, but it is useful to remind ourselves also of how far we have come in our knowledge. Look at the diet used to treat diabetes in the British army in the 1790s.

Breakfast: 1½ pint of milk and ½ pint of lime water, mixed together; bread and butter.
Noon: Plain blood pudding, blood and suet only.
Dinner: Game or old meats; fat and rancid old meats "as much fat as the stomach may bear."
Supper: Same as breakfast.

Back then, diabetes was thought to be a disease of the stomach, so all fruits and vegetables were eliminated from the diet. Today there is great emphasis on eliminating dietary fat, consuming no more than the RDA for protein, and reducing sodium intake. The lesson from this is that refinement in the treatment of diabetes, and other nutrition-related diseases, is constantly taking place.

Arthritis: Inflammation of a joint, usually accompanied by pain and frequently by changes in bone structure.

Arthritis. This may be relieved with supplements of omega-3 fatty acids, which are found mainly in fish oils. Some evidence suggests that they also help to reduce morning stiffness and tenderness in the joints. However, the disease is not eliminated; the original arthritic condition returns when the supplements are no longer taken. The optimal dose and duration of treatment with fish oils remains to be worked out.

■ Nutrition and the elderly

Think beyond Figure 16-7. Are some nutrition problems more common among the elderly? Is our knowledge of nutrient requirements for the elderly as complete as it is for younger age groups?

Lewis Thomas was one of the most elegant writers on biomedical research. In his book *The Fragile Species* he has this to say about research on aging:

> In spite of today's ignorance about so many diseases, including most of the chronic illnesses associated with aging, there is the most surprising optimism, amounting to something like exhilaration, within the community of basic biomedical researchers . . . . We are learning some facts about nutrition and longevity that we never understood before.

Couple this information with the following quotation from the *New York Times* (October 10, 1992):

> The extent of malnutrition among the elderly in general is a murky battleground for their advocates, public health officials and assorted experts. While some nutritionists estimate that 50% of all elderly Americans open themselves up to a host of diseases by not eating enough of the foods they need, very little is known about the problem.

We need to learn more about nutrition and aging because the elderly population in most countries is growing at a rapid rate (and we will all be in this age group some day!). By the year 2030, there will be twice as many elderly people in the United States as there are today, and by the second half of the 21st century, that proportion will have changed so that almost half of the population is over 50 years of age.[13] Research shows that we are reaching the maximum in terms of life span, and the chances of extension of life by various means, including nutrition, are limited.[14]

Nutrition problems exist among the elderly in the United States. Surveys of elderly people, including appropriate representation from low-income groups, provided the following information.[15,16]

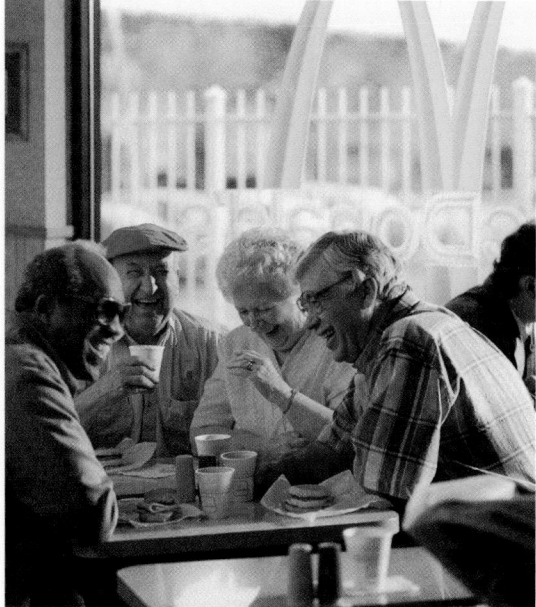

Figure 16-7. Fast-food eating places offer older people, and others who live alone, a convenient location to enjoy the social aspects of eating.

Think beyond these numbers to determine how the situations they describe may be corrected:

- One in five didn't have enough money to buy the food they need.
- One in three always had enough money to buy food.
- One in three ate less than three meals per day.
- One in 20 had been without food for more than three days in a row in the past month.
- One in five had lost weight without trying over the last month.
- One in 10 had eaten less than five kinds of food the day before.
- One in three had no one to help them if sick in bed.

- One in four of eligible low-income elderly people received food stamps.
- One in four were overweight.
- One in three lived alone, possibly increasing the tendency to skip meals and not cook.
- One in two used multiple prescription drugs, which can alter appetite and the absorption and metabolism of nutrients.

Why do these problems exist in our elderly community? One or more of the characteristics or problems shown in Table 16-3 can be contributing factors to poor nutritional status in the elderly.

Notice how a number of economic, social, and medical problems influence the quantity and quality of the diet. Let's look at some of the physiological and medical causes of nutrition problems in the elderly.

Table 16-3. Nutrition Risk Characteristics Likely to Be Associated with Increased Risk of Poor Nutritional Status and Health in Older Americans

Characteristic or Problem	Examples
Inappropriate, inadequate, or excessive food intake	Quantity, quality, or both with respect to intake of: milk and milk products, meat and meat substitutes, fruits and vegetables, breads and cereals, fat, sweets, and alcohol
	Dietary modification (prescribed or self-imposed)
	Alcohol abuse
Poverty	Low income
	Low food expenditures or inadequate food resources
	Reliance on economic assistance programs for food or other basic needs
Social isolation	Reduced social contact resulting from limited availability or use of support systems
	Living arrangements isolated or inadequate in respect to cooking, food storage, transportation, etc.
Chronic use of medication	Many different prescribed or self-administered drugs, especially those affecting nutritional status
	Quackery
	Excessive use or overreliance on nutritional supplements
Dependency and disability	Little activity, even for daily routines
	Disabling conditions present or lack of manual dexterity; use of assistive devices
Acute or chronic diseases or conditions	Abnormalities of body weight
	Alcohol abuse
	Cognitive or emotional impairment (such as depression, dementia)
	Pressure sores
	Sensory impairment
Advanced age, e.g., above 80 years	

Four significant changes have taken place since youth that affect the nutritional needs of the elderly. First, body composition and the physiological functioning of many tissues change significantly in the elderly, which can cause difficulties in obtaining food and utilizing nutrients. These changes are discussed in the next section. Second, chronic diseases and disabilities are more common–coronary heart disease, cancer, diabetes, hypertension, and others–and usually necessitate dietary changes that may be difficult for some elderly people to follow. Third, intake of prescription medications is also high for some people, and these may interfere with the absorption and utilization of some nutrients. Fourth, elderly people eat less, so they are less able to choose the wide variety of foods that constitute a nutritious diet. We will deal with the specifics of food intake by the elderly in the "People are Different" and the "Nutrition and Food Science in Action" sections at the end of this chapter.

Nutrition-Related Changes in Body Functions

At about 30 years of age, significant changes in body composition and decreases in the physiological functions of most tissues begin to occur. Table 16-4 and the discussion that follows list some of these changes, those that have significant impact on nutritional status. Their extent varies among people because this age group contains people from 60 to 100 or more years of age. Spend a moment to determine how many of these functions may be influenced by lifestyles or diet throughout life.

Decrease in sensory abilities

The elderly are less able to see, hear, smell, and taste food and less able than young people to detect bitter and spicy tastes or smooth and crunchy textures in foods. Loss of vision makes it difficult to get to stores and to read food labels and menus. Poor hearing can make the elderly less inclined to eat with others. Because of their decreased ability to smell food, odors are not well detected and their sense of taste is diminished. They may not be able to smell food well enough to know whether it has gone bad. All of these factors may make older people less interested in food. Zinc deficiency, which decreases the sense of taste, may be a problem for some. A further complication is loss of appetite, resulting in lowered food intake.[17] Elderly people have decreased sensitivity to thirst, at a time when maintaining appropriate fluid intake is particularly important.

Decrease in nerve-muscle coordination

Lack of coordination makes it difficult for some older people to cut their food. This decline may make eating difficult.

Decrease in chewing and swallowing ability

This is a problem because many elderly people (half of all Americans) have lost all of their teeth by age 65. A Canadian study found that only half of the people with dentures could chew their food properly, even though the nutritive value of the diet consumed seemed to be satisfactory.[18] "Dysphagia" is the medical term for difficulty in swallowing; this af-

Table 16-4. Nutritional Implications of Loss of Tissue Function During Aging

Tissue	Functional Change	Nutritional Implications
Lean body mass	Loss of muscle and other soft tissue	Decreased energy requirements because of decreased basal requirements
Heart	Decreased output	Decreased oxygen delivered for tissue metabolism
Lungs	Decreased maximum breathing capacity	Decreased oxygen delivered for tissue metabolism
Muscles	Decreased strength and endurance	Difficulty in cutting some foods
Nerves	Decreased conduction velocity	Decreased muscle coordination—difficulty in cutting some foods
Kidneys	Decreased filtration rates	Possible difficulty in eliminating some end products of metabolism (e.g., nitrogen from protein metabolism); water and electrolyte balance more difficult to control
Bones	Brittle and soft, leading to increased incidence of broken bones	Immobility and inability to buy or prepare food
Mouth	Decreased saliva flow; loss of taste discrimination	Loss of ability to chew and taste food; may lead to different food choices
Teeth	Loss	Inability to chew certain foods; dentures may cause the same problem, and lack of lubrication resulting from decreased saliva may cause infections under dentures
Digestive system	Decreased digestive juices; decreased muscle activity	Difficulty in digesting some foods; constipation because of loss of muscles in digestive system; decreased efficiency in absorbing some nutrients—fat, iron, vitamin B-12—and some medication
Eyes	Deterioration	Decreased ability to shop, prepare, and appreciate food
Hearing	Deterioration	May prevent people from using food as a means of social interaction

fects about 20 million Americans of all ages[19] and is a particularly serious problem for the elderly.

Decreases in the functioning of the GI tract and related tissues

These decreases have major nutritional implications.[20] Changes include decreased functioning of the liver and pancreas, decreased production of gastric juice, a thinning of the walls of the stomach, and decreased muscular activity in the GI tract, resulting in constipation. Elderly people seem to have a difficult time digesting and absorbing dietary fat, calcium, vitamin B-12, and vitamin C. Iron absorption may be reduced because less hydrochloric acid is secreted in the stomach.[16]

Older people may suffer from intestinal gas, which some try to avoid by eliminating such gas-producing foods as cabbage and legumes. But in reality, much of the problem is from swallowing air along with the food.

Decreases in immune function

Impaired immune responses may be critical for the elderly. They are ill much more often than the young, in part because of impaired immune responses.[21] The immune system protects against microorganisms–including viruses, bacteria, fungi, and occasionally parasites–and against allergens, toxins, and malignant cells. Nutritionists and immunologists have learned much about the immune system from work on undernourished children in developing countries, and this is now being applied to studies on the elderly. There are many similarities as well as differences between the young and the old. Both age groups have less than optimum immune responses; both are at a high risk of developing infections; and adequate diets are critical for both.

The elderly get infections more frequently, especially respiratory diseases. Infections result in loss of appetite, poor dietary intake, and malnutrition, which weaken the patient's resistance to further infection.[22] Nutrition is important for proper functioning of the immune system. Protein-energy malnutrition and deficiencies of various nutrients impair several immune responses. When elderly people take supplements of vitamins and trace elements in amounts similar to RDA values, immunity improves and the risk of infection decreases. The use of a single nutrient in large doses is *not* recommended, because an impaired immune response may result, and large doses may hinder the absorption of other nutrients.[21]

Decrease in lean body mass

This results in lower energy requirements per unit of body weight. The consequences of this decrease in lean tissue, especially muscle,[23] may include decreased strength and physical activity, altered energy metabolism, and impaired resistance to infection.[24] Fewer calories are required in the diet to meet energy needs, but nutrient requirements are still high (see the RDA table inside the back cover). This means that the elderly must choose food with a high nutrient density to meet those requirements. Therefore, alcohol and foods high in fat and sugar should be avoided.

Decreased kidney function

This decrease makes the elderly less able to produce urine, which makes it more difficult for them to maintain water and electrolyte balance. Older people should avoid diets high in protein and sodium because these nutrients place an added strain on the excretory functions of the aging kidneys. We have already noted that perception of thirst is poor in many older people.[22] They should be advised to maintain adequate fluid intake even though they may not feel thirsty. Adequate fluid intake during and after exercise is important.

Other Health Problems

Dietary changes are usually prescribed for people with CHD, hypertension, diabetes, obesity, osteoporosis, and other nutrition-related medical problems. These and the following ailments mean that elderly people may have many dietary adjustments to make. This may not be easy if they live alone, are on a limited income, or are a long way from stores.

Constipation

We suspect that up to 20% of the elderly suffer from constipation. One of the causes is *irritable bowel syndrome*, which is an alteration in normal bowel habits accompanied by abdominal pain that is influenced by psychological and stressful situations.[25] Diets low in fiber contribute to the

Irritable bowel syndrome: A group of symptoms including diarrhea, heartburn, flatulence, loss of appetite, nausea, vomiting, and/or abdominal distention after meals. Causes are unknown, but emotional stress may be a factor.

problem. Nerve function decreases in aging, and this affects the activity of muscles needed to push the feces along the GI tract.

Diarrhea

An article in the journal *Geriatric Medicine* says,

> Acute diarrhea is one of the commoner complaints in elderly medicine and represents a particular risk to the frail elderly and to those in institutional care.[26]

We saw in Chapter 5 that oral rehydration therapy (ORT) (feeding a sugar, salt, and water solution) was effective in correcting dehydration in under-nourished children. This procedure can also be applied successfully to the elderly with acute diarrhea. It must be done under medical supervision because many of the elderly may be on drugs that have a diuretic effect, which makes it necessary to carefully monitor the extent of dehydration.

Drugs

Prescription and over-the-counter drug use by elderly people is significant and increasing.[22] Elderly people living at home take an average of four different drugs a day, but in nursing homes they might receive up to eight medications daily.[22] Think about the implications of the drugs in Table 16-5 on nutritional status.

■ People are different–Some elderly people become victims of quackery and faddism

The Japanese Ministry of Health and Welfare recently provided the following eating habit guidelines for the elderly. If these guidelines were followed, few people would be victims of quackery and faddism, which are common problems for the elderly.

- Beware of undernutrition. A decrease in weight is a warning sign.
- Devise cooking schemes that add variety to the menu. Eat every kind of food, but avoid overeating.
- Eat side dishes first. Side dishes are important when you get older.
- Adopt regularity into your eating habits. Eat slowly; don't miss any meals.
- Get enough exercise. The feeling of an empty stomach is the best seasoning.
- Learn wise eating habits. Eating habit wisdom will point the way to preserving a healthy and youthful condition.
- Enjoy delicious and enjoyable meals. A rich spirit will foster healthy golden years.

The American Council on Science and Health's report *Quackery and the Elderly* tells us that health charlatans bilk elderly Americans out of over $10 billion each year. Some of this is spent in treatments not recommended by medical authorities to correct various illnesses, while some is spent to reverse the undesirable effects of aging and to retain the vigor of youth. The

Table 16-5. Some Drugs Commonly Used by the Elderly, and Their Nutritional Side Effects

Drug	Nutritional Side Effects
Influencing appetite and food intake	
Antipsychotics and sedatives	Somnolence; disinterest in food
Digoxin[a]	Marked anorexia; nausea; vomiting; weakness
Cancer chemotherapies	Nausea; vomiting; aversion to food
Affecting absorption of nutrients	
Laxatives and cathartics	Malabsorption of fat-soluble vitamins; fluid and electrolyte loss
Corticosteroids[b]	Decreased vitamin D activity
Anticonvulsants	Decreased vitamin D activity
Aluminum or magnesium antacids	Phosphate depletion
Cholestyramine[c]	Decreased absorption of lipids, folic acid, iron, vitamin B-12, and fat-soluble vitamins; gastrointestinal side effects
Affecting metabolism of nutrients	
Isoniazid,[d] L-dopa[e]	Vitamin B-6 antagonism
Salicylates[f]	Iron loss from gastrointestinal bleeding
Anticoagulants	Vitamin K antagonism

[a] A heart stimulant.
[b] Steroid hormones.
[c] Used to control blood cholesterol levels.
[d] Used in treatment of tuberculosis.
[e] Used in treatment of Parkinson's disease (a nervous disease including tremors and muscular weakness).
[f] Used in making aspirin.

report lists the following methods used to sell unproven products and to make sometimes dangerous diagnoses.

- **Extraordinary promises** are sometimes made, along with claims that the product being offered is the only available cure for the health problem. The false promises that fool many elderly people include the claim that the use of the amino acid L-cysteine will protect against environmental contaminants that damage DNA; that the amino acids arginine and ornithine will improve immune function; and that the enzyme *superoxide dismutase* (SOD) slows the aging process by destroying free radicals. SOD is an enzyme and therefore a protein, which is digested in the GI tract along with other dietary proteins and is totally useless when taken in this manner.

- **The term "alternative,"** which is commonly associated with therapies such as chiropractic and acupuncture, is used sometimes to promote questionable therapies.

- **False prevention** includes spreading the idea that taking a nutritional supplement or other product even when the person has no medical problem is good practice "just in case" the problem should arise.

Superoxide dismutase: An enzyme preventing oxidative damage in body tissues.

Kinesiology: The study of muscles and muscular movement.

- **Fantasy and science fiction** are often used to sell nutritional supplements. Scientific data are sometimes misused, or disproven findings are used. The food supply is portrayed as unhealthy, and supplements are said to be needed to improve nutrient intake and protect against toxicants and contaminants in foods. Attempts are made to place doubt in the minds of consumers about the food, nutrition, and health advice given by legitimate medical and scientific organizations such as the American Medical Association and the American Dietetic Association, by federal agencies such as the FDA and the USDA, and by the food and pharmaceutical industries. Of course, people should always ask questions and be fully informed about the background sources for nutrition information coming from these organizations. But to say or imply that they conspire to mislead the public is irresponsible.

- **Unproven diagnostic methods** include the detection of supposed nutritional deficiencies and diseases by applied *kinesiology*. A person's extremities are pushed and felt, and then various nutritional supplements are recommended. Another method is hair analysis, which has long been discredited as a means of detecting nutritional deficiencies. Values may vary widely between different testing laboratories, but nutritional supplements are usually recommended when results of the hair analysis are returned. A third method is live cell analysis, which uses red blood cells examined under a special microscope to diagnose nutrient deficiencies and some diseases. No recognized experts use this procedure.

- **Products sold to treat specific conditions** include special dietary cures and products for arthritis. This is a large market because about 97% of the people over the age of 60 have arthritis in some form. It is an attractive market for nutritional con artists because most forms of arthritis are incurable. People with arthritis are sold special diets, herbs, large doses of cod liver oil, combinations of vitamins and minerals, green-lipped mussel extract, and desiccated liver tablets. Waters from special sources given in unusual ways, such as by injection, are touted as cures for arthritis. Food allergy is said to cause arthritis. There is no scientific evidence to confirm any of the above claims.

The complete list of nutrition frauds is long–specialty diets or nutrition supplements are sold for Alzheimer's disease, CHD, cancer, and other medical problems. Many elderly people are vulnerable and alone and frequently have little help in obtaining creditable information.

■ Nutrition and food science in action–Why are no foods made specifically for the elderly?

Think beyond Figure 16-8. Why are no foods manufactured specifically for the elderly?

This is an appropriate question considering the amount of misinformation and number of useless products just reviewed that are offered (and sold) to the elderly. There are other reasons why this is a puzzle–one in six people (over 43 million) in North America is elderly. By the year 2025, one in four will be elderly–a huge market.[27] Think about your local supermarket and the size of the sections selling baby and infant food, junior food for toddlers, meals for young children, food for teenagers, for "yuppies," for "people on the go," for dieters, and for just about everybody except the elderly. Why? The answer is a fascinating mixture of psychology and economics. The United States is seen as a youth-oriented society, and foods specifically for the elderly would probably be a commercial disaster. That can be corrected only by changing the psychological attitudes of consumers. The huge size of the potential market for products for the elderly suggests that this situation may not remain static much longer. The technology to make foods that meet the nutritional, sensory, and convenience needs of the elderly exists, but that important psychological barrier must be broken first before commercial success is possible.

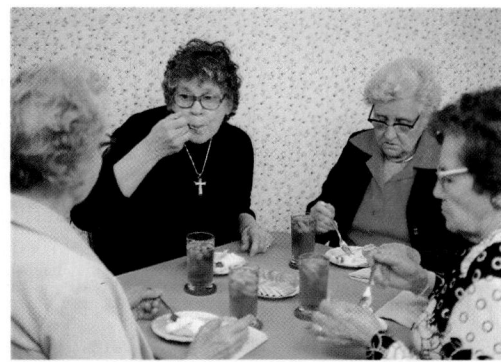

Figure 16-8. Older adults have different nutritional needs than younger ones. This is a market that the food industry will probably develop in the near future.

There are indications that elderly people are beginning to make significant changes in their diets.[28] In Table 16-6, notice the increased consumption of low-fat and high-fiber foods, fruits, and grains and the decreased consumption of eggs, bacon, and high-fat foods. The medical profession is realizing the importance of these dietary changes in preventing many problems in the elderly.[29] The food industry also has an opportunity to respond to these changing attitudes.

Food science and technology have contributed to the quality, safety, convenience, nutritional content, and economic value of our food supply.[30] All of these factors are important in designing foods for the elderly. Nutritious foods can now be made that meet the texture requirements of people with dentures and that can remedy the loss of taste and smell by elderly people. Because many of the elderly reduce their food intake as a result of decreased sensitivity to the taste and aroma of food, foods designed for them generally must have enhanced flavors. (This may not apply to those on chemotherapy or radiation treatment for cancer, or to those who lack a sense of smell or are obese or anorexic. Anorexic patients often reduce food consumption when flavors are added to foods.) Technology can also remove undesirable natu-

Table 16-6. Changes in the Proportion of U.S. Elderly People Consuming Selected Food Groups, 1977–1978 to 1987–1988 (weighted)

Size and Direction of Change (percentage of population)	New Consumption Pattern
>10% increase	Low-fat poultry products
	Low-fat milk and milk products
	Diet soft drinks
	Low-fat fish products
5–10% increase	Fruits
	Regular soft drinks
	Low-fat, high-fiber breads
	High-fat, grain-based mixed dishes
	High-fat, low-fiber breads
	Low-fat, grain-based mixed dishes
	Low-fat beef and pork
5–10% decrease	Eggs and egg dishes
	Coffee
	Bacon
	Tea
>10% decrease	Low-fat, low-fiber breads
	High-fat milk and milk products
	High-fat beef and pork

rally occurring constituents in food, such as those that cause intestinal distress and gas.

Elderly people are also relatively less sensitive to salt and to sugar than other consumers.[30] This might suggest that foods for them should have higher concentrations of salt and sugar to improve palatability. However, this is *not* recommended because of the high incidence of hypertension and diabetes in the elderly. About 45% of the 30 million Americans over 65 have hypertension, with African-Americans having higher incidences than whites.[31] So *salty peptides* and non-nutritive sweeteners should be used instead of salt and sugar, respectively. But there are limitations to the use of non-nutritive sweeteners because sugar provides several benefits not provided by non-nutritive sweeteners–preservation, flavor and aroma, bulk, texture, and control of water activity. In addition, sugar is a fermentable substrate. This is yet another example of the fact that components of food have both functional and nutritive values and that these sometimes interact and conflict. Because of this, not all of the sugar in foods for the elderly can be replaced by non-nutritive sweeteners.

It has been suggested that the color of food can be manipulated to provide increased perceptions of sweetness in foods and drinks.[30] Red and yellow colors seem to fool us into perceiving more sweetness. Perhaps we associate these colors with ripeness in sweet foods such as strawberries, raspberries, and bananas. By making beverages more appealing, creative use of color may solve the problem of fluid intake for older people who have lost much of the sensation of thirst.

The physical properties of polyunsaturated oils can be manipulated by food technology so that they form with water a thick, emulsified butter-like spread. This preserves the polyunsaturated nature of the fat, while allowing the incorporation of fat into a food to increase its caloric density. In addition, fats carry flavors and bring a tender and juicy sensation to many foods. Additional information on the importance of fat is given in Chapter 7, and you are encouraged to determine why these are important in designing foods for the elderly. Foods may now contain fat substitutes made from protein and other sources, and in the future soybeans and other oilseeds may be genetically engineered to produce the fatty acid composition most needed in foods for the elderly and other population groups.

The protein needs of the elderly are poorly understood.[32] There are suggestions that the requirement for several amino acids may be different in the elderly than in younger people. For example, the requirement for the essential amino acid lysine is about three times higher in older people. Lysine is the limiting amino acid in nearly all cereals (see Chapter 8). These differences may affect elderly people's response to stresses from physical, infectious, and psychological injuries and to burns, all of which have negative effects on amino acid and protein metabolism.

One solution to the problem of constipation among older people is to incorporate "nature's natural laxative," fiber, in a palatable form into foods designed for them. Genetic engineering could change the carbohydrate composition of plants. Chemical changes to starches and/or fiber could change their rate of passage through the GI tract.

Food fortified with vitamins and minerals will be increasingly important

Salty peptide: A group of specific amino acids forming a peptide that gives a salty flavor.

to the elderly as more convenience foods become available. We must improve our understanding of the bioavailability of these nutrients in elderly people. They are of zero value if they are in a form that is not absorbed into the body from the GI tract.

Foods for the elderly must be safe, easy to prepare, and in packages that are easy to read, easy to open, and with easily understandable nutrition labels and preparation instructions. In the future, we will see more use of sensors on packages to indicate the keeping quality and moisture content of the food. These food safety considerations are especially important for elderly people.[30]

■ Now you know

- Adolescent girls tend to have diets low in calcium, magnesium, iron, zinc, copper, and manganese.

- Adolescent girls avoid foods high in fat more often than boys do.

- Compared to adolescents of 100 years ago, nutrition-related characteristics of adolescents today include earlier onset of puberty; larger body size; more concern with weight-loss and eating disorders; and better access to a more nutritious diet as well as to snacks, fast foods, soft drinks, nutrient supplements, alcohol, and drugs. Foods contain more additives; people are exposed to advertising of food and drink in the media; teen pregnancy is higher; working hours differ; and athletics are given more emphasis.

- Nutrition-related problems often found among college students include dental caries, obesity, anemia (in women), acne, and alcohol and drug abuse.

- Middle-aged women have a higher incidence than men of obesity, certain cancers, osteoporosis, anemia, and goiter. In addition, they have premenstrual syndrome. Men have higher incidences of coronary heart disease and of certain cancers. Nutrition-related problems common to both genders include hypertension, dental and gum disorders, diabetes, and arthritis.

- The risk of an elderly person having poor nutritional status is increased by these factors: inappropriate, inadequate, or excessive food intake; poverty; social isolation; chronic use of medication; dependency and disability; acute or chronic diseases or conditions; and advanced age (over 80).

- Nutrition-related changes in body function with aging include decreases in these areas: sensory abilities, nerve-muscle coordination, chewing and swallowing ability, GI tract function, immune function, lean body mass, and kidney function.

- Other nutrition-related problems common in the elderly include constipation, diarrhea, and excessive use of prescription and over-the-counter drugs.

- Many elderly people are victims of nutritional quacks and fads.

- Food scientists can design foods to meet specific nutrient requirements for the elderly, but psychological and economic barriers prevent this from being done at present.

Further Reading

1. Millstein, S. G., and others. Health-risk behaviors and health concerns among young adolescents. *Pediatrics* 89:422, 1992.
2. Fisher, M. Parents' views of adolescent health issues. *Pediatrics* 90:335, 1992.
3. Wharton, B. Food and biological clocks. *Proceedings of the Nutrition Society* 51:145, 1992.
4. Farthing, M. C. Current eating patterns of adolescents in the United States. *Nutrition Today* 26(2):35, 1991.
5. Finn, S., and Kass, L. S. *The Real Life Nutrition Book: Making the Right Food Choices Without Changing Your Life-style*. Penguin Books, New York, 1992.
6. Wardle, J., and others. Eating style and eating behaviour in adolescents. *Appetite* 18:167, 1992.
7. Lender, M. E., and Martin, J. K. *Drinking in America*, The Free Press, New York, page 109, 1987.
8. Anonymous. Selected tobacco-use behaviors, dietary patterns among high school students–United States, 1991. *Journal of the American Medical Association* 268:448, 1992.
9. Foulke, J. E. On the teen scene. Good news about good nutrition. *FDA Consumer* 26(3):36, 1992.
10. Philen, R. M., and others. Survey of advertising for nutritional supplements in health and bodybuilding magazines. *Journal of the American Medical Association* 268:1008, 1992.
11. Hertzler, A. A., and Frary, R. Dietary status and eating out practices of college students. *Journal of the American Dietetic Association* 92:867, 1992.
12. Liddell, J. A., and others. Effects of a nutrition education programme on the dietary habits of a population of students and staff at a centre for higher learning. *Journal of Human Nutrition and Dietetics* 5:23, 1992.
13. Senauer, B., and others. *Food Trends and the Changing Consumer.* Eagan Press, St. Paul, MN, page 199, 1991.
14. Lohman, P. H. M., and others. Choosing the limits to life. *Nature* 357:185, 1992.
15. Parker, S. L. A national survey of nutritional risk among the elderly. *Journal of Nutrition Education* 24:23S, 1992.
16. Dwyer, J., and others. Screening older Americans' nutritional health: Future possibilities. *Nutrition Today* 26(5):21, 1991.
17. Rolls, B. J. Aging and appetite. *Nutrition Reviews* 50:422, 1992.
18. Lachapelle, D., and others. Masticatory ability and dietary adequacy of elderly denture wearers. *Journal of the Canadian Dietetic Association* 53:145, 1992.
19. Williams, M. Dysphagia–The new frontier. *Nutrition Today* 27(3):26, 1992.
20. Hosoda, S., and others. Age-related changes in the gastrointestinal tract. *Nutrition Reviews* 50:374, 1992.
21. Chandra, R. K. Effect of vitamin and trace-element supplementation on immune responses and infection in elderly subjects. *Lancet* 340:1124, 1992.
22. Kerstetter, J. E., and others. Malnutrition in the institutionalized older adult. *Journal of the American Dietetic Association* 92:1109, 1992.
23. Rosenberg, I. H., and Miller, J. W. Nutritional factors in physical and cognitive

functions of elderly people. ***American Journal of Clinical Nutrition*** 55:1237S, 1992.

24. Roubenoff, R., and Rall, L. C. Humoral mediation of changing body composition during aging and chronic inflammation. ***Nutrition Reviews*** 51:1, 1993.

25. Murray, F. E., and Bliss, C. M. Constipation: An update on a common problem. ***Geriatric Medicine*** 22(3):55, 1992.

26. Black, D. A. Diarrhoea deserves diagnosis. ***Geriatric Medicine*** 23(2):15, 1993.

27. Dichter, C. R. Designing foods for the elderly: An American view. ***Nutrition Reviews*** 50:480, 1992.

28. Anonymous. Are older Americans making better food choices to meet diet and health recommendations? ***Nutrition Reviews*** 51:20, 1993.

29. Johnson, K., and Kligman, E. W. Preventive nutrition: An 'optimal' diet for older adults. ***Geriatrics*** 47:56, 1992.

30. Clydesdale, F. M. Meeting the needs of the elderly with the foods of today and tomorrow. ***Nutrition Today*** 26(5):13, 1991.

31. Elnicki, M., and Kotchen, T. A. Hypertension: Patient evaluation, indications for treatment. ***Geriatrics*** 48(4):47, 1993.

32. Young, V. R. Macronutrient needs in the elderly. ***Nutrition Reviews*** 50:454, 1992.

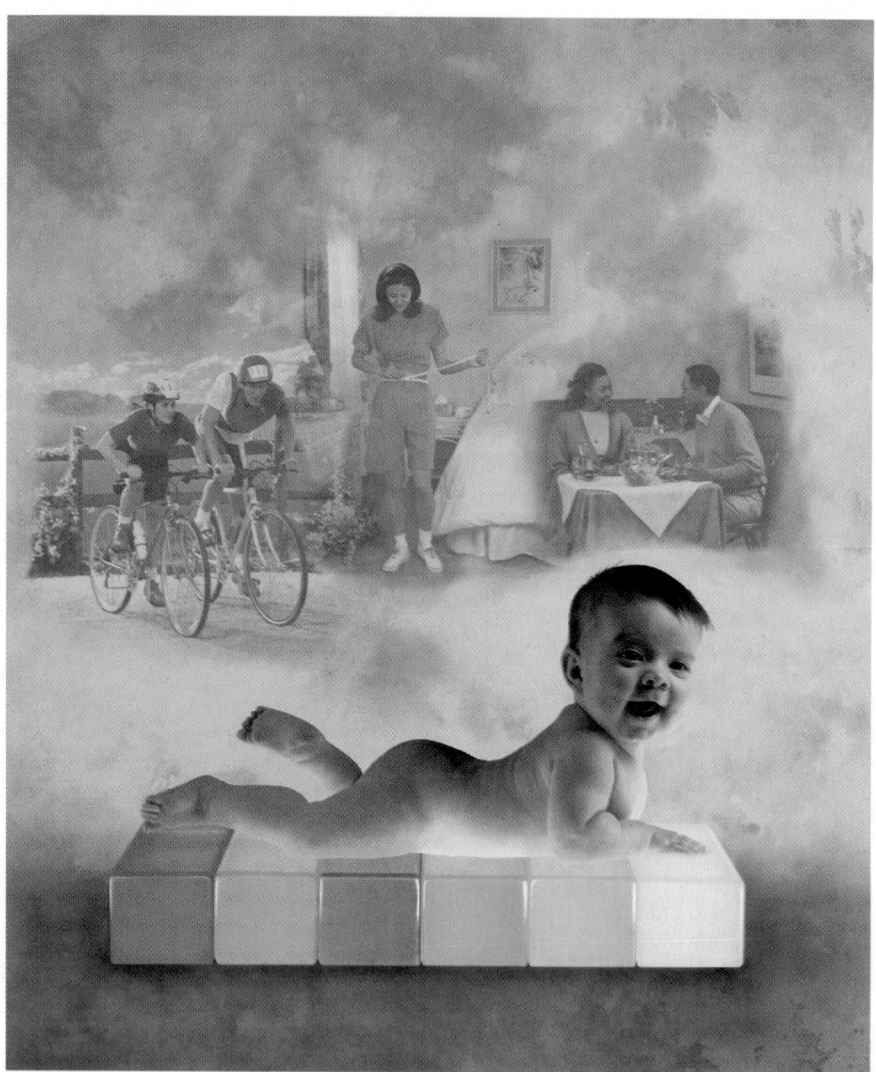

Figure 17-1. Changing lifestyles throughout life, as well as the varied lifestyles found in different places in the world, have a major effect on what and how people eat.

## CHAPTER 17

Nutrition, Food, and Lifestyles

■ Nutrition in our lives–Lifestyle plays a major role in nutrition

Dictionaries define "lifestyle" as a way of living; a person's typical mode of conduct or behavior. A large part of each of our lifestyles is determined for us by a number of factors, which are discussed below. They are the result of being born into a particular family, ethnic group, country, and time in history. But each of us also makes choices that affect our lifestyle–we can choose behaviors that contribute to a healthy, productive life. The focus in this chapter is on the way that lifestyle influences nutrition, particularly the foods we eat, and on the nutritional choices that we can make to improve our lifestyles.

In the picture above, the people may have stressful lives that influence their intake of food and nutrients. Maybe they have a sound knowledge of nutrition, or maybe they are misled by misinformation, faddism, and quackery. Religious belief may or may nor have an influence on their food choices. The picture does not tell us whether they have some nutrition-related diseases, maybe even unknown to them, such as cancer, coronary heart disease, diabetes, or others. All of these things influence the way they live, the nutrients they consume, and therefore their nutritional status. The picture shows people from a developed country–it does not account for other lifestyles from various parts of the world. Also missing from it are the homeless, the elderly, people starving from famine, the hospitalized, people with low income and, in the case of the adults, the uneducated. These conditions are also factors in lifestyle that influence nutritional status.

In this chapter we will think about some of the many different lifestyles of the approximately 5.5 billion people in the world. This is no easy task. For instance, here are two contrasting lifestyles that have nutritional implications.

Major Topics in This Chapter

Your lifestyle has an important influence on food choices and nutrient intake.

Adequate income for food is essential for satisfactory nutritional status.

■

Homelessness is associated with nutrient deficiencies.

Day care centers must be evaluated carefully for safe food handling and nutritious diets.

Education is an important factor in influencing nutrient intake.

Ethnic identity influences food choices by immigrants and refugees.

Religious beliefs may influence food choices.

Lifestyles have important influences on relationships among nutrition and health and physiological characteristics.

The Masai tribe in Kenya in eastern Africa live mainly as herders of their cattle. Tourist postcards from Kenya feature the very tall, red-robed Masai men with their cattle. Medical researchers from around the world have studied them in detail over a 20-year period. The reason for such interest is that the Masai diet contradicts the dietary guidelines of developed countries, including the United States, yet the incidence of coronary heart disease among the Masai is low. They eat large quantities of meat and butter, and even drink their cattle's blood after slaughter, resulting in a high intake of cholesterol and saturated fat. One explanation for this contradiction is that they get an enormous amount of physical exercise while herding their cattle. Their lifestyle seems untroubled, but it is not stress-free because of the threat from wild animals.

> To the Masai . . . the wild animals are a nuisance, at best. Predators . . . occasionally attack cattle and, less frequently, their keepers. (*Scientific American*, page 38, September 1989)

Contrast the way the Masai live with the following description in the *Economist* (May 4, 1991).

> Americans spend $20 billion a year on food and drink served by mechanical dispensers. Now they are about to be offered the most ubiquitous of junk-food staples, French fries–chips to Britons–via a vending machine . . . . Soon 'Prize Frize' machines will appear at shops, schools, and even car-washes all over the Los Angeles area.

Certain lifestyles and cultural attitudes may hurt people's nutritional status. This is true for women in some parts of the world. In poor rural households in Nepal, north of India, a woman may have lower nutrient intake because she is usually the last family member to eat.[1] Preferential distribution of food is given to the elderly and the young of both sexes. Women receive special foods only when they are pregnant or breast feeding.

The food industry is a careful observer of changing lifestyles. *Food Engineering* (May 1991) carried an editorial under the heading "Rethink demographics. Focus on lifestyle and basic science." The editor writes,

> my suggestion to product development people at the food companies is to pay more attention to what may be changing lifestyle factors, regardless of age, income, marital status, etc.

This acknowledges that, if new foods are to have commercial success, they must meet the needs of differing lifestyles. The editor goes on to say that factors basic to lifestyle considerations should be health, personal image (not just "looks," but also self-image), interpersonal values including family interaction, and finally, work habits and attitudes toward leisure.

Think beyond the diagram in Figure 17-2. How is food a part of your lifestyle? How does lifestyle influence your food habits?

Each of us will have different answers to these two questions. The diagram serves as a framework to provide an answer for your specific lifestyle as well as guiding us in the following discussion.

Notice the important location of the box labeled "lifestyle" at the bottom of the diagram and the many factors that lead to it. It is worth the journey through this diagram a few times to see where you fit into each of these categories. How important is each one to you? Did one or more of these factors have a significant influence on your food intake during the last few years? Are these lifestyle factors likely to change in the near future or throughout your life? How do you think other people might fit into these lifestyle factors? Consider a family member or friend, or somebody from the other side of the country or another culture, or a European, African, or Asian person. Countries throughout the world have different food production and distribution systems and socioeconomic-political systems that influence their peoples' food choices and nutritional status. We will use this diagram to guide us through discussion of the influences of various lifestyle factors on nutrition and health and the role of food in lifestyle, starting with the role of income as it relates to nutrient intake.

■ Income

People with high incomes generally have access to many different foods and can easily obtain balanced diets if they understand the principles of good nutrition and have the desire to use them. On the other hand, they may overeat or choose diets that contain too much of some types of foods, especially those with fats and sugars. We have noted that "diseases of affluence" (coronary heart disease, cancer, diabetes, hypertension, and obesity, among others) tend to be more prevalent in the developed countries, in which average incomes are high. Research on these diseases and education about nutrition may make them less prevalent in the future. More complex problems stem from the effects of lack of income on nutritional status.

The World Declaration on Nutrition was signed in Rome, Italy, in December 1992 by representatives of most countries.[2] The following statement from the declaration shows the importance of personal income as an influence on people's nutritional status.

> We recognize that poverty and lack of education, which are often the effects of underdevelopment, are the primary causes of hunger and undernutrition. There are poor people in most societies who do not have adequate access to food, safe water and sanitation, health services and education, which are the basic requirements for nutritional well-being.

Food as a Human Right is the title of a book published by the United Nations University in which arguments are presented that the citizens of every nation have a human right to food (as well as to work, education, and health). This raises a critical question: Who is to pay for the food?

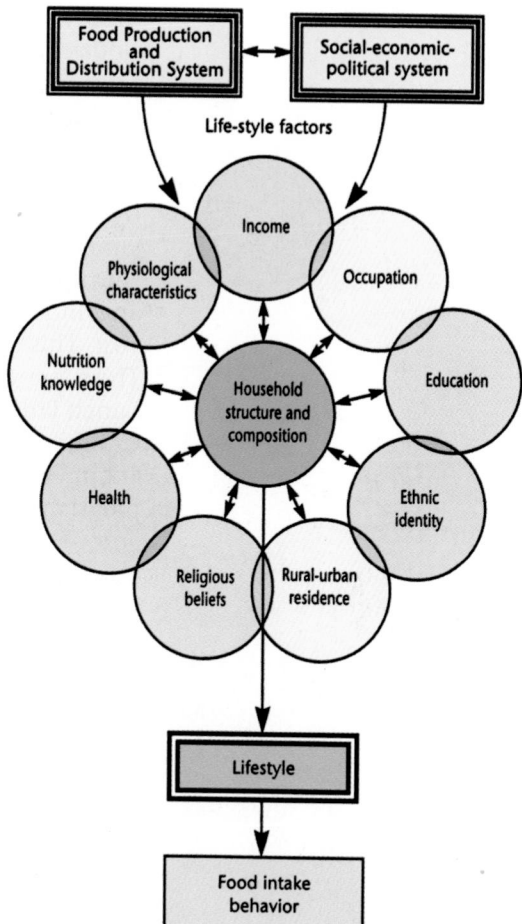

Figure 17-2. Lifestyle factors influencing food intake behavior.

Clearly, food is a commodity to be traded like automobiles, cameras, or clothes. Throughout the world it is a source of income for farmers, processors, distributors, and shopkeepers. It is to governments, therefore, that the hungry in most countries turn for food assistance programs.

In the United States, the various federal food assistance programs evolved from the farm support programs developed during the Great Depression of the 1930s.[3] These were set up to provide food to low-income families using surplus food produced by farmers. One of them, the Family Nutrition Program, includes the Food Stamp Program, which operates at an annual cost of over $22 billion and serves about 25 million people each year. This means that about one in every 10 Americans is in the program. There are five child nutrition programs, of which the National School Lunch Program is the largest. Others are the School Breakfast program, the Child and Adult Care Food Program, the Special Milk Program, and the Summer Food Service Program. The best known of the supplemental food programs is the Special Supplemental Food Program for Women, Infants, and Children (WIC), which we discussed in Chapter 15. The government purchases surplus food from farmers and distributes it through the Temporary Emergency Food Assistance Program (TEFAP), the Nutrition Program for the Elderly, and charitable institutions. The number of people dependent on one or more of these programs is increasing at a time when budget problems at the national and local level are also increasing.

Hunger among the homeless is a reality.[4] Many feeding programs provide about 1,000 calories, with some meals low in fruits, vegetables, grains, and dairy products. In Chapter 11 we learned that most adults with an intake of 1,000 calories per day will lose weight because this energy intake is not sufficient to meet resting energy expenditure. That is exactly what was found in a study in Miami, Florida, where one in five homeless men studied had wasting malnutrition.[5] One researcher in this study noted that

> . . . the threat and reality of homelessness crosses both genders and all races, marital backgrounds, and professions.

Estimates of homeless people in the United States are as high as 3 million, most of whom are single adults or families headed by single women. Their food is often obtained from soup kitchens and shelters, family or friends, or from garbage cans. Homeless people begging for money or food are a common sight in many cities. Most experts agree that the homelessness problem has four main causes–lack of available housing, poverty, alcohol and drugs, and mental illness. Social workers are concerned that donated money may be spent on alcohol and/or drugs rather than on food. A few years ago, the city of Berkeley, California, introduced the "Berkeley Cares" program, which distributes vouchers to homeless people in the city. Written on each voucher is the statement: "Good for food, bus or laundry at locations listed on the back" and in bolder print: "Not good for alcohol or tobacco. Not redeemable in cash."

Children are the most rapidly expanding component of the homeless population. Homeless children have multiple health problems, including increased incidences of delayed growth and mental development and of diarrhea. Single homeless women and their children in a study in Kansas

City, Missouri, had iron deficiency anemia, were obese (probably from consumption of high-fat foods), and had high blood-cholesterol levels and inadequate intake of some minerals and vitamins, as seen in Table 17-1.[6]

Think about the reasons why these are problem nutrients for the homeless.

Refer back to the list of nutrients and their food sources in Chapter 1. Further input for your answer can come from thinking of the cost of these foods and of their storage and preparation. Some nutrition problems can be solved with improved nutrition education, a fact recognized all over the world (Figure 17-3).

Income is also a factor for the approximately 17 million refugees in the world who are dependent on food aid and to a further 15 million people displaced by war in their own countries.[7] Vitamin deficiency diseases–scurvy, pellagra, beriberi, and blindness due to vitamin A deficiency–are common, as is iron-deficiency anemia. Relief programs often fail to provide foods high in these nutrients, usually because of difficulties with food distribution.

Discussions on food relief and nutrient deficiencies in developing countries often give the idea that the situation in these countries is hopeless. But it is not, as evidenced in a history of dietary changes in The Netherlands as it became a developed country in Western Europe.[8] The change from a poor and monotonous diet to one of abundance was not linear but was a series of corrections from various setbacks. The same situation exists in some of the developing countries today.

Table 17-1. Inadequate Intake of Some Minerals and Vitamins by Single Homeless Women and Their Children

| Nutrient | Mean Intake Less than 70% RDA | | |
| | Children | | |
	0.5–1 Years	7–10 Years	Mothers
Calcium			x
Magnesium	x	x	x
Zinc	x	x	x
Iron	x	x	x
Vitamin A	x	x	
Folacin	x	x	x

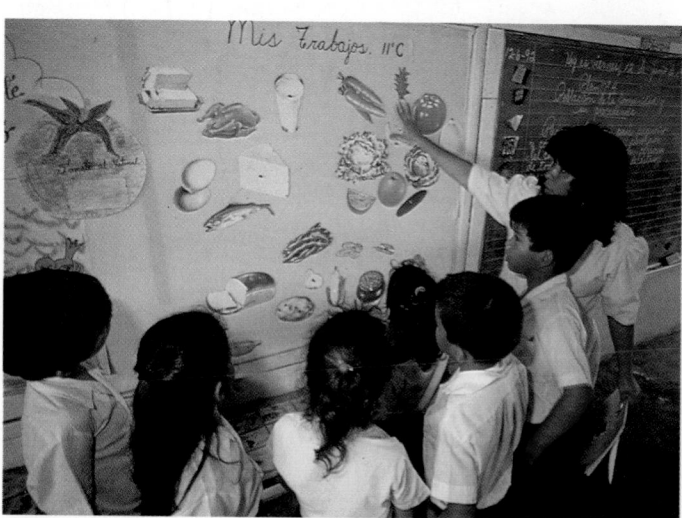

Figure 17-3. Better access to nutrition education can solve many nutritional problems in all parts of the world.

■ Occupation

Your job frequently dictates your eating pattern–you have to deal with business lunches, travel, or being too far from home for a midday lunch. One person's occupation may influence the food intake of other people. For example, eating patterns of young children placed in child care centers may influence food intake in some two-income families.

Children at some child care facilities may have low intake levels of energy, iron, zinc, magnesium, vitamins A and C, and folacin.[9] This list of inadequate nutrients is similar to the list we saw for children in homeless shelters. However, one of the federal food assistance programs, the Child and Adult Care Program, subsidizes meals for children in licensed child

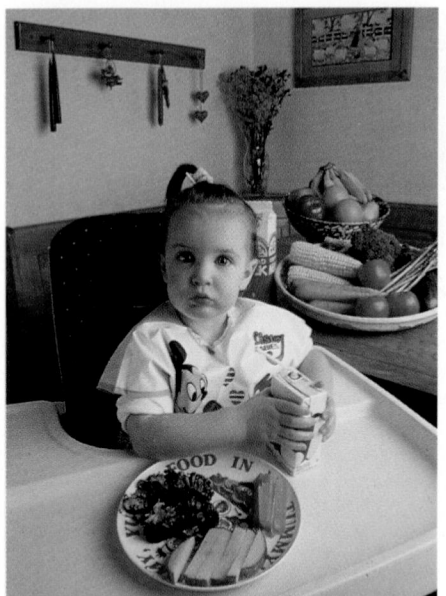

Figure 17-4. A child having lunch in a child care center. Child care arrangements may have a significant influence on a child's nutrient intake during the preschool years. Dietary quality and safety in food handling should be factors examined before deciding on a child care facility.

care homes and centers and also provides nutritional education and guidelines. Food safety is a major problem in some child care facilities because of unhygienic handling and storage of food. Transmission of the harmful bacteria is sometimes through the fecal-oral route. This does not imply that all children in child care are exposed to nutritional and food safety problems or that similar problems do not occur with some children who are fed at home. It does illustrate the importance of paying attention to nutrition and food safety when making decisions about which child care program to use.

The following precautions should be observed to decrease the likelihood of transmission of diarrheal disease in child care facilities, as well as in the home:[10]

- Staff, parents, and children should wash their hands well with soap and running water. This should be done after using the toilet and before handling, preparing, and eating food.
- Preparers of food (including bottles) should not change diapers or assist children in using the toilet. If they must do these activities, rigorous handwashing is required.
- Surfaces and hard-surface toys should be decontaminated regularly.
- Children with diarrhea should be excluded from the day care facility until they are well.

Stress is another factor associated with occupation, as it seems to go with the job in most countries. Some stresses in the work environment may influence the quantity, quality, and speed at which food is consumed. Job-related stress can impair the physiological functioning of the body, including the digestion and metabolism of food (producing acid-indigestion, for example). Stress can also interfere with physical activity and relaxation patterns and may be a factor in ill health because it is a risk factor in coronary heart disease, hypertension, and stomach ulcers. Some studies show that people with a type A personality–people who are impatient, highly competitive, and obsessed with details–have a higher risk for heart attacks. What is still unsolved is whether stress causes this type of behavior or whether the behavior causes stress. A further complication is that type A people are usually heavy cigarette smokers and coffee drinkers, both of which are categories of people with risk factors for coronary heart disease. On the other hand, some people actually thrive on stress (and to relax would probably kill them!).

> Most women turn to eating in times of stress. It can be sweet and tender or tough and chewy–it's there for you to choose,

writes Dr. Judith Rodin of Yale University.[11] She describes food as a friend and eating as a way of loving oneself.

The commercialization of stress relief is to be expected, given the amount of it that supposedly exists in most people's lives. The "stress segment" of drugstore vitamin sales is large and expanding. Supplements with trade names such as Stresstabs, Stressgard, Megastress, Superstress, and Ultrastress are available in most supermarkets. These are multivitamin and mineral preparations. Do they work? There is no evidence that these nutrient supplements will correct minor stresses. Furthermore, some manufacturers play games with the word "stress" to increase sales of their multinutrient products. This is possible because there are two types of stress, physical and psychological. Physical stress occurs after injury, burns, infections, trauma, surgery, and temperature extremes. Nutrients are important in the repair of tissues from these stresses. Psychological stresses include emotional tension and anxiety, for which nutrients are not directly helpful. Advertisements for multinutrient products may just mention the word "stress," assuming that consumers will relate the word to the psychological stress in their lives. Some manufacturers admit that their products are effective for physical stress only, but this is rarely stated in advertisements.

It is best to cope with psychological stress by eating an adequate diet to prevent nutrient deficiencies, finding time to relax, avoiding high salt intake because of salt's relationship to hypertension in some people, and avoiding caffeine, which makes some people nervous. However, these recommendations are not very useful for millions of people in the developing world, where stress is caused by the struggle for food and survival.

■ Education

Education is usually related to other lifestyle factors influencing food intake, such as income and nutrition knowledge. However, knowing what is "good for you" does not always translate into eating what is "good for you." Consumers are often misinformed about healthful eating, despite the millions of dollars spent on nutrition education programs.[12] Many people are interested in nutrition education but are not prepared to spend time to get reliable nutrition information.[13] This was observed in the response of supermarket shoppers to five videotapes, each lasting just 1 minute. Each tape focused on the role of nutrition in reducing cancer risks, with topics on dietary fat, vitamin A, fiber, vitamin C, and cruciferous vegetables (broccoli, brussels sprouts, cabbage, and cauliflower). Only one in four shoppers viewed these 1-minute videos, and lack of time was given as the reason for nonviewing. "Quest for Convenience: A Matter of Time" is the title of an article that best summarizes some of the influences of our lifestyle on nutrient intake.[14] Busy lifestyles don't allow some people the time to be educated about the purchase and preparation of healthy foods.

Think about the numbers in Table 17-2. Do you know the nutritional facts about fast foods?

Look at the variation in percent calories from fat, the amount and type of fat, and the amount of sodium. Your choice of fast food could be important if you are watching your intake of calories, fat, and/or sodium.

Table 17-2. "Low-Fat" Fast Foods

Food	Percent Calories from Fat	Calories	Total Fat (g)	Saturated Fat (g)	Sodium (mg)	Quality[b]
Poultry sandwiches						
Arby's light roast turkey deluxe	21	260	6	2	1,262	★★★
Wendy's grilled chicken[c]	22	290	7	1	670	★★★★
Arby's light roast chicken deluxe	23	276	7	2	777	★★★★
Burger King's BK broiler chicken	32	280	10	2	770	★★★
Beef sandwiches						
McDonald's McLean deluxe[c]	28	320	10	4	670	★★★
Wendy's Jr. hamburger	30	270	9	3	590	★★★
Arby's light roast beef deluxe	31	294	10	4	826	★★★★
Chicken salads[a]						
McDonald's chunky chicken salad[c]	24	150	4	1	230	★★★
Burger King chunky chicken salad	25	142	4	1	443	★★★
Hardee's grilled chicken salad[c]	30	120	4	1	520	...[d]
Arby's roast chicken salad	32	204	7	3	508	★★★★
Wendy's grilled chicken salad	36	200	8	1	690	★★★★
Side salads[a]						
Arby's side salad	...[e]	25	≤1	0	30	★★★
Burger King side salad	...[e]	20	≤1	0	10	★★★
Hardee's side salad	...[e]	20	≤1	≤1	20	★★★
McDonald's side salad	...[e]	30	≤1	0	35	★★★
Wendy's side salad	45	60	3	≤1	200	★★★
Vanilla shakes						
McDonald's low-fat milk shake	4	290	1	1	170	★★
Burger King shake	17	310	6	4	230	...[d]
Hardee's shake	22	370	9	6	210	★★★
Arby's shake	31	330	12	4	281	★★★
Chocolate shakes						
McDonald's low-fat milk shake	5	320	2	1	240	★★
Burger King shake	20	400	9	5	350	...[d]
Arby's shake	23	451	12	3	341	★★★
Hardee's shake	23	390	10	6	220	★★★
Wendy's frosty dairy dessert	25	460	13	7	260	★★★
Sundaes						
McDonald's hot fudge low-fat frozen yogurt sundae	11	240	3	2	170	★★★
Hardee's cool twist hot fudge sundae	28	320	10	5	260	★★★

[a] Tested without dressing.
[b] In decreasing order of quality: ★★★★★, ★★★★, ★★★, ★★, ★.
[c] Contains 60 milligrams of cholesterol or more per serving (20% of the recommended daily limit).
[d] Not ranked for quality.
[e] Insignificant amount of fat.

■ Ethnic identity

Recent immigrants frequently maintain the eating patterns of "the old country." For instance, the Hmong people come from Southern China, Vietnam, Thailand, Burma, and Northern Laos. Many have settled in California and Minnesota, where they maintain their specific eating patterns, staple foods, methods of food preparation and food handling, their perceptions and beliefs about body size and health, and their food and nutrition needs and interests.[15] But the food patterns of immigrants tend to be modified over the generations. For example, while new immigrants from Asia maintain their traditional eating patterns, third and fourth generation Asian-Americans have much lower preferences for traditional Asian cuisine. Nutrition educators must be sensitive to the cultural beliefs and traditions of the groups they work with.

■ Rural-urban residence

Think beyond the picture in Figure 17-6. What are two heads of lettuce doing in a section examining the impact of rural or urban residence on nutritional status?

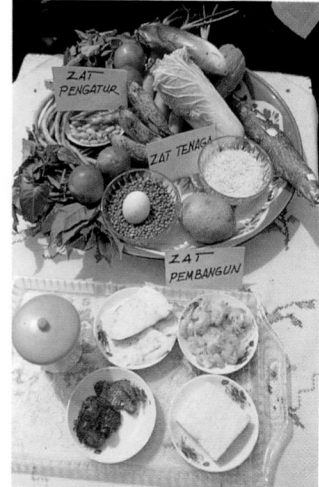

Figure 17-5. Ethnic foods are now available to everyone, as the food industry adapts to the needs of busy lifestyles.

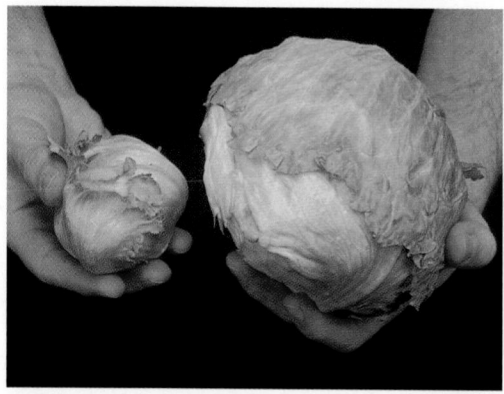

Figure 17-6. Genetics is playing a part in adapting food for changing lifestyles. The head of lettuce on the left has been genetically selected to be smaller to meet the needs of smaller families and people living alone.

Think about why the USDA has spent money and time to genetically develop a smaller head of lettuce. One reason is that family size is smaller now than it used to be. Also, people tend to have less available refrigerator space because of the many other foods also requiring refrigeration. Smaller heads should also increase the demand for lettuce, thus providing more work for farmers.

A poor farmer may have more access to fresh foods than a person with the same income living in the inner city. Nevertheless, some poor people living in rural America have a limited selection of food that is sold in high-priced small and medium-sized stores. Because these food prices are higher than those in the city, food stamp benefit allotments may not purchase as much food for them.[16] Nutrient intake also can differ among urban dwellers, as seen in a Canadian study in several different cities.[17] Income was a significant factor associated with lower intake in all the cities, but the findings were not the same everywhere. For instance, in the province of Quebec, people spent more money on food for home preparation and less on eating out than people in the rest of Canada.

It is in the developing world that rural-urban differences in nutrient intake are seen most dramatically.

Think beyond Figure 17-7 to understand some of the relationships between nutrition, food, and the environment in developing countries.

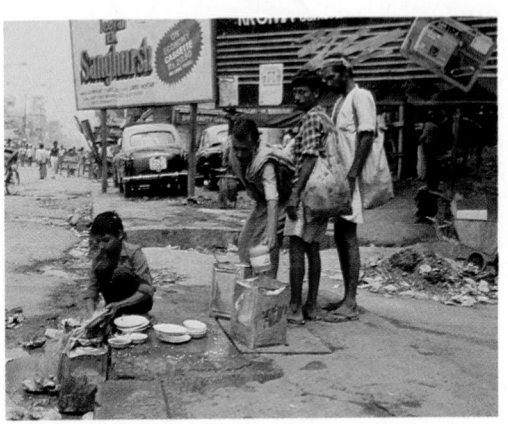

In Bangladesh, one of the poorest countries in the world, the urban poor are at greater nutritional risk than the rural poor.[18] Children living in these slums showed a higher prevalence of wasting than children living with rural families. Researchers describe the situation as "alarming" because of low intake of almost all foods and nutrients, especially cereals, fish, milk, and other dairy products. Low nutrient intake is made worse by living conditions that include inadequacy in water supply, housing, sewage and drainage facilities, paved roads, clearance of garbage, and general hygienic and sanitary conditions.

Figure 17-7. Street foods offer convenience in cities all over the world. Food safety and environmental standards are not always observed.

Think beyond Table 17-3 and compare the problems, interventions, and constraints listed with those in your city or community.

The table was developed by the Food and Agricultural Organization of the United Nations after a survey of many cities in Africa, Asia, and Latin America in the 1980s. The information in the table illustrates how nutrition interacts with economics and politics, urban planning, environmental studies, education, engineering, and medicine.

Street food vendors are common sights in cities in developing countries. The demand for relatively inexpensive, ready-to-eat food has increased as the population increased and people have had less time to prepare meals.[19] "Street foods" refers to a wide range of ready-to-eat foods and beverages sold and sometimes prepared in public places, notably streets (Figure 17-8).

Street foods are important in the economy of many cities and a significant part of the diet of many citizens. Some Asian countries experience problems with street foods,[19] including: the unauthorized use of food coloring and sweetening agents, lead contamination of food, peanuts contaminated with aflatoxin, and high pesticide residues, especially in vegetable products. (Pesticide residues are problems in home-cooked meals also.) Microbiological standards are difficult to enforce, especially for cold meals such as rice and vegetable dishes. The risks and benefits of

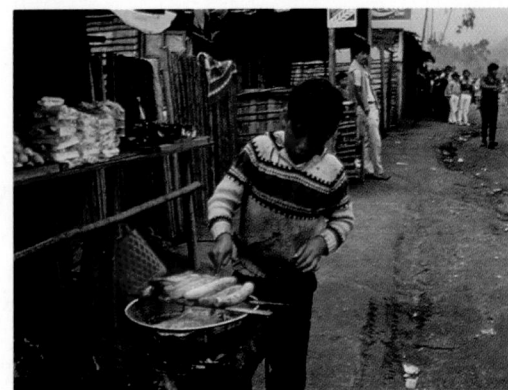

Figure 17-8. The risks and benefits of street foods are based on nutritional, social, economic, and regulatory (including food safety) factors.

Table 17-3. Reports and Results of FAO Missions to Urban Centers in Africa, Asia, and Latin America[a]

Problems	Interventions	Constraints
Prices of food too high for the poor; food value/packaging ratio	Fair price shops; simpler packaging, communal buying, consumer cooperatives	Economic and political decisions required
Prices of staples fluctuate at times of scarcity and prices at parallel markets soar	Have city stocks especially for the poor, placed in poor areas for easy access	Political and economic decisions required
Time shortage for breast feeding, infant food preparation, reduced child care; nutritional problems of the old	Day care centers at work places, formulated cheap weaning foods, communal kitchens	Lack of relevant legislation for working mothers; lack of technology and resources
Unbalanced food intake, micronutrient deficiencies, lack of household food safety	Urban agriculture for fresh vegetables and fruit; fortification and production of cheap nutrient-dense food mixes; fish ponds and small animal raising	Legal restriction for city agriculture; lack of space and extension services; lack of fruit-tree nurseries
Poor environment; scarcity of cooking fuel; insufficient safe drinking-water sources; poor health	Piped water at street outlets; urban fuel wood plots; expansion of health services to slum areas; education on environmental hygiene	Cost-effective interventions but requiring political decisions
Long distances to markets	Establishment of controlled and serviced markets in poor areas	Needs careful planning and execution, may require subsidies
Lack of knowledge regarding nutrition	Nutrition education	Illiteracy; program funding; misleading advertising
Lack of statistics on the urban poor and nutrition status, and of programs for planning and monitoring	Mandate the collection of data to urban statistical offices	Legal problem as slum areas not considered to be part of city administration
Scarcity of manpower for program implementation	In-service training for staff, volunteers, and youth	Difficulty in finding sufficient literate volunteers; high drop-out rate
Insufficient nutritional aspects within existing community development activities	Awareness-raising among urban leaders and planners	Need for greater political awareness
Waste of resources and efforts due to lack of program and coordination by public sector and NGOs[b]	Establish coordinating mechanism	Danger of diluting commitment and initiative of NGOs through formalized action

[a] Nairobi, Lusaka, Lagos, Dhakka, Jakarta, Bangkok and cities in Argentina, Brazil, Colombia, Chile, Ecuador, Mexico, Peru, Uruguay, and Venezuela.
[b] Nongovernment organizations.

street food are further examples of the mix of nutrition with social, economic, and regulatory factors, as summarized in Table 17-4 (next page).

■ Religious and ethical beliefs

The influence of religious beliefs on food intake depends on the religion and the religious intensity of the believer. Many Christian groups have few or no restrictions on food. Exceptions include Seventh-Day Adventists, who do not prepare food on the Sabbath (Saturday) and do not consume meat, spices, tea, coffee, alcohol, or tobacco. Mormons (Latter-day Saints) emphasize vegetables and herbs, with meat used sparingly. Orthodox

Table 17-4. Current Benefits and Problems of Street Foods in Many Developing Countries

Benefits	Problems
Use of local resources	Contamination; poor hygiene
Employment opportunities	Not a recognized industry
Adequate earnings for vendors; varied and nutritious food; inexpensive, accessible service	Lack of social status; complex or nonexistent licensing systems
Quality upgraded by licensing and inspection	Ineffective and arbitrary inspection
Social needs met	Traffic congestion aggravated

Judaism prohibits consumption of pork and shellfish and consumption of meat and dairy products at the same meal.

All religions and all legal codes have long upheld the principle that life is sacred and ought to be preserved. However, advances in medical technology have created a conflict–should people be kept alive who, without intervention, would surely die? This is a complex question and is discussed here only because nutrition support for terminally ill patients is a problem for dietitians and nutritionists. The issue of feeding the terminally ill patient raises questions involving medicine, law, ethics, and philosophy, as well as nutrition.

Terminal illness is defined as

> the end or stage of a specific, progressive, normally irreversible lethal disease when physicians have 'determined, through objective medical validation, that medical treatment of that disease is futile' and the disease will cause the patient's death in the foreseeable future.[20]

The American Dietetic Association issued the following position statement on feeding the terminally ill person:

> . . . that the dietitian take an active role in developing criteria for feeding the terminally ill adult within the practice setting and collaborate with the health care team in making recommendations on each case.

This can be interpreted to mean that each individual case is special, and it raises some further questions, especially regarding cases where the disease is advanced and the patient is in a vegetative state. Doctors withhold medical treatment, such as antibiotics and cardiopulmonary resuscitation, from vegetative patients after consultation with family and nursing staff.[21] Should they also withhold artificial feeding because it is a form of medical treatment? Most medical and legal opinion in the United States holds that feeding nutrients through the nose or into the stomach is medical treatment. An important question is whether withdrawal of food and fluids will cause the patient the pain and suffering that usually accompany starvation and dehydration. Medical evidence suggests that the vegetative patient has lost the nervous activity to make pain or suffering possible. A working group on medical ethics has said:

> . . . giving food and water to the sick has symbolic significance as a mark of continuing care and an expression of humanity. But the symbolic significance of an act cannot be divorced from its purpose and context. In vegetative patients the normal purpose of sustaining life and easing the ravages of hunger and thirst do not apply, and feeding does not benefit the patient.[21]

This is a difficult nutrition question to which you may bring your own interpretation.

■ Health

Think about the pictures in Figures 17-9 and 17-10. Are we relying on unusual foods to correct some lifestyle-related diseases?

The food industry continues to search for combinations of foods and for ingredients to satisfy our tastes as well as our requirements for healthy food. Expect to hear more about the health-giving or curative properties of specific foods. Garlic–the "stinking rose"– is a good example. It "wards off tumors as well as vampires," according to the title of an article in a Penn State University publication. Garlic is one of the oldest cultivated plants and is an essential

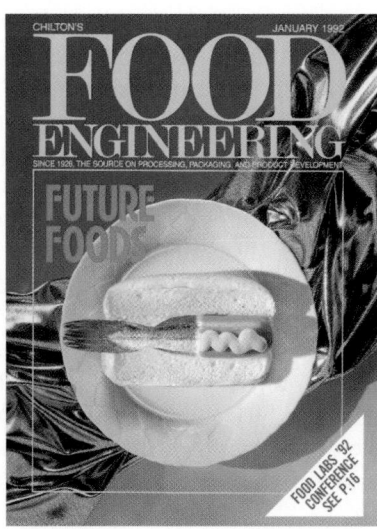

Figure 17-9. Although, in the future, you may not get fish and hot dogs combined into one food, you can expect many other interesting combinations.

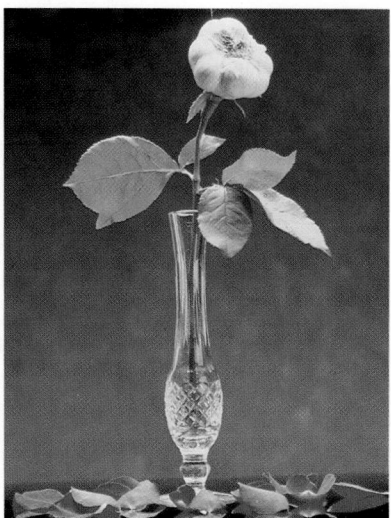

Figure 17-10. A depiction of garlic as "the stinking rose." Garlic, along with other foods, has been said to have health-giving or curative properties.

culinary ingredient in many countries. Besides its use as a flavoring, it is studied for its medicinal properties. Some studies suggest that garlic helps prevent cancer, coronary heart disease, and hypertension. Much research remains to be done to show why and how it may prevent these diseases.

We have met numerous examples of the positive and negative effects on health given by specific foods. Now let's take a brief look at some issues not previously covered.

Food for travelers

Diet and food preference considerations have taken to the air, literally. Air travel is such a part of many people's lives that airlines provide (on request) low-cholesterol, vegetarian, kosher, and other specific food requirements. There is also increasing emphasis on food safety during travel by air, rail, bus, or sea.[22] "You are our extra eyes and ears" is how an FDA official describes the help provided by the public in reporting food poisoning and other food-related problems while traveling. Contrast this with a writer's view of food served during air travel in the past:

> For the first 45 years of commercial air travel, the food served at 30,000 feet was always good for a laugh–unless you had to eat it. Indescribable, indestructible, and tasteless at best, the standard passenger fuel was often unfriendly to the waistline and the coronary arteries as well (*Newsweek*, November 26, 1990).

Two problems regarding children

Here's a brief look at two examples, selected from many, that show the effects of lifestyle on the nutritional status of children in developing and developed countries. Hookworms, roundworms, and whipworms are common infections in developing countries, especially among children. They are transmitted by the improper disposal of feces from infected individuals. Children suffering from protein-energy malnutrition have reduced growth rates because of these infections. One or two doses of a chemical that kills these parasites improves the nutritional status of infected children.[23] This remedy is inexpensive and easy to administer.

A problem for children in some developed countries is candy cigarettes, which are easily available to young children and often preferred over other snacks.[24] Candy cigarettes are packaged to resemble cigarette brands and are considered important in causing children to develop a positive attitude toward cigarette smoking. This is a nutritional problem because many studies show the negative effects of smoking on food intake and nutritional status. For example, one study reports that adult smokers have lower intake of vegetables, fruits, and cereals and higher consumption of coffee and alcohol as compared with nonsmokers.[25]

Health concerns in specific populations

Let's return one last time to the emphasis on "people are different" in this book. Various ethnic groups may have different views and concerns about specific nutritional problems. In a study of two ethnic groups, African-American parents had greater concern than Hispanic parents about children's dental caries and less concern about anemia and high lead. Both groups had equal concern about underweight, overweight, and growth delay.[26] Regarding health problems in adults, African-Americans had greater concern about anemia, high blood pressure, cancer, and overweight, whereas Hispanics had greater concern about diabetes. Current preferences for sources of nutrition information suggest how health education about these nutrition-related problems can best be conducted.

Think about the data in Table 17-5. Where do you get *your* nutrition information?

Table 17-5. Current and Preferred Sources of Nutrition Information in Two Ethnic Groups

Source of Nutrition Information	Percent Agreement	
	African-American	Hispanic
Current		
WIC	55	61
Physician	44	43
Magazines	21	24
Food labels	32	23
Child's school	28	21
Newspaper	21	11
Family (mother)	36	25
Preferred		
Nutrition handouts	50	43
Individual meeting	24	14
Cooking and tasting demonstration	39	32
Videos, films, and slides	27	18

■ Nutrition knowledge

The future presents an exciting challenge regarding nutrition knowledge as our diet becomes more complex. Supermarket shoppers must balance knowledge about nutrition with concerns about price, quality, health, food safety, and environmental issues, while taking into consideration culture and religion, family structure, the social status of food, and allergies. Consumers are being encouraged to disclose their nutrition and food concerns.[27] We should see more corporate and hospital wellness programs that include a significant nutrition component providing nutrition assessment, individual counseling on nutrition problems, and activities to increase awareness of nutrition-related diseases.[28]

The role of "junk food" versus "healthy food" in the diet is an ongoing debate. Some nutritionists hold that there are no junk foods, only junk diets. They contend that a low intake of low-nutrient foods is not damaging to health, provided that the overall nutrient intake is adequate. But it seems that people adopt their own interpretation of the effects of junk food–in one study, they associated it with weight gain, pleasure, friends, independence, and guilt.[29] Consumption of health food was associated with weight loss, parents, and being at home. The general public seems to have its own definitions of "junk" and "health" foods. Much work remains to be done on improving the public's knowledge about nutrition.

■ Physiological characteristics

We have discussed physiological characteristics throughout this book–age, gender, and state of health–and you are invited to think about the interaction of these factors with lifestyles.

■ Household structure and composition

Lifestyles are influenced by the family unit–nuclear, extended, single-parent, couples with no children, groups of unrelated adults, or people living alone. The way that lifestyle affects food intake, nutritional status, and health and the impact this has on the environment are unique for each family and each person in the family. Lifestyles within nations may determine the future condition of the world and its food supply.

Think beyond these photographs. What proportion of your food in the future will be prepared by traditional methods in your home, and what proportion will you buy in processed form?

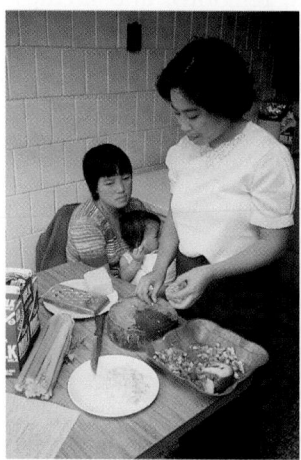 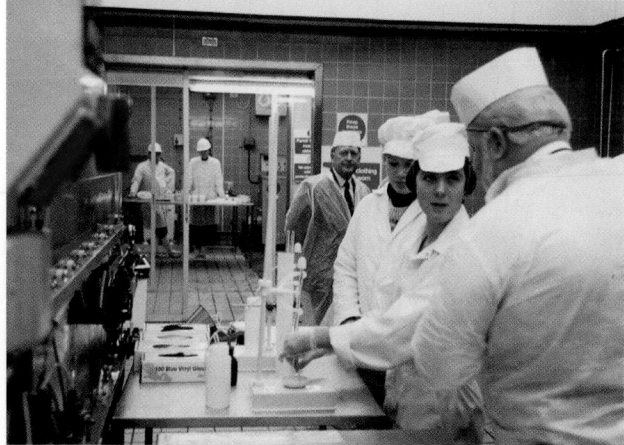

Figures 17-11 and 17-12. Learning about food preparation. Left, the specifics of food preparation are passed on from generation to generation within the home. Right, students preparing to work in food industries are trained in methods that will ensure a nutritious, safe, healthy, economical, and satisfying food supply in the future.

Nutrition will always be both a personal concern and a concern of governments and industry. We want to provide, both on family and societal levels, a wide variety of foods that meet our nutritional and social needs while protecting the source of that food, the natural environment.

Understanding the complex interactions of lifestyle, food supply, environmental issues, and the intriguing way our bodies use nutrients is a challenge for all of us. I hope it was made a little easier for you by reading this book.

■ Now you know

- Lifestyle has an important influence on food choices and nutrient intake.
- Income is a leading factor in determining food choices. High incomes may lead to "diseases of affluence" and low incomes to undernutrition.
- Food assistance programs serve about one in 10 Americans at an annual cost of about $22 billion.
- Homelessness is associated with nutrition deficiencies in zinc, iron, folacin, magnesium, and vitamin A in children and adults.
- Day care centers should be evaluated carefully for safe food handling and nutritious diets.
- Both physiological and psychological stresses influence food intake.
- Education is an important factor influencing nutrient intake.
- Nutritionists should be sensitive to the influence of ethnic identity on food choices by immigrants and refugees.
- Parts of the world have people living in extreme poverty in both the cities and the country, with high incidences of undernutrition.
- Food choices are important in some religions. Termination of feeding the terminally ill may involve ethical, moral, religious, and medical considerations.
- Lifestyle has an important influence on the interrelationships of nutrition with health, nutrition knowledge, and physiological characteristics.

Further Reading

1. Anonymous. Women on the short end of the loaf: Intrahousehold food allocation among members of poor Nepalese families. **Nutrition Reviews** 50:236, 1992.
2. Anonymous. World declaration on nutrition. **Nutrition Reviews** 51:41, 1993.
3. Sims, L. S. Public policy in nutrition: A framework for action. **Nutrition Today** 28(2):10, 1993.
4. Cohen, B. E., and others. Food sources and intake of homeless persons. **Journal of Nutrition Education** 24:45S, 1992.
5. Wolgemuth, J. C., and others. Wasting malnutrition and inadequate nutrient intakes identified in a multiethnic homeless population. **Journal of the American Dietetic Association** 92:834, 1992.

6. Drake, M. A. The nutritional status and dietary adequacy of single homeless women and their children in shelters. *Public Health Reports* 107:312, 1992.

7. Toole, M. J. Micronutrient deficiencies in refugees. *Lancet* 339:1214, 1992.

8. Den Hartog, A. P. Dietary change and industrialization: The making of the modern Dutch diet (1850–1985). *Ecology of Food and Nutrition* 27:307, 1992.

9. Drake, M. A. Menu evaluation, nutrient intake of young children, and nutrition knowledge of menu planners in child care centers in Missouri. *Journal of Nutrition Education* 24:145, 1992.

10. Anonymous. Shigellosis in child day care centers–Lexington-Fayette County, Kentucky, 1991. *Journal of the American Medical Association* 268:860, 1992.

11. Rodin, J. *Body Traps*. William Morrow and Company, Inc., New York, 1992.

12. Hudnall, M., and Wellman, N. S. Missing the nutrition message of balance, variety and moderation. *Journal of Nutrition Education* 24:320, 1992.

13. Cotugna, N., and Vickery, C. E. Development and supermarket field testing of videotaped nutrition messages for cancer risk reduction. *Public Health Reports* 107:691, 1992.

14. Kinsey, J. Quest for convenience: A matter of time. *Cereal Foods World* 37:305, 1992.

15. Ikeda, J. P., and others. Food habits of the Hmong living in Central California. *Journal of Nutrition Education* 23:168, 1991.

16. Morris, P. M., and others. Food security in rural America: A study of the availability and costs of food. *Journal of Nutrition Education* 24:52S, 1992.

17. Horton, S., and Campbell, C. Regional variations in apparent nutrient intake in urban Canada. *Journal of the Canadian Dietetic Association* 53:19, 1992.

18. Hassan, N., and Ahmad, K. The nutrition profile of the slum dwellers: A comparison with the rural poor. *Ecology of Food and Nutrition* 26:203, 1991.

19. Winarno, F. G., and Allain, A. Street foods in developing countries: Lessons from Asia. *Food, Nutrition, and Agriculture* 1:11, 1991.

20. The American Dietetic Association. Position of The American Dietetic Association: Issues in feeding the terminally ill adult. *Journal of the American Dietetic Association* 92:996, 1992.

21. Institute of Medical Ethics Working Party on the Ethics of Prolonging Life and Assisting Death. Withdrawal of life-support from patients in a persistent vegetative state. *Lancet* 337:96, 1991.

22. Foulke, J. E. Foods in transit. Who's watching the kitchen? *FDA Consumer* 27(2):6, 1993.

23. Stephenson, L. S., and others. Weight gain of Kenyan school children infected with hookworm, *Trichuris trichiura* and *Ascaris lumbricoides* is improved following once- or twice-yearly treatment with albendazole. *Journal of Nutrition* 123:656, 1993.

24. Klein, J. D., and others. Candy cigarettes: Do they encourage children's smoking? *Pediatrics* 89:27, 1992.

25. Morabia, A., and Wynder, E. L. Dietary habits of smokers, people who never smoked, and exsmokers. *American Journal of Clinical Nutrition* 52:933, 1990.

26. Pestano-Binghay, E., and others. Nutrition education issues for minority parents: A needs assessment. *Journal of Nutrition Education* 25:144, 1993.

27. McNutt, K. Market research data: Consumers' contribution to improved nutrition education. *Nutrition Today* 28(2):37, 1993.

28. Hickerson, M., and Gregoire, M. B. Characteristics of the nutrition provider in corporate and hospital wellness programs. *Journal of the American Dietetic Association* 92:339, 1992.

29. Chapman, G., and Maclean, H. "Junk food" and "healthy food": Meanings of food in adolescent women's culture. *Journal of Nutrition Education* 25:108, 1993.

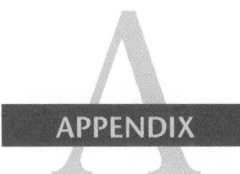

Table of Food Composition

From the Database of Diet Easy for Windows™

This table of food composition was compiled as part of the database for the Diet Easy for Windows™ nutrition and fitness software. It includes more than 2,400 selected foods, grouped by category and given in common household units. Each foods is analyzed for 24 nutritional components. The nutritional data has been verified by recognized sources, such as the USDA and articles in scientific journals, as well as data from fast food companies and food manufacturers where appropriate.

This table is a part of the Diet Easy for Windows™ database and is copyrighted. It may not be reprinted without permission from First DataBank—The Hearst Corporation (N-Squared Computing), San Bruno, CA.

Appendix A - Table of Food Composition

Item	Food name	Portion	Weight (g)	Food Energy (Kcal)	Protein (gm)	Carbohydrates (gm)	Fiber (gm)	Total Fat (gm)	Saturated Fat (gm)	Cholesterol (mg)	Sodium (mg)	Potassium (mg)	Magnesium (mg)	Iron (mg)	Zinc (mg)	Vitamin A (RE)	Vitamin C (mg)	Thiamin (mg)	Riboflavin (mg)	Niacin (mg)	Vitamin B6 (mg)	Folates (µg)	Vitamin B12 (µg)	Calcium (mg)	Phosphorus (mg)
Baby foods																									
761	Baby food-cereal-oatmeal-milk	oz	28.4	33	1	4	0.7	1	0.4	0	13	58	10	3.4	0.3	6	tr	0.14	0.16	1.7	0.02	3	0.09	62	45
762	Baby food-cereal-rice-milk	oz	28.4	33	1	5	0.3	1	tr	0	13	54	13	3.5	0.2	6	tr	0.13	0.14	1.5	0.03	2	0.09	68	50
779	Baby food-dessert-bananas & tapioca	oz	28.4	16	tr	4	0.7	0	0	0	3	25	3	0.1	tr	1	5	tr	0.01	0.1	0.03	2	0	1	2
763	Baby food-dessert-custard chocolate-USDA	oz	28.4	24	1	5	0.1	tr	0.3	0	7	24	3	0.1	0.1	1	tr	tr	0.03	tr	tr	1	tr	17	14
766	Baby food-dessert-custard-vanilla	oz	28.4	24	tr	5	0.1	tr	0.3	0	8	19	2	0.1	0.1	1	tr	tr	0.02	tr	0.01	2	tr	16	13
780	Baby food-dessert-mango/tapioca	oz	28.4	23	tr	6	0	tr	0	0	3	17	1	tr	tr	19	35	0.01	0.01	0.1	0.03	1	0	1	2
765	Baby food-dessert-orange pudding	oz	28.4	23	tr	5	0.1	tr	0.2	0	6	24	2	tr	tr	3	3	0.01	0.02	tr	0.01	2	0	9	8
781	Baby food-dessert-papaya/apple/tapioca	oz	28.4	20	tr	5	0.1	0	0	0	1	22	1	0.1	tr	2	32	tr	0.01	tr	0.01	1	0	2	2
785	Baby food-dessert-plums & tapioca	oz	28.4	20	0	6	0.3	0	0	0	2	24	1	0.1	tr	3	tr	tr	0.01	tr	0.01	tr	0	2	2
786	Baby food-dessert-prunes & tapioca	oz	28.4	20	tr	5	0.7	0	0	0	11	50	3	0.1	tr	13	tr	0.01	0.02	0.1	0.02	tr	0	4	4
794	Baby food-egg yolks	serv	28.4	58	3	tr	0	5	1.5	223	11	22	2	0.8	0.5	107	tr	0.02	0.08	0.1	0.05	26	0.44	22	81
787	Baby food-fruit juice-apple	fl oz	31	14	tr	4	0.3	0	0	0	1	28	1	0.2	tr	1	18	0.01	0.01	0.1	0.01	0	0	1	2
777	Baby food-fruit juice-apple blueberry	oz	28.4	17	tr	5	0.1	tr	0	0	0	20	1	0.1	tr	1	8	0.01	0.01	tr	0.01	tr	0	1	2
788	Baby food-fruit juice-apple peach-USDA	fl oz	31	13	0	3	0.3	tr	0	0	tr	30	1	0.2	tr	2	18	tr	tr	0.1	0.01	tr	0	1	1
789	Baby food-fruit juice-apple prune-USDA	fl oz	31	23	tr	6	0.5	0	0	0	2	46	2	0.3	tr	1	21	tr	tr	0.1	0.01	0	0	3	5
790	Baby food-fruit juice-mixed fruit-USDA	fl oz	31	14	0	4	0.3	0	0	0	0	31	2	0.1	tr	2	20	0.01	0.01	tr	0.01	2	0	2	2
791	Baby food-fruit juice-orange	fl oz	31	14	tr	3	0.3	tr	0	0	0	57	3	0.1	0.1	2	19	tr	tr	0.1	0.02	8	0	4	3
778	Baby food-fruit-applesauce	oz	28.4	12	tr	3	0.7	0	0	0	1	20	1	0.1	tr	0	11	tr	0.01	tr	0.01	1	0	2	3
782	Baby food-fruit-peaches	oz	28.4	20	tr	5	0.7	0	0	0	2	46	2	0.1	tr	5	9	tr	0.01	0.2	tr	1	0	2	3
783	Baby food-fruit-pears	oz	28.4	12	tr	3	0.3	0	0	0	1	37	2	0.1	tr	1	7	tr	0.01	0.1	tr	1	0	2	3
784	Baby food-fruit-pears & pineapple	oz	28.4	12	tr	3	0.3	0	0	0	2	33	2	0.1	tr	1	8	tr	0.01	0.1	0.01	1	0	3	2
792	Baby food-meat-beef	oz	28.4	30	4	0	0	2	0.7	4	2	62	5	0.4	0.7	16	1	0.01	0.04	0.8	0.04	1	0.4	3	24
137	Baby food-meat-beef & egg noodles-strained	oz	28.4	15	1	2	0.1	1	0.2	2	8	13	3	0.1	0.1	31	1	0.01	0.01	0.1	0.01	1	0.03	3	8
768	Baby food-meat-beef stew	oz	28.4	14	1	2	0.3	tr	0.2	4	98	40	3	0.2	0.2	95	1	tr	0.02	0.4	0.02	2	0.15	3	12
173	Baby food-meat-chicken stew-strained	oz	28.4	22	2	2	0.2	1	0.3	8	114	26	3	0.2	0.1	50	1	0.01	0.02	0.3	0.01	tr	0.04	10	14
796	Baby food-meat-lamb	oz	28.4	29	4	0	0	1	0.7	52	18	58	4	0.4	0.8	7	tr	0.01	0.06	0.8	0.04	1	0.62	2	27
797	Baby food-meat-liver	oz	28.4	29	4	tr	0	1	0.4	52	21	64	4	1.5	0.8	3247	6	0.01	0.51	2.4	0.1	96	0.61	1	58
798	Baby food-meat-pork	oz	28.4	35	4	0	0	2	0.7	11	12	63	3	0.3	0.6	3	1	0.04	0.06	0.6	0.06	1	0.28	1	27
800	Baby food-meat-veal	oz	28.4	29	4	0	0	1	0.7	11	18	61	3	0.4	0.6	1	1	0.01	0.05	1	0.04	1	0.37	2	28
801	Baby food-vegetables-beans-green	oz	28.4	7	tr	2	0.4	0	0	0	1	45	7	0.2	0.1	13	2	0.01	0.02	0.1	0.01	10	0	11	6
137	Baby food-vegetables-beans-green/bu-strained	fl oz	28.4	9	tr	2	0.7	tr	tr	0	1	45	7	0.4	0.1	13	2	0.01	0.03	0.1	0.01	8	0	18	6
604	Baby food-vegetables-carrots-strained-USDA	fl oz	30	8	tr	2	0.7	0	0	0	11	56	3	0.1	tr	325	2	0.01	0.01	0.1	0.02	4	0	6	6
803	Baby food-vegetables-garden	oz	28.4	11	1	2	0.7	tr	0	0	10	48	6	0.2	0.1	172	2	0.02	0.02	0.2	0.03	11	0	8	8
804	Baby food-vegetables-peas	oz	28.4	11	1	2	0.7	tr	0	0	1	32	4	0.3	0.1	16	2	0.02	0.02	0.3	0.02	7	0	6	12
805	Baby food-vegetables-squash	oz	28.4	7	tr	2	0.7	tr	0	0	1	51	3	0.1	tr	57	2	0.02	0.02	0.1	0.02	4	0	7	4
806	Baby food-vegetables-sweet potatoes	oz	28.4	16	tr	4	0.7	0	0	0	6	75	4	0.1	0.1	183	3	0.01	0.01	0.1	0.03	3	0	4	7
Beverages																									
800	Ale-mild-American	cup	230	98	1	8	0	0	0	0	16	*	*	0.2	*	0	0	0	0.07	0.5	*	*	*	30	41
802	Beer-Budweiser	fl oz	30	13	tr	1	0.2	0	0	0	2	7	2	tr	0	0	0	tr	0.01	0.1	0.02	2	0.01	1	4
803	Beer-light	fl oz	29.5	8	tr	tr	0	0	0	0	1	5	1	tr	0	0	0	tr	0.01	0.1	0.01	1	tr	1	4
804	Beer-Michelob	fl oz	30	13	tr	1	0.1	0	0	0	2	7	2	tr	tr	0	0	tr	0.01	0.1	0.02	2	0.01	1	4
805	Beer-natural light	fl oz	30	8	tr	1	0	0	0	0	2	5	1	tr	tr	0	0	tr	0.01	0.1	0.01	1	0.01	1	4
685	Beer-regular	fl oz	29.7	12	tr	1	0.1	0	0	0	1	7	2	tr	tr	0	0	tr	0.01	0.1	0.02	2	0.01	1	4
787	Brandy-California	item	30	73	*	*	0	0	0	0	tr	*	*	*	*	*	*	*	*	*	*	*	*	*	*
788	Brandy-cognac-pony	item	30	73	0	0	0	0	0	0	tr	1	0	tr	tr	*	0	tr	tr	tr	0	0	0	0	1
345	Carnation instant breakfast-chocolate	item	36	130	7	23	*	1	*	*	136	422	80	4.5	3	525	27	0.3	0.07	5	0.4	*	0.6	100	150
344	Carnation instant breakfast-eggnog	item	34	130	7	23	0	0	0	0	196	266	80	4.5	3	525	27	0.3	0.07	5	0.4	0	0.6	100	150
343	Carnation instant breakfast-vanilla	item	35	130	7	24	*	0	0	0	145	382	80	4.5	3	525	27	0.3	0.07	5	0.4	0	0.6	100	150
792	Champagne-domestic-glassful	item	120	84	tr	3	0	0	0	0	6	*	*	*	*	*	0	tr	tr	*	*	*	*	*	*	*

Code	Food	Unit																									
546	Chocolate beverage powder-dry milk added	oz	28.4	100	5	20	0.5	1	0.5	2	147	227	23	0.5	0.3	0.3	3	1	0.04	0.04	0.21	0.2	tr	12	0.68	167	155
547	Chocolate beverage powder-no dry milk	oz	28.4	99	1	26	12	1	0.5	0	60	168	28	0.9	0.4	0.4	1	tr	0.01	0.04	0.04	0.1	tr	2	0	11	36
789	Cider-fermented	fl oz	30	12	tr	tr	0	tr	0	0	0	36	2	0.1	tr	tr	tr	tr	0.01	0.01	0.01	tr	0.01	tr	0	2	2
807	Cocktail-daiquiri	item	100	186	tr	7	0	16	1.8	94	5	21	2	0.2	0.1	0.1	1	2	0.01	tr	tr	tr	0.01	2	0.57	3	6
808	Cocktail-eggnog	item	123	335	4	18	0	16	1.8	94	75	178	16	0.7	0.6	0.6	25	0	0.04	0.11	0.11	0.04	0.07	15	0.57	44	74
809	Cocktail-gin rickey	item	120	150	0	1	0	0	0	0	19	12	1	0	0.1	0.1	tr	4	0.01	0	0	0	tr	1	0	2	1
810	Cocktail-highball	fl oz	29	26	0	0	0	0	0	0	4	1	tr	tr	tr	tr	0	0	tr	0	0	tr	0	0	0	1	1
811	Cocktail-manhattan	fl oz	28.5	64	0	tr	0	tr	0	0	1	7	1	tr	tr	tr	0	0	tr	0	0	tr	tr	tr	0	1	2
812	Cocktail-martini	fl oz	28.2	63	0	tr	0	0	0	0	1	5	1	tr	tr	tr	0	0	0	tr	tr	tr	tr	0	0	1	1
813	Cocktail-mint julep	item	300	212	0	3	0	0	0	0	0	6	tr	0.1	0.1	0.1	0	0	0.02	0.01	0.01	tr	tr	0	tr	tr	10
814	Cocktail-old fashioned	item	100	180	0	4	0	0	0	0	1	2	0	tr	tr	tr	0	0	0.01	tr	tr	tr	tr	0	0	0	4
1702	Cocktail-pina colada-home recipe	fl oz	31.4	58	tr	9	0.1	1	0.3	0	2	22	3	0.1	tr	tr	1	0	0.01	0.01	0.01	0.01	0.01	3	0	3	2
815	Cocktail-planters punch	item	100	175	tr	8	0	0	0	0	*	*	10	0.1	*	*	8	0	0.1	0	0	tr	*	*	*	4	3
816	Cocktail-rum sour	item	100	165	0	0	0	0	0	0	1	2	0	tr	tr	tr	0	0	0.01	0.01	0.01	tr	tr	0	0	0	4
817	Cocktail-Tom Collins	fl oz	29.6	16	0	tr	0	0	0	0	5	2	tr	0.1	tr	tr	1	0	tr	tr	tr	tr	tr	0	0	1	tr
1307	Coffee substitute-prepared	fl oz	30.3	2	tr	tr	0	0	0	0	1	7	1	tr	tr	tr	0	0	tr	tr	0	0.1	tr	0	0	1	2
730	Coffee-brewed	fl oz	29.6	1	tr	tr	0	tr	0	0	1	16	1	tr	tr	tr	0	0	0	0	0.01	0.1	0	tr	0	1	tr
731	Coffee-instant-prepared	cup	239	5	tr	1	0	tr	0	0	10	86	10	0.1	0.1	0.1	1	0	tr	0	tr	0.7	tr	0	0	7	7
735	Cordials/liqueur-54 proof	fl oz	34	97	12	12	0	0	0	0	1	1	tr	tr	tr	tr	0	0	tr	0	0	tr	0	1	0	0	0
1541	Fruit punch drink-canned	fl oz	31	15	0	4	0	0	0	0	7	8	1	0.1	tr	tr	9	0	0.01	0.01	0.01	tr	tr	tr	0	2	tr
1364	Fruit punch-powdered-prepared with water	cup	262	97	25	25	*	0	0	0	37	3	3	0.1	0.1	0.1	31	1	0	0.01	0.01	tr	0	tr	0	42	52
1700	Gatorade-thirst quenching drink	fl oz	30.1	8	0	2	0	0	0	0	12	3	tr	tr	tr	tr	0	96	tr	0	0	0	0	0	0	0	3
842	Hot cocoa-prepared with milk-home recipe	cup	250	218	9	26	3	9	5.6	33	123	480	56	0.8	1.2	1.2	2	2	0.1	0.44	0.44	0.4	0.11	12	0.87	298	270
782	Liqueurs-anisette	item	20	74	0	7	0	0	0	0	*	*	*	*	*	*	*	*	*	*	*	*	*	1	*	*	*
783	Liqueurs-apricot brandy	item	20	64	6	6	0	0	0	0	2	11	1	tr	0.01	0.01	3	0	tr	tr	tr	tr	tr	1	0	1	1
784	Liqueurs-benedictine	item	20	69	7	7	0	0	0	0	*	8	*	*	*	*	7	0	*	*	*	*	*	*	*	*	*
785	Liqueurs-creme de menthe	fl oz	33.6	125	0	14	0	0	0	0	2	3	0	tr	tr	tr	0	0	tr	0	0	tr	0	0	0	7	0
786	Liqueurs-curacao	item	20	54	*	6	0	0	0	0	0	0	0	tr	tr	tr	1	0	0	0	0	tr	0	0	0	0	0
1306	Ovaltine-chocolate flavor-prepared/milk	cup	265	227	10	29	0.2	9	5.5	34	228	600	52	4.8	1.1	1.1	29	9	0.63	0.97	0.97	12.7	0.77	29	0.87	392	302
1305	Ovaltine-malt flavor-prepared with milk	cup	265	228	10	29	0.1	8	5.4	37	201	576	47	4.5	1.1	1.1	30	8	0.67	1.16	1.16	11.9	0.75	29	0.87	371	308
1361	Postum-instant grain beverage-dry mix	oz	28.4	103	2	24	0	0	0	0	28	896	*	1.9	*	*	107	0	0.17	0.08	0.08	6.8	*	*	*	77	189
1369	Sanka-decaffeinated coffee-prepared	fl oz	29.8	0	0	0	0	0	0	0	6	10	tr	tr	tr	tr	9	0	0	0	0	tr	0	0	0	1	1
691	Soda-club-carbonated	fl oz	29.6	0	0	0	0	0	0	0	6	tr	0	tr	tr	tr	0	0	0	0	0	0	0	0	0	1	0
692	Soda-cola type-carbonated	fl oz	30.8	13	0	3	0	0	0	0	1	tr	tr	tr	tr	tr	0	0	0	0	0	0	0	0	0	1	4
1301	Soda-cream flavored-carbonated	fl oz	30.9	16	0	4	0	0	0	0	4	tr	tr	tr	tr	tr	0	0	0	0	0	0	0	0	0	2	3
1304	Soda-diet cola-Nutrasweet-carbonated	fl oz	29.6	0	0	0	0	0	0	0	2	0	tr	tr	tr	tr	0	0	0	0	0.01	0	0	0	0	0	0
1303	Soda-Dr. Pepper type cola-carbonated	fl oz	30.8	13	0	3	0	0	0	0	3	tr	tr	tr	tr	tr	0	0	0	0	0	0	0	0	0	1	3
694	Soda-ginger ale-carbonated	fl oz	30.5	10	0	3	0	0	0	0	2	tr	tr	tr	tr	tr	0	0	0	0	0	0	0	0	0	1	0
693	Soda-grape-carbonated	fl oz	31	13	0	3	0	0	0	0	5	tr	tr	tr	tr	tr	0	0	0	0	0	0	0	0	0	1	0
695	Soda-root beer-carbonated	fl oz	30.8	13	0	3	0	0	0	0	4	tr	tr	tr	tr	tr	0	0	0	0	0	0	0	0	0	2	0
1349	Soda-Tab-low calorie cola-carbonated	cup	236	0	0	0	0	0	0	0	30	tr	tr	tr	tr	tr	0	0	0	0	0	0	0	0	0	*	30
1701	Soda-tonic water/quinine-carbonated	fl oz	30.5	10	0	3	0	0	0	0	0	0	0	tr	tr	tr	0	0	0	0	0	0	0	0	0	tr	0
1363	Tang-instant breakfast drink-orange-dry	oz	28.4	104	0	26	*	0	0	0	13	81	*	tr	tr	tr	0	535	0	0	0	0	0	0	0	71	76
732	Tea-brewed	fl oz	29.6	tr	0	0	0	0	0	0	1	11	1	tr	tr	tr	0	0	0	tr	tr	tr	0	2	0	0	tr
1699	Tea-herbal-brewed	fl oz	29.6	tr	0	tr	0	0	0	0	tr	3	tr	tr	tr	tr	0	0	0	0	0	0	0	tr	0	1	0
734	Tea-instant-prepared-sweetened	cup	259	88	tr	22	0	0	0	0	8	49	5	0.1	0.1	0.1	0	0	tr	0.05	0.05	0.1	0.01	10	0	5	3
733	Tea-instant-prepared-unsweetened	cup	237	2	0	tr	0	0	0	0	7	47	5	tr	0.1	0.1	0	0	tr	0.01	0.01	0.1	0.01	1	0	5	2
1302	Water-mineral-Perrier	cup	237	0	0	0	0	0	0	0	3	0	2	0	0	0	0	0	0	0	0	0	0	0	0	32	0
1643	Water-municipal tap	cup	237	0	0	0	0	0	0	0	7	1	2	0.1	0.1	0.1	0	0	0	0	0	tr	0	0	0	5	0
791	Whiskey/gin/rum/vodka-100 proof	fl oz	27.8	82	0	0	0	0	0	0	0	0	tr	tr	tr	tr	0	0	0	0	tr	tr	0	0	0	0	1
686	Whiskey/gin/rum/vodka-80 proof	fl oz	27.8	64	0	0	0	0	0	0	1	0	0	tr	tr	tr	0	0	0	0	0	tr	tr	0	0	0	1

* indicates that no data was available.

©1994 First DataBank—The Hearst Corporation (N-Squared Computing).

Appendix A - Table of Food Composition (continued)

Item	Food name	Portion	Weight (g)	Food Energy (Kcal)	Protein (gm)	Carbohydrates (gm)	Fiber (gm)	Total Fat (gm)	Saturated Fat (gm)	Cholesterol (mg)	Sodium (mg)	Potassium (mg)	Magnesium (mg)	Iron (mg)	Zinc (mg)	Vitamin A (RE)	Vitamin C (mg)	Thiamin (mg)	Riboflavin (mg)	Niacin (mg)	Vitamin B6 (mg)	Folates (µg)	Vitamin B12 (µg)	Calcium (mg)	Phosphorus (mg)
687	Whiskey/gin/rum/vodka-86 proof	fl oz	27.8	70	0	tr	0	0	*	0	tr	1	0	tr	0	0	0	tr	0	tr	0	0	0	0	1
688	Whiskey/gin/rum/vodka-90 proof	fl oz	27.7	73	0	0	0	0	0	0	1	0	0	0	0	0	0	tr	0	0	0	0	0	0	1
790	Whiskey/gin/rum/vodka-94 proof	fl oz	27.8	77	0	0	0	0	0	0	1	0	0	tr	0	0	0	tr	tr	tr	0	0	0	0	1
1633	Wine cooler-white wine and 7Up	serv	102	55	tr	6	0	0	0	0	7	41	5	0.2	0.1	0	2	tr	tr	tr	0.01	tr	0	6	7
795	Wine-California/red-glassful	item	102	85	tr	3	0	0	0	0	10	116	11	1	0.1	0	0	0.01	0.03	0.1	0.04	1	0.01	8	13
689	Wine-dessert	fl oz	30	46	tr	4	0	0	0	0	3	28	3	0.1	tr	0	0	0.01	0.01	0.1	0	tr	0	2	3
793	Wine-madeira-glassful	item	100	105	tr	1	0	0	0	0	5	92	9	0.2	0.1	0	0	0.02	0.02	0.2	0	tr	0	8	9
794	Wine-muscatel/port-glassful	item	100	158	tr	14	0	0	0	0	19	75	4	1.6	0.1	0	0	0.01	0.01	0.2	0.05	2	0	8	9
690	Wine-red-table	fl oz	29.5	21	tr	1	0	0	0	0	1	41	4	0.1	0.1	0	0	tr	0.01	tr	0.01	1	0	2	4
1703	Wine-rose-table	fl oz	29.5	21	tr	tr	0	0	0	0	1	29	3	0.1	tr	0	0	tr	0.01	tr	0.01	0	tr	2	4
796	Wine-sauterne-glassful	item	100	84	tr	4	0	0	0	0	2	89	10	0.4	0.1	0	0	tr	0.02	0.1	0.02	1	0.01	8	14
797	Wine-sherry-dry-glassful	item	60	84	tr	5	0	0	0	0	2	45	6	0.2	tr	0	0	0.01	0.01	0.1	0.01	1	0.01	5	8
798	Wine-vermouth-dry-glassful	item	100	105	0	1	0	0	0	0	4	75	10	0.4	0.1	0	0	0.01	0.01	0.2	0.02	1	0.01	8	14
799	Wine-vermouth-sweet-glassful	item	100	167	0	12	0	0	0	0	9	92	9	0.2	0.1	0	0	0.02	0.02	0.2	tr	tr	0	2	9
1370	Wine-white-table	fl oz	29.5	20	tr	tr	0	0	0	0	1	24	3	0.1	0.1	0	0	tr	tr	tr	tr	0	0	3	4

Breads

Item	Food name	Portion	Weight (g)	Food Energy (Kcal)	Protein (gm)	Carbohydrates (gm)	Fiber (gm)	Total Fat (gm)	Saturated Fat (gm)	Cholesterol (mg)	Sodium (mg)	Potassium (mg)	Magnesium (mg)	Iron (mg)	Zinc (mg)	Vitamin A (RE)	Vitamin C (mg)	Thiamin (mg)	Riboflavin (mg)	Niacin (mg)	Vitamin B6 (mg)	Folates (µg)	Vitamin B12 (µg)	Calcium (mg)	Phosphorus (mg)
319	Bagel-egg-3 inch diameter	item	55	163	6	31	1.2	1	*	8	198	41	11	1.5	0.3	24	0	0.21	0.16	1.9	0.02	13	0.05	23	37
320	Bagel-water-3 inch diameter	item	55	163	6	31	1.2	1	0.2	0	198	41	11	1.5	0.3	0	0	0.21	0.16	1.9	0.02	13	0	23	37
322	Biscuits-baking powder-from home recipe	item	28.4	105	2	13	0.4	5	1.2	0	175	33	6	0.4	*	0	0	0.08	0.08	0.7	*	*	*	34	49
1560	Biscuits-baking powder-prepared from mix	item	35	104	2	13	0.5	5	3.3	1	221	33	3	0.6	0.1	37	0	0.1	0.07	1.8	0.01	2	0.04	34	99
325	Bread sticks-Vienna type	slice	35	106	2	20	1	5	*	0	548	33	*	0.3	*	*	0	0.02	0.03	0.3	*	*	*	16	31
327	Bread-Boston brown-canned	slice	45	95	2	21	2.1	1	0.1	0	112	131	9	0.9	0.3	0	0	0.06	0.04	0.7	*	*	*	41	72
1757	Bread-cracked wheat-enriched	slice	25	66	2	13	1.3	1	0.1	0	108	33	*	0.7	*	*	0	0.1	0.1	0.8	0.02	*	*	16	32
1753	Bread-crisp-breakfast-Wasa	slice	13.9	54	2	9	0.5	2	*	0	70	35	*	*	*	*	0	*	*	*	*	1	*	*	6
329	Bread-crisp-whole grain-Wasa	slice	6.25	22	1	5	0.5	0	*	0	4	6	1	0.3	tr	0	0	0.03	0.02	0.3	tr	1	0	1	6
332	Bread-french-enriched	slice	35	98	3	18	0.8	1	0.2	0	193	30	7	1.1	0.2	0	0	0.16	0.12	1.4	0.02	13	0	39	28
1756	Bread-italian-enriched	slice	30	85	3	17	0.8	0	*	0	152	22	6	0.7	*	0	0	0.12	0.07	1	0.02	11	0	5	23
1755	Bread-melba toast-plain	slice	4.67	16	1	3	0.3	0	0	0	30	11	2	0.1	0.1	0	0	0.01	0.01	0.1	0.01	1	0	5	10
1754	Bread-melba toast-wheat	slice	4.67	16	1	3	0.3	0	0	0	30	11	3	0.1	0.1	0	0	0.01	0.01	0.1	0.01	1	0	5	10
1283	Bread-melba toast-wheat-unsalted	slice	4.67	16	1	3	0.3	0	0	0	5	11	3	0.1	0.1	0	0	0.01	0.01	0.1	0.01	1	0	5	10
1282	Bread-mixed grain-toasted	slice	22	66	3	12	0.9	1	0.2	0	105	56	13	0.8	0.3	0	0	0.08	0.1	1.1	0.03	17	0	27	54
1762	Bread-mixed grain-untoasted	slice	25	64	2	12	1.6	1	0.2	0	103	55	12	0.8	0.3	*	0	0.1	0.1	*	0.03	16	*	26	53
1767	Bread-oat bran-no cholesterol-Monterey	slice	45.4	99	4	18	3.3	1	*	0	204	55	*	0.8	0.3	*	0	0.1	0.1	*	0.03	*	*	26	53
1298	Bread-oatmeal and bran-Oatmeal Goodness	slice	35.5	90	4	15	1	2	0.4	0	140	64	13	1.1	0.4	0	0	0.15	0.1	1.6	0.02	11	0.02	40	50
338	Bread-pita	item	38	105	4	21	0.6	1	0.1	0	215	45	8	0.9	0.3	0	0	0.17	0.08	1.4	0.04	22	0	31	38
334	Bread-pumpernickel	slice	32	82	3	15	1.9	1	*	0	173	139	22	0.9	0.4	0	0	0.11	0.17	1.1	0.05	*	0	23	70
336	Bread-raisin-enriched	slice	25	70	2	13	0.6	1	0.2	0	94	60	6	0.8	0.2	0	0	0.08	0.16	1	0.01	9	0	26	23
330	Bread-rye-American-light	slice	25	66	2	12	1.6	1	0.1	0	174	51	6	0.7	0.3	0	0	0.1	0.08	0.8	0.02	10	0	20	36
362	Bread-Vienna-enriched	slice	25	70	2	13	0.8	1	0.2	0	138	22	5	0.8	0.2	0	0	0.12	0.09	1	0.01	*	0	28	20
359	Bread-wheat-firm-enriched-toasted	slice	21	59	2	11	2.4	1	0.1	0	153	42	23	0.8	0.4	11	0	0.07	0.05	0.9	0.05	13	0	17	63
1285	Bread-wheat-soft-enriched-toasted	slice	24	67	3	13	2.7	1	*	0	175	49	26	0.9	0.5	0	0	0.08	0.06	1.1	0.05	15	0	20	72
352	Bread-wheat-soft-enriched-toasted-from home recipe	slice	22	68	2	12	2.5	2	0.2	0	91	87	24	0.7	0.6	tr	0	0.06	0.04	0.8	0.05	13	0.03	20	64
353	Bread-white-firm-enriched	slice	23	61	2	11	0.4	1	0.2	0	118	26	5	0.7	0.1	0	0	0.11	0.07	0.9	0.01	8	0	29	25
340	Bread-white-firm-enriched-toasted	slice	20	65	2	12	0.5	1	0.2	0	117	28	5	0.6	0.1	0	0	0.07	0.06	0.8	0.01	8	0	22	23
350	Bread-white-soft	cup	25	67	2	12	0.7	1	0.2	0	129	28	5	0.7	0.2	0	0	0.12	0.08	0.9	0.01	9	0	32	27
349	Bread-white-soft-enriched-cubes	cup	30	120	4	22	1.2	2	0.3	0	231	50	9	1.3	0.3	0	0	0.21	0.14	1.7	0.02	16	0	57	49
341	Bread-white-soft-enriched-crumbs	cup	30	80	2	15	0.8	2	0.2	0	154	34	6	0.9	0.2	0	0	0.14	0.09	1.1	0.01	11	0	38	32
361	Bread-white-soft-toasted	slice	22	67	2	12	0.6	1	0.2	0	129	28	5	0.7	0.2	0	0	0.1	0.08	0.9	0.01	9	0	32	27
1284	Bread-whole wheat-firm-enriched	slice	25	61	2	11	2.8	1	0.1	0	159	44	23	0.9	0.4	0	0	0.09	0.05	1	0.05	14	0	18	65
358	Bread-whole wheat-from home recipe	slice	28.4	69	3	13	3.2	1	*	0	178	49	26	1	0.6	11	0	0.1	0.04	0.8	0.05	12	0.03	20	63
324	Bread-whole wheat-enriched	slice	25	67	3	13	3.2	1	1	0	178	49	26	1	0.5	0	0	0.1	0.06	1.1	0.05	15	0	20	73
	Breadcrumbs-dry-grated-enriched	cup	100	390	13	73	3.7	5	1	0	736	152	32	3.6	*	0	0	0.35	0.35	4.8	0.05	*	*	122	141

Code	Food	Measure	Wt	Cal																				
1274	Cornbread-home recipe	slice	45	108	2	16	1.2	4	1.5	0	126	42	8	0.7	0.2	7	0	0.08	0	0.08	0.7	0.03	5	0.08	49	44
1311	Crackers-animal-Ralston	item	1.9	9	tr	1	tr	tr	0.1	0	8	2	tr	0.1	tr	0	0	0.01	0	0.01	0.1	0	tr	tr	tr	1
1312	Crackers-cheddar snacks-Ralston	item	1.6	7	tr	1	0.1	tr	*	0	14	2	tr	0.1	tr	0	0	0.01	0	0.01	0.1	tr	tr	0.01	1	2
1275	Crackers-cheese	item	1	5	tr	1	tr	tr	0.1	tr	12	2	tr	tr	tr	0	0	tr	0	tr	0.1	tr	tr	0.01	1	2
1319	Crackers-cheese and chives-Ralston	item	1.6	7	tr	1	0.1	tr	*	*	14	2	tr	0.1	tr	0	0	0.01	0	0.01	0.1	tr	tr	0.01	1	2
1313	Crackers-cheese snacks-Ralston	item	1.13	6	tr	1	tr	tr	0.1	0	10	2	tr	0.1	tr	0	0	0.01	0	0.01	tr	tr	tr	0.04	tr	1
430	Crackers-graham-plain	item	7	28	1	5	0.2	1	0.1	0	33	28	4	0.3	0.1	0	0	0.01	0	0.01	0.3	0.01	1	0	3	11
1276	Crackers-graham-sugar-honey	item	7	30	1	5	0.1	1	0.1	0	33	12	2	0.2	0.1	0	0	0.02	0	0.02	0.2	0.01	1	0	3	8
1314	Crackers-oyster-Ralston	item	0.45	2	tr	tr	tr	tr	0	0	5	1	tr	tr	tr	0	0	tr	0	tr	tr	0	*	0	tr	tr
1315	Crackers-rich and crisp-Ralston	item	3.2	16	tr	2	0.1	1	*	0	21	3	tr	0.1	tr	0	0	0.02	*	0.02	0.1	*	tr	0	2	4
1691	Crackers-Ritz	item	3.33	18	tr	2	0.1	1	0.1	*	32	3	1	0.1	tr	*	*	0.01	*	0.01	0.1	*	*	*	5	8
1308	Crackers-Ry Krisp-natural-Ralston	item	2.1	8	tr	2	0.3	tr	0	0	19	10	3	0.1	0.1	*	*	0.01	*	0.01	0.1	0.01	tr	0.01	1	7
1309	Crackers-Ry Krisp-seasoned-Ralston	item	2.2	8	tr	2	0.4	tr	*	0	27	11	3	0.1	0.1	0	*	0.01	0	0.01	0.1	tr	1	*	1	6
1310	Crackers-Ry Krisp-sesame-Ralston	item	2.5	8	tr	2	0.4	tr	*	0	29	12	3	0.1	0.1	1	0	0.01	0	0.01	0.1	0.01	1	*	1	8
1316	Crackers-Rye Snacks-Ralston	item	1.9	9	tr	1	0.3	tr	*	0	14	3	1	0.1	tr	0	0	0.01	0	0.01	0.1	*	tr	0.01	tr	2
431	Crackers-rye wafers	item	6.5	23	1	5	1.1	0	0	0	57	39	*	0.3	*	0	0	0.02	0	0.02	0.1	*	*	0	4	25
432	Crackers-saltines	item	2.75	13	tr	2	0.1	tr	0.1	1	37	4	1	0.1	tr	0	0	0.13	0	0.13	0.1	tr	*	0	3	3
1320	Crackers-Sesame and Wheat-Ralston	item	1.9	18	tr	2	0.2	tr	0.1	1	17	4	1	0.1	tr	0	0	0.01	0	0.01	0.1	tr	*	0.01	1	3
1317	Crackers-Snackers-Ralston	item	3.5	18	tr	2	0.1	1	*	0	24	4	tr	0.1	tr	0	0	0.01	0	0.01	0.2	tr	tr	tr	1	3
1473	Crackers-Triscuits	item	4.5	21	1	3	0.2	1	0.2	0	24	6	3	0.2	0.2	0	0	0.02	0	0.02	0.2	0.01	1	0.04	1	9
1318	Crackers-Wheat Snacks	item	1.9	9	tr	1	0.1	tr	0.2	0	12	3	1	0.1	0.1	0	0	0.01	0	0.01	0.1	0.01	tr	0.01	1	3
1474	Crackers-Wheat Thins	item	1.8	9	tr	1	0.1	tr	*	*	31	4	*	*	*	0	0	*	0	*	*	*	*	*	*	14
1747	Crackers-whole wheat-low sodium	serv	7.53	30	1	7	2.8	0	0	0	31	33	4	0.3	0.1	0	0	0.04	0	0.04	0.4	0.01	2	0	2	14
1748	Crackers-whole wheat-sodium free	serv	7.53	30	1	7	2.8	0	0	0	1	35	5	0.2	0.1	0	0	0.04	0	0.04	0.3	0.01	2	0.07	2	14
1336	French toast-from frozen-Campbells	slice	50	94	4	11	1.6	5	*	*	235	54	*	1.1	*	15	0	0.09	0	0.04	0.7	*	34	*	34	*
1277	French toast-from home recipe	slice	65	153	6	17	2	7	0.5	tr	257	86	12	1.3	0.6	22	0	0.16	0	0.12	1	0.04	18	0.29	72	85
1716	French toast-with butter	slice	67.5	178	5	18	0.9	9	3.9	59	257	89	8	0.9	0.3	60	tr	0.25	0	0.29	2	0.03	15	0.18	37	73
1765	Muffin-blueberry oat bran-Health Valley	item	57	140	4	27	4.7	4	*	0	95	260	50	1.4	0.8	0	5	0.09	5	0.23	0.1	0.08	14	0.29	27	144
443	Muffin-blueberry-from home recipe	item	40	110	3	17	0.9	4	1.1	21	252	46	10	0.6	0.7	18	0	0.09	*	0.09	0.7	*	*	*	34	53
444	Muffin-bran-from home recipe	item	40	112	3	17	2.5	5	1.2	21	168	99	35	1.3	1.1	40	2	0.1	0	0.1	1.3	0.11	17	0.09	54	111
445	Muffin-corn-from home recipe	item	40	125	3	19	1	4	1.2	21	192	54	18	0.7	*	25	0	0.1	0	0.1	0.7	*	*	*	42	68
447	Muffin-corn-from mix-with egg and milk	item	40	130	3	20	1	4	1.2	21	191	44	*	0.6	*	20	0	0.08	0	0.08	0.7	*	*	*	96	152
1271	Muffin-english-plain-toasted	item	53	154	5	30	1.5	1	0.3	0	414	364	12	1.8	0.5	0	0	0.24	0	0.24	2.4	0.03	21	0	105	73
1270	Muffin-english-plain-untoasted	item	56	133	4	26	1.3	2	1.9	0	358	314	11	1.6	0.4	0	0	0.26	0	0.26	2.1	0.02	18	0	91	63
446	Muffin-plain-from home recipe	item	40	120	3	17	0.9	4	1	21	176	50	11	0.6	0.2	8	0	0.09	0	0.09	0.9	0.01	*	*	42	38
1764	Muffin-raisin oat bran-Health Valley	item	57	140	3	31	5.2	3	0.4	0	100	290	55	1.7	0.9	0	4	0.25	0	0.25	0.5	0.09	15	0	33	160
1553	Muffin-soy	item	40	119	4	17	0.8	4	*	0	*	54	52	0.9	*	40	0	0.08	0	0.08	0.5	*	*	*	35	56
450	Pancakes-buckwheat-from mix	item	27	55	2	6	0.6	2	0.8	20	160	66	5	0.4	0.2	12	0	0.04	5	0.04	0.2	0.06	3	0.36	59	91
451	Pancakes-plain-from home recipe	item	27	60	2	9	0.5	2	0.5	20	160	33	5	0.4	0.2	6	0	0.06	0	0.06	0.5	0.06	3	0.36	27	38
452	Pancakes-plain-from mix	item	27	59	2	8	0.4	2	0.7	20	160	43	5	0.3	0.2	8	0	0.06	0	0.04	0.3	0.06	3	0.36	36	71
1551	Pancakes-soybean-25% soy flour	item	45	68	3	10	0.5	2	*	29	160	37	55	0.6	*	18	0	0.07	0	0.07	0.4	*	*	0.01	26	42
487	Roll-Brown & Serve-enriched	item	26	85	2	14	1	2	0.4	0	144	25	12	0.8	0.3	0	0	0.1	0	0.1	0.9	0.02	10	0	20	23
1724	Roll-cinnamon	item	26	100	2	14	0.7	4	0.6	tr	96	36	5	0.5	0.1	4	tr	0.07	0	0.07	0.4	0.02	6	tr	8	22
492	Roll-cloverleaf-from home recipe	item	35	120	3	20	1.3	3	0.8	6	193	41	7	0.7	0.3	6	0	0.12	0	0.12	1.2	0.02	13	0.36	16	36
488	Roll-cloverleaf/pan-commercial-enriched	item	28.4	85	2	15	1.1	2	0.4	0	155	27	6	0.8	0.2	0	0	0.11	0	0.11	0.9	0.02	11	0.36	21	24
1552	Roll-croissant-Sara Lee	item	26	109	2	11	0.6	6	3.3	29	140	40	7	1	0.2	8	0	0.28	0	0.1	1.2	0.02	9	0.05	12	32
489	Roll-hamburger/hotdog-commercial	item	40	114	3	20	1	4	0.5	0	241	37	8	1.2	0.2	18	0	0.2	0	0.2	1.6	0.01	15	*	54	33
490	Roll-hard-commercial-enriched	item	50	155	5	30	1.5	5	0.4	0	312	49	12	1.2	0.3	0	0	0.2	0	0.2	1.7	0.02	30	0	24	46
491	Roll-submarine/hoagie-enriched	item	135	390	12	75	3.8	4	0.9	0	761	122	*	3	*	0	0	0.54	0	0.54	4.5	0.05	*	*	58	115
1476	Roll-whole wheat-homemade	item	35	90	4	18	1.8	1	0.4	0	197	102	40	0.8	0.6	0	0	0.12	0	0.12	1.1	0.08	16	0.05	34	98
500	Waffles-enriched-from home recipe	item	75	245	7	26	1.1	13	2.3	45	445	129	17	1.5	0.7	28	0	0.18	0	0.24	1.5	0.05	14	0.37	154	135

A 5

* indicates that no data was available.
©1994 First DataBank—The Hearst Corporation (N-Squared Computing).

Item	Food name	Portion	Weight (g)	Food Energy (Kcal)	Protein (gm)	Carbohydrates (gm)	Fiber (gm)	Total Fat (gm)	Saturated Fat (gm)	Cholesterol (mg)	Sodium (mg)	Potassium (mg)	Magnesium (mg)	Iron (mg)	Zinc (mg)	Vitamin A (RE)	Vitamin C (mg)	Thiamin (mg)	Riboflavin (mg)	Niacin (mg)	Vitamin B6 (mg)	Folates (µg)	Vitamin B12 (µg)	Calcium (mg)	Phosphorus (mg)
501	Waffles-enriched-from mix-egg & milk	item	75	205	7	27	1.1	8	2.8	45	514	146	*	1	*	34	0	0.14	0.22	0.9	*	*	*	179	257
1281	Waffles-frozen	item	37	103	2	16	0.9	4	*	0	256	78	8	1.8	0.3	95	0	0.17	0.2	1.9	0.1	1	*	30	141
1761	Waffles-oat bran-no cholesterol-Eggo	item	39	110	3	16	2	4	0.7	0	220	194	39	1.8	0.7	100	0	0.15	0.17	0.8	0.2	16	0.6	20	135
	Breakfast cereals																								
1147	Cereal-100% bran	cup	66	178	8	48	19.5	3	0.6	0	457	824	312	8.1	5.7	0	63	1.6	1.8	20.9	2.1	47	6.3	46	801
1148	Cereal-100% natural-plain	cup	104	489	12	65	3.8	22	15.1	0	45	514	125	3.1	2.4	6	0	0.31	0.56	2.4	0.19	31	0.13	181	383
1126	Cereal-40% bran flakes-Kelloggs	cup	39	127	5	31	5.5	1	0	0	363	248	71	11.2	5.1	516	0	0.5	0.6	6.9	0.7	138	2.1	19	192
1127	Cereal-40% bran flakes-Post	cup	47	152	5	37	6.5	1	0	0	431	251	102	7.5	2.5	622	0	0.6	0.7	8.3	0.8	166	2.5	21	296
1105	Cereal-All Bran	cup	85.2	212	12	63	25.5	2	0.2	0	961	1051	318	13.5	11.2	1125	45	1.11	1.28	15	1.53	301	0	69	794
1106	Cereal-Alpha Bits	cup	28.4	111	2	25	0.3	1	0.1	0	219	110	17	1.8	1.5	375	15	0.4	0.4	5	0.5	100	1.5	8	51
1107	Cereal-Apple Jacks	cup	28.4	110	2	26	0.2	tr	0	0	125	23	6	4.5	3.7	375	15	0.4	0.4	5	0.5	100	0	8	30
1108	Cerea-Bran Buds	cup	85.2	220	12	65	23.6	2	0.3	0	523	1425	271	13.5	11.2	1125	0	1.11	1.28	15	1.53	301	0	57	740
1109	Cerea-Bran Chex	cup	49	156	5	39	7.9	1	0.2	0	455	394	126	7.8	2.1	11	26	0.6	0.26	8.6	0.9	173	2.6	29	327
369	Cereal-bran flakes-Ralston	cup	49	159	6	39	6	1	0	0	456	191	118	7.8	2	649	26	0.6	0.7	8.6	0.9	173	2.6	27	273
1110	Cereal-C. W. Post-plain	cup	97	432	9	69	2.2	15	11.3	0	167	198	67	15.4	1.6	1284	0	1.3	1.5	17.1	1.7	342	5.1	47	224
1111	Cereal-C. W. Post-with raisins	cup	103	446	9	74	2	15	11	0	160	260	74	16.4	1.6	1364	0	1.3	1.5	18.1	1.9	364	5.5	51	232
1112	Cereal-Cap'n Crunch	cup	37	156	2	30	0.4	3	2.2	0	278	48	15	9.8	4	5	0	0.66	0.71	8.6	1	238	2.34	6	47
1113	Cereal-Cap'n Crunch-Crunchberries	cup	35	146	2	29	0.4	3	1.9	0	243	49	14	9	3.6	5	0	0.59	0.67	8.1	0.93	128	2.51	11	47
1114	Cereal-Cheerios	cup	22.7	89	3	16	0.9	1	0.3	0	246	81	31	3.6	0.6	300	12	0.3	0.34	4	0.41	5	1.2	39	107
1115	Cereal-Cocoa Krispies	cup	36	139	2	32	0.2	2	1	0	275	53	12	2.3	1.9	477	19	0.5	0.5	6.3	0.6	127	0.02	6	47
1116	Cereal-Cocoa Pebbles	cup	32.5	133	2	28	0.2	2	0	0	155	54	13	2.1	1.7	430	0	0.42	0.49	5.7	0.59	115	1.72	6	25
1117	Cereal-corn bran	cup	36	125	2	30	6.8	1	*	0	310	70	18	12.2	4	8	0	0.37	0.7	10.9	0.86	232	1.39	41	52
1118	Cereal-Corn Chex	cup	28.4	111	2	25	0.5	tr	0	0	271	23	4	1.8	0.1	14	15	0.4	0.07	5	0.5	100	1.5	3	11
1119	Cereal-corn flakes-Kelloggs	cup	22.7	88	2	20	0.5	tr	0	0	281	21	3	1.4	0.1	300	12	0.3	0.34	4	0.41	80	1.5	1	14
1120	Cereal-corn flakes-low sodium	cup	25	100	2	22	0.3	tr	0	0	3	18	3	0.6	0.1	10	0	tr	0.05	0.1	0.02	2	0	11	12
371	Cereal-corn flakes-Ralston	cup	25	98	2	22	0.5	tr	0	0	239	22	3	0.6	0.2	10	13	0.1	0	1.1	0.02	2	0	2	10
363	Cereal-corn grits-regular-enriched-hot	cup	242	145	3	32	0.6	tr	0.1	0	0	53	10	1.6	0.2	*	*	0.24	0.15	2	0.06	2	0	0	29
364	Cereal-corn grits-regular-unenriched-hot	cup	242	145	3	32	0.6	tr	0.1	0	0	53	10	1.6	0.2	0	*	0.24	0.15	2	0.06	2	0	0	29
374	Cereal-corn-shredded-added sugar	cup	25	95	2	22	1.5	0	0	0	247	*	4	0.6	0.1	0	13	0.33	0.05	4.4	0.45	88	1.33	1	10
1121	Cereal-Cracklin Bran	cup	60	229	6	41	9.1	9	5.6	0	487	355	116	3.8	3.2	794	32	0.8	0.9	10.6	1.1	212	0	40	241
1759	Cereal-Cracklin Oat Bran-Kelloggs	serv	28.4	110	3	20	2	4	1	0	140	160	60	1.8	1.5	180	15	0.38	0.43	5	0.5	100	1.5	20	150
1166	Cereal-Cream of Rice-cooked	cup	244	127	2	28	0.4	tr	0	0	6	49	7	0.5	0.4	0	0	0	0	1	0.07	7	0	7	42
1168	Cereal-Cream of Wheat-instant	cup	241	153	4	32	2.2	tr	0	0	6	48	14	12	0.2	0	0	0.2	0.1	1.8	0.03	11	0	59	43
1079	Cereal-Cream of Wheat-packet size	item	150	132	3	29	2	tr	0	0	241	55	9	8.1	0.2	1250	0	0.4	0.2	5	0.5	100	0	40	20
1167	Cereal-Cream of Wheat-regular-hot	cup	251	133	4	28	1.9	1	0	0	2	43	10	10.3	0.3	0	0	0.25	0	1.5	0.04	10	0	50	42
1122	Cereal-crisp rice-low sodium	cup	26	105	1	24	0.4	tr	0	0	3	20	10	0.8	0.4	0	0	0	0.05	0.4	0.04	3	0	17	27
1123	Cereal-Crispy Rice	cup	28.4	112	2	25	1	tr	0	0	208	27	12	0.7	0.5	0	0	0.11	0.03	2	0.04	3	0.08	5	31
1124	Cereal-Crispy Wheats and Raisins	cup	43	150	3	35	2	1	0	0	204	174	35	6.8	0.5	569	4	0.6	0.6	7.6	0.8	15	2.3	71	117
365	Cereal-farina-cooked-enriched-hot	cup	233	117	3	25	3.3	tr	tr	0	0	30	5	1.2	0.2	0	0	0.19	0.12	1.3	0.02	5	0	5	28
1125	Cereal-fortified oat flakes	cup	48	177	9	35	1.2	1	0	0	429	343	58	13.7	1.5	636	0	0.73	0.7	8.4	0.9	169	2.5	68	176
1128	Cereal-Froot Loops-General Mills	cup	28.4	111	2	25	0.3	1	0	0	145	26	7	4.5	3.7	375	15	0.4	0.4	5	0.5	100	0	3	24
372	Cereal-frosted flakes-Kellogg	cup	35	133	2	32	0.8	tr	0	0	284	22	3	2.2	0.1	463	19	0.5	0.5	6.2	0.6	124	0	1	26
373	Cereal-frosted flakes-Ralston	cup	38	149	2	34	0.8	1	0	0	247	24	3	1	0.8	503	20	0.5	0.6	6.7	0.7	3	2	4	9
1129	Cereal-frosted Mini Wheats-Kelloggs	item	7.1	26	1	6	0.5	tr	0	0	3	24	56	0.4	0.4	94	4	0.09	0.11	1.3	0.13	25	0	2	19
1130	Cereal-frosted Rice Krispies-Kelloggs	cup	28.4	109	1	26	0.1	tr	0	0	240	21	5	1.8	0.3	375	15	0.4	0.4	5	0.5	100	0	1	27
1131	Cereal-granola-homemade	cup	122	594	15	67	12.8	33	5.8	0	12	612	141	4.8	4.5	10	1	0.73	0.31	2.1	0.43	99	0	76	494
1142	Cereal-granola-Nature Valley	cup	113	503	12	76	4.2	20	13	0	232	389	116	3.8	2.2	94	4	0.39	0.19	0.8	0.09	85	0	71	354
1133	Cereal-Grape Nuts Flakes-Post	cup	32.5	116	3	27	2.1	tr	0	0	250	113	36	5.2	0.7	430	0	0.42	0.49	5.7	0.59	115	1.72	13	97
1132	Cereal-Grape Nuts-Post	cup	114	407	13	94	5.5	tr	0	0	792	381	76	5	2.5	1500	0	1.48	1.71	20.1	2.05	402	6.04	43	286
1134	Cereal-Heartland Natural-plain	cup	115	499	12	79	5.4	18	9.5	0	294	385	147	4.3	3	7	1	0.36	0.16	1.6	0.19	64	0	75	416
1136	Cereal-honey bran	cup	35	119	3	29	3.9	1	0	0	202	151	46	5.6	0.9	463	19	0.4	0.5	6.2	0.6	23	1.9	16	132
1135	Cereal-Honey Nut Cheerios-General Mills	cup	33	125	4	27	1.3	1	0.1	0	299	115	39	5.2	0.9	437	17	0.4	0.5	5.8	0.6	22	1.7	23	122

#	Food	Portion																						
1137	Cereal-Honeycomb-Post	cup	22	86	20	0.3	1	tr	tr	0	166	70	8	1.4	1.2	291	0	0.3	0.3	3.9	0.4	78	1.2	4	22
1138	Cereal-King Vitaman	cup	21	85	18	0.3	1	0.7	0.7	0	161	26	7	12.7	0.2	717	33	0.92	1.06	12.9	1.18	286	4.13	2	27
1139	Cereal-Kix	cup	18.9	74	16	0.3	2	0.1	0.1	0	226	30	8	5.4	0.2	250	10	0.25	0.28	3.3	0.34	67	1	24	26
1140	Cereal-Life-plain/cinnamon	cup	44	162	32	1.4	8	0	1	0	229	197	14	11.6	1.5	3	1	0.95	1	11.6	0.08	37	0	154	238
1141	Cereal-Lucky Charms	cup	32	125	26	0.6	3	0.2	1	0	227	66	27	5.1	0.6	424	17	0.4	0.5	5.6	0.6	6	1.7	36	88
1169	Cereal-Malt o Meal-cooked	cup	240	122	26	0.6	4	0	tr	0	2	31	5	9.5	0.2	0	0	0.4	0.3	5.9	0.02	6	0	5	23
1170	Cereal-Maypo-cooked-hot	cup	240	170	32	1.2	6	*	2	0	9	211	51	8.4	1.5	702	28	0.5	0.8	9.4	0.9	9	2.8	125	248
1143	Cereal-Nutri Grain-barley	cup	41	153	34	2.4	5	0	tr	0	277	108	32	1.5	5.4	543	22	0.5	0.6	7.2	0.7	145	2.2	11	126
1144	Cereal-Nutri Grain-corn	cup	42	160	36	2.6	3	0.1	1	0	276	98	27	0.9	5.5	556	22	0.5	0.6	7.4	0.8	148	2.2	1	120
1145	Cereal-Nutri Grain-rye	cup	40	144	34	2.6	4	0	tr	0	272	72	31	1.1	5.3	530	21	0.5	0.6	7	0.7	141	2.1	8	104
1146	Cereal-Nutri Grain-wheat	cup	44	158	37	2.8	4	0	1	0	299	120	34	1.2	5.8	583	23	0.6	0.7	7.7	0.8	155	2.3	12	164
1792	Cereal-oat bran-cooked	cup	219	88	25	1.8	7	0.4	2	0	2	201	27	1.9	1.2	2	0	0.35	0.07	0.3	0.06	13	0	22	261
1758	Cereal-oat bran-Kelloggs	serv	28.4	100	22	1.5	6	*	1	0	270	115	40	4.5	3.8	180	*	0.38	0.43	5	0.5	*	1.5	*	150
1723	Cereal-oat bran-Quaker	cup	85	270	51	12.3	18	0.8	6	0	15	540	180	5.4	3.6	1028	0	0.9	0.31	15	1.49	48	5.18	60	600
1763	Cereal-oat bran-raisin/spice-hot	oz	28.4	100	19	3.8	3	*	1	0	10	100	43	0.7	0.8	0	tr	0.06	0.05	1.2	0.08	24	0	16	148
366	Cereal-oatmeal-cooked	cup	234	145	25	2.1	6	0.4	2	0	1	132	56	1.6	1.2	7	*	0.26	0.05	0.3	0.05	9	0	20	178
1693	Cereal-oatmeal-raw	cup	81	311	54	4.6	13	0.9	5	0	3	284	120	3.4	2.5	10	0	0.59	0.11	0.6	0.1	26	0	42	384
1081	Cereal-oats-apple/cinnamon-Quaker-packet	item	149	135	26	1.4	4	0.3	2	0	222	107	57	6.1	0.7	435	0	0.48	0.28	5.1	0.7	137	0	158	117
1082	Cereal-oats-bran/raisin/cinnamon-Quaker-packet	item	195	158	30	1.8	5	0.3	tr	0	247	236	57	7.6	1.4	479	0	0.56	0.63	8.1	0.76	155	0	173	206
1083	Cereal-oats-cinnamon/spice-Quaker-packet	item	161	177	35	1.5	5	0.3	2	0	280	104	51	6.7	1	475	0	0.56	0.34	5.7	0.77	153	0	172	146
1084	Cereal-oats-maple/sugar-Quaker-packet	item	155	163	32	1.4	5	0.3	2	0	280	102	42	6.4	0.9	451	0	0.53	0.32	5.4	0.74	145	0	162	143
1080	Cereal-oats-plain-Quaker-instant-packet	item	177	104	18	1.6	4	0.3	2	0	286	100	43	6.3	0.9	455	13	0.53	0.29	5.5	0.74	150	0	163	133
375	Cereal-oats-puffed-added sugar	cup	25	100	19	2.7	3	0.2	1	0	294	*	28	4	0.7	275	70	0.33	0.38	4.4	0.45	6	1.33	44	102
377	Cereal-Product 19-Kelloggs	cup	33	126	27	0.4	3	0	tr	0	378	51	12	21	0.5	1748	70	1.7	2	23.3	2.3	466	7	4	47
1150	Cereal-raisin bran-Kelloggs	cup	49.2	154	37	5.3	5	0.1	2	0	359	256	64	6	5	500	0	0.49	0.59	6.7	0.69	133	2.02	17	183
1151	Cereal-raisin bran-Post	cup	56.8	174	43	6	5	0.2	1	0	370	350	97	9	3	750	0	0.74	0.85	10	1.02	201	3.01	27	238
370	Cereal-raisin bran-Ralston	cup	56	178	47	7.1	4	0	tr	0	486	287	84	6.7	1.7	556	2	0.6	0.6	7.4	0.7	148	2.2	27	247
1085	Cereal-Ralston-cooked-hot	cup	253	134	28	4.2	6	0	1	0	4	153	59	1.6	1.4	0	0	0.2	0.18	2.1	0.11	18	0.11	14	148
1152	Cereal-Rice Chex	cup	25.2	100	23	0.2	1	0	tr	0	211	29	6	1.6	0.3	2	13	0.33	0.01	4.4	0.45	89	1.34	4	25
1153	Cereal-Rice Krispies-Kelloggs	cup	28.4	112	25	0.1	2	0	tr	0	340	30	18	1.8	0.5	375	15	0.4	0.5	5	0.5	100	0	4	34
377	Cereal-rice-puffed-added sugar	cup	14	56	13	0.1	1	0	tr	0	21	43	8	2.1	1.5	300	15	0.31	0.36	4.2	0.43	9	1.27	3	14
376	Cereal-rice-puffed-plain	cup	14	56	13	0.1	1	0	tr	0	tr	16	4	0.1	0.1	0	0	0	0.01	0.4	0.01	3	0	1	14
1171	Cereal-Roman Meal-cooked	cup	241	147	33	2.3	7	*	1	0	3	302	109	2.1	1.8	0	0	0.24	0.12	3.1	0.11	24	0	30	215
1154	Cereal-Special K-Kelloggs	cup	21.3	83	16	0.2	4	tr	tr	0	199	37	12	3.4	2.8	280	11	0.28	0.32	3.8	0.38	75	0.01	6	41
1155	Cereal-Sugar Corn Pops-Kelloggs	cup	28.4	108	26	0.2	1	tr	tr	0	103	17	2	1.8	1.5	375	15	0.4	0.4	5	0.5	100	1	1	28
1156	Cereal-Sugar Smacks-Kelloggs	cup	37.9	141	33	0.5	2	0	tr	0	100	56	18	2.4	0.4	500	20	0.49	0.57	6.7	0.68	134	0	4	41
1157	Cereal-Super Sugar Crisp-Post	cup	33	123	30	0.5	2	tr	0	0	29	123	20	2.1	1.7	437	13	0.4	0.5	5.8	0.6	116	1.7	7	60
1158	Cereal-Tasteeos	cup	24	94	19	0.8	3	0	1	0	183	71	26	3.8	3.8	318	13	0.31	0.36	4.2	0.43	9	1.27	11	96
1159	Cereal-Team	cup	42	164	36	0.4	3	0	tr	0	259	71	19	2.6	0.7	556	22	0.5	0.6	7.4	0.8	7	2.2	6	65
1160	Cereal-Toasties-Post	cup	22.7	88	20	0.4	2	tr	tr	0	238	26	3	0.6	0.1	300	0	0.3	0.34	4	0.41	80	1.2	1	10
1161	Cereal-Total-General Mills	cup	33	116	26	2.4	3	0.1	1	0	409	123	37	21	0.8	1748	70	1.7	2	23.3	2.3	466	7	56	137
1162	Cereal-Trix-General Mills	cup	28.4	109	25	0.3	2	0	tr	0	181	27	6	4.5	0.1	371	15	0.37	0.43	5	0.51	27	1.51	6	19
1163	Cereal-Wheat Chex	cup	46	169	38	3.4	5	0.5	1	0	308	174	58	7.3	1.2	0	24	0.6	0.17	8.1	0.8	162	2.4	18	182
378	Cereal-wheat flakes-added sugar	cup	30	105	24	2.7	3	0	0	0	368	81	33	4.8	0.7	330	16	0.4	0.45	5.3	0.54	9	1.59	12	83
1164	Cereal-wheat germ-brown sugar and honey	cup	113	426	69	5.7	25	1.6	9	0	3	803	272	7.7	14.1	0	0	1.41	0.7	4.7	0.83	298	0	38	971
382	Cereal-wheat germ-toasted	serv	113	432	56	14.6	33	2.1	12	0	5	1070	362	10.3	18.8	50	7	1.89	0.93	6.3	1.11	398	0	51	1295
380	Cereal-wheat-puffed-added sugar	serv	38	138	30	2.1	6	*	tr	0	2	132	55	1.8	0.9	0	0	0.08	0.09	4.1	0.07	12	0	11	135
379	Cereal-wheat-puffed-plain	cup	12	44	10	0.4	2	0	0	0	tr	42	17	0.6	0.3	0	0	0.02	0.03	1.3	0.02	4	0	3	43
367	Cereal-wheat-rolled-cooked-hot	cup	240	180	41	2.9	5	0.2	1	0	535	202	53	1.7	1.2	0	0	0.17	0.07	2.2	*	26	*	19	182
381	Cereal-wheat-shredded-biscuit	item	23.6	83	19	2.2	3	0	tr	0	tr	77	40	0.7	0.6	0	0	0.07	0.06	1.1	0.06	12	0	10	86
368	Cereal-wheat-whole meal-cooked-hot	cup	245	110	23	1.6	4	0.2	1	0	535	118	54	1.2	1.2	0	0	0.15	0.05	1.5	*	27	*	17	127

* indicates that no data was available.
©1994 First DataBank—The Hearst Corporation (N-Squared Computing).

Appendix A - Table of Food Composition
(continued)

Combination foods (beginning after cereals)

Item	Food name	Portion	Weight (g)	Food Energy (Kcal)	Protein (gm)	Carbohydrates (gm)	Fiber (gm)	Total Fat (gm)	Saturated Fat (gm)	Cholesterol (mg)	Sodium (mg)	Potassium (mg)	Magnesium (mg)	Iron (mg)	Zinc (mg)	Vitamin A (RE)	Vitamin C (mg)	Thiamin (mg)	Riboflavin (mg)	Niacin (mg)	Vitamin B6 (mg)	Folates (µg)	Vitamin B12 (µg)	Calcium (mg)	Phosphorus (mg)
1172	Cereal-Wheatena-cooked	cup	243	136	5	29	2.6	1	*	0	5	187	49	1.4	1.7	0	0	0.02	0.05	1.3	0.05	17	0	10	146
1165	Cereal-Wheaties	cup	29	200	3	23	2	1	0.1	0	363	108	32	4.6	0.7	384	15	0.4	0.4	5.1	0.5	9	1.5	44	100
1173	Cereal-whole wheat natural	cup	242	150	5	33	2.7	1	0.2	0	1	171	54	1.5	1.2	0	0	0.17	0.12	2.2	0.18	27	0	17	167
1793	Oats-rolled or oatmeal-dry	cup	81	311	13	54	3.8	5	0.9	0	3	284	120	3.4	2.5	20	0	0.59	0.11	0.6	0.1	26	0	42	384
Combination foods																									
2179	ABC's & 123's in sauce-Chef Boyardee	serv	213	160	5	31	3	1	1	2	830	341	27	1.4	0.6	40	0	0.3	0.17	2	0.18	13	0	0	78
###	ABC's & 123's-Chef Boyardee	serv	244	200	6	42	*	1	1	2	1020	*	*	1.4	*	60	0	0.3	0.17	3	*	*	*	20	*
2194	ABC's & 123's/meatballs-Chef Boyardee	serv	244	280	9	35	3	11	2.1	23	1090	425	36	2.7	1.7	100	0	0.15	0.17	3	0.17	26	0.6	0	142
2178	ABC's/123's/mini meatballs-Chef Boyardee	serv	213	240	8	33	*	9	0.6	18	920	*	20	1.8	*	80	0	0.15	0.17	3	*	*	*	0	133
###	Anchovy-dried-fried-chili (ikan bilis)	oz	28.3	90	8	1	tr	6	*	24	121	93	20	0.3	0.7	24	0	0.03	0.08	0.7	0.06	4	0.25	12	133
###	Beans & onions-pinto-seasoned/pork-Luck's	serv	213	250	11	37	15	6	2	6	560	465	55	3.6	3.7	0	1	0.15	0.1	0.8	0.09	59	0	60	206
2217	Beans & weiners-7 oz-Luck's	serv	198	300	15	37	13.7	12	4.7	12	1210	*	*	2.7	*	0	0	0.15	0.14	2	*	*	0	40	23
###	Beans & weiners-microwave-Luck's	serv	213	320	15	40	10	15	5	30	1145	tr	0	2.7	11.8	0	4	0.09	0.17	2	946	669	574	60	290
###	Beans-lima-giant-seasoned/pork-Luck's	serv	213	240	12	36	9	5	2	6	500	995	124	2.7	1.7	0	0	0.15	0.1	0.8	0.44	72	*	20	*
###	Beans-lima-green-seasoned/pork-Luck's	serv	213	240	11	37	8	5	0.4	6	590	*	75	2.7	*	0	0	0.15	0.1	0.8	*	*	0	40	249
###	Beans-navy-seasoned/pork-Luck's	serv	213	230	12	33	11	6	2	6	560	*	75	3.6	*	0	0	0.12	0.1	0.8	0.15	48	*	80	59
###	Beans-october-seasoned/pork-7.5 oz-Luck's	serv	213	230	12	32	9	5	0.8	15	600	639	75	3.6	12.5	0	0	0.09	0.14	0.8	*	48	0	40	249
2215	Beans-pinto-seasoned/pork-Luck's	serv	198	200	10	29	9	4	2	0	550	216	30	2.7	0.5	0	0	0.09	0.14	0.4	0.1	36	0.04	40	286
###	Beans/pork-butter-Luck's	serv	213	230	10	38	9	4	0.8	15	570	639	75	2.7	12.5	0	0	0.12	0.14	0.8	0.15	48	0	40	249
###	Beans/pork-kidney-red-Luck's	serv	213	240	11	33	10	7	5.1	15	550	797	89	3.6	2.2	0	0	0.12	0.14	1.2	0.24	253	0.04	40	286
###	Beans/pork-northern-Luck's	serv	213	230	11	34	10	5	2	9	550	639	75	2.7	12.5	0	0	0.09	0.1	0.8	0.15	48	0	80	249
2218	Beans/pork-yelloweye-Luck's	serv	213	240	12	35	10	6	0.8	15	530	639	75	3.6	12.5	0	0	0.12	0.1	1.2	0.15	48	0	60	249
###	Beef burger (burger daging lembu)	oz	28.3	67	3	7	tr	3	2	25	87	68	8	2.8	1.7	110	0	0.01	0.04	0.7	0.09	2	0.68	13	7
###	Beef chow mein/chop suey w/ noodles	oz	28.4	53	4	4	0.4	3	0.7	6	116	65	8	0.5	0.4	17	3	0.02	0.03	0.5	0.05	4	0.21	5	29
###	Beef curry (kari daging lembu)	oz	28.3	41	4	2	0.1	2	0.9	8	21	42	7	0.7	0.7	137	0	0.01	0.01	0.3	0.06	2	0.37	6	99
###	Beef in tomato sauce (lembu-masak merah)	oz	28.3	44	3	4	0.1	2	1.3	13	66	57	6	0.7	0.8	120	0	0.05	0.07	0.6	0.06	2	0.37	14	43
178	Beef potpie-home recipe-1/3 of 9" pie	slice	210	515	21	39	3.9	30	7.9	44	596	334	33	3.8	*	344	6	0.3	0.3	5.5	0.25	*	*	29	149
###	Beef ravioli in meat sauce-Chef Boyardee	serv	213	220	8	35	2.3	5	2	15	1120	437	33	1.8	2.8	100	0	0.12	0.17	2	0.26	22	1.39	0	179
2195	Beef ravioli/sauce-8 oz-Chef Boyardee	serv	227	220	8	35	2.4	5	2.4	15	1190	465	36	1.8	3	100	0	0.09	0.17	2	0.26	23	1.48	0	190
###	Beef rendang (rendang daging lembu)	oz	28.3	72	5	2	0.1	5	*	*	90	72	*	0.7	*	112	0	0.02	0.03	0.4	*	*	*	6	31
###	Beef satay (satay daging lembu)	oz	28.3	68	6	6	0.1	2	*	*	26	57	*	1.1	*	20	0	0.04	0.06	1.5	*	*	*	5	131
###	Beef stew-chef style-Legout	oz	28.4	20	2	2	*	1	*	*	125	73	*	0.3	*	0	0	*	0.03	0.3	*	*	*	3	*
177	Beef stew-with vegetables	cup	245	220	16	15	3.2	11	4.9	72	1006	613	40	2.9	*	480	17	0.15	0.17	4.7	*	*	tr	29	184
2261	Beef-creamed-sliced-cured-Legout	oz	28.4	25	1	3	*	1	*	14	223	43	27	0.6	0.8	118	0	0	0.02	0.1	*	*	*	3	*
###	Beef-fried (goreng daging lembu)	oz	28.3	96	9	5	0.1	6	1.9	27	35	119	28	1.1	1.4	117	0	0.04	0.08	0.8	0.14	2	0.93	11	211
###	Beef-liver rendang (rendang hati lembu)	oz	28.3	72	5	1	0.2	6	0.8	136	41	97	14	5.2	1.5	205	0	0.09	0.24	1	0.4	62	31.5	13	171
###	Beef-lung-fried (paru lembu goreng)	oz	28.3	138	11	tr	0.2	10	*	*	4	104	14	1.8	*	26	0	0.04	0.06	0.9	*	2	*	11	141
2195	Beef-o-getti-Chef Boyardee	serv	213	220	7	29	*	9	*	20	1240	*	*	1.8	*	60	0	0.15	0.17	2	*	*	*	0	*
77	Beef-raviolios-canned with meat sauce	oz	28.4	28	1	4	0.2	2	*	*	131	46	*	0.3	0.2	50	tr	0.03	0.02	0.4	*	*	*	5	*
###	Beef-spleen rendang (rendang limpa lembu)	oz	28.3	67	5	6	0.3	4	*	19	12	105	29	3.9	1.6	27	0	0.04	0.06	0.7	*	*	*	11	145
2196	Beefaroni-7.5 oz-Chef Boyardee	serv	213	220	8	29	*	8	4.8	*	1070	*	*	1.8	*	60	0	0.12	0.12	3	*	*	*	0	*
2173	Bowties/vegetables-Pasta Perfect	cup	227	220	10	38	*	6	1	0	110	340	*	2.9	*	160	48	0.45	0.34	3.2	*	*	*	40	80
1719	Burrito-beans and cheese	item	93	189	8	28	8.3	6	3.4	14	583	248	*	1.1	0.8	118	1	0.11	0.36	1.8	0.13	41	0.45	107	90
###	Capati-green gram gravy	oz	28.3	27	1	3	0.3	1	*	5	123	7	*	0.4	*	1	0	0.04	0.04	0.6	*	3	*	5	46
2251	Cheese ravioli in sauce-Chef Boyardee	serv	213	200	7	33	4	6	1	11	990	337	*	1.8	1.2	150	0	0.12	0.17	2	0.16	23	0.32	60	176
2210	Cheese ravioli/beef sauce-Chef Boyardee	serv	213	200	7	34	1.8	7	6	11	1205	352	*	1.8	1.8	80	0	0.12	0.17	2	0.18	22	0.68	20	186
1500	Cheese souffle-home recipe	cup	95	207	9	6	0.1	16	6.6	137	346	115	14	1	1	152	0	0.05	0.23	0.2	0.06	14	0.35	191	185
2251	Chicken & dumplings-canned-Swanson	oz	28.4	30	2	3	0.1	2	0.7	11	135	35	*	0.1	0.2	11	tr	tr	0.01	0.3	0.04	1	0.04	3	29
###	Chicken & dumplings-Luck's	serv	206	260	15	22	4	12	4.8	65	680	253	29	1.1	1.6	0	0	0.09	0.17	4	0.26	8	0.27	60	206
###	Chicken & dumplings-microwave-Luck's	serv	213	170	17	20	2	2	1	25	1550	261	30	1.1	1.7	0	4	0.06	0.17	4	0.27	8	0.28	20	213

A 8

2231	Chicken & potatoes-microwave-Luck's	serv	213	190	16	22	3	4	1	20	1085	373	41	1.1	1.8	0	6	0.03	0.17	5	0.3	12	0.24	20	214
###	Chicken & rice-microwave-Luck's	serv	213	150	17	17	2	2	1	30	1170	169	30	0.7	2	0	9	0.03	0.14	4	0.26	7	0.16	40	147
###	Chicken a la king-canned-Swanson	oz	28.4	36	2	2	*	2	*	*	131	*	*	0.1	*	0	0	0.01	0.03	0.4	*	*	*	8	*
214	Chicken a la king-cooked-home recipe	cup	245	470	27	12	1.2	34	12.9	186	759	404	*	2.5	*	226	12	0.1	0.42	5.4	*	*	*	127	358
###	Chicken a la king-Legout	oz	28.4	30	3	2	*	1	*	*	183	63	*	0.6	*	0	0	0	0.03	0.2	*	*	*	3	*
215	Chicken and noodles-cooked-home recipe	cup	240	365	22	26	1.3	18	5.9	96	600	149	*	2.2	*	80	0	0.05	0.17	4.3	*	*	*	26	247
216	Chicken chow mein-canned	cup	250	95	7	18	0.9	0	0	98	722	418	*	1.3	*	30	13	0.05	0.1	1	*	*	*	45	85
2168	Chicken chow mein-canned-La Choy	cup	300	132	7	15	0.6	6	3.7	18	999	491	61	3.2	2.4	17	17	0.06	0.12	2.3	0.44	36	0.27	48	235
217	Chicken chow mein-home recipe	cup	250	255	31	10	0.5	10	2.4	98	717	473	*	2.5	*	56	10	0.08	0.23	4.3	*	*	*	58	293
###	Chicken chow mein/chop suey w/ noodles	oz	28.4	37	3	3	0.3	2	0.3	6	147	46	6	0.3	0.2	2	1	0.02	0.03	0.8	0.04	3	0.03	5	22
###	Chicken curry (kari ayam)	oz	28.3	58	5	1	tr	4	0.4	10	33	54	6	0.7	0.3	39	0	0.01	0.03	0.7	0.06	2	0.04	13	66
1911	Chicken Helper-cheesy broccoli-skillet	serv	43.9	160	4	32	*	2	*	*	720	160	*	1.1	*	0	0	0.15	0.07	1.2	*	*	*	40	*
1912	Chicken Helper-creamy chicken-skillet	serv	41	170	6	26	*	5	*	*	720	150	*	1.1	*	150	0	0.23	0.14	1.6	*	*	*	20	*
1913	Chicken Helper-creamy mushroom-skillet	serv	41	170	5	28	*	4	*	*	720	150	*	1.1	*	0	0	0.23	0.14	2	*	*	*	20	*
1914	Chicken Helper-fettucini alfredo-skillet	serv	41	170	6	27	*	4	*	*	730	105	*	1.1	*	0	0	0.3	0.17	1.6	*	*	*	40	*
1915	Chicken Helper-stirfried chicken-skillet	serv	46.8	170	4	36	*	1	*	*	800	130	*	1.1	*	0	0	0.15	0.03	1.6	*	*	*	40	*
2148	Chicken pieces with fried rice	oz	28.3	51	2	7	0.5	2	0.2	7	36	38	6	0.6	0.2	7	tr	0.02	0.01	0.3	0.07	3	0.03	5	58
218	Chicken potpie-baked-home recipe	slice	232	545	23	42	4.2	31	11	72	593	343	*	3	*	618	5	0.34	0.31	5.5	*	*	*	70	232
2213	Chicken ravioli-Chef Boyardee	serv	213	180	7	29	*	4	*	13	1100	*	*	1.8	*	20	0	0.15	0.17	1.6	*	*	*	60	*
###	Chicken satay (satay ayam)	oz	28.3	69	5	4	0.5	4	*	*	38	63	*	0.8	*	24	0	0.01	0.03	1.9	*	*	*	8	95
2149	Chicken soto	oz	28.3	30	tr	3	0.1	2	*	*	49	79	*	0.2	*	9	tr	0.01	0.03	0.2	*	*	*	3	79
###	Chicken'n'dumplings-Legout	oz	28.4	17	2	1	*	1	*	*	125	25	*	0.3	*	0	*	*	0.03	0	*	*	*	0	*
###	Chicken-chunk style mixin-canned-Swanson	oz	28.4	52	5	tr	*	3	*	*	92	*	*	0.3	*	0	0	0	0.03	0.8	*	*	*	8	*
###	Chicken-liver rendang (rendang hati ayam)	oz	28.3	78	8	1	0.1	5	0.8	162	43	80	7	1.1	1.2	141	0	0.02	0.05	0.9	0.17	232	6.77	7	330
2175	Chili & beans-chili bowl	oz	28.4	30	2	3	0.6	2	1	5	100	110	6	0.7	0.5	0	0	0.03	0.03	0.4	0.03	5	0.16	0	25
###	Chili con carne-w/beans-Legout	oz	28.4	38	3	3	*	2	*	*	160	62	*	0.6	*	0	*	0.01	0.04	0.5	*	*	*	10	*
179	Chili con carne-with beans-canned	cup	255	340	19	31	5	16	7.5	38	1354	594	*	4.3	*	30	*	0.08	0.18	3.3	0.26	*	*	82	321
###	Chili concarne w/beans-Legout	oz	28.4	43	2	4	*	2	*	*	193	133	*	1.5	*	0	0	0.02	0.04	0.1	*	*	*	7	*
2212	Chili mac-Chef Boyardee	serv	213	230	8	26	4	11	3.4	20	1410	501	41	1.8	3	150	1	0.15	0.17	3	0.19	30	0.98	0	177
1631	Chili with beans-canned	cup	255	286	15	30	6.9	14	6	43	1330	932	115	8.8	5.1	86	4	0.12	0.27	0.9	0.34	58	0.03	119	393
2174	Chili-homestyle-chili bowl	oz	28.4	50	2	2	0.6	4	2	10	135	90	6	0	0.5	0	0	0.06	0.03	0.8	0.03	5	0.16	0	25
2157	Chili-mild vegetarian-lowfat-H Valley	oz	28.4	28	2	5	2.4	tr	0.1	0	6	116	9	0.4	0.3	120	tr	0.02	0.05	0.3	0.04	22	0	0	58
2156	Chili-mild vegetarian/3 bean-H Valley	oz	28.4	18	2	2	1.8	tr	*	0	36	88	*	0.4	*	120	tr	0.03	0.02	0.2	*	*	*	8	*
2154	Chili-mild vegetarian/beans-H Valley	oz	28.4	28	2	5	2.4	tr	0.1	0	58	116	9	0.5	0.3	120	tr	0.02	0.05	0.3	0.04	22	0	0	58
2158	Chili-mild vegetarian/lentils-H Valley	oz	28.4	28	2	3	1.4	1	*	0	58	98	*	0.7	*	40	2	0.02	0.03	0.4	*	*	*	12	*
2167	Chili-no beans-Hunt's	fl oz	32	53	3	2	0.5	4	0.8	10	153	46	6	0.6	0.6	64	1	0.03	0.03	0.6	0.04	3	0.25	10	28
2163	Chili-plain-Gebhardt	fl oz	32	59	3	2	0.7	5	0.6	8	157	70	7	0.5	0.5	87	1	0.03	0.04	0.4	0.03	5	0.18	7	29
2155	Chili-spicy vegetarian/beans-H Valley	oz	28.4	28	2	5	2.4	tr	0.1	0	58	116	9	0.5	0.3	120	tr	0.02	0.05	0.3	0.04	22	0	0	58
2162	Chili/beans-Gebhardt	fl oz	35	76	4	8	*	3	*	*	163	136	*	1	*	51	tr	0.1	0.04	0.5	*	*	*	17	*
2166	Chili/beans-Hunt's	fl oz	35	45	3	3	*	2	*	*	164	76	*	0.7	*	33	1	0.03	0.03	0.5	*	*	*	11	*
2164	Chili/beans-longhorn-Gebhardt	fl oz	35	85	4	8	*	4	*	*	155	148	*	1	*	127	tr	0.1	0.05	0.5	*	*	*	18	*
1720	Chimichanga-beef	item	174	425	20	43	4.3	20	8.5	9	910	587	62	4.6	5	15	5	0.48	0.64	5.8	0.27	31	1.52	63	123
180	Chop suey-with beef and pork-home recipe	cup	250	300	26	13	*	17	8.5	64	1052	425	*	4.8	*	120	33	0.28	0.38	5	*	*	*	60	248
2169	Chow mein-meatless-canned-La Choy	cup	300	69	2	15	0.2	tr	13.7	0	999	219	207	10.5	3.3	7	20	0.06	0.12	1	0.24	21	0	41	270
2221	Collard greens/pork-chopped-Luck's	serv	213	90	2	8	2	5	*	*	500	*	*	1.8	*	100	60	0	0.14	0.8	*	*	*	200	*
1847	Corn dog-plain	item	175	460	17	56	2.8	19	5.2	79	972	262	17	6.2	1.3	36	0	0.29	0.71	4.2	0.1	60	0.44	101	166
###	Corned beef hash-Legout	oz	28.4	48	6	4	*	3	*	*	193	90	*	0.9	*	0	0	0	0	0.2	*	*	*	3	*
###	Cucur badak	oz	28.3	72	2	10	0.3	3	*	*	105	82	*	0.3	*	23	tr	0.02	0.01	0.3	*	*	*	6	17
###	Currypuff (karipap)	oz	28.3	90	1	12	0.1	4	*	*	48	47	*	0.4	*	14	tr	0.03	0.02	0.2	*	*	*	7	17
###	Currypuff-mini (karipap mini)	oz	28.3	155	3	14	0.3	10	*	*	45	60	*	0.6	*	15	0	0.03	0.01	0.2	*	*	*	24	35
###	Currypuff-twisted (karipap pusing)	oz	28.3	61	1	3	0.2	5	*	*	81	60	*	0.5	*	16	0	0.07	0.06	0.3	*	*	*	11	16

* indicates that no data was available.

©1994 First DataBank—The Hearst Corporation (N-Squared Computing).

Item	Food name	Portion	Weight (g)	Food Energy (Kcal)	Protein (gm)	Carbohydrates (gm)	Fiber (gm)	Total Fat (gm)	Saturated Fat (gm)	Cholesterol (mg)	Sodium (mg)	Potassium (mg)	Magnesium (mg)	Iron (mg)	Zinc (mg)	Vitamin A (RE)	Vitamin C (mg)	Thiamin (mg)	Riboflavin (mg)	Niacin (mg)	Vitamin B6 (mg)	Folates (µg)	Vitamin B12 (µg)	Calcium (mg)	Phosphorus (mg)
2191	Dinosaurs-7.5 oz-Chef Boyardee	serv	213	160	4	33	3	1	1	1	790	*	*	1.1	*	60	0	0.3	0.17	2	*	*	*	20	*
2192	Dinosaurs/meatballs-Chef Boyardee	serv	244	280	9	36	*	11	1	21	1130	*	32	2.7	*	100	0	0.23	0.17	3	*	*	*	0	*
2185	Dinosaurs/mini meatballs-Chef Boyardee	serv	213	230	7	32	1.8	8	9.2	19	960	326	32	1.8	3.5	100	0	0.15	0.14	3	0.26	15	1.55	20	198
##	Dumpling-chicken (kuih pau ayam)	oz	28.3	68	3	12	0.2	3	0.7	11	28	4	3	0.8	0.2	25	1	0.03	0.03	0.3	0.04	1	0.04	6	18
##	Dumpling-red gram (kuih pau kacang merah)	oz	28.3	79	2	16	0.2	2	0.3	1	3	2	3	1.8	0.1	20	1	0.03	0.02	0.2	0.01	1	0.02	7	3
##	Egg banjo (banjo telur)	oz	28.3	59	2	7	0	3	*	*	65	45	4	0.5	*	104	1	0.03	0.05	0.4	*	*	*	12	41
1295	Enchilada-cheese	item	163	320	10	29	3.2	19	10.6	44	784	240	50	1.3	2.5	186	1	0.09	0.42	1.9	0.39	34	0.74	324	133
1726	Enchirito-cheese/beef/bean	item	193	344	18	34	3.4	16	8	49	1251	560	71	2.4	2.8	134	5	0.18	0.69	3	0.21	254	1.63	217	224
2151	Fast menu-amaranth/vegetables-H Valley	oz	28.4	19	1	2	1.1	tr	*	0	19	13	*	3.6	*	133	0	0.02	0.02	0.2	*	*	*	3	*
2152	Fast menu-hearty lentil-H Valley	oz	28.4	20	2	2	2.1	tr	0.7	0	27	48	12	3.6	0.3	133	0	0.02	0.02	0.1	0.02	20	0.01	8	29
2153	Fast menu-western black bean-H Valley	oz	28.4	20	2	2	1.9	tr	*	0	23	37	12	0.4	*	13	0	0.02	0.02	0.1	0.02	20	0.01	13	29
##	Fish-bream-coconut milk (ikan tilapia)	oz	28.3	54	4	tr	0	4	6	*	24	118	11	0.9	0.2	75	0	0.01	0.06	0.7	0.01	5	0	9	71
2101	Fish-bream-fried-chili (ikan tilapia)	oz	28.3	83	7	3	tr	5	*	*	105	177	*	0.6	*	99	0	0.01	0.07	0.2	*	*	*	15	186
2102	Fish-cuttlefish-fried-chili (sotong)	oz	28.3	42	7	2	0	2	*	57	45	23	*	0.8	*	37	0	0.03	0.05	0.1	*	*	*	13	51
##	Fish-hairtail scad-chili (cincaru-berlad)	oz	28.3	61	5	2	0.1	4	*	*	24	98	*	0.7	*	52	0	0.01	0.01	0.7	*	*	*	17	187
2105	Fish-Indian mackerel-chili (kembong-berl)	oz	28.3	95	6	tr	*	8	*	*	25	127	*	0.8	*	11	0	0.01	0.01	1.1	*	*	*	17	141
2103	Fish-Indian mackerel-curry (kembong kari)	oz	28.3	30	5	tr	0	3	*	*	39	110	*	0.7	*	16	0	0.02	0.04	0.8	*	*	*	10	154
2104	Fish-Indian mackerel-soy (kembong-kicap)	oz	28.3	74	5	3	tr	5	*	*	26	115	*	0.8	*	11	0	0.01	0.1	0.9	*	*	*	12	164
2100	Fish-pomfret-fried-chili (bawal-berlada)	oz	28.3	69	7	1	0	4	*	*	53	67	*	0.6	*	20	0	0.11	0.05	0.2	*	*	*	13	127
2107	Fish-red snapper-coconut milk (merah)	oz	28.3	71	5	2	tr	5	*	*	66	92	*	0.7	*	92	0	0.03	0.05	0.8	*	*	*	15	49
2106	Fish-red snapper-fried-tamarind	oz	28.3	65	6	2	0	4	*	*	26	131	*	0.6	*	60	0	0.05	0.05	0.6	*	*	*	11	68
2108	Fish-shrimp-cooked-chili (udang-sambal)	oz	28.3	57	5	tr	0.1	4	0.1	57	91	134	12	0.8	0.4	31	0	tr	0.01	0.1	0.04	1	0.26	156	188
2109	Fish-snakehead-salted-fried (haruan)	oz	28.3	116	13	7	0	4	*	*	113	157	1	0.9	*	37	0	0.1	0.05	0.3	*	*	*	11	68
##	Ham croquette	cup	225	565	37	26	151	34	13.5	157	769	187	1	4.7	0.6	175	0	0.63	0.5	5.6	0.37	12	0.81	155	360
1879	Hamburger Helper-beef noodle-dry	cup	39.7	150	4	29	0.6	2	0.4	16	920	50	7	0.7	1.2	0	0	0.23	0.1	1.6	0.06	6	0.41	0	46
1880	Hamburger Helper-beef romanoff-dry	cup	45.4	180	7	31	*	3	*	*	1030	200	7	1.4	*	0	0	0.38	0.26	2	*	*	*	60	*
1881	Hamburger Helper-beef taco-dry	cup	42.5	160	4	33	0.3	1	2.4	21	930	120	7	1.1	1.1	60	1	0.23	0.1	1.6	0.07	6	0.56	20	57
1882	Hamburger Helper-cheddar/bacon-dry	cup	43.9	190	6	27	*	6	*	*	900	125	*	0.7	*	0	0	0.23	0.17	1.6	*	*	*	60	*
1883	Hamburger Helper-cheeseburger macaroni	cup	45.4	190	6	28	*	6	*	*	980	190	*	1.1	*	40	0	0.23	0.17	2	*	*	*	60	*
1884	Hamburger Helper-cheesy italian-dry	cup	39.7	170	6	27	*	3	*	*	970	175	*	1.1	*	20	0	0.23	0.14	2	*	*	*	40	*
1885	Hamburger Helper-chili macaroni-dry	cup	42.5	150	4	32	*	1	*	*	920	210	*	0.7	*	60	0	0.23	0.1	1.6	*	*	*	20	*
1886	Hamburger Helper-hamburger hash-dry	cup	34	140	3	27	*	2	*	*	1070	110	*	1.1	*	0	1	0.23	0.07	1.6	*	*	*	20	*
1887	Hamburger Helper-hamburger stew-dry	cup	31.2	120	3	26	0.5	1	*	14	960	330	9	1.4	0.8	150	0	0	0.07	0.8	0.08	4	0.45	40	37
1888	Hamburger Helper-lasagna-dry	cup	43.9	160	4	33	*	1	*	*	860	220	*	1.1	*	80	0	0.23	0.14	2	*	*	*	20	*
1889	Hamburger Helper-meat loaf-dry	serv	17	70	2	13	*	2	*	*	620	120	*	0.7	*	0	0	0.06	0	0.8	*	*	*	20	*
1890	Hamburger Helper-nacho cheese-dry	cup	42.5	160	4	32	*	2	*	*	980	80	*	0.7	*	60	0	0.23	0.1	1.6	*	*	*	20	*
1891	Hamburger Helper-pizza dish-dry	cup	48.2	180	6	37	*	1	*	*	960	290	*	1.8	*	100	1	0.38	0.17	4	*	*	*	20	*
1892	Hamburger Helper-pizzabake-dry	serv	38.9	150	4	29	*	2	*	*	800	180	*	1.4	*	40	0	0.15	0.1	2	*	*	*	40	*
1894	Hamburger Helper-potato stroganoff-dry	cup	36.3	140	3	26	*	3	*	*	930	350	*	0.4	*	0	0	0	0.03	1.6	*	*	*	40	*
1893	Hamburger Helper-potatoes au gratin-dry	cup	36.9	140	4	27	*	2	*	*	820	340	*	0.7	*	60	0	0.03	0.07	1.6	*	*	*	20	*
1895	Hamburger Helper-rice oriental-dry	cup	45.4	180	4	38	*	1	*	*	1070	110	*	1.1	*	0	0	0.15	0.03	1.6	*	*	*	20	*
1896	Hamburger Helper-sloppy joe bake-dry	serv	44.9	180	5	33	0.5	3	1.6	14	1060	220	9	1.4	0.8	150	0	0.23	0.14	1.6	0.08	4	0.45	40	37
1897	Hamburger Helper-spaghetti-dry	cup	42.5	160	6	32	*	1	*	*	1060	300	*	1.4	*	20	0	0.23	0.17	3	*	*	*	20	*
1898	Hamburger Helper-stroganoff-dry	cup	45.4	190	5	30	*	5	*	*	800	100	*	1.1	*	40	0	0.23	0.14	2	*	*	*	20	*
1899	Hamburger Helper-tacobake-dry	serv	42.5	170	4	31	*	4	*	*	920	160	*	1.8	*	60	0	0.23	0.17	2	*	*	*	40	*
1900	Hamburger Helper-zesty italian-dry	cup	46.8	170	6	35	0.1	1	*	*	940	290	*	1.4	*	60	0	0.23	0.14	2	*	*	*	20	*
1299	Hamburger-bacon and cheese-generic	item	150	464	25	29	1.8	27	5.3	68	660	339	35	3.7	5.3	75	2	0.15	0.27	4.9	0.24	26	1.8	116	302
1300	Hot dog-plain with bun-generic	item	98	242	10	11	0.9	13	1.6	44	671	143	13	2.3	2	0	tr	0.24	0.27	3.7	0.05	30	0.51	24	97
2061	Kuih bawang	oz	28.3	138	2	18	0.1	6	*	*	154	30	*	0.4	*	1	0	0.02	0.02	2	*	*	*	6	24
2197	Lasagna-7.5 oz-Chef Boyardee	serv	213	240	8	31	3.2	8	5.3	18	1010	414	38	1.8	1.7	60	2	0.09	0.17	2	0.21	17	0.16	116	244
##	Lobster-salad with tomato and egg	cup	256	211	13	11	2.1	13	1.6	176	637	468	32	1.6	1.6	214	23	0.16	0.18	0.9	0.19	37	0.53	65	175

Code	Food	Unit																			
###	Lor-mai-fan	oz	28.3	63	1	12	0	1	*	86	6	1.1	*	0	0.01	0.01	0.3	*	*	5	9
###	Macaroni & cheese-baked-home recipe	cup	200	430	17	40	*	22	68	1086	240	1.6	1.8	258	0.31	0.15	1.5	17	0.46	362	322
###	Macaroni & cheese-canned	cup	240	228	9	26	*	10	24	730	139	1	2.2	79	0.24	0.12	1	20	*	199	182
441	Macaroni & cheese-enriched-canned	cup	240	230	9	26	1.4	10	42	729	139	1	*	52	0.12	0.12	1	*	*	199	182
442	Macaroni & cheese-enriched-home recipe	cup	200	430	17	40	1.2	22	42	1086	240	1.8	*	172	0.2	0.2	1.8	*	*	362	322
###	Macaroni & cheese-Franco	oz	28.4	23	1	3	0.3	1	6	118	38	0.1	0.3	14	0.02	0.03	0.3	2	0.02	11	59
2177	Macaroni shells-Chef Boyardee	serv	213	150	6	31	1.7	1	0	930	129	1.4	0.8	20	0.14	0.15	3	13	0.15	0	106
###	Maw satay (satay perut lembu)	oz	28.3	62	6	2	0.1	3	*	53	46	1.6	*	7	0.03	0.01	0.4	*	*	5	91
2091	Maw-coconut gravy (perut lembu masak)	oz	28.3	41	4	1	0	2	*	69	23	0.5	*	20	0.09	0.04	0.5	*	*	10	110
1692	Meat loaf-with celery and onions	serv	87.6	213	16	5	0.1	14	107	103	182	1.9	3.1	12	0.15	0.05	3.2	11	0.16	23	112
2180	Mini bites-Chef Boyardee	serv	213	260	8	30	1	12	17	1020	*	1.8	1.8	80	0.17	0.12	1.8	*	*	20	*
2181	Mini cannelloni-Chef Boyardee	serv	213	230	9	33	5	7	14	1050	197	1.8	1.3	60	0.15	0.15	3	15	0.12	20	213
2214	Mini chicken ravioli-Chef Boyardee	serv	213	220	7	29	*	8	*	1090	*	1.8	*	100	0.12	0.12	1.6	*	*	40	*
###	Mini ravioli-beef-7.5 oz-Chef Boyardee	serv	213	210	7	31	1.5	5	12	1140	327	1.8	4.7	80	0.15	0.15	2	29	0.27	0	267
936	Mixed fruit-canned-heavy syrup pack	cup	255	184	1	48	2.9	tr	0	10	214	0.9	0.2	49	0.1	0.04	1.5	8	0.09	3	26
937	Mixed fruit-frozen-sweetened	cup	250	245	4	61	3	tr	0	8	327	0.7	0.1	81	0.09	0.04	1	19	0.06	18	30
2150	Murtabak	oz	28.3	45	2	5	0.3	2	*	99	35	0.3	*	19	0.02	0.03	0.7	*	*	5	73
1721	Nachos-cheese	serv	113	345	9	36	2.2	19	18	816	172	1.3	1.8	92	0.37	0.19	1.5	10	0.2	272	276
2184	Pac man in chicken sauce-Chef Boyardee	serv	213	170	6	22	*	7	*	905	*	1.4	*	20	0.17	0.15	2	*	*	0	14
2182	Pac man in tomato sauce-Chef Boyardee	serv	213	150	6	30	1	1	2	830	*	1.1	*	60	0.15	0.15	2	*	*	20	35
2183	Pac man with meatballs-Chef Boyardee	serv	213	230	7	32	3	9	17	880	*	1.4	*	80	0.17	0.12	2	*	*	0	116
###	Pasta in cheese sauce-circuso's-Franco	oz	28.4	23	1	4	0.4	tr	1	117	45	0.1	0.1	14	0.02	0.03	0.3	2	0.02	3	14
###	Pasta/meatballs-circuso's-Franco	oz	28.4	29	1	3	0.4	1	13	129	79	0.8	0.8	14	0.02	0.02	0.4	5	0.05	3	35
1519	Peas & carrots-canned-dietary-low sodium	cup	255	96	6	22	7.1	1	0	10	256	1.9	1.5	1471	0.14	0.19	1.5	47	0.22	58	116
1016	Peas and carrots-canned	cup	255	97	6	22	8.6	1	0	663	255	1.9	1.5	1471	0.19	0.19	1.5	47	0.22	59	117
1017	Peas and carrots-frozen-boiled	cup	160	77	5	16	7.1	1	0	109	253	1.5	0.7	1242	0.36	0.1	1.9	42	0.14	37	78
1018	Peas and onions-canned	cup	120	61	4	10	4.3	tr	0	530	115	1	0.7	19	0.12	0.08	1.5	32	0.23	20	61
1019	Peas and onions-frozen-boiled	cup	180	81	5	16	4.7	tr	0	67	211	1.6	0.5	63	0.27	0.12	1.9	36	0.16	25	61
2216	Peas-blackeye-seasoned/pork-7 oz-Luck's	serv	198	230	9	28	6	9	0	600	805	2.7	1.5	0	0.03	0.1	0.8	200	0.1	20	229
2219	Peas-crowder-seasoned/pork-Luck's	serv	213	210	10	33	7	4	*	600	*	1.8	*	0	0.06	0.1	0.8	*	*	20	*
###	Peppers-sweet-red & green-beef & crumbs	cup	140	238	18	24	2.2	8	53	440	361	2.9	0.3	39	0.24	0.13	3.5	23	0.3	59	169
475	Pizza-cheese-baked	slice	63	140	8	21	1.6	3	9	336	110	0.6	0.8	74	0.16	0.18	2.5	59	0.04	116	113
1718	Pizza-cheese/meat/vegetable	slice	79	184	13	21	1.8	5	21	382	178	1.5	1.1	101	0.17	0.21	2	27	0.09	101	131
1491	Pizza-pepperoni-baked	slice	71	181	10	20	1.5	7	14	267	153	0.9	0.5	54	0.23	0.14	3.1	53	0.05	65	75
###	Plate dinner-beef pot roast-potatoes/pea	oz	28.4	30	4	2	0.3	1	14	73	69	0.5	0.2	3	0.03	0.02	0.6	7	0.08	3	22
###	Plate dinner-chicken-fried-potatoes	oz	28.4	49	4	3	0.3	2	14	98	32	0.3	0.2	17	0.05	0.02	1.5	5	0.04	12	41
###	Plate dinner-meat loaf-potatoes-peas	oz	28.4	37	2	3	0.5	2	9	111	33	0.4	0.3	12	0.04	0.03	0.5	3	0.03	5	33
2041	Plate dinner-turkey-potatoes-peas	oz	28.4	32	2	4	*	1	9	113	50	0.3	*	4	0.03	0.02	0.7	4	*	7	25
###	Pork & beans in tomato sauce-Luck's	serv	213	240	11	44	11	2	0	980	1160	2.7	2	0	0.1	0.15	0.8	109	0.29	80	189
###	Pork & beans/sauce-Campbell's	oz	28.4	25	1	5	*	tr	*	96	*	0.3	*	13	0.01	0.02	0.1	13	*	13	*
511	Pork and beans with frankfurters-canned	cup	257	365	17	40	12.8	17	15	1105	604	4.5	4.8	39	0.14	0.15	2.3	77	0.12	123	267
513	Pork and beans with sweet sauce-canned	cup	253	281	13	53	14	4	18	850	673	4.2	3.8	28	0.12	0.12	0.9	95	0.22	154	266
512	Pork and beans with tomato sauce-canned	cup	253	248	13	49	13.8	3	17	1113	759	8.3	14.8	62	0.12	0.13	1.3	57	0.18	141	297
###	Pork chow mein/chop suey w/ noodles	oz	28.4	56	3	4	0.4	3	7	117	61	0.4	0.4	17	0.04	0.07	0.6	4	0.05	6	30
###	Pulut panggang/udang	oz	28.3	63	1	10	0.2	2	*	127	43	0.7	*	9	0.02	0.01	0.3	3	*	3	8
###	Raviolios-beef in meat sauce-Franco	oz	28.4	33	1	5	*	1	*	123	*	0.2	*	13	0.02	0.03	0.4	25	*	3	*
###	Rawadosai	oz	28.3	68	1	11	0.1	2	*	66	5	0.3	*	3	0.01	0.01	0.3	*	*	3	43
###	Rice noodle-bandung (kuih-teow bandung)	oz	28.3	34	1	4	tr	2	0	72	37	1.9	0.1	70	0.01	0.01	0.3	tr	*	7	20
2071	Rice noodle-fried (kuih-teow goreng)	oz	28.3	31	1	4	0.1	1	1	63	51	0.1	0.1	71	0.03	0.01	0.3	tr	0.01	6	23
###	Rice noodle-fried (kuih-teow goreng)	oz	28.3	54	2	6	tr	3	3	142	38	0.1	0.1	18	0.04	0.01	0.1	3	0.02	5	13
###	Rice noodle-fried (mee-hoon goreng)	oz	28.3	49	1	7	0.1	2	0	120	11	0.1	0.5	16	0.02	0.01	0.2	tr	0.01	5	18

* indicates that no data was available.
©1994 First DataBank—The Hearst Corporation (N-Squared Computing).

Appendix A - Table of Food Composition
(continued)

Item	Food name	Portion	Weight (g)	Food Energy (Kcal)	Protein (gm)	Carbohydrates (gm)	Fiber (gm)	Total Fat (gm)	Saturated Fat (gm)	Cholesterol (mg)	Sodium (mg)	Potassium (mg)	Magnesium (mg)	Iron (mg)	Zinc (mg)	Vitamin A (RE)	Vitamin C (mg)	Thiamin (mg)	Riboflavin (mg)	Niacin (mg)	Vitamin B6 (mg)	Folates (µg)	Vitamin B12 (µg)	Calcium (mg)	Phosphorus (mg)
###	Rice-chicken (nasi ayam)	oz	28.3	34	2	6	tr	2	0.3	8	87	17	4	0.1	0.3	11	tr	0.01	0.02	0.3	0.03	1	0.02	3	17
###	Rice-coconut milk (nasi lemak)	oz	28.3	48	1	7	0.1	2	4.6	1	96	34	10	0.5	0.2	15	tr	0.03	0.02	0.2	0.02	4	0	7	15
###	Rice-dagang (nasi dagang)	oz	28.3	58	1	10	0.1	1	*	*	49	6	*	0.4	*	0	0	0.05	0.09	0.1	*	*	*	2	17
2081	Rice-fried (nasi goreng)	oz	28.3	55	1	7	tr	2	0.3	7	126	41	4	2.2	0.1	70	30	0.01	0.01	0.5	0.02	3	0.02	6	15
2176	Roller coaster-Chef Boyardee	serv	213	230	7	28	3	10	3	19	1070	*	*	1.8	*	40	0	0.15	0.17	3	*	3	*	0	*
###	Roti telur	oz	28.3	75	3	10	0	3	*	*	111	40	*	0.5	*	39	0	0.04	0.05	0.9	*	*	*	9	44
2171	Rotini-spinach/vegetables-Pasta Perfect	cup	227	200	8	38	*	0	0	0	30	300	*	2.2	*	1400	30	0.45	0.34	3.2	*	58	*	0	40
2170	Rotini/vegetables-Pasta Perfect	cup	227	220	10	40	5.2	2	0.1	0	120	340	39	2.9	0.9	800	42	0.6	0.34	3.2	0.24	58	0	40	80
1597	Salad-carrot raisin-home recipe	cup	268	306	4	56	16.7	12	6.8	33	377	928	42	3	0.5	1100	12	0.16	0.16	1	0.68	28	0.14	96	130
1709	Salad-chef-with ham and cheese	serv	200	196	13	7	2.4	13	7	46	567	415	28	1.2	1.7	740	24	0.34	0.24	2.2	0.21	46	0.47	227	251
1600	Salad-chicken	cup	205	502	26	17	2.2	36	4.3	67	1395	521	40	3.7	2	30	2	0.47	0.42	7.7	0.34	39	0.2	128	207
996	Salad-coleslaw	tbsp	8	6	tr	1	0.3	tr	tr	1	14	9	3	tr	tr	7	3	0.01	0.01	tr	0.01	2	0	4	3
1398	Salad-crab	serv	100	145	12	5	0.3	9	1	69	487	260	26	0.6	2.8	9	2	0.06	0.06	1.3	0.12	35	4.74	38	129
914	Salad-fruit-canned-juice pack	cup	249	125	1	33	1.6	tr	tr	0	13	288	21	0.6	0.4	149	8	0.03	0.04	0.9	0.07	6	0	28	36
913	Salad-fruit-canned-water pack	cup	245	74	1	19	4.5	tr	tr	0	7	191	12	0.7	0.2	108	5	0.04	0.05	0.9	0.08	6	0	17	22
1648	Salad-green salad-tossed	serv	207	22	3	5	2.1	tr	tr	0	53	356	22	1.3	0.4	235	48	0.06	0.1	1.2	0.16	77	0	26	80
1596	Salad-macaroni	serv	28.4	51	3	7	0.3	3	0.2	1	148	21	3	0.3	0.1	4	1	0.03	0.02	0.2	0.02	2	0.01	5	12
1599	Salad-mandarin orange gelatin	serv	28.4	23	tr	6	0.6	3	0	0	14	9	3	0.3	tr	7	3	*	*	tr	*	2	*	4	3
654	Salad-potato	cup	250	358	7	28	5.3	21	3.6	171	1323	635	39	1.6	0.8	82	25	0.19	0.15	2.2	0.35	17	0.39	48	130
1722	Salad-taco	serv	198	279	13	24	2.8	15	6.8	44	763	416	52	2.3	2.7	78	4	0.1	0.35	2.5	0.21	40	0.64	192	143
1598	Salad-three bean-Alex	serv	28.4	33	1	7	2.1	tr	*	*	107	63	*	0.2	*	5	tr	0.02	0.03	0.7	*	*	*	10	28
121	Salad-three bean-canned-Del Monte	oz	28.4	22	2	5	1.5	tr	0	0	101	38	6	0.3	0.1	8	1	0.01	0.01	0.1	0.01	10	0.01	10	16
1601	Salad-waldorf gelatin	serv	28.4	27	2	12	0.2	2	0	0	16	14	5	0.1	0.1	5	1	0.01	0.01	tr	0.02	2	0.01	5	10
###	Salmon rice loaf	cup	210	256	25	15	0.7	9	2.1	44	577	271	61	1.9	1.9	241	0	0.19	0.11	6.1	0.44	38	4.7	111	223
1567	Sandwich-BLT-with mayonnaise	item	148	282	7	29	2.9	16	6.8	44	1222	274	27	1.5	1.8	174	13	0.16	0.14	1.6	0.23	26	0.55	53	89
2146	Sandwich-chicken/salad/cheese/potato	oz	28.3	55	5	5	0.8	2	0.6	9	155	47	6	0.2	0.3	13	tr	0.02	0.04	0.9	0.05	5	0.03	34	36
2145	Sandwich-chicken/salad/mayonnaise	oz	28.3	81	5	5	0.4	5	0.6	9	75	27	6	0.3	0.3	11	tr	0.02	0.04	0.8	0.05	5	0.03	7	26
1568	Sandwich-club	item	315	590	36	42	4.2	21	14.5	93	2601	583	58	4.3	3.9	350	27	0.38	0.41	10.2	0.5	55	1.17	103	394
1728	Sandwich-ham and cheese	item	146	353	21	33	3.3	16	6.4	58	772	290	16	3.3	1.4	77	3	0.31	0.49	2.7	0.2	71	0.54	130	152
2147	Sandwich-pepperoni/salad/salami/cheese	oz	28.3	52	5	6	0.7	1	*	*	105	31	*	0.2	*	5	tr	0.02	0.03	0.7	*	*	*	10	28
1732	Sandwich-roast beef-plain	item	139	346	22	34	3.4	14	3.6	52	792	316	31	4.2	3.4	21	2	0.38	0.31	5.9	0.27	40	1.22	54	239
1733	Sandwich-roast beef-with cheese	item	176	402	32	27	2.7	18	9	77	1634	345	40	5.1	5.4	46	0	0.38	0.46	5.9	0.34	41	2.05	183	401
###	Sandwich-sardine (sandwic sardin)	oz	28.3	71	9	12	0.2	2	0.6	29	130	26	5	0.5	0.2	21	0	0.03	0.04	0.3	0.04	7	0.88	27	23
1729	Sandwich-steak	item	204	459	30	52	5.2	14	3.8	73	798	525	49	2.7	4.5	44	6	0.4	0.37	7.3	0.37	89	1.57	91	297
1731	Sandwich-submarine-roast beef	item	216	411	29	44	4.4	13	7.1	73	845	330	67	2.8	4.4	50	6	0.42	0.42	6	0.32	45	1.82	41	193
1730	Sandwich-submarine-with coldcuts	item	228	456	22	51	5.1	19	6.8	35	1650	394	68	2.5	2.6	79	12	1	0.8	5.5	0.13	54	1.09	189	287
2143	Sandwich-tuna/pineapple/cheese/sauce	oz	28.3	49	6	6	0.7	tr	*	3	139	68	6	0.2	*	16	tr	0.02	0.04	0.8	*	*	*	24	40
2144	Sandwich-tuna/salad/mayonnaise	oz	28.3	64	6	5	0.3	3	0.4	3	93	31	4	0.4	0.1	11	tr	0.02	0.04	0.9	0.03	6	0.21	10	34
2172	Seashells/vegetables-Pasta Perfect	cup	227	260	12	50	*	2	1	*	130	400	*	3.6	*	900	48	0.6	0.34	4	*	*	*	40	120
###	Sharks-Chef Boyardee	serv	213	170	4	34	0.3	tr	0.4	8	780	57	6	0.2	0.3	40	tr	0.3	0.17	2	0.04	3	*	20	40
###	Sharks/meatballs-Chef Boyardee	serv	213	230	8	32	1.8	7	9.2	15	890	326	32	1.8	3.5	80	0	0.15	0.17	3	0.26	15	1.55	0	198
2188	Smurf pasta/meatballs-Chef Boyardee	serv	213	240	8	31	2	9	2	19	900	707	45	1.1	5.5	80	0	0.12	0.17	2	0.35	21	2.23	0	300
2186	Smurf ravioli/pasta/sauce-Chef Boyardee	serv	213	230	9	38	6.3	5	8	11	1160	407	97	2.7	2.5	80	6	0.12	0.17	2	0.23	35	0.23	27	366
2187	Smurf-Chef Boyardee	serv	213	150	6	29	3	1	*	2	830	*	*	1.4	*	60	6	0.15	0.17	2	*	*	*	20	*
2241	Spaghetti in sauce/cheese-Franco	serv	28.4	11	tr	5	*	2	0.4	*	114	*	*	0.2	*	11	tr	0.03	0.02	0.3	*	*	*	3	*
2139	Spaghetti-cheese/meat	oz	28.3	29	4	3	0.3	tr	0.4	8	99	57	6	0.2	0.3	4	tr	0.01	0.01	0.8	0.04	3	0.11	3	11
2141	Spaghetti-chicken/mushroom/sauce/cheese	oz	28.3	25	5	1	tr	tr	0.3	3	92	17	4	0.4	0.3	4	tr	0.03	0.01	0.3	0.03	3	0.08	3	8
###	Spaghetti-meat balls-tomato sauce-canned	cup	250	257	12	29	7.8	10	2.2	23	1220	245	60	3.3	1.4	300	5	0.15	0.18	2.3	0.88	26	0.49	53	112
###	Spaghetti-meat balls-tomato sauce-cooked	cup	248	332	19	39	*	12	3.3	74	1009	665	97	3.7	*	476	22	0.25	0.3	4	0.31	20	0.47	124	236
2140	Spaghetti-shrimp/mushroom/cheese	oz	28.3	26	5	1	0	tr	0.7	28	77	10	7	0.4	0.3	3	tr	0.02	0.03	0.3	0.02	2	0.2	3	9
###	Spaghetti-tomato sauce-cheese-canned	cup	250	190	6	39	7.8	2	0.4	8	955	302	15	2.8	1.3	58	10	0.35	0.28	4.5	0.13	13	0	40	88

Item	Food	Unit	Wt	1	2	3	4	5	6	7	8	9	10	11	12	13	14	15	16	17	18	19	20	21
###	Spaghetti-tomato sauce-cheese-cooked	cup	250	9	37	*	9	2	8	955	407	*	2.3	*	322	13	0.25	0.18	2.3	0.19	13	0.05	80	135
2199	Spaghetti/beef/sauce-Chef Boyardee	serv	213	7	30	3.6	9	4	18	1120	929	53	1.8	2.9	60	0	0.06	0.17	2	0.45	20	1.22	0	146
###	Spaghetti/meatballs in sauce-Franco	oz	28.4	1	4	0.4	1	1	13	118	79	6	0.2	0.8	11	0	0.02	0.01	0.3	0.05	5	0.42	3	35
###	Spaghetti/meatballs-7.5 oz-Chef Boyardee	serv	213	8	27	3	9	7.8	19	970	594	47	1.8	6.1	60	0	0.12	0.17	3	0.4	35	3.18	0	260
2201	Spaghetti/meatballs-7.8 oz-Chef Boyardee	serv	221	7	30	3.1	10	8.1	19	1140	616	48	1.8	6.4	60	0	0.09	0.17	2	0.41	36	3.3	0	270
###	Spaghetti/meatballs-8.5 oz-Chef Boyardee	serv	241	8	30	4	11	4	19	1210	672	53	1.8	7	60	0	0.09	0.17	2	0.45	39	3.59	0	294
496	Spaghetti/tomato/cheese-canned	cup	250	6	39	2.5	2	0.5	4	955	303	28	2.8	*	186	10	0.35	0.28	4.5	0.28	*	*	40	88
495	Spaghetti/tomato/cheese-from home recipe	cup	250	9	37	2.5	9	2	4	955	408	*	2.3	*	216	13	0.25	0.18	2.3	0.18	*	*	80	135
498	Spaghetti/tomato/meat-canned	cup	250	12	29	2.8	10	2.2	39	1220	245	28	3.3	*	200	5	0.15	0.18	2.3	0.18	*	*	53	113
497	Spaghetti/tomato/meat-from home recipe	cup	248	19	39	2.7	12	3.3	75	1009	665	*	3.7	*	1590	22	0.25	0.3	4	0.3	*	*	124	236
###	Spaghettio's in cheese sauce-Franco	oz	28.4	1	4	0.3	1	*	2	115	*	*	0.1	*	13	0	0.03	0.02	0.3	0.02	3	0.07	3	*
###	Spaghettio's/meatballs-Franco	oz	28.4	1	4	0.3	1	0.2	2	129	50	4	0.2	0.2	11	0	0.02	0.02	0.3	0.03	2	0.07	3	17
###	Spaghettio's/sliced franks-Franco	oz	28.4	1	3	0.3	1	0.6	3	136	49	4	0.2	0.2	11	3	0.02	0.02	0.5	0.12	2	*	230	14
1044	Spinach souffle	cup	136	11	3	0.8	18	7.2	184	763	201	38	1.3	1.3	675	0	0.09	0.31	0.5	*	62	1.36	230	231
###	Sportyo's in cheese sauce-Franco	oz	28.4	1	4	0.4	1	*	13	115	*	6	0.1	*	13	tr	0.02	0.02	0.4	0.05	3	0.42	5	*
###	Sportyo's pasta/meatballs/sauce-Franco	oz	28.4	2	7	0.4	2	1	13	129	79	4	0.3	0.8	14	0	tr	0.02	0.2	0.04	1	0.06	5	35
###	Spring roll (popia)	oz	28.3	1	10	0.3	3	0.7	2	106	27	4	0.3	0.2	6	3	0.02	0.1	0.3	0.04	1	0.19	6	11
###	Spring roll-fried (popia goreng)	oz	28.3	1	10	0.3	3	3.2	20	111	44	3	0.3	0.5	7	0	tr	0.02	0.3	0.04	1	0.19	6	17
###	Stew-brunswick-microwave-Luck's	serv	213	10	25	3	1	1	10	960	541	45	1.1	2.4	100	4	0.03	0.1	3	0.34	25	0.34	20	200
2211	Stew-meatball-Chef Boyardee	serv	227	10	22	0	23	18.3	40	1470	570	47	1.8	16.9	250	4	0.03	0.17	3	0.64	16	5.57	20	496
1490	Taco	item	171	21	27	2.7	21	11.4	57	802	473	71	2.4	3.9	147	2	0.15	0.45	3.2	0.24	23	1.04	221	203
2165	Tamales-beef-Gebhardt	item	64	3	8	2.2	8	3.4	22	542	65	26	0.6	1	239	tr	0.05	0.03	0.4	0.11	5	0.16	9	73
###	Teddyo's in cheese sauce-Franco	oz	28.4	1	4	0.4	tr	0.2	1	120	45	4	0.2	0.1	13	0	0.03	0.01	0.3	0.02	2	0.01	5	14
###	Teddyo's pasta/meatballs-Franco	oz	28.4	3	3	*	1	*	tr	129	*	2	0.2	*	14	tr	0.02	0.02	0.4	*	3	*	3	28
2189	Tic Tac Toes-7.5 oz-Chef Boyardee	serv	213	5	31	3	5	1	1	870	*	45	1.1	1.1	40	0	0.15	0.17	2	0.17	*	*	0	*
2193	Tic Tac Toes-8.6 oz-Chef Boyardee	serv	244	5	41	*	1	1	1	1080	*	47	1.8	1.8	60	0	0.3	0.17	3	0.3	*	20	20	*
2190	Tic Tac Toes/meatballs-Chef Boyardee	serv	213	8	31	2.7	9	2.3	18	1000	*	71	2	*	80	0	0.15	0.26	3	0.15	*	0	0	*
2159	Tofu fast menu-baked beans-Health Valley	oz	28.4	1	2	2.1	tr	0.2	0	19	35	29	0.6	0.2	133	0	0.07	0.07	0.9	0.07	4	0	13	*
2160	Tofu fast menu-black beans-Health Valley	oz	28.4	2	2	1.8	tr	*	0	33	35	*	1.2	*	133	0	0.03	0.03	0.2	0.03	20	*	20	*
2161	Tofu fast menu-lentils-Health Valley	oz	28.4	2	2	2	tr	*	0	35	45	*	1.9	*	133	tr	0.03	0.02	0.2	0.02	*	*	5	*
1901	Tuna Helper-au gratin-dry	serv	41.1	6	27	*	5	1	*	800	100	*	1.1	*	0	0	0.6	0.17	2	0.17	*	40	40	*
1902	Tuna Helper-buttery rice-dry	serv	42.5	4	32	*	2	*	*	830	125	*	0.7	*	100	0	0.12	0.07	1.2	0.07	*	60	60	*
1903	Tuna Helper-cheesy noodle-dry	serv	41.1	7	26	*	3	*	*	810	140	*	1.1	*	0	0	0.23	0.17	1.6	0.17	*	60	60	*
1904	Tuna Helper-creamy mushroom-dry	serv	38.3	5	28	*	1	*	*	580	180	*	1.1	*	20	0	0.23	0.17	2	0.17	*	20	20	*
1905	Tuna Helper-creamy noodle-dry	serv	46.8	6	28	*	9	*	*	790	140	*	1.1	*	60	0	0.3	0.17	2	0.17	*	20	20	*
1906	Tuna Helper fettucini alfredo-dry	serv	41.1	6	28	*	3	*	*	760	120	*	1.1	*	0	0	0.3	0.17	2	0.17	*	40	40	*
1907	Tuna Helper-romanoff-dry	serv	52.4	7	38	*	3	*	*	660	180	*	1.1	*	0	0	0.3	0.26	2	0.26	*	40	40	*
1910	Tuna Helper-tetrazzini-dry	serv	39.7	6	26	*	3	*	*	620	90	*	0.7	*	0	0	0.45	0.14	1.6	0.14	*	40	40	*
1908	Tuna Helper-tuna pot pie-dry	serv	55.5	4	31	0.6	17	2.3	7	730	120	9	1.4	0.3	100	0	0.15	0.14	1.2	0.14	5	0.26	20	61
1909	Tuna Helper-tuna salad-dry	serv	35.4	5	28	0.2	1	0.3	*	580	110	7	1.1	0.1	0	0	0.23	0.1	1.6	0.1	2	0.43	0	39
160	Tuna-salad-celery/mayonnaise/pickle/egg	cup	205	30	7	1	22	4.3	68	434	474	26	2.7	*	118	2	0.08	0.23	10.3	0.23	41	*	41	291
###	Turkey potpie-baked-home-prepared	cup	240	25	44	2.8	32	10.8	74	655	308	35	3.4	1.8	958	5	0.34	0.36	6.7	0.11	65	0.1	65	242
###	Turkey potpie-frozen-unheated-commercial	cup	240	14	48	2.7	25	9.6	22	886	274	42	2.2	2	641	5	0.22	0.19	3.8	0.42	23	0.31	29	134
###	Vadai-kacang dal kuning	oz	28.3	4	8	0.1	5	*	*	128	9	*	0.7	0.2	4	0	0.01	0.09	0.7	0.09	*	*	5	86
###	Vadai-kacang hitam	oz	28.3	3	7	0.1	5	*	*	92	8	*	0.9	*	3	0	0.03	0.04	0.8	0.04	*	*	9	58
###	Vegetables-jellied salad	cup	256	3	29	*	tr	0	0	85	112	9	0.3	0.1	17	11	0.03	0.02	*	0.02	15	0	13	60
1066	Vegetables-mixed-canned-drained	cup	163	4	15	8.1	tr	0.1	0	243	474	26	1.7	0.7	1899	8	0.08	0.08	0.9	0.13	39	0.13	44	69
679	Vegetables-mixed-frozen-boiled	cup	182	5	24	6.9	tr	0.1	0	64	308	40	1.5	0.9	778	6	0.13	0.22	1.6	0.14	35	0.14	46	93
###	Welsh-rarebit	cup	232	18	14	0.1	30	14.8	73	694	350	41	0.6	2.2	316	1	0.09	0.51	0.2	0.09	15	0.59	557	415
###	Wheat noodle-bandung (mee bandung)	oz	28.3	1	3	0.1	2	tr	2	140	114	11	2.3	0.2	70	0	0.02	0.03	0.1	0.02	5	0	7	23
###	Wheat noodle-curry (mee kari)	oz	28.3	3	3	0.1	3	*	3	170	57	*	0.5	*	33	0	0.01	0.03	0.3	*	5	*	4	3

* indicates that no data was available.

©1994 First DataBank—The Hearst Corporation (N-Squared Computing).

Appendix A - Table of Food Composition (continued)

Item	Food name	Portion	Weight (g)	Food Energy (Kcal)	Protein (gm)	Carbohydrates (gm)	Fiber (gm)	Total Fat (gm)	Saturated Fat (gm)	Cholesterol (mg)	Sodium (mg)	Potassium (mg)	Magnesium (mg)	Iron (mg)	Zinc (mg)	Vitamin A (RE)	Vitamin C (mg)	Thiamin (mg)	Riboflavin (mg)	Niacin (mg)	Vitamin B6 (mg)	Folates (µg)	Vitamin B12 (µg)	Calcium (mg)	Phosphorus (mg)
###	Wheat noodle-fried (mee goreng)	oz	28.3	47	2	7	0.1		tr	0	185	13	11	0.4	0.2	11	tr	0.01	0.02	0.2	0.02	5	*	5	9
2198	Zooroni/meatballs in sauce-Chef Boyardee	serv	213	240	8	33	*	8		17	970	*	*	1.8	*	80	0	0.15	0.17	3	*	*	*	0	*
	Dairy products																								
24	Cheese food-American-pasteurized process	oz	28.4	93	6	2	0	7	4.4	18	337	79	9	0.2	0.9	78	0	0.01	0.13	tr	0.04	2	0.32	163	130
25	Cheese spread-American-processed	oz	28.4	82	5	2	0	6	3.8	16	381	69	8	0.1	0.7	67	0	0.01	0.12	tr	0.03	2	0.11	159	202
22	Cheese-American-pasteurized process	oz	28.4	106	6	tr	0	9	5.6	16	406	46	8	0.1	0.9	103	0	0.01	0.1	tr	0.02	2	0.2	174	211
1	Cheese-blue	oz	28.4	100	6	tr	0	8	5.3	21	396	73	7	0.1	0.8	61	0	0.01	0.11	0.3	0.05	10	0.35	150	110
1322	Cheese-blue-crumbled-unpacked	cup	135	477	29	3	0	39	25.2	102	1884	346	31	0.4	3.6	292	0	0.04	0.52	1.4	0.22	49	1.64	712	523
818	Cheese-brick	oz	28.4	105	7	1	0	8	5.3	27	159	38	7	0.1	0.7	92	0	tr	0.1	tr	0.02	6	0.36	191	128
819	Cheese-brie	oz	28.4	95	6	tr	0	8	4.9	28	178	43	6	0.1	0.7	57	0	0.02	0.15	0.1	0.07	18	0.47	52	53
2	Cheese-camembert-wedge	item	38	114	8	tr	0	9	5.8	27	320	71	8	0.1	0.9	105	0	0.01	0.19	0.2	0.09	24	0.49	147	132
820	Cheese-caraway	oz	28.4	107	7	1	0	8	5.3	26	196	26	6	0.2	0.8	90	0	0.01	0.13	0.1	0.02	5	0.08	191	139
3	Cheese-cheddar-cut pieces	oz	28.4	114	7	tr	0	9	6	30	176	28	8	0.2	0.9	90	0	tr	0.11	tr	0.02	5	0.23	204	145
4	Cheese-cheddar-inch cubes	item	17.2	69	5	tr	0	6	3.6	18	107	17	5	0.1	0.5	55	0	tr	0.07	tr	0.01	3	0.14	124	88
1751	Cheese-cheddar-lowfat-low sodium-Pauly	oz	28.4	83	9	1	0	5	1.3	14	68	32	8	0.2	0.9	18	0	0.01	0.01	0.1	0.02	5	0.24	200	137
5	Cheese-cheddar-shredded	cup	113	455	28	1	0	38	23.8	119	701	111	31	0.8	3.5	359	0	0.03	0.42	0.1	0.08	21	0.94	815	579
821	Cheese-cheshire	oz	28.4	110	7	1	0	9	5.5	29	198	27	6	0.1	0.8	84	0	0.01	0.08	tr	0.02	5	0.23	182	131
822	Cheese-colby	oz	28.4	112	7	1	0	9	5.7	27	171	36	7	0.2	0.9	88	0	tr	0.11	tr	0.02	5	0.23	194	129
9	Cheese-cottage-1% lowfat-unpacked	cup	226	164	28	6	0	2	1.5	10	918	193	12	0.3	0.9	25	0	0.05	0.37	0.3	0.15	28	1.43	138	302
8	Cheese-cottage-2% lowfat-unpacked	cup	226	203	31	8	0	4	2.8	19	918	217	14	0.4	1	47	0	0.05	0.42	0.3	0.17	30	1.61	155	340
6	Cheese-cottage-4% fat-large curd-unpacked	cup	225	232	28	6	0	10	6.4	34	911	189	11	0.3	0.8	110	0	0.05	0.37	0.3	0.15	27	1.4	135	297
7	Cheese-cottage-4% fat-small curd-unpacked	cup	210	217	26	6	0	9	6	31	850	177	11	0.3	0.8	103	0	0.04	0.34	0.3	0.14	26	1.31	126	277
10	Cheese-cottage-dry curd-uncreamed	cup	145	123	25	3	0	1	0.4	10	19	47	6	0.3	0.7	13	0	0.04	0.21	0.2	0.12	21	1.2	46	151
16	Cheese-cottage-with fruit-unpacked	cup	226	279	22	30	0	8	4.9	25	915	151	9	0.3	0.7	84	0	0.04	0.29	0.2	0.12	22	1.12	108	236
11	Cheese-cream	oz	28.4	100	2	1	0	10	6.3	31	85	34	2	0.3	0.2	122	0	0.01	0.06	tr	0.01	4	0.12	23	30
823	Cheese-edam	oz	28.4	101	7	tr	0	8	5	25	274	53	8	0.1	1.1	78	0	0.01	0.11	tr	0.02	5	0.44	207	152
824	Cheese-feta	oz	28.4	75	4	1	0	6	4.2	25	316	18	5	0.2	0.8	36	0	0.04	0.24	0.3	0.12	9	0.48	140	96
825	Cheese-fontina	oz	28.4	110	7	tr	0	9	5.4	33	227	18	4	0.1	1	100	0	0.01	0.06	tr	0.02	2	0.48	156	98
1750	Cheese-garlic-lowfat-low sodium-Pauly	oz	28.4	80	8	0	0	6	3	20	95	*	20	*	*	*	*	0.09	0.39	*	0.08	1	0.69	113	126
826	Cheese-gjetost	oz	28.4	132	3	12	0	8	5.4	27	170	399	20	0.1	0.3	78	0	0.02	0.39	0.2	0.02	2	0.44	198	155
827	Cheese-gouda	oz	28.4	101	7	tr	0	8	5	32	232	34	8	0.1	1.1	55	0	0.01	0.1	tr	0.02	6	0.44	198	155
828	Cheese-gruyere	oz	28.4	117	8	tr	0	9	5.4	31	95	23	10	tr	1.1	104	0	0.02	0.08	tr	0.02	3	0.45	287	172
829	Cheese-limburger	oz	28.4	93	6	tr	0	8	4.8	26	227	36	6	tr	0.6	109	0	0.02	0.14	tr	0.02	16	0.3	141	111
830	Cheese-monterey jack	oz	28.4	106	7	tr	0	9	5.4	25	152	23	8	0.2	0.9	81	0	tr	0.11	tr	0.02	5	0.23	212	126
1749	Cheese-monterey jack-lowfat-low sodium	oz	28.4	80	8	0	0	6	3	25	95	*	8	*	*	*	*	0.01	0.09	tr	0.02	2	0.23	183	131
13	Cheese-mozzarella-made from skim milk	oz	28.4	72	7	1	0	5	2.9	16	132	24	7	0.1	0.8	50	0	0.01	0.09	tr	0.02	2	0.23	147	105
12	Cheese-mozzarella-made from whole milk	oz	28.4	80	6	1	0	6	3.7	22	106	19	5	0.1	0.6	68	0	tr	0.07	tr	0.02	2	0.19	147	133
831	Cheese-muenster	oz	28.4	104	7	tr	0	9	5.4	27	178	38	8	0.1	0.8	96	0	tr	0.09	tr	0.02	3	0.42	203	133
832	Cheese-neufchatel	oz	28.4	74	3	1	0	7	4.2	22	113	32	2	0.1	0.2	96	0	0.01	0.06	tr	0.01	3	0.08	21	39
14	Cheese-parmesan-grated	cup	100	456	42	4	0	30	19.1	79	1862	107	51	1	3.2	211	0	0.05	0.39	0.3	0.11	8	1.4	1376	807
836	Cheese-pimento-processed	oz	28.4	106	6	tr	0	9	5.6	27	405	46	6	0.1	0.8	108	1	0.01	0.1	tr	0.02	2	0.2	174	211
833	Cheese-port du salut	oz	28.4	100	7	tr	0	8	4.7	35	151	39	7	0.1	0.7	114	0	tr	0.07	tr	0.02	5	0.43	184	102
17	Cheese-provolone	oz	28.4	100	7	1	0	8	4.8	20	248	39	8	0.2	0.9	69	0	0.01	0.09	tr	0.02	3	0.42	214	141
19	Cheese-ricotta-made with part skim milk	cup	246	340	28	13	0	20	12.1	76	307	308	36	1.1	3.3	319	0	0.05	0.46	0.2	0.05	32	0.72	669	449
18	Cheese-ricotta-made with whole milk	cup	246	428	28	7	0	32	20.4	124	207	257	28	0.9	2.9	362	0	0.03	0.48	0.3	0.11	30	0.83	509	389
20	Cheese-romano	oz	28.4	110	9	1	0	8	4.9	29	340	25	12	0.2	0.7	49	0	0.01	0.11	tr	0.02	3	0.32	302	215
834	Cheese-roquefort	oz	28.4	105	6	1	0	9	5.5	26	513	26	8	0.2	0.6	89	0	0.01	0.17	0.2	0.04	14	0.18	188	111
21	Cheese-swiss	oz	28.4	107	8	1	0	8	5	26	74	31	10	0.1	1.1	72	0	0.01	0.1	tr	0.02	2	0.48	272	171
1752	Cheese-swiss-lowfat-low sodium-Pauly	oz	28.4	97	9	1	0	7	5.1	19	32	32	10	tr	1.1	72	0	0.01	0.11	tr	0.02	2	0.48	273	172
23	Cheese-swiss-pasteurized process	oz	28.4	95	7	1	0	7	4.6	24	388	61	8	0.2	1	69	0	tr	0.08	tr	0.01	2	0.35	219	216
835	Cheese-tilsit	oz	28.4	96	7	1	0	7	4.8	29	213	18	4	0.1	1	89	0	0.02	0.1	0.1	0.02	6	0.6	198	142

No.	Food	Measure	1	2	3	4	5	6	7	8	9	10	11	12	13	14	15	16	17	18	19	20	21	22	23
28	Cream-coffee-table-light-fluid	cup	240	469	6	9	0	46	28.9	159	95	292	21	0.1	0.7	519	2	0.08	0.36	0.1	0.08	6	0.53	231	192
26	Cream-half & half-milk and cream-fluid	cup	242	315	7	10	0	28	17.3	89	98	314	25	0.2	1.2	315	2	0.09	0.36	0.2	0.09	6	0.8	254	230
38	Cream-imitation-liquid-non dairy-frozen	cup	245	333	2	28	0	24	4.8	0	194	466	4	0.1	tr	66	0	0	0	0	0	0	0	22	157
40	Cream-imitation-non dairy-powdered	cup	94	514	5	52	0	33	30.6	0	170	763	*	1.1	0.5	57	*	*	0.16	*	*	*	0	21	397
1841	Cream-mocha mix-non dairy	tbsp	15	20	1	1	tr	2	0.8	102	5	20	26	0.1	0.6	546	2	0.08	0.34	0.2	0.04	25	0.69	*	*
36	Cream-sour-cultured	cup	230	493	7	10	0	48	30	0	123	331	2	0.1	0.1	20	0	0.01	0.02	tr	tr	2	0.05	268	195
837	Cream-sour-half & half	tbsp	15	20	1	1	0	2	2	6	6	19	*	tr	0.1	6	0	0	0	tr	tr	0	0	16	14
838	Cream-sour-imitation	oz	28.4	59	1	11	0	6	5	0	29	46	1	0.1	0.3	194	2	0.09	0.38	0.2	0	0	*	1	13
48	Cream-sour-imitation-nonfat dry milk	cup	235	415	8	17	0	39	31.2	0	240	380	8	0.1	*	87	0	0	0.38	0	0.09	0	0	266	205
42	Cream-whipped-imitation-non dairy-frozen	cup	75	239	1	13	0	19	16.3	0	19	14	6	0.1	tr	165	0	0.05	0.26	0.1	0.06	3	0	5	6
44	Cream-whipped-imitation-non dairy-powder	cup	80	151	3	13	0	10	8.6	8	53	121	1	0.1	0.2	99	1	0.06	0.3	0.1	0.07	2	0.21	72	69
34	Cream-whipped-imitation-pressurized	cup	60	154	2	7	0	13	8.3	46	78	88	17	0.1	0.2	1051	1	0.02	0.04	tr	0.03	2	0.18	61	54
46	Cream-whipped-imitation-pressurized	cup	70	184	1	11	0	16	13.2	0	43	13	17	tr	tr	809	1	0	0	0	0	0	0	4	13
32	Cream-whipping-heavy-unwhipped-fluid	cup	238	821	5	7	0	88	54.8	326	89	179	34	0.1	0.6	24	1	0.06	0.26	0.1	0.06	9	0.43	154	149
30	Cream-whipping-light-unwhipped-fluid	cup	239	699	5	7	0	74	46.2	265	82	231	35	0.1	0.6	79	1	0.07	0.3	0.1	0.07	9	0.47	166	146
54	Milk-1% fat-lowfat-fluid	cup	244	102	8	12	0	3	1.6	10	123	381	39	0.1	1	150	2	0.1	0.41	0.2	0.11	12	0.9	300	235
55	Milk-1% fat-nonfat milk solids added	cup	245	104	9	12	0	2	1.5	10	128	397	40	0.1	1	150	2	0.1	0.42	0.2	0.11	13	0.94	313	245
56	Milk-1% fat-protein fortified	cup	246	119	10	14	0	3	1.8	10	143	444	33	0.2	1.1	150	3	0.11	0.47	0.2	0.12	15	1.05	349	273
53	Milk-2% fat-fluid-protein fortified	cup	246	137	10	12	0	5	3	19	145	447	35	0.2	1.1	150	2	0.11	0.48	0.2	0.13	15	1.05	352	276
51	Milk-2% fat-lowfat-fluid	cup	244	121	8	12	0	5	2.9	18	122	377	27	0.2	1	150	2	0.1	0.4	0.2	0.11	12	0.89	297	232
52	Milk-2% fat-nonfat milk solids added	cup	245	125	9	12	0	5	2.9	18	128	397	131	0.1	1	150	2	0.1	0.42	0.1	0.11	13	0.94	313	245
60	Milk-buttermilk-cultured-fluid	cup	245	99	8	12	0	2	1.3	9	257	371	33	0.1	1	24	2	0.08	0.38	0.1	0.08	12	0.54	285	219
64	Milk-buttermilk-dried-sweet cream	cup	120	464	41	59	0.2	7	4.3	83	621	1910	33	0.4	4.8	79	7	0.47	1.9	1.1	0.41	57	4.59	1421	1119
69	Milk-chocolate-1% fat-fluid	cup	250	158	8	26	0.2	3	1.5	7	152	426	78	0.6	1	150	2	0.1	0.42	0.3	0.16	12	0.86	287	256
68	Milk-chocolate-2% fat-fluid	cup	250	179	8	26	0.2	5	3.1	17	150	422	47	0.6	1	150	2	0.09	0.41	0.3	0.13	12	0.85	284	254
67	Milk-chocolate-whole-fluid	cup	250	208	8	26	0.2	8	5.3	30	149	417	69	0.6	1	91	2	0.09	0.41	0.3	0.14	12	0.84	280	251
63	Milk-condensed-sweetened-canned	cup	306	982	24	166	0	27	16.8	104	389	1136	61	0.6	2.9	302	8	0.28	1.27	0.6	0.13	34	1.36	868	775
70	Milk-eggnog-commercial	cup	254	342	10	34	0	19	11.3	149	138	420	34	0.5	1.2	268	4	0.09	0.48	0.3	0.11	2	1.14	330	278
62	Milk-evaporated-skim-canned	cup	255	199	19	29	0	1	0.3	10	293	847	78	0.7	2.3	300	3	0.12	0.79	0.4	0.14	23	0.61	740	497
61	Milk-evaporated-whole-canned	cup	252	338	17	25	0	19	11.6	73	267	764	47	0.5	1.9	184	5	0.12	0.8	0.5	0.13	20	0.41	658	509
843	Milk-goat-whole-fluid	cup	244	168	8	11	0	10	6.5	28	122	499	34	0.1	0.7	135	3	0.12	0.34	0.7	0.11	1	0.16	326	270
844	Milk-human-whole-mature	cup	246	171	3	17	0	11	4.9	34	42	126	33	0.1	0.4	178	12	0.03	0.09	0.4	0.03	13	0.11	79	34
839	Milk-imitation	cup	244	150	4	15	3.1	8	1.9	0	191	279	61	1	2.9	0	0	0.03	0.22	0	0.06	0	0	79	181
845	Milk-Indian buffalo-whole	cup	244	236	9	13	0	17	11.2	46	127	434	78	0.3	0.5	130	5	0.13	0.33	0.2	0.14	14	0.89	412	286
71	Milk-malted-chocolate flavor-prepared	cup	265	229	9	30	0.1	9	5.5	34	172	499	76	0.5	1.1	80	3	0.13	0.44	0.6	0.19	16	0.91	304	265
	Milk-malted-natural flavor-prepared	cup	265	237	10	27	0.2	10	6	37	223	529	47	0.5	1.1	94	3	0.2	0.59	1.3	0.19	22	1.03	354	303
57	Milk-nonfat/skim-fluid	cup	245	86	8	12	0	tr	0.3	4	126	406	52	0.1	1.1	150	3	0.09	0.34	0.2	0.1	22	0.93	302	247
66	Milk-nonfat/skim-instantized-dried	cup	68	244	24	36	0	tr	0.3	12	373	1160	28	0.1	3	484	4	0.28	1.19	0.6	0.24	34	2.72	837	670
65	Milk-nonfat/skim-instantized-envelope	item	91	326	32	48	0	1	0.4	17	499	1552	45	0.3	4	648	5	0.38	1.59	0.8	0.31	45	3.63	1120	896
58	Milk-nonfat/skim-milk solids added	cup	245	90	9	12	0	1	0.4	5	130	418	36	0.1	1	150	2	0.1	0.43	0.2	0.11	13	0.95	316	255
59	Milk-nonfat/skim-protein fortified	cup	246	100	10	14	0	1	0.4	5	144	446	40	0.2	1.1	150	3	0.11	0.48	0.2	0.12	15	1.05	352	275
846	Milk-sheep-whole-fluid	cup	245	264	15	13	0	17	11.3	66	108	334	45	0.2	1.3	108	10	0.16	0.87	1	0.15	17	1.74	474	387
1635	Milk-soy-fluid	cup	240	79	7	4	0	5	0.5	0	29	338	12	0.2	0.6	7	tr	0.39	0.17	0.4	0.16	4	0.07	10	118
841	Milk-whole-dry	cup	128	635	34	49	0	34	21.4	124	475	1702	33	0.6	4.3	354	11	0.36	1.54	0.8	0.39	47	4.16	1168	993
840	Milk-whole-low sodium	cup	244	149	8	11	0	8	5.3	33	6	617	48	0.1	0.9	95	2	0.05	0.26	0.1	0.08	12	0.88	246	209
50	Milk-whole-regular-3.3% fat-fluid	cup	244	150	8	11	0	8	5.1	33	120	370	37	0.1	0.9	92	2	0.09	0.4	0.2	0.1	12	0.87	291	228
73	Milkshake-chocolate-thick	item	300	356	9	64	0.8	8	5	32	333	672	48	0.9	1.4	78	0	0.14	0.67	0.4	0.08	15	0.95	396	378
74	Milkshake-vanilla-thick	item	313	350	12	56	0.2	9	5.9	37	299	572	37	0.3	1.2	107	0	0.09	0.61	0.5	0.13	21	1.63	457	361
849	Whey-acid-dry	tbsp	2.9	10	tr	2	0	tr	tr	1	28	66	6	0.2	0.2	1	tr	0.02	0.06	tr	0.02	1	0.07	59	39
847	Whey-acid-fluid	cup	246	59	2	13	0	tr	0.1	tr	118	352	24	0.2	1.1	5	tr	0.1	0.34	0.2	0.1	5	0.44	253	191
850	Whey-sweet-dry	tbsp	7.5	26	1	6	0	tr	0.1	tr	80	155	13	0.1	0.2	1	tr	0.04	0.17	0.1	0.04	1	0.18	59	70

A 15

* indicates that no data was available.
©1994 First DataBank—The Hearst Corporation (N-Squared Computing).

Appendix A - Table of Food Composition
(continued)

Item	Food name	Portion	Weight (g)	Food Energy (Kcal)	Protein (gm)	Carbohydrates (gm)	Fiber (gm)	Total Fat (gm)	Saturated Fat (gm)	Cholesterol (mg)	Sodium (mg)	Potassium (mg)	Magnesium (mg)	Iron (mg)	Zinc (mg)	Vitamin A (RE)	Vitamin C (mg)	Thiamin (mg)	Riboflavin (mg)	Niacin (mg)	Vitamin B6 (mg)	Folates (µg)	Vitamin B12 (µg)	Calcium (mg)	Phosphorus (mg)
848	Whey-sweet-fluid	cup	246	66	2	13	0	1	0.6	5	132	396	20	0.2	0.3	12	tr	0.09	0.39	0.2	0.08	2	0.68	115	112
92	Yogurt-fruit flavors-lowfat-added solids	cup	227	231	10	43	0.8	2	1.6	10	133	442	33	0.2	1.7	31	2	0.08	0.4	0.2	0.09	21	1.06	345	271
1760	Yogurt-original coffee-lowfat-Dannon	serv	227	200	10	34	1.3	3	1.8	11	140	498	37	0.2	1.9	30	2	0.1	0.46	0.6	0.1	24	1.2	389	306
93	Yogurt-plain-lowfat-milk solids added	cup	227	144	12	16	0	tr	2.3	14	159	531	40	0.2	2	45	4	0.1	0.49	0.3	0.11	25	1.28	415	326
94	Yogurt-plain-nonfat-milk solids added	cup	227	127	13	17	0	tr	0.3	4	174	579	43	0.2	2.2	5	2	0.11	0.53	0.3	0.12	28	1.39	452	355
95	Yogurt-plain-whole milk-no solids	cup	227	139	8	11	0	7	4.8	29	105	351	26	0.1	1.3	84	1	0.07	0.32	0.2	0.07	17	0.84	274	215
Desserts																									
412	Brownies with nuts-home recipe	item	20	95	1	10	0.5	6	1.5	0	50	38	3	0.4	*	7	0	0.04	0.03	0.2	*	*	*	8	30
414	Brownies-chocolate icing-from frozen	item	25	105	1	15	0.5	5	2	13	59	44	10	0.4	0.4	8	0	0.03	0.03	0.2	0.04	3	0.05	10	31
413	Brownies-commercially prepared	item	60	243	3	39	1.3	10	3.1	9	153	83	16	1.3	0.6	3	3	0.07	0.13	0.6	0.03	4	0.15	4	87
386	Cake-angel food-prepared from mix	slice	53	142	4	32	tr	tr	*	0	142	52	6	0.5	0.1	0	0	0.06	0.12	0.6	0.01	5	0.02	50	63
1288	Cake-cheesecake-commercial	slice	85	257	5	24	1.8	16	6.7	57	189	83	9	0.4	0.4	43	4	0.03	0.11	0.4	0.05	15	0.42	48	75
388	Cake-coffee-prepared from mix	slice	72	230	5	38	2.4	7	2	*	310	78	*	1.2	*	24	0	0.14	0.15	1.3	*	*	*	44	125
392	Cake-devils food with icing-from mix	slice	69	235	3	40	1.5	8	3.1	33	180	90	14	1	0.3	20	0	0.07	0.1	0.6	0.05	4	0.07	41	72
395	Cake-gingerbread-prepared from mix	slice	63	175	2	32	1.8	5	1.1	*	90	173	12	0.9	0.4	0	0	0.09	0.11	0.8	0.04	5	0.06	57	63
1286	Cake-pineapple upside down-home recipe	slice	70	221	2	35	1.2	9	1.9	20	167	119	*	1.1	*	54	4	0.11	0.08	0.7	0.04	2	*	8	44
409	Cake-pound-home recipe	slice	33	160	2	16	0.1	10	5.9	68	58	20	12	0.5	*	16	0	0.05	0.06	0.4	0.02	6	0.09	6	24
405	Cake-sheet-no icing-home recipe	slice	86	315	3	48	1	12	3.3	1	382	68	7	0.9	0.3	30	0	0.13	0.15	1.1	*	7	0.09	55	88
407	Cake-sheet-plain-uncooked white icing	slice	121	445	4	77	0	14	4.7	1	274	74	7	0.8	*	48	0	0.14	0.16	1.1	*	*	*	61	91
411	Cake-sponge-home recipe	slice	66	188	5	36	0.9	3	1.1	162	164	59	7	1.1	0.8	25	0	0.09	0.13	0.7	0.04	15	0.33	25	65
1569	Cake-strawberry shortcake	serv	175	344	5	61	2.1	9	*	*	214	55	7	2	*	86	89	0.17	0.21	1.3	*	5	0.1	73	84
1287	Cake-streusel type-with icing-from mix	slice	50	172	2	25	0.9	8	*	*	200	7	7	0.7	0.2	6	0	0.06	0.06	0.5	0.02	*	*	27	99
397	Cake-white/chocolate icing-from mix	slice	71	271	3	42	0.8	11	3	3	191	77	14	0.7	0.3	4	0	0.07	0.11	0.7	0.02	4	0.06	70	127
399	Cake-yellow/chocolate icing-home recipe	slice	69	268	3	40	0.6	11	3	36	157	73	13	0.8	0.3	10	0	0.08	0.1	0.7	0.02	6	0.12	57	61
1429	Cheesecake-Weight Watchers-frozen	slice	113	180	6	25	1.5	6	5.2	23	366	192	17	1.8	0.6	90	tr	0.05	0.31	1.1	0.05	13	0.25	60	106
1430	Cobbler-Weight Watchers-frozen	slice	124	160	1	26	0.9	6	0.7	*	109	14	3	0.2	0.1	25	*	0.09	*	0.2	0.04	15	*	3	7
415	Cookie-chocolate chip-baked from mix	item	10.5	50	1	7	0.3	3	0.6	6	38	21	4	0.2	tr	6	0	0.02	0.02	0.2	tr	1	*	3	8
416	Cookie-chocolate chip-from home recipe	item	10	46	1	6	0.3	3	0.6	5	21	7	2	0.2	tr	1	0	0.01	0.02	0.1	tr	tr	0.01	2	6
1538	Cookie-chocolate chip-low sodium	item	5.2	25	1	3	0.1	1	0.5	5	5	7	2	0.1	tr	2	0	0.01	0.01	0.1	tr	tr	0	10	8
417	Cookie-fig bar-commercial	item	14	53	1	11	0.6	1	0.2	0	45	41	4	0.3	0.1	3	0	0.02	0.02	0.2	0.02	1	0.01	3	7
1539	Cookie-fudge-low sodium	item	5.2	25	1	3	0.1	1	0.2	0	5	7	2	0.2	tr	2	0	0.01	0.01	0.1	tr	tr	*	2	4
418	Cookie-gingersnap-from home recipe	item	7	34	1	5	0.3	2	0.5	*	20	14	2	0.4	0.1	1	0	0.01	0.01	0.1	0.01	1	0.01	5	16
419	Cookie-macaroon	item	19	90	1	13	1	5	2	0	10	88	3	0.2	*	0	0	0.02	0.03	0.1	*	*	*	4	14
420	Cookie-oatmeal/raisin-prepared from mix	item	13	62	1	9	0.4	2	0.6	6	37	23	4	0.3	0.1	2	0	0.02	0.02	0.2	0.01	2	*	12	24
1479	Cookie-peanut butter-from mix	item	10	50	1	6	0.2	3	0.8	5	57	19	4	0.2	0.8	3	0	0.03	0.02	0.4	0.01	2	0.01	4	9
421	Cookie-plain-prepared from mix	item	12	60	1	8	0.2	3	0.6	0	65	6	1	0.2	tr	8	0	0.03	0.02	0.2	0.01	1	*	4	24
422	Cookie-sandwich-chocolate/vanilla	item	10	50	1	7	0.2	2	0.6	0	63	4	5	0.2	0.1	0	0	0.02	0.03	0.2	tr	tr	0	3	7
1273	Cookie-sugar-from mix	item	20	99	1	13	0.3	5	1.6	*	109	14	2	0.4	0.1	3	0	0.04	0.02	0.5	0.01	2	0.01	2	38
423	Cookie-vanilla wafer	item	4	19	tr	3	1	1	0.3	10	10	10	1	0.1	*	1	0	0.01	0.01	0.1	0.01	*	*	3	3
390	Cupcake with chocolate icing	item	36	130	2	21	0.4	5	1.6	15	120	42	4	0.4	*	12	0	0.05	0.06	0.4	*	*	*	47	71
393	Cupcake-devils food with chocolate icing	item	35	120	2	20	0.7	4	0.8	3	91	46	4	0.5	0.3	10	0	0.03	0.05	0.3	0.01	2	0.01	21	37
389	Cupcake-no icing	item	25	90	1	14	0.3	3	0.8	0	113	21	5	0.3	0.1	8	0	0.05	0.05	0.4	tr	1	0	40	59
86	Custard-baked	cup	265	305	14	29	1	15	6.8	278	209	387	24	1.1	0.8	87	1	0.11	0.5	0.3	0.11	*	0.5	297	310
1713	Danish pastry-cheese	item	91	353	6	29	0.6	25	5.1	20	320	116	16	1.9	0.6	43	3	0.27	0.21	2.6	0.06	15	0.23	70	80
1714	Danish pastry-cinnamon	item	88	349	5	47	1.1	17	3.5	28	333	96	14	1.8	0.5	5	3	0.26	0.19	2.2	0.06	14	0.22	37	74
1715	Danish pastry-fruit	item	94	335	5	45	1.8	16	3.3	19	333	110	14	1.4	0.5	24	2	0.29	0.21	1.8	0.06	15	0.23	22	69
434	Danish pastry-plain	item	65	250	4	29	0.6	14	4.7	10	249	61	10	1.2	0.5	11	0	0.16	0.15	1.5	*	*	*	69	66
436	Doughnuts-cake-plain	item	25	104	1	12	0.3	6	1.2	13	139	27	6	0.4	0.1	2	0	0.06	0.05	0.4	0.01	2	*	11	55
437	Doughnuts-yeast-glazed	item	50	205	3	22	1.1	11	3	13	117	34	10	0.6	*	5	0	0.1	0.1	0.8	*	11	*	16	33
1504	Eclair-custard with chocolate icing	item	100	239	6	23	0.5	14	4	*	82	82	24	0.7	*	68	0	0.04	0.16	0.1	*	*	*	80	112
1570	Frozen yogurt-fruit varieties	cup	226	216	7	42	*	2	1.2	0	5	122	40	0	*	0	0	0.01	0.26	0	*	*	*	200	200
1766	Fruit bar-oat bran-nuts-Health Valley	item	43	150	4	28	2.9	4	0.5	0	10	230	40	1.4	0.8	0	10	0.19	0.06	0.7	0.06	19	0	25	134

Code	Food	Measure	g																							
1717	Fruit pie-fried	item	85	266	2	33	2	14	6.5	13	325	51	8	0.9	0.2	33	1	1	0.1	0.08	1	0.03	4	0.08	12	38
403	Fruitcake-dark-home recipe	slice	15	57	1	9	0.3	2	0.5	7	24	74	4	0.4	*	4	tr	tr	0.02	0.02	0.2	*	*	*	11	17
1272	Granola bar	item	24	109	2	16	1	4	*	*	67	78	*	0.8	*	6	*	*	0.07	0.03	*	*	0	0	14	67
672	Granola clusters-Nature Valley	item	34	150	2	28	1.7	3	5.3	0	115	126	38	0.9	0.7	6	tr	0.1	0.03	0.03	0.1	0	26	0.64	24	96
1289	Ice cream sundae-caramel	item	165	323	8	53	*	10	4.8	26	208	338	30	0.2	0.9	56	4	0.07	0.31	0.05	0.31	0.07	13	0.68	201	231
1290	Ice cream sundae-hot fudge	item	165	297	6	50	1.2	9	5.3	13	190	413	35	0.2	1	46	2	0.07	0.31	0.13	0.31	0.07	10	0.68	216	238
1291	Ice cream-strawberry	item	165	289	7	48	0.7	8	5.3	10	99	292	26	0.3	0.7	48	1	0.07	0.3	0.08	0.3	0.07	20	0.69	173	167
78	Ice cream-french vanilla-soft serve	cup	173	377	7	38	0	23	13.5	153	153	338	25	0.4	2	199	1	0.08	0.3	0.1	0.45	0.08	9	1	236	199
76	Ice cream-vanilla-hardened-10% fat	cup	133	269	5	32	0	14	8.9	59	116	257	18	0.1	1.4	133	1	0.05	0.33	0.06	0.33	0.05	3	0.63	176	134
80	Ice cream-vanilla-rich-hardened-16% fat	cup	148	349	4	32	0	24	14.7	88	108	221	16	0.1	1.2	207	1	0.04	0.28	0.05	0.28	0.04	2	0.54	151	115
82	Ice milk-vanilla-hardened-4.3% fat	cup	131	184	5	29	0	6	3.5	18	105	265	19	0.2	0.6	52	1	0.08	0.35	0.09	0.35	0.08	3	0.88	176	129
83	Ice milk-vanilla-soft serve-2.6% fat	cup	175	223	8	38	0	6	2.9	13	163	412	29	0.3	0.9	44	1	0.12	0.54	0.13	0.54	0.12	5	1.37	274	202
454	Pie-apple-from home recipe	slice	135	323	3	49	2.2	14	3.9	0	207	115	11	1.2	0.2	5	2	0.15	0.11	0.04	1.2	0.04	7	0	82	31
456	Pie-banana cream-from home recipe	slice	130	285	6	40	1.4	12	3.8	40	252	264	*	1	*	66	1	0.11	0.22	*	1	*	*	*	86	107
458	Pie-blueberry-from home recipe	slice	135	325	3	47	1.7	15	3.5	0	361	88	9	1.4	*	8	4	0.15	0.11	*	1.4	*	*	0	15	31
401	Pie-Boston cream-home recipe	slice	69	210	3	34	1	6	1.9	0	128	61	*	0.7	*	28	0	0.09	0.11	*	0.8	*	7	*	46	70
460	Pie-cherry-from home recipe	slice	135	350	4	52	1.1	15	4	0	410	142	9	0.9	*	118	0	0.16	0.12	0.05	1.4	*	9	0.37	19	34
1480	Pie-chocolate cream-from home recipe	slice	100	264	5	30	2	5	5.4	55	273	142	25	1.1	0.7	53	0	0.1	0.17	*	0.7	*	*	*	84	109
462	Pie-custard-from home recipe	slice	130	285	8	30	2.1	14	4.8	0	373	178	*	1.2	*	60	4	0.11	0.27	*	0.8	*	11	*	125	147
464	Pie-lemon meringue-from home recipe	slice	120	300	4	47	1.4	11	3.7	0	223	53	7	0.9	0.3	33	0	0.1	0.12	0.03	0.7	0.03	*	0.19	16	48
466	Pie-mince-from home recipe	slice	135	365	3	56	2	16	4	0	604	240	24	1.9	*	0	4	0.14	0.12	*	1.4	*	*	*	38	51
468	Pie-peach-from home recipe	slice	135	345	3	52	1.8	14	3.5	0	361	21	9	1.2	*	198	4	0.15	0.14	*	2	*	*	0	14	39
470	Pie-pecan-from home recipe	slice	118	495	6	61	4.1	27	5.4	*	260	145	*	3.7	*	40	1	0.26	0.14	*	1	*	*	*	55	122
472	Pie-pumpkin-from home recipe	slice	130	275	5	32	3.5	15	5.4	*	278	208	17	1	*	320	*	0.11	0.18	*	1	*	*	*	66	90
473	Piecrust-baked-from home recipe	item	180	900	11	79	4.7	60	14.8	0	1099	89	25	3.1	*	0	5	0.47	0.4	0.4	5	*	*	*	25	90
474	Piecrust-baked-prepared from mix	item	160	743	10	71	4.2	47	11.4	0	1300	90	*	3.1	*	0	5	0.54	0.4	0.4	5	*	*	*	66	136
1365	Pudding-banana cream-instant mix-Jello	oz	28.4	106	0	27	0	0	0	0	190	1	*	tr	*	0	0	0	0	0	0	*	*	1	1	111
1366	Pudding-butterscotch-instant mix-Jello	oz	28.4	105	0	27	0	0	0	0	244	1	*	tr	*	0	0	0	0	0	0	*	*	1	1	102
90	Pudding-chocolate-cooked-from mix & milk	cup	260	320	9	59	0	8	4.3	32	335	354	38	0.8	*	68	2	0.05	0.39	0.3	0.3	0.05	*	*	265	247
87	Pudding-chocolate-home recipe-starch	cup	260	385	9	67	1.3	12	7.6	32	145	445	22	1.3	*	78	1	0.05	0.36	0.36	0.3	0.05	*	*	250	255
91	Pudding-chocolate-instant from mix	cup	260	325	8	71	0	7	3.6	28	322	335	18	1.3	*	68	2	0.08	0.39	0.3	0.3	0.08	*	*	374	237
1745	Pudding-chocolate-sugar free-2% milk	serv	133	100	5	14	0.3	3	*	3	310	*	*	0.7	*	40	0	0.06	0.26	*	0.3	0.06	*	*	150	300
1368	Pudding-coconut cream-instant mix-Jello	oz	28.4	117	0	23	0.5	3	0.6	3	186	55	3	0.2	0.1	0	0	tr	tr	*	*	tr	1	0.08	9	10
998	Pudding-corn	cup	250	273	11	32	1.1	13	6.3	250	138	402	38	1.4	1.3	90	7	1.03	0.32	0.3	2.5	0.3	63	0.23	100	143
1367	Pudding-lemon-instant mix-Jello	oz	28.4	105	tr	27	0.3	0	0	0	190	1	9	tr	0.3	96	0	tr	0.17	0.19	0	0.19	40	0.23	1	111
1545	Pudding-rice with raisins	cup	265	387	10	71	1.4	8	4.1	8	188	469	3	tr	0.1	14	tr	0.08	0.37	0.08	0.5	0.01	1	0.03	260	249
89	Pudding-tapioca cream-home recipe-starch	cup	165	220	8	28	0.6	8	4.1	80	257	223	20	0.7	*	60	2	0.07	0.3	0.2	0.2	0.07	*	*	173	180
88	Pudding-vanilla (blancmange)-home recipe	cup	255	285	9	41	0	10	6.2	36	165	352	14	0	*	82	2	0.08	0.41	0.3	0.3	0.08	*	*	298	232
1746	Pudding-vanilla-sugar free-with 2% milk	serv	133	90	4	12	0.2	2	*	3	380	*	3	*	*	40	0	0.03	0.17	*	*	0.03	*	0.08	150	200
85	Sherbet-orange-2% fat	cup	193	270	2	59	0.7	4	2.4	14	198	198	15	0.3	1.3	39	4	0.03	0.09	0.09	0.1	0.03	14	0.16	103	74
499	Toaster pastries/Pop Tarts	item	50	196	2	35	0.7	6	*	0	230	85	9	2.1	0.3	96	2	0.16	0.17	0.17	2.1	0.19	40	0	97	97
1292	Turnover-apple	oz	28.4	85	1	11	0.2	5	1.3	0	109	14	3	0.3	0.1	14	tr	0.03	0.02	0.03	0.3	0.01	1	0.03	4	11
1293	Turnover-cherry	oz	28.4	84	1	11	0.2	5	1.1	4	124	20	3	0.2	0.1	12	tr	0.02	0.02	0.02	0.2	0.01	5	0	4	14
1294	Turnover-lemon	oz	28.4	93	1	12	0.2	5	1.1	7	95	14	3	0.4	0.1	12	tr	0.06	0.03	0.06	0.6	0.01	5	0.06	4	18
1584	Twinkie-Hostess	item	42	143	1	26	*	4	*	21	189	*	*	0.5	*	8	0	0.06	0.06	0.06	0.5	*	4	*	19	*

Eggs

Code	Food	Measure	g																							
854	Egg substitute-frozen	cup	240	384	27	8	0	27	4.6	5	479	512	36	4.8	2.4	324	1	0.29	0.93	0.32	0.3	0.32	39	0.81	175	172
852	Egg substitute-liquid	cup	251	211	30	2	0	8	1.7	3	444	828	22	5.3	3.3	542	0	0.28	0.75	0.01	0.3	0.01	37	0.75	133	304
853	Egg substitute-powder	serv	28.4	126	16	6	0	6	1.1	162	227	211	18	0.9	0.5	105	tr	0.06	0.5	0.04	0.2	0.04	35	1	92	136
851	Egg-duck-whole-fresh-raw	item	70	130	9	1	0	10	2.6	619	102	156	12	2.7	1.5	279	0	0.11	0.28	0.18	0.1	0.18	56	3.78	45	154
99	Egg-fried in butter-whole-large-chicken	item	46	92	6	1	0	7	1.9	211	162	61	5	0.7	0.5	114	0	0.03	0.24	0.07	tr	0.07	18	0.42	25	89
100	Egg-hard cooked-no shell-large-chicken	item	50	77	6	1	0	5	1.6	213	62	63	5	0.6	0.5	84	0	0.03	0.26	0.06	tr	0.06	22	0.56	25	86

* indicates that no data was available.

©1994 First DataBank—The Hearst Corporation (N-Squared Computing).

Appendix A - Table of Food Composition
(continued)

Item	Food name	Portion	Weight (g)	Food Energy (Kcal)	Protein (gm)	Carbohydrates (gm)	Fiber (gm)	Total Fat (gm)	Saturated Fat (gm)	Cholesterol (mg)	Sodium (mg)	Potassium (mg)	Magnesium (mg)	Iron (mg)	Zinc (mg)	Vitamin A (RE)	Vitamin C (mg)	Thiamin (mg)	Riboflavin (mg)	Niacin (mg)	Vitamin B6 (mg)	Folates (µg)	Vitamin B12 (µg)	Calcium (mg)	Phosphorus (mg)
101	Egg-poached-whole-large-chicken	item	50	74	6	1	0	5	1.5	212	140	60	5	0.7	0.6	95	0	0.03	0.22	tr	0.06	18	0.4	25	89
97	Egg-raw-white-large-chicken	item	33.4	17	4	tr	0	0	0	0	55	48	4	tr	0	0	0	tr	0.15	tr	tr	1	0.07	2	4
96	Egg-raw-whole-large-chicken	item	50	75	6	1	0	5	1.6	213	63	60	5	0.7	0.5	95	0	0.03	0.25	tr	0.07	23	0.5	25	89
98	Egg-raw-yolk-large-chicken	item	16.6	59	3	tr	0	5	1.6	213	7	16	1	0.6	0.6	323	0	0.03	0.11	tr	0.07	24	0.52	23	81
102	Egg-scrambled-with milk & butter-chicken	item	61	101	7	1	0	7	2.2	215	171	84	7	0.7	0.6	119	tr	0.03	0.27	tr	0.07	18	0.47	44	104
1296	Omelet-two egg-ham and cheese	item	120	266	19	2	0	20	7.3	445	598	182	17	1.7	1.8	273	4	0.18	0.57	0.8	0.19	38	1.08	153	286
Fast foods																									
750	Arby's-beef and cheese sandwch	item	176	402	32	27	1.1	18	9	77	1634	345	40	5.1	5.4	58	0	0.38	0.46	5.9	0.34	41	2.05	183	401
1830	Arby's-chicken breast sandwich	item	184	493	23	48	1.6	25	5.1	91	1019	330	46	3.5	1.7	15	0	0.45	0.39	14.8	0.65	32	0.34	111	290
753	Arby's-club sandwich	item	252	560	30	43	2.3	30	11.6	100	1610	466	46	3.6	3.1	127	28	0.68	0.43	7	0.4	44	0.94	200	433
751	Arby's-ham and cheese sandwich	item	146	353	21	33	1	16	6.4	58	772	290	16	3.3	1.4	96	3	0.31	0.49	2.7	0.2	71	0.54	130	152
749	Arby's-roast beef sandwich	item	139	346	22	34	1	14	3.6	52	792	316	31	4.2	3.4	63	2	0.38	0.31	5.9	0.27	40	1.22	54	239
1831	Arby's-super roast beef sandwich	item	234	501	25	50	1.6	22	8.5	40	798	503	58	6.4	10.7	0	2	0.53	0.6	9.4	0.48	41	4.29	115	402
752	Arby's-turkey deluxe	item	236	510	28	46	*	24	*	70	1220	*	*	2.7	*	*	*	0.45	0.34	8	*	*	*	80	*
###	Arbys-soup-Boston clam chowder	serv	227	207	10	18	1.4	11	4	28	1157	319	20	1.4	0.7	100	4	0.06	0.22	0.9	0.12	9	9.38	170	143
###	Arbys-soup-cream of broccoli	serv	227	180	9	18	1.8	8	5	3	1113	455	55	0.8	0.6	50	9	0.11	0.42	0.8	0.18	46	0.59	237	193
2010	Arbys-soup-french onion	serv	227	67	2	7	0.9	7	2	0	1248	106	2	0.6	0.6	10	2	0.03	0.02	0.6	0.05	14	0	25	11
2011	Arbys-soup-lumberjack mixed vegetable	serv	227	89	2	13	1.3	4	2	4	1075	268	6	1.9	2.7	250	9	0.06	0.1	1.9	0.15	14	0.3	41	91
2012	Arbys-soup-old fashioned chicken noodle	serv	227	99	6	15	0.7	2	1	25	929	78	5	0.7	0.4	200	1	0.05	0.06	1.3	0.03	2	0.14	16	34
2013	Arbys-soup-pilgrim clam chowder	serv	227	193	10	18	1.9	11	4	28	1157	379	19	2	1.1	350	4	0.06	0.16	1.3	0.15	9	9.67	134	126
###	Arbys-soup-roast beef and vegetable	serv	227	96	5	14	0.5	3	1	10	996	211	5	1	1.4	300	5	0.03	0.05	1	0.07	10	0.3	16	39
2014	Arbys-soup-split pea and ham	serv	227	200	8	21	3.9	10	5	30	1029	272	36	2	1.4	300	1	0.11	0.09	2.4	0.2	4	0.23	32	168
2015	Arbys-soup-tomato florentine	serv	227	84	3	15	0.5	2	1	2	910	221	10	1.6	0.2	100	12	0.09	0.09	1.3	0.12	15	0.1	45	58
2016	Arbys-soup-Wisconsin cheese	serv	227	287	9	19	1.8	19	8	31	1129	441	7	1.3	1.1	90	2	0.03	0.24	0.7	0.05	7	0	252	241
1561	Arthur Treacher-chicken sandwich	item	156	413	16	44	*	19	*	*	708	279	27	1.7	*	37	19	0.17	0.24	8.1	*	*	*	59	147
2122	Beef burger-fast food	oz	28.3	72	5	7	tr	3	*	*	55	46	*	0.3	*	8	tr	0.02	0.04	0.8	*	*	*	3	25
2113	Bun-hamburger/hotdog-fast food	oz	28.3	98	3	16	1.1	3	*	*	22	31	*	0.2	*	0	tr	0.07	0.02	0.4	*	*	*	9	13
1983	Burger King-bacon double cheese-deluxe	serv	195	592	33	28	1.1	39	16	111	804	463	38	4	6.4	71	8	0.3	0.39	8.1	0.37	31	3.24	156	373
1917	Burger King-barbecue bacon double cheese	item	174	536	32	31	0.8	31	14	105	795	429	36	4	6.5	49	4	0.29	0.39	8.3	0.35	27	3.34	158	379
1918	Burger King-BK broiler	item	168	379	24	31	1.8	18	3	53	764	324	29	3.2	3.2	44	6	0.27	0.26	5.2	0.24	38	1.52	74	153
1919	Burger King-BK broiler sauce	serv	14	90	0	0	0	10	1	7	95	*	*	*	*	*	0	*	*	*	*	*	*	*	*
1975	Burger King-chicken tenders	piece	90	39	3	2	0.3	2	0.5	8	90	249	22	1	0.7	25	0	0.14	0.12	6.2	0.32	9	0.3	9	234
1711	Burger King-croissant-egg and cheese	item	127	369	13	24	2.1	25	14.1	216	551	174	22	2.2	1.8	300	tr	0.19	0.38	1.5	0.1	36	0.78	244	349
1712	Burger King-croissant-egg/cheese/ham	item	152	475	19	24	1.4	34	17.5	100	1080	272	26	2.1	2	135	1	0.52	0.3	3.2	0.23	36	1.01	144	336
1976	Burger King-double cheeseburger	item	172	483	30	29	1.4	27	13	100	851	344	31	3	4	100	6	0.22	0.31	4.9	0.24	31	1.81	189	305
1920	Burger King-fish tenders	serv	99	267	12	18	1.1	16	3	28	870	176	33	1.7	0.6	20	0	0.23	0.17	2.3	0.06	23	1.05	60	191
1921	Burger King-mushroom swiss double cheese	item	176	473	31	27	*	27	12	95	746	*	*	4.1	*	*	tr	*	*	*	*	*	*	*	*
1977	Burger King-ranch dip sauce	serv	28	171	0	2	tr	18	3	0	208	*	*	0.1	*	8	tr	*	*	1.9	tr	tr	0	1	3
1978	Burger King-sweet & sour sauce	serv	28	45	0	11	tr	0	0	0	52	9	2	0.1	tr	0	0	tr	tr	0.1	tr	2	0.06	7	8
1979	Burger King-tartar dip sauce	serv	28	174	0	3	*	18	3	16	302	14	1	0.3	*	26	0	0.01	0.01	tr	0.08	2	*	*	*
1980	Burger King-tater tenders	serv	71	213	2	25	*	12	3	3	318	*	*	*	*	*	13	*	*	*	*	*	*	*	*
1559	Burger King-whopper hamburger	item	261	630	26	50	2.5	36	16.5	104	990	520	50	6	5.3	192	13	0.02	0.03	5.2	0.31	31	2.81	104	312
2123	Cheeseburger-fast food	oz	28.3	78	6	7	0.1	3	1.7	12	198	68	6	0.6	0.7	9	tr	0.02	0.05	0.6	0.04	7	0.31	25	33
1697	Chicken-breast and wing-breaded-fried	serv	163	494	36	20	0.3	30	7.8	149	975	566	38	1.5	1.6	58	0	0.14	0.3	12	0.57	9	0.67	60	307
2117	Chicken-breast-fast food	oz	28.3	73	8	3	0	4	0.6	24	142	85	8	0.2	0.3	9	1	0.02	0.05	2	0.16	9	0.09	4	52
1356	Chicken-drumstick & thigh-breaded-fried	serv	148	430	30	16	0.2	27	7.1	165	756	446	37	1.6	3.2	67	0	0.14	0.43	7.2	0.33	10	0.83	36	240
2119	Chicken-drumstick-fast food	oz	28.3	59	7	4	0	2	0.9	26	133	74	6	0.3	0.8	7	tr	0.02	0.06	1.4	0.1	2	0.09	4	41
2110	Chicken-fried-fast food-various portions	oz	28.3	82	5	6	0	5	1.1	25	153	71	7	0.3	0.6	7	tr	0.02	0.05	1.6	0.12	2	0.09	4	39
2111	Chicken-meat-shaped-fried-fast food	oz	28.3	82	5	5	0	5	*	*	141	40	*	0.3	*	6	tr	0.01	0.01	0.8	*	*	*	4	34
2121	Chicken-shoulder-fast food	oz	28.3	92	5	3	0	6	*	*	150	74	*	0.1	*	4	tr	0.02	0.04	1.9	*	*	*	4	32
2120	Chicken-thigh-fast food	oz	28.3	104	7	3	0	7	1.2	26	139	68	6	0.1	0.7	6	tr	0.02	0.07	1.4	0.09	2	0.08	4	37
2118	Chicken-wing-fast food	oz	28.3	92	7	3	0	5	*	*	198	54	*	0.2	*	7	1	0.02	0.04	1.5	*	*	*	5	31

Nutritional data table (fast food items). Columns are not labeled on this page (headers cut off). Values are transcribed left-to-right as printed; `*` indicates no data available, `tr` indicates trace.

Ref.	Food	Unit	1	2	3	4	5	6	7	8	9	10	11	12	13	14	15	16	17	18	19	20	21	22	23	24
1562	Churchs chicken-white meat	item	100	327	21	10	*	23	*	*	498	186	*	4	*	1	*	tr	48	1	0.1	0.18	7.2	*	*	94
2114	Coleslaw-fast food	oz	28.3	24	1	3	0	1	0.2	*	77	45	4	0.5	tr	8	tr	0.01	0.01	tr	0.02	tr	9	*	10	*
1355	Dairy Queen-banana split	item	383	540	10	91	*	15	*	30	*	*	*	1.8	*	225	18	0.6	0.6	0.8	0.9	*	350	*	*	250
1351	Dairy Queen-dip ice cream cone-regular	item	156	300	7	40	*	13	*	20	*	*	*	0.4	*	90	0	0.09	0.34	0	0.6	*	200	*	*	200
1354	Dairy Queen-float	item	397	330	6	59	*	8	*	20	*	*	*	0	*	30	0	0.12	0.17	0	0.6	*	200	*	7	200
1350	Dairy Queen-ice cream cone-regular	item	142	226	5	33	*	8	4.9	38	126	233	21	0.2	0.8	87	2	0.07	0.36	0.4	0.28	0.6	212	*	7	192
1352	Dairy Queen-ice cream sundae-regular	item	177	319	6	53	2.2	10	5.6	23	204	443	37	0.7	1.1	75	4	0.07	0.34	1.2	0.34	0.73	232	1.8	11	255
1353	Dairy Queen-malt-regular	item	418	600	15	89	*	20	*	50	*	*	*	3.6	*	225	4	0.12	0.6	0.8	0.6	1.8	500	*	*	400
2124	Double cheese burger-fast food	oz	28.4	66	4	7	0.1	3	2.2	17	50	85	6	0.3	0.9	8	tr	0.02	0.04	0.8	0.04	0.42	3	0.42	5	31
2051	Fast food-pizza with cheese	oz	28.4	63	3	9	0.6	1	0.7	4	151	49	7	0.3	0.4	33	1	0.08	0.07	1.1	0.07	0.15	52	0.15	26	51
##	Fast food-pizza with pepperoni	oz	28.4	72	4	8	0.6	3	0.9	6	107	61	3	0.4	0.2	22	1	0.05	0.09	1.2	0.07	0.07	26	0.07	21	30
2125	Fish cake-fried-with bun-fast food	oz	28.3	85	3	8	0.4	5	*	15	167	52	8	0.5	0.7	6	tr	0.02	0.04	1.4	0.04	0.85	14	0.85	12	34
2126	Frankfurter-coney dog-fast food	oz	28.3	69	3	7	0	3	3.1	15	242	49	3	1	0.6	7	tr	0.07	0.07	1.1	0.03	0.33	12	0.33	1	30
2127	Frankfurter-hot dog-fast food	oz	28.3	78	3	7	0	3	3.1	15	219	48	3	0.6	0.6	5	tr	0.01	0.01	0.6	0.03	0.33	6	0.33	6	33
###	Hamburger-double patty-everything on it	oz	28.4	68	4	5	0.3	3	1.3	15	99	71	6	0.7	0.7	1	tr	0.05	0.05	1	0.05	0.51	13	0.51	6	39
1922	Hardee-bacon and egg biscuit	serv	124	410	15	35	0.6	24	5	155	990	180	25	2.2	1.4	116	3	0.33	0.45	3	0.14	0.47	253	0.47	14	358
1923	Hardee-bacon egg and cheese biscuit	serv	137	460	17	35	0.7	28	8	165	1220	200	27	2.4	1.5	129	3	0.37	0.49	3.3	0.15	0.52	279	0.52	15	396
1925	Hardee-big country breakfast-country ham	serv	254	670	29	52	*	38	*	345	2870	710	*	*	*	*	*	*	*	*	*	*	*	*	*	*
1927	Hardee-big country breakfast-sausage	serv	274	850	33	51	16	57	16	340	1980	670	44	3	2.5	333	0	0.31	0.8	4.2	0.34	1.5	78	53	347
1924	Hardee-big country breakfast-with bacon	serv	217	660	24	51	10	40	10	305	1540	530	23	2.5	*	333	0	0.31	0.8	1.8	0.31	1.5	78	53	347
1926	Hardee-big country breakfast-with ham	serv	251	620	28	51	7	33	*	325	1780	620	*	*	*	*	*	*	*	*	*	*	*	*	*	*
1928	Hardee-big roast beef sandwich	serv	134	300	18	32	5	11	5	45	880	320	33	3.7	6.1	0	0	0.3	0.34	5.4	0.28	2.45	66	0.47	24	230
1929	Hardee-big twin hamburger	serv	173	450	23	34	11	25	11	55	580	280	35	4	4.6	17	3	0.28	0.31	6.7	0.27	2.27	80	0.52	34	197
1930	Hardee-biscuit n gravy	serv	221	440	9	45	24	24	6	15	1250	210	*	*	*	*	*	*	*	*	*	*	*	*	*	*
1931	Hardee-chicken n pasta salad	serv	414	230	27	23	3	3	1	55	380	620	*	9	*	0	0	*	*	*	*	*	*	*	*	*
1932	Hardee-crispy curls	serv	85	300	4	36	16	16	3	0	840	370	*	*	*	*	3	0.28	*	*	*	*	*	*	*	*
1933	Hardee-grilled chicken sandwich	serv	192	310	24	34	9	9	1	60	890	410	44	3	2.7	413	tr	0.43	0.59	4.2	0.1	0.47	542	0.47	31	611
1934	Hardee-ham & egg biscuit	serv	138	370	15	35	15	19	4	160	1050	210	26	2.8	1.6	127	9	0.56	0.54	3.9	0.21	0.73	95	0.73	39	234
1935	Hardee-ham egg & cheese biscuit	serv	151	420	18	35	23	23	6	170	1270	230	30	2.7	1.7	142	4	0.4	0.54	3.7	0.17	0.57	308	0.57	17	436
1936	Hardee-mushroom n swiss hamburger	serv	186	490	30	33	27	27	13	70	940	370	44	4.5	4.2	74	4	0.47	0.34	11.6	0.3	2.68	134	*	*	261
1937	Hardee-regular roast beef sandwich	serv	114	260	15	31	9	9	4	35	730	260	30	1.7	1.1	72	1	0.3	0.21	4.5	0.12	1.1	167	0.33	20	263
1981	Jack in the Box-the lean one sandwich	item	220	420	27	37	18	18	8	85	760	510	15	0.9	0.4	2	1	0.09	0.1	7.7	0.06	0.12	73	0.06	11	86
1938	Hardee-three pancakes	serv	137	280	8	56	2	2	1	15	890	240	22	1.5	0.9	63	1	0.05	0.15	1.4	0.1	0.42	18	0.49	4	175
1563	Jack in the Box-breakfast jack sandwich	item	121	301	18	28	13	13	*	182	1037	297	41	3.1	1.8	133	3	0.4	0.35	13.4	0.14	1.1	341	0.59	29	411
1358	Jack in the Box-jumbo jack cheeseburger	item	272	628	32	45	35	35	15	110	1666	499	40	1.6	4.8	220	5	0.52	0.38	18.4	0.31	3.05	177	0.77	39	310
1357	Jack in the Box-jumbo jack hamburger	item	246	551	28	45	29	29	11.4	80	1134	492	44	4.5	4.2	74	4	0.47	0.34	4.1	0.16	2.68	273	0.24	5	411
1680	Jack in the Box-moby jack sandwich	item	141	455	17	38	26	26	8	56	837	246	30	1.7	1.1	72	1	0.3	0.21	8.2	0.29	1.1	134	0.4	6	261
1359	Jack in the Box-onion rings-bag	item	83	275	4	31	19	19	7	14	430	129	15	0.9	0.4	25	5	0.09	0.1	4.3	0.09	0.12	167	0.36	10	221
1944	KFC-chicken hot wings	piece	119	63	3	3	5	5	0.8	25	113	94	22	1.5	2.1	63	tr	0.05	0.15	7.7	0.49	0.33	10	0.5	2	97
1939	KFC-chicken sandwich	serv	166	482	21	39	27	27	6	47	1060	297	41	3.1	1.5	63	0	0.4	0.35	13.4	0.59	1.1	100	0.5	34	764
1940	KFC-crispy chicken-breast	piece	135	342	33	12	20	20	5	114	790	347	40	1.6	1.5	14	0	0.11	0.17	11.6	0.58	3.05	252	0.43	39	899
1941	KFC-crispy chicken-drumstick	piece	69	204	14	6	14	14	tr	71	324	157	16	0.9	0.9	20	0	0.06	0.16	9.7	0.77	2.68	200	0.87	67	1017
1942	KFC-crispy chicken-thigh	piece	119	406	20	14	30	30	8	129	688	280	29	1.8	3	17	0	0.11	0.29	8.2	0.36	2.68	8	0.4	10	120
1943	KFC-crispy chicken-wing	piece	65	254	12	9	19	19	4	67	422	115	12	0.8	1.1	25	2	0.04	0.09	4.3	0.27	0.18	10	0.09	2	221
1960	Long John Silver-battered shrimp-9 piece	piece	357	95	3	10	5	5	1.1	14	163	94	132	10.3	4.2	242	5	0.3	0.5	9.9	0.36	3.4	214	0.33	34	97
1945	Long John Silver-breaded shrimp	serv	420	51	1	6	2	2	0.5	6	85	41	156	12.1	5	285	6	0.35	0.58	11.6	0.43	3.99	252	0.31	39	764
1946	Long John Silver-catfish fillet	serv	373	860	28	90	42	42	10	65	990	1180	121	4.6	3.4	317	11	0.2	0.49	9.7	0.87	9.41	200	0.46	5	312
1952	Long John Silver-chicken plank-4 piece	serv	415	940	39	94	44	44	10	70	1660	1320	95	4.6	2.1	63	11	0.2	0.15	7.7	0.22	9.41	134	0.24	6	120
2019	Long John Silver-chicken-light herb	serv	498	630	35	85	3	85	3	85	2170	790	95	4.8	3.6	120	0	0.32	0.65	26.3	1.05	0.75	214	0.36	10	782
1947	Long John Silver-clam chowder with cod	serv	198	140	11	10	6	6	2	20	590	380	17	1.7	0.9	74	4	0.05	0.14	1.2	0.13	8.44	117	0.18	8	110
1948	Long John Silver-clam dinner	serv	363	980	21	122	45	45	10	15	1200	870	41	6.2	6.2	365	47	0.34	0.91	7.2	0.26	201	209	0.26	54	572

* indicates that no data was available.

©1994 First DataBank—The Hearst Corporation (N-Squared Computing).

A 19

Appendix A - Table of Food Composition
(continued)

Item	Food name	Portion	Weight (g)	Food Energy (Kcal)	Protein (gm)	Carbohydrates (gm)	Fiber (gm)	Total Fat (gm)	Saturated Fat (gm)	Cholesterol (mg)	Sodium (mg)	Potassium (mg)	Magnesium (mg)	Iron (mg)	Zinc (mg)	Vitamin A (RE)	Vitamin C (mg)	Thiamin (mg)	Riboflavin (mg)	Niacin (mg)	Vitamin B6 (mg)	Folates (µg)	Vitamin B12 (µg)	Calcium (mg)	Phosphorus (mg)
1949	Long John Silver-cole slaw	serv	98	140	1	20	2.3	6	1	15	260	190	13	0.5	0.1	225	30	0.04	0.03	0.3	0.13	37	0.03	36	23
1950	Long John Silver-fish & chicken entree	serv	398	870	35	91	*	40	9	70	1520	1290	*	3.3	2.1	*	5	*	0.5	12.3	0.72	46	5.17	133	769
1951	Long John Silver-fish & more entree	serv	381	800	31	88	1.7	37	8	70	1390	1260	131	3.3	2.1	71	5	0.39	0.5	12.3	0.72	46	5.17	133	769
1969	Long John Silver-fish and fryes-3 piece	serv	358	810	42	77	*	38	9	85	1630	1050	94	6.4	2.3	65	2	0.87	0.65	11.1	0.42	89	2.29	238	488
1957	Long John Silver-fish sandwich platter	serv	379	870	26	108	4.1	38	8	55	1110	1050	94	6.4	2.3	65	2	0.87	0.65	11.1	0.42	89	2.29	238	488
1953	Long John Silver-fries	serv	85	220	3	30	2.9	10	3	5	60	390	29	0.6	0.3	0	9	0.15	0.02	2.8	0.2	25	0.27	16	79
1954	Long John Silver-garden salad	serv	246	170	9	13	2.1	9	0.8	5	380	20	40	1.7	1.1	239	26	0.14	0.15	11.4	0.56	66	0.27	42	217
1955	Long John Silver-gumbo-cod & shrimp bobs	serv	198	120	9	4	3	8	2	25	740	310	41	2.3	0.8	300	21	0.12	0.08	2	0.17	47	0.24	100	105
1956	Long John Silver-homestyle fish sandwich	serv	196	510	22	58	2.1	22	5	45	780	470	48	18	1.1	33	1	0.45	0.34	5.7	0.22	46	1.19	123	252
1968	Long John Silver-homestyle fish-3 piece	serv	456	960	43	97	2	44	10	100	1890	1540	157	3.9	2.6	85	6	0.47	0.59	14.7	0.87	56	6.19	159	920
1967	Long John Silver-homestyle fish-6 piece	serv	513	1260	49	124	2.3	64	14	130	1590	1660	177	4.4	2.9	96	7	0.53	0.67	16.6	0.98	62	6.97	179	1035
1958	Long John Silver-hushpuppies	piece	24	70	2	10	*	2	1	5	25	65	*	*	*	*	*	*	*	*	*	*	*	*	56
2018	Long John Silver-light fish-lemon	serv	291	320	24	49	2.4	4	1	75	900	470	56	2.3	1.4	80	10	0.29	0.15	3.4	0.34	46	0.58	40	238
2017	Long John Silver-light fish-paprika	serv	284	300	24	45	1.3	2	1	70	650	460	98	2.4	1.6	53	4	0.29	0.37	9.2	0.54	35	3.86	99	573
1959	Long John Silver-mixed vegetables	serv	113	60	2	9	5.9	2	1	0	330	120	24	0.9	0.5	75	4	0.08	0.13	0.9	0.08	21	tr	29	56
1961	Long John Silver-ocean chef salad	serv	321	250	24	19	*	9	2	80	1340	160	*	1.8	0.6	60	1	0.15	0.02	1.5	0.08	5	0.01	17	45
2021	Long John Silver-rice pilaf	serv	142	210	5	43	0.8	2	1	0	570	140	17	1.8	2.2	59	13	0.42	0.37	8.2	0.88	37	1.68	109	484
1962	Long John Silver-seafood platter	serv	400	970	30	109	5.3	46	10	70	1540	1100	114	4.1	5.2	129	20	0.42	0.37	8.2	0.88	47	2.89	148	444
1963	Long John Silver-seafood salad	serv	337	270	16	36	1.3	7	1	90	670	100	86	3.2	5.2	129	8	0.13	0.16	3.7	0.27	20	1.22	63	187
1964	Long John Silver-seafood salad-scoop	serv	142	210	14	26	0.6	7	1	90	570	100	36	1.4	1.6	250	8	0.05	0.07	1.6	0.11	20	1.22	63	187
1965	Long John Silver-shrimp & fish dinner	serv	348	770	25	85	7.3	37	8	80	1250	1030	82	3.5	1.6	28	17	0.37	0.21	6.6	0.64	35	1.06	54	422
1966	Long John Silver-shrimp fish & chicken	serv	380	840	31	89	*	40	9	80	1450	1170	*	1	*	411	14	0.31	0.29	3.6	*	*	*	*	*
##	Long John Silver-shrimp scampi	serv	529	610	25	87	0	18	3	220	2120	560	203	13.6	6.2	364	11	0.13	0.2	13.6	0.55	10	5.57	299	1156
1853	McDonalds-apple bran muffin	serv	85	190	5	46	4.5	0	0	0	230	202	55	0.6	1.2	1	1	0.02	0.08	0.4	0.37	77	0.78	31	178
1828	McDonalds-apple danish	serv	115	390	6	51	1.6	18	3.5	26	370	69	8	1.4	0.2	35	16	0.28	0.2	2.2	0.03	3	0	14	31
1871	McDonalds-apple pie	slice	83	260	2	30	1.1	15	4.8	0	240	50	6	0.7	0.2	0	11	0.06	0.02	0.3	0.02	2	0	11	22
1851	McDonalds-bacon and egg biscuit	serv	156	440	18	33	0.8	26	8.2	253	1230	237	31	2.6	1.7	160	0	0.36	0.33	2.5	0.17	18	0.59	185	451
1864	McDonalds-bacon bits	serv	3	16	1	tr	0	1	0.1	0	95	4	3	0	0.1	0	0	0.01	0	0	tr	4	0.04	0	7
1856	McDonalds-barbeque (barbecue) sauce	serv	32	50	tr	12	1.9	1	0.1	0	340	56	6	0.3	0.1	30	2	0.01	0.01	0.2	0.02	1	0	13	6
736	McDonalds-big Mac hamburger	item	215	560	25	43	*	32	10.1	103	950	237	38	4	4.7	106	2	0.48	0.41	6.8	0.27	21	1.8	256	314
1850	McDonalds-biscuit with spread	item	75	260	5	32	1	13	3.4	1	730	100	14	1.3	0.7	0	0	0.23	0.11	1.7	0.03	6	0.1	75	168
737	McDonalds-cheeseburger	item	116	310	15	31	0.6	14	5.2	53	750	223	21	2.3	2.1	118	2	0.29	0.21	3.9	0.12	18	0.94	199	177
1859	McDonalds-chef salad	serv	283	230	21	8	*	13	5.9	128	490	*	*	1.5	2.1	411	14	0.31	0.29	3.6	*	*	*	256	*
1695	McDonalds-chicken Mcnuggets-6 piece	serv	113	290	19	17	0.5	16	4.1	65	520	213	5	0.4	0.1	0	tr	0.05	0.03	0.4	0.01	3	0.8	13	15
1873	McDonalds-chocolate milkshake-lowfat	serv	293	320	12	66	1.4	2	0.8	10	240	*	33	2.8	1.8	92	1	0.13	0.5	3.7	0.16	44	0.8	332	319
1861	McDonalds-chunky chicken salad	serv	250	140	23	5	1	3	0.9	78	230	436	37	1	0.4	366	20	0.22	0.17	8.5	0.6	27	0.63	34	257
1842	McDonalds-cinnamon and raisin danish	item	110	440	6	58	1.1	21	4.2	35	430	150	27	1.8	0.9	33	3	0.32	0.24	2.8	0.1	51	tr	35	229
1876	McDonalds-cookie-chocolaty	serv	56	330	4	42	1.1	16	5	4	280	72	20	2.2	0.5	0	0	0.18	0.21	2.5	0.03	5	0.07	24	71
1875	McDonalds-cookie-Mcdonaldland	serv	56	290	4	47	0.6	9	1.9	0	300	38	13	2.1	0.3	0	0	0.25	0.18	2.5	0.03	4	0.07	9	91
1863	McDonalds-croutons	serv	11	50	1	7	0.5	2	0.5	0	140	20	5	0.4	0.1	0	tr	0.05	0.03	0.4	0.01	3	0	6	15
742	McDonalds-egg Mcmuffin	item	138	290	18	28	1.4	11	3.8	226	740	213	33	2.8	1.8	150	1	0.47	0.33	3.7	0.16	44	0.8	256	319
1849	McDonalds-english muffin	item	59	170	5	27	1.6	5	2.4	9	270	74	12	1.6	0.4	37	tr	0.33	0.14	2.5	0.1	51	tr	151	60
741	McDonalds-filet o fish	item	142	440	14	38	1.1	26	5.2	50	1030	150	27	1.8	0.9	44	tr	0.3	0.15	2.7	0.1	20	0.82	165	229
1866	McDonalds-french fries-large	serv	122	400	6	46	4.2	22	9.1	16	200	866	40	0.9	0.5	0	15	0.24	0	3.3	0.32	40	0.15	18	162
1865	McDonalds-french fries-medium	serv	97	320	4	36	3.4	17	7.2	12	150	692	32	0.7	0.5	0	12	0.19	0	2.6	0.25	32	0.12	14	129
1694	McDonalds-french fries-regular order	serv	68	220	3	26	*	12	5.1	9	110	484	22	0.5	0.4	8	8	0.14	0	1.8	0.18	22	0.08	10	90
1860	McDonalds-garden salad	serv	213	110	7	6	1.8	7	2.9	83	160	450	35	1.3	1	391	14	0.1	0.16	0.6	0.49	57	0.23	149	188
738	McDonalds-hamburger	item	102	260	12	31	*	10	3.6	37	500	215	23	2.3	2.1	46	2	0.28	0.16	3.8	0.12	17	0.84	122	110
1825	McDonalds-hashbrown potato	serv	55	130	1	15	1.1	7	3.2	9	330	238	9	0.3	0.2	0	2	0.06	0.02	0.9	0.07	4	0	6	39
1858	McDonalds-honey sauce	serv	14	45	0	12	0	0	0	0	0	*	*	0.1	0	0	tr	0	0.01	tr	*	*	*	*	*
1696	McDonalds-hot cakes with syrup	serv	176	410	8	74	*	9	3.7	21	640	187	25	2.1	0.6	52	5	0.32	0.33	2.8	0.12	9	0.19	114	501

A 20

Code	Food	Unit																						
1870	McDonalds-hot caramel sundae	serv	174	270	7	59	1	3	1.5	13	180	51	0.1	1.1	87	0	0.08	0.35	0.3	0.38	19	0.66	222	198
1869	McDonalds-hot fudge sundae	serv	169	240	7	51	1.3	3	2.4	6	170	32	0.5	1.3	64	0	0.08	0.35	0.3	0.07	7	0.6	235	178
1855	McDonalds-hot mustard sauce	serv	30	70	1	8	0.3	4	0.5	5	250	5	0.2	0.1	2	tr	0.01	0.01	0.2	0.01	1	0	15	7
1852	McDonalds-iced cheese danish	serv	110	390	7	42	*	22	6	47	420	47	1.4	*	38	1	0.29	0.23	2.1	*	*	*	33	*
1854	McDonalds-Mcchicken sandwich	serv	190	490	19	40	1.6	29	5.4	43	780	340	2.6	1.7	31	2	0.96	0.21	8.9	0.67	33	0.35	143	299
1823	McDonalds-McDLT hamburger	item	234	580	26	36	11.5	37	11.5	109	990	*	3.9	*	226	7	0.39	0.36	6.9	*	*	*	225	*
##	McDonalds-Mclean deluxe hamburger	serv	206	320	22	35	2.4	10	4	60	670	290	3.8	3.2	67	10	0.35	0.31	5.8	0.26	48	1.48	93	170
1970	McDonalds-milkshake-chocolate-lowfat	serv	293	320	12	66	*	2	1	10	240	*	*	*	*	*	*	*	*	*	*	*	332	*
1971	McDonalds-milkshake-strawberry-lowfat	serv	293	320	11	67	*	1	1	10	170	*	*	*	*	*	*	*	*	*	*	*	327	*
1972	McDonalds-milkshake-vanilla-lowfat	serv	293	290	11	60	0	1	1	10	170	48	0.2	2.4	38	2	0.12	0.59	0.3	0.13	31	1.54	327	394
1848	McDonalds-pork sausage	serv	48	180	8	0	0	16	5.9	48	350	*	0.7	*	0	0	0.27	0.1	2.3	*	40	*	8	*
740	McDonalds-quarter pound cheeseburger	item	194	520	29	35	*	21	11.2	118	1150	341	3.7	5.7	211	3	0.37	0.39	6.7	0.23	23	2.15	295	382
739	McDonalds-quarter pounder hamburger	item	166	410	23	34	*	21	8.1	86	660	322	3.7	5.1	67	3	0.36	0.29	6.7	0.27	23	1.88	142	249
1829	McDonalds-raspberry danish	item	117	410	6	62	*	16	3.1	26	310	*	1.5	*	35	3	0.33	0.21	2.1	*	14	*	14	*
1973	McDonalds-salad dressing-peppercorn	oz	28.4	160	0	2	0	18	2	14	170	22	0	tr	6	0	tr	0.01	tr	tr	1	0.04	4	*
1974	McDonalds-salad dressing-red french	oz	28.4	80	0	10	0	4	0	0	220	22	0.1	tr	6	0	0.05	0.01	tr	tr	1	0.04	3	4
1710	McDonalds-sausage and egg biscuit	item	180	520	20	33	*	35	11.2	275	1250	319	3.2	2.2	88	tr	0.53	0.35	4	0.2	40	1.37	116	490
1826	McDonalds-sausage biscuit	item	123	440	13	32	1.4	22	9.3	49	1080	196	2	1.5	64	0	0.49	0.21	4	0.11	9	0.5	83	443
1832	McDonalds-sausage Mcmuffin	item	117	370	17	27	1.1	27	7.8	64	830	179	2.3	1.7	72	1	0.6	0.29	4.8	0.13	48	0.5	235	273
1827	McDonalds-sausage Mcmuffin with egg	item	167	440	23	28	1.6	27	9.5	263	980	255	3.3	2.4	150	0	0.64	0.42	4.8	0.19	68	0.72	263	390
1824	McDonalds-scrambled eggs	serv	98	140	12	1	0	10	3.3	399	290	102	2.1	1.1	156	0	0.07	0.26	0.1	0.08	27	1.68	57	136
1862	McDonalds-side salad	serv	115	60	4	3	1.2	3	1.5	41	85	219	0.7	0.3	217	7	0.05	0.08	0.3	0.06	40	0	76	26
1874	McDonalds-strawberry milkshake-lowfat	serv	293	320	11	67	*	1	0.6	10	170	*	0.1	*	92	0	0.13	0.48	0.3	*	3	*	327	*
1868	McDonalds-strawberry sundae	serv	171	210	6	49	0.7	6	0.6	5	95	263	0.2	1.2	64	1	0.07	0.29	0.3	0.07	9	0.54	190	127
1857	McDonalds-sweet and sour sauce	serv	32	60	tr	14	tr	tr	0.6	2	190	10	0.2	tr	65	1	0	0.01	0.1	tr	tr	0	11	3
1872	McDonalds-vanilla milkshake-lowfat	serv	293	290	11	60	*	1	0.6	10	170	*	0.1	*	92	0	0.13	0.48	0.3	*	*	*	327	*
1867	McDonalds-vanilla-frozen yogurt	serv	80	100	4	22	*	1	0.4	3	80	*	0.2	0.2	38	0	0.04	0.18	0.4	0.18	27	*	112	*
2130	Pizza-beef/chicken/onion	oz	28.3	73	6	7	tr	2	*	*	267	49	0.7	*	23	1	0.03	0.02	1.3	0.02	7	0.08	73	53
2133	Pizza-beef/onion	oz	28.3	73	4	8	0.1	3	*	*	132	50	0.9	*	23	tr	0.01	0.02	0.9	0.06	2	0.37	21	36
2131	Pizza-chicken curry/peas	oz	28.3	82	4	9	0.2	3	*	*	146	45	1.7	*	30	tr	0.02	0.03	1.7	*	*	*	19	37
2135	Pizza-chicken/mushroom/tomato	oz	28.3	61	5	7	0.1	4	*	*	167	44	0.8	*	23	tr	0.01	0.01	0.8	*	*	*	24	37
2129	Pizza-chicken/pineapple	oz	28.3	81	4	6	0.1	6	*	*	267	37	2.1	*	25	1	0.03	0.03	2.1	*	*	*	86	114
2138	Pizza-combination supreme	oz	28.3	51	7	7	0.2	7	1.3	6	165	45	1.8	0.3	10	1	0.02	0.02	1.8	0.04	7	0.08	27	39
2132	Pizza-curry beef/peas	oz	28.3	71	5	7	0.2	3	0.9	8	130	47	3.6	0.7	29	1	0.02	0.02	3.6	0.06	2	0.37	24	38
2134	Pizza-onion/tomato/green pepper/mushroom	oz	28.3	45	3	5	0.2	1	*	*	136	43	1.6	*	9	tr	0.01	0.02	1.6	0.02	25	*	25	33
2128	Pizza-pepperoni/beef/salami/mushroom/etc	oz	28.3	83	5	5	0.1	5	*	*	367	61	3.1	*	22	tr	0.02	tr	3.1	*	*	*	76	59
2136	Pizza-shrimp/cucumber	oz	28.3	69	4	7	0.1	4	*	*	143	46	0.8	0.2	12	tr	0.01	0.01	2.3	0.01	25	*	25	48
2137	Pizza-shrimp/squid/mushroom	oz	28.3	70	5	7	0.1	5	*	*	160	33	0.9	0.2	13	1	0.01	0.01	0.9	0.01	22	*	22	38
2116	Potatoes-french fried-fast food	oz	28.3	91	1	10	0	5	1.8	3	17	130	0.6	0.1	6	tr	0.02	0.01	0.4	0.07	8	0	2	20
2112	Potatoes-mashed-fast food	oz	28.3	26	1	5	0	tr	0.3	1	82	48	0.8	0.1	15	tr	0.02	0.01	0.2	0.06	2	0.02	3	14
1982	Rax-grilled chicken sandwich	item	190	440	24	36	1.6	19	2.9	88	1050	340	3.6	1.7	16	0	0.46	0.4	15.3	0.67	33	0.35	114	299
2115	Salad-fast food	oz	28.3	34	tr	3	0	tr	*	*	128	40	0.7	*	4	1	0.02	0.01	tr	*	*	*	5	14
2142	Spaghetti-vegetables/sauce/cheese	oz	28.3	28	4	3	0.3	tr	*	*	84	52	0.3	*	4	tr	0.01	0.01	0.2	*	*	*	4	10
385	Subway sandwich-ham and cheese-on wheat	item	194	673	39	86	6	22	7	73	2508	918	2.9	2.7	87	17	0.36	0.33	3.8	0.2	39	1.23	227	315
1877	Subway-bmt sandwich-on honey wheat roll	item	220	1011	45	88	6	57	20	133	3199	1002	3	2.8	174	17	0.53	0.39	3.6	0.34	45	0.76	304	527
##	Subway-bmt sandwich-on italian roll	item	213	982	44	83	5	55	20	133	3139	917	4.3	6.1	67	5	0.27	0.34	5.1	0.48	63	2.33	64	308
2031	Subway-club sandwich-on honey wheat	item	220	722	47	89	5	23	7	84	2777	1055	3.2	1.4	83	15	0.49	0.35	9.3	0.46	43	0.44	96	247
1878	Subway-club sandwich-on italian roll	item	213	693	46	83	5	22	7	84	2717	971	3.1	2.5	74	20	0.48	0.33	12.5	0.58	47	0.95	58	384
##	Subway-cold cut combo sandwich-italian	item	184	853	46	83	5	40	12	166	2218	876	2.9	2.7	87	17	0.36	0.33	3.8	0.2	39	1.23	227	315
##	Subway-cold cut combo sandwich-on wheat	item	191	883	48	88	6	41	12	166	2278	1010	3	2.8	90	18	0.37	0.35	3.9	0.21	41	1.28	235	327
##	Subway-ham & cheese sandwich-on italian	item	184	643	38	81	5	18	7	73	1710	834	2.2	2.8	174	17	0.53	0.39	3.6	0.34	45	0.76	304	527

* indicates that no data was available.

©1994 First DataBank—The Hearst Corporation (N-Squared Computing).

A 21

Appendix A - Table of Food Composition (continued)

Item	Food name	Portion	Weight (g)	Food Energy (Kcal)	Protein (gm)	Carbohydrates (gm)	Fiber (gm)	Total Fat (gm)	Saturated Fat (gm)	Cholesterol (mg)	Sodium (mg)	Potassium (mg)	Magnesium (mg)	Iron (mg)	Zinc (mg)	Vitamin A (RE)	Vitamin C (mg)	Thiamin (mg)	Riboflavin (mg)	Niacin (mg)	Vitamin B6 (mg)	Folates (µg)	Vitamin B12 (µg)	Calcium (mg)	Phosphorus (mg)
###	Subway-meatball sandwich-on italian roll	item	215	918	42	96	3	44	17	88	2022	1210	47	5	6.2	72	19	0.33	0.39	9.4	0.4	35	3.21	78	263
###	Subway-meatball-on honey wheat roll	item	224	947	44	101	*	45	17	88	2082	1498	*	3.7	5.3	58	*	0.23	0.29	4.4	0.42	54	2.01	55	266
###	Subway-roast beef sandwich-italian roll	item	184	689	42	84	5	23	8	83	2288	910	57	3.8	5.4	58	5	0.24	0.3	4.5	0.43	56	2.07	56	273
1984	Subway-roast beef sandwich-on wheat roll	item	189	717	41	89	6	24	8	75	2348	994	59	3.8	5.4	59	5	0.24	0.3	4.5	*	*	*	*	*
1985	Subway-salad dressing-buttermilk ranch	serv	56.7	348	1	2	0	37	5	6	492	17	1	0.1	0.1	48	5	0.01	0.01	tr	0.01	4	0.12	8	15
###	Subway-salad dressing-lite italian	serv	56.7	23	1	4	0	1	4	0	952	13	tr	0.1	0.1	14	5	0.01	0.01	tr	0.01	3	0.09	6	3
###	Subway-seafood/crab sandwich-on italian	item	210	986	29	94	*	57	11	56	1967	557	62	4.4	5.3	107	*	0.51	0.38	7	0.26	91	6.54	230	336
###	Subway-seafood/crab sandwich-on wheat	item	219	1015	31	100	2.5	58	11	56	2027	641	*	*	*	*	5	*	*	*	*	*	*	*	*
###	Subway-spicy italian sandwich-on italian	item	213	1043	42	83	6	63	23	137	2282	880	43	4.2	6.8	119	6	0.33	0.46	5.1	0.38	36	2.54	231	456
1916	Subway-steak & cheese sandwich-italian	item	213	765	43	83	6	32	12	82	1556	909	tr	*	*	*	*	*	*	*	*	*	*	*	*
###	Subway-turkey breast sandwich-wheat roll	item	192	674	17	88	7	20	6	67	2520	605	*	3.8	3	240	3	0.28	0.6	3.9	0.21	73	1	144	143
743	Taco Bell-bean burrito	item	168	332	13	43	6.4	12	5.6	79	1030	405	41	3.1	2.4	42	1	0.12	0.46	3.2	0.16	20	0.99	88	88
744	Taco Bell-beef burrito	item	110	262	16	29	1.3	10	5.2	33	746	370	*	2.5	2.5	383	4	0.09	0.5	2.9	0.26	tr	1.13	42	173
745	Taco Bell-beefy tostada	serv	225	334	21	30	5.2	17	11.5	75	870	490	68	3.8	5.9	216	8	0.45	0.92	6.2	0.27	43	1.53	190	245
748	Taco Bell-burrito supreme	item	225	457	21	43	5	22	7.7	126	367	350	52	3.8	5.9	286	9	0.43	2.19	3.7	0.35	132	2.18	146	548
1840	Taco Bell-double beef burrito supreme	item	255	457	24	42	5.7	22	10.1	57	1053	431	87	4	5.9	290	28	0.26	0.42	2.3	0.27	*	*	145	*
1846	Taco Bell-enchirito	item	213	382	20	31	*	20	9.3	54	1243	*	*	2.8	2.3	295	31	0.32	0.33	3	*	113	0.2	269	360
1843	Taco Bell-Mexican pizza	serv	223	575	21	40	5.8	37	11.4	52	1031	408	63	3.7	2.6	169	2	0.01	0.16	0.7	0.12	16	0.62	257	439
1833	Taco Bell-nachos	serv	106	346	7	38	1.4	19	5.7	9	399	159	43	0.9	1.1	341	58	0.1	0.34	2.2	*	98	0.08	191	175
1834	Taco Bell-nachos Bellgrande	serv	287	649	22	61	7	35	12.3	36	997	674	*	3.5	1.4	132	51	0.05	0.15	0.4	0.19	40	0.31	297	132
1845	Taco Bell-pintos & cheese	serv	128	190	9	22	4.9	16	3.6	16	642	399	50	1.4	2.4	64	5	0.39	0.22	2.7	0.16	71	0.55	156	234
1836	Taco Bell-soft taco	item	92.1	228	12	18	2.6	12	5.4	32	516	178	31	2.3	*	254	5	0.11	0.29	2	0.28	*	*	116	203
1835	Taco Bell-taco Bellgrande	item	163	355	18	18	4.5	23	10.9	56	472	334	54	1.9	9.1	199	5	0.2	0.33	2.5	0.24	23	1.04	182	116
1844	Taco Bell-taco light	item	170	410	19	18	*	29	11.6	56	594	316	63	2.4	2.3	908	76	0.26	0.45	3.2	0.17	75	2.26	155	1015
1838	Taco Bell-taco salad with salsa/no shell	serv	530	520	31	30	7	31	14.4	80	1431	1151	111	5.1	9.1	888	77	0.51	0.64	4.8	1.94	99	2.92	367	567
1837	Taco Bell-taco salad with salsa/shell	serv	595	941	36	63	7	61	18.7	80	1662	1212	125	7.1	10.3	572	74	0.25	0.75	3.2	0.38	51	0.3	398	637
1839	Taco Bell-taco salad-no salsa-no shell	serv	530	502	30	26	7	61	14.4	80	1056	988	111	4.5	9.1	257	1	0.15	0.5	3.2	0.24	31	0.22	331	567
746	Taco Bell-taco-regular	item	171	370	21	27	1.2	21	11.4	57	802	473	71	2.4	3.9	187	16	0.1	0.33	1.3	0.48	45	0.17	221	259
747	Taco Bell-tostada-regular	serv	144	223	10	27	4	10	5.4	30	543	403	59	1.9	1.9	266	1	0.36	0.81	14.5	0.13	6	0.14	211	58
1986	Wendys-bacon and cheese potato	serv	347	450	27	57	9.9	18	37.1	10	1125	1580	167	15.3	7	162	34	1.04	0.39	7.6	0.23	41	1.46	713	1015
1987	Wendys-big classic-quarter pound burger	serv	277	570	27	46	2.3	33	15.9	85	1075	590	49	4.8	6.4	266	9	0.35	0.5	8	0.54	27	4.07	304	491
1988	Wendys-broccoli and cheese potato	serv	377	400	9	59	*	16	*	0	470	1555	*	4.8	*	162	77	*	*	2.2	0.32	39	0	417	398
1989	Wendys-cheese potato	serv	348	470	13	57	3.6	2	12.1	0	580	1435	72	2.3	2.4	288	34	0.22	0.43	3.5	0.57	31	0.3	417	398
1990	Wendys-cheese sauce	serv	56	40	1	5	0.2	2	1.9	0	300	70	10	0.1	0.2	24	tr	0.03	0.11	0.1	0.03	3	0.22	114	88
1991	Wendys-cheese tortellini/spaghetti sauce	serv	112	120	4	24	1	1	2.8	5	280	110	14	1.3	0.6	110	4	0.12	0.18	1.2	0.09	12	0.17	75	92
1992	Wendys-chicken club sandwich	item	231	500	30	42	2.3	24	5.5	75	950	515	42	14.4	1.5	87	16	0.51	0.37	16	0.48	45	0.46	101	259
1993	Wendys-chicken salad	serv	56	120	7	4	0.2	8	3	45	215	60	8	0.5	0.7	22	1	0.02	0.08	1.8	0.13	6	0.14	13	58
1994	Wendys-chili	serv	255	220	21	23	4.6	6	3	45	750	495	53	6.3	4.1	146	19	0.16	0.26	4.8	0.23	41	1.46	55	228
755	Wendys-double hamburger	item	226	540	34	40	2.3	27	10.5	122	791	569	49	6	5.7	31	3	0.36	0.39	7.6	0.54	27	4.07	102	314
1995	Wendys-french fries-regular size	serv	134	440	5	53	4.6	23	8.5	25	265	855	46	1	0.5	0	14	0.24	0.04	4.4	0.32	39	0	26	125
1996	Wendys-kids meal hamburger	item	104	260	14	30	1.3	9	3.5	35	545	205	22	2.5	2.2	7	1	0.23	0.2	3.8	0.14	25	1	63	110
1997	Wendys-refried beans	serv	56	70	4	10	3	3	1	0	215	210	25	1.2	0.5	0	2	0.08	0.04	0.2	0.09	71	0	25	72
1998	Wendys-seafood salad	serv	56	110	4	7	0.2	1	0.1	0	455	40	14	0.5	0.9	21	3	0.02	0.03	0.6	0.05	8	0.48	74	74
1999	Wendys-single cheeseburger/everything	serv	252	490	29	35	2.7	27	10.8	90	1155	495	44	4.3	4.3	136	11	0.4	0.42	6.5	0.3	55	1.8	234	348
754	Wendys-single hamburger	item	218	511	26	29	2.8	27	10.4	86	825	479	43	4.9	4.9	93	11	0.42	0.38	7.3	0.33	36	2.38	96	233
###	Wendys-single hamburger/everything	serv	234	420	25	35	2.7	21	6.7	70	865	495	40	4.3	3.7	76	11	0.4	0.35	6.6	0.29	54	1.68	105	193
2001	Wendys-spanish rice	serv	56	70	2	13	0.7	1	0.1	0	440	130	9	0.7	0.2	24	9	0.05	0.02	0.6	0.06	4	0	15	17
###	Wendys-taco salad with taco chips	serv	791	660	40	46	10.5	37	28.8	35	1110	1330	166	9.2	13.6	1478	67	0.4	0.93	15.2	1.16	147	6.41	532	847
756	Wendys-triple hamburger	item	259	693	50	29	*	42	15.9	142	713	785	55	8.3	10.8	47	1	0.31	0.56	11	0.62	31	4.92	65	393
###	Wendys-tuna salad	serv	56	100	8	4	0.3	6	1	0	290	90	10	0.6	0.2	15	1	0.02	0.04	3.8	0.05	4	0.68	9	62

Fats & oils

No.	Fats & oils	Unit																									
105	Butter-regular-pat	item	5	36	tr	tr	0	0	4	2.5	11	41	1	tr	tr	8	0	tr	tr	0.01	tr	0	tr	0.01	1	1
103	Butter-regular-stick	item	113	813	tr	1	0	0	92	57.3	248	937	29	2	0.2	0.1	855	0	tr	0.04	0.01	tr	tr	3	0.14	27	26
104	Butter-regular-tablespoon	tbsp	14	100	tr	tr	0	0	11	7.1	31	116	4	tr	tr	tr	105	0	tr	0.01	0.02	tr	0	tr	0.02	3	3
855	Butter-unsalted-pat	item	5	36	tr	tr	0.1	0	4	2.5	11	1	1	tr	tr	tr	38	0	0	tr	0.01	tr	tr	tr	0.01	1	1
108	Butter-whipped-pat	item	3.8	27	tr	tr	0	0	3	1.9	8	31	tr	tr	tr	tr	29	0	tr	tr	0.01	tr	0	tr	0.01	1	1
106	Butter-whipped-stick	item	75.6	542	tr	1	0	0	61	38.2	165	625	20	2	0.1	tr	570	0	tr	0.03	0.1	tr	2	2	0.1	18	17
107	Butter-whipped-tablespoon	tbsp	9	65	tr	tr	0	0	7	4.5	20	74	2	tr	tr	tr	68	0	0	tr	0.01	tr	0	tr	0.01	2	2
878	Butter-whipped-unsalted-pat	item	3.8	27	tr	tr	0	0	3	1.9	8	tr	1	tr	0	0	29	0	0	tr	0.01	tr	0	0	0.01	1	1
856	Fat-animal-chicken-for cooking	tbsp	12.8	115	0	0	0	0	13	3.8	11	tr	tr	0	0	0	29	0	0	0	0	tr	0	0	0	1	0
111	Fat-animal-lard (pork)	cup	205	1849	0	0	0	0	205	80.4	195	tr	tr	0	0	0.2	0	0	tr	0	0	0	0	0	0	tr	0
858	Margarine-corn-regular-hydrogenated-hard	tsp	4.7	34	0	0	0	0	4	0.6	0	44	2	tr	tr	*	47	tr	tr	tr	tr	tr	0	tr	tr	1	1
863	Margarine-corn-regular-soft	tsp	4.7	34	0	0	0	0	4	0.7	0	51	2	tr	tr	0	47	tr	tr	tr	tr	tr	0	tr	tr	1	1
859	Margarine-corn/soybean-unsalted	tsp	4.7	34	0	0	0	0	4	0.7	0	tr	1	tr	0	0	47	tr	tr	tr	tr	tr	0	tr	tr	1	1
110	Margarine-diet/low calorie-Mazola	tbsp	14	50	0	0	0	0	6	1	0	130	1	tr	0	0	130	0	0	tr	0	0	0	0	0	0	tr
868	Margarine-imitation-40% fat	tsp	4.8	17	0	0	0	0	2	0.4	0	46	tr	tr	0	0	48	tr	0	tr	0	tr	0	0	0	1	tr
869	Margarine-imitation-spread-60% fat	tsp	4.8	26	0	0	0	0	3	0.6	0	48	1	tr	0	0	48	tr	0	tr	tr	tr	0	tr	tr	1	1
867	Margarine-liquid-regular-soybean	tsp	4.7	34	tr	tr	0	0	4	0.6	0	37	4	tr	0	0	47	tr	0	tr	0.01	tr	0	tr	0.01	3	2
112	Margarine-no stick-spray-Mazola	serv	0.72	6	0	0	0	0	1	0.1	0	0	*	*	0	*	0	*	*	*	*	*	*	*	*	0	0
862	Margarine-regular-hard-unsalted	tsp	4.7	34	0	0	0	0	4	0.7	0	tr	1	tr	0	0	47	tr	0	tr	tr	tr	0	tr	tr	1	1
866	Margarine-regular-soft-unsalted	tsp	4.7	34	0	0	0	0	4	0.6	0	1	2	tr	0	0	47	tr	0	tr	tr	tr	0	tr	0.01	1	1
115	Margarine-regular-unspecified oils-pat	item	5	36	tr	tr	0	0	4	0.8	0	47	2	tr	0	0	15	tr	tr	tr	0.01	tr	0	tr	0.01	2	tr
113	Margarine-regular-unspecified oils-stick	item	113	812	1	1	0	0	91	17.9	0	1066	48	3	0.1	0.1	338	tr	0.01	0.04	0.11	tr	1	1	0.11	34	26
114	Margarine-regular-unspecified oils-tbsp	tbsp	14	101	0	tr	0	0	11	2.2	0	132	6	tr	0	0	139	tr	tr	0.01	0.01	tr	tr	tr	0.01	4	3
864	Margarine-safflower-regular-soft-tub	tsp	4.7	34	0	0	0	0	4	0.4	0	51	2	tr	0	0	47	tr	0	tr	tr	tr	0	tr	tr	1	1
860	Margarine-safflower/soybean-hydrogenated	tsp	4.7	34	0	0	0	0	4	0.6	0	44	2	tr	0	0	47	tr	0	tr	tr	tr	0	tr	tr	1	1
865	Margarine-soybean-soft-tub-unsalted	tsp	4.7	34	0	0	0	0	4	0.6	0	1	2	tr	0	0	47	tr	0	tr	tr	tr	0	tr	0.01	4	3
117	Margarine-unspecified oils-soft-tbsp	tbsp	14	100	0	tr	0	0	11	1.9	0	151	5	tr	0	0	139	tr	0	tr	0.01	tr	0	4	0.01	4	3
116	Margarine-unspecified oils-soft-tub	cup	227	1626	2	1	0	0	183	31.3	0	2449	86	5	0.4	0.4	675	tr	0.02	0.07	0.19	2	2	60	0.19	60	46
119	Margarine-whipped	tbsp	9	70	0	0	0	0	8	1.4	0	97	2	tr	0	0	310	0	tr	0.01	0.01	tr	0	2	0.01	2	2
870	Mayonnaise-imitation-milk cream	tbsp	15	15	tr	2	0	0	1	0.4	6	76	15	1	0.1	0	tr	tr	tr	0.02	0.04	tr	tr	11	0.04	11	9
871	Mayonnaise-imitation-soybean	tbsp	15	35	0	2	0	0	3	0.5	4	75	2	tr	tr	0	0	0	0	0	0	0	0	tr	0	tr	tr
872	Mayonnaise-imitation-soybean-chol free	tbsp	14	68	0	2	0	0	7	1.1	0	49	1	tr	tr	0	0	0	0	0	0.01	0	0	0	0	tr	tr
1463	Mayonnaise-light-low calorie-Kraft	tbsp	14	40	1	1	0	0	4	0.5	5	15	0	0	tr	0	1	0	0	0	0.01	0	0	0	0.01	1	0
138	Mayonnaise-soybean-commercial	tbsp	14	99	tr	tr	0	0	11	1.6	8	78	5	tr	0.1	tr	12	tr	0.04	0.04	0.04	0	1	1	0.04	2	4
120	Oil-vegetable-corn	cup	218	1927	0	0	0	0	218	27.7	0	tr	0	0	0	0	0	0	0	0	0	0	0	0	0	0	0
122	Oil-vegetable-olive	cup	216	1909	0	0	0	0	216	30.7	0	tr	tr	tr	0.8	0.1	0	0	0	0	0	0	0	tr	0	tr	3
124	Oil-vegetable-peanut	cup	216	1909	0	0	0	0	216	36.4	0	tr	tr	tr	0.1	0.1	0	0	0	0	0	0	0	tr	0	tr	0
861	Oil-vegetable-rice bran	cup	13.6	120	0	0	0	0	14	2.7	0	0	0	0	tr	tr	0	0	0	0	0	0	0	0	0	0	0
126	Oil-vegetable-safflower	cup	218	1927	0	0	0	0	218	20.5	0	0	0	0	tr	tr	0	0	0	0	0	0	0	0	0	0	0
857	Oil-vegetable-sesame	tbsp	13.6	120	0	0	0	0	14	1.9	0	0	0	0	0	0	0	0	0	0	0	0	0	0	0	0	0
128	Oil-vegetable-soybean	cup	218	1927	0	0	0	0	218	31.8	0	0	0	0	0.1	0	0	0	0	0	0	0	0	0	0	0	0
130	Oil-vegetable-soybean/cottonseed	cup	218	1927	0	0	0	0	218	38.2	0	0	0	0	0	0	0	0	0	0	0	0	0	0	0	tr	0
132	Salad dressing-blue cheese	tbsp	15.3	77	1	1	0.1	1	8	1.5	9	167	6	tr	0	tr	10	tr	0.02	0.02	0.01	0	1	12	0.04	12	11
133	Salad dressing-blue cheese-low calorie	tbsp	16	10	0	1	0	1	1	0.5	4	177	5	tr	tr	*	9	0	0.01	0.01	*	*	*	tr	*	10	8
1586	Salad dressing-caesar	cup	15	70	0	1	tr	7	7	*	*	*	*	*	*	*	tr	*	*	*	*	*	*	*	*	*	*
134	Salad dressing-french	tbsp	15.6	67	tr	3	0.1	6	6	1.5	2	214	12	tr	0.1	tr	3	0	tr	tr	0.02	tr	0	1	0.02	2	2
135	Salad dressing-french-low calorie	tbsp	16.3	22	tr	4	0.1	1	1	0.1	1	128	13	0	0.1	0	0	0	0	0	0	0	0	0	0	2	2
1589	Salad dressing-garlic-prepared from mix	tbsp	16	83	tr	1	tr	9	9	1.4	0	222	6	1	0.1	tr	7	0	0	0	0	*	*	3	0	3	3
1588	Salad dressing-Green Goddess	tbsp	14	68	1	1	0	7	7	1	0	150	9	tr	tr	0	10	tr	tr	0.01	0.04	tr	1	2	0.04	2	1
144	Salad dressing-home recipe-cooked	tbsp	16	25	1	2	0	2	2	0.5	8	117	19	1	0.1	0	20	tr	0.02	0.02	0	0.01	1	13	0.02	13	14
136	Salad dressing-italian	tbsp	14.7	69	0	2	0.1	7	7	1	0	116	2	tr	0	tr	4	0	0	0	0.02	tr	1	1	0.02	1	1

* indicates that no data was available.

©1994 First DataBank—The Hearst Corporation (N-Squared Computing).

Appendix A - Table of Food Composition
(continued)

Item	Food name	Portion	Weight (g)	Food Energy (Kcal)	Protein (gm)	Carbohydrates (gm)	Fiber (gm)	Total Fat (gm)	Saturated Fat (gm)	Cholesterol (mg)	Sodium (mg)	Potassium (mg)	Magnesium (mg)	Iron (mg)	Zinc (mg)	Vitamin A (RE)	Vitamin C (mg)	Thiamin (mg)	Riboflavin (mg)	Niacin (mg)	Vitamin B6 (mg)	Folates (µg)	Vitamin B12 (µg)	Calcium (mg)	Phosphorus (mg)
137	Salad dressing-italian-low calorie	tbsp	15	16	0	1	0.1	2	0.2	1	118	2	0	0	tr	0		0	0	0	0	0	0	0	1
139	Salad dressing-mayonnaise type	tbsp	14.7	57	0	4	0	5	0.7	4	104	1	tr	0	tr	10		0	0	0	tr	1	0.03	2	4
140	Salad dressing-mayonnaise-low calorie	tbsp	16	20	0	2	0	2	0.4	4	44	1	*	0	*	12	*	0	0	0	*	*	*	3	4
1532	Salad dressing-Miracle Whip light	tbsp	14	45	0	2	0	4	*	5	95	1	0	0	0	0		0	0	0	0	0	0	2	*
876	Salad dressing-oil/vinegar-home recipe	tbsp	15.6	70	0	tr	0	8	1.4	0	tr	1	tr	0	0	0		0	0	0	0	0	0.03	2	1
1587	Salad dressing-ranch style	tbsp	15	54	tr	1	0	6	0.7	4	97	1	tr	0.1	0.1	13		0.01	0.01	0.1	tr	1	0.05	3	4
874	Salad dressing-russian	tbsp	15.3	76	tr	2	tr	8	1.1	0	133	24	tr	0.1	0.1	32		0.01	0.01	0.1	0.01	2	0.02	3	6
873	Salad dressing-russian-low calorie	tbsp	16.3	23	tr	5	0.2	tr	0.1	0	141	26	tr	0.1	tr	3		tr	tr	tr	tr	tr	0	3	6
875	Salad dressing-sesame seed	tbsp	15.3	68	1	1	0.2	7	0.9	0	153	24	tr	0.1	tr	32		tr	tr	tr	tr	0	0.03	3	*
1594	Salad dressing-sweet and sour	tbsp	15	29	tr	7	0.3	tr	0	0	68	14	tr	tr	tr	15		tr	0	tr	tr	tr	0	1	1
142	Salad dressing-thousand island	tbsp	15.6	59	0	2	0.6	6	0.9	5	109	18	tr	0.1	0.1	15		0	0	0	0	1	0.03	2	3
143	Salad dressing-thousand-low calorie	tbsp	15.3	24	tr	3	0.3	5	0.2	2	153	17	tr	0.1	tr	15		0	0	0	0	1	0.03	2	3
877	Sandwich spread-commercial	tbsp	15.3	60	0	3	tr	5	0.8	12	153	5	0	0	tr	0		0	0	0	0	0	0	0	0
109	Shortening-vegetable-soybean/cottonseed	cup	205	1812	0	0	0	205	51.2	0	0	0	0	0	0	0	0	0	0	0	0	0	0	0	0
356	Vegetable spray-Pam-butter flavored	serv	0.9	7	0	0	0	1	0.1	0	0	0	*	*	*	0	*	*	*	*	*	*	*	0	0
357	Vegetable spray-Pam-unflavored	serv	0.9	7	0	0	0	1	0.1	0	0	0	*	*	*	0	0	*	*	*	*	*	*	0	0
Fish																									
1416	Fish eggs-carp/cod/pike/shad-roe-raw	oz	28.4	39	6	tr	0	2	0.4	106	26	63	6	0.2	0.3	22	5	0.07	0.21	0.5	0.05	23	2.84	6	114
1395	Fish eggs-caviar-sturgeon-granular	tbsp	16	40	4	1	0	3	0.7	94	240	29	48	1.9	0.2	90	0	0.03	0.1	tr	0.05	8	3.2	44	57
149	Fish sticks-breaded-frozen-cooked	oz	28.4	77	4	7	0.7	3	0.9	32	165	74	7	0.2	0.2	9	0	0.04	0.05	0.6	0.02	5	0.51	5	51
1679	Fish-abalone-cooked-fried	serv	85	161	17	9	0.3	6	1.4	80	502	241	47	3.2	0.8	2	2	0.19	0.11	1.6	0.13	4	0.59	32	184
1678	Fish-abalone-raw	serv	85	89	15	5	0	1	0.1	72	256	213	41	2.7	0.7	2	2	0.16	0.09	1.3	0.13	1	0.62	26	162
1391	Fish-anchovy-fillet-canned	item	4	8	1	0	0	tr	0.1	3	147	22	3	0.2	0.1	1	0	tr	0.02	0.8	0.01	*	0.04	9	10
1392	Fish-bass-black-baked	oz	28.4	32	5	0	0	1	0.2	19	20	101	9	0.4	0.2	*	*	*	*	*	*	*	*	23	57
1393	Fish-bass-striped-broiled	serv	159	154	28	0	0	4	0.8	127	110	501	79	1.3	0.6	170	3	0.19	0.22	2.9	0.69	10	6.07	22	373
1525	Fish-bass-striped-oven fried	item	200	392	43	13	0.3	17	1.8			*	16	1.1	*	24	*	0.17	0.16	2.9	*	*		45	
145	Fish-bluefish-baked with butter	item	155	246	41	0	0	8	1.8	108	161	558	43	1.1	1.2	179	tr	0.09	0.12	2.9	0.6	2	1.64	10	445
1394	Fish-bluefish-broiled	serv	150	186	30	0	0	6	1.4	88	90	363	50	0.7	1.6	8	1	0.12	0.06	8.9	0.19	15	8.09	44	341
1641	Fish-carp-cooked-dry heat	serv	85	138	19	0	0	6	1.2	72	54	289	32	1.4	0.7	7	0	0.06	0.11	1.8	0.16	14	1.25	37	451
1642	Fish-catfish-breaded-fried	serv	85	195	15	7	0.8	11	2.8	69	238	277	23	1.2	1.2	7	0	0.09	0.21	1.9	0.05	16	1.62	54	184
1681	Fish-clams-breaded-fried	serv	85	172	12	9	0.3	9	2.3	52	309		12	11.8	1.2	77	9	0.09	0.03	1.8	*	*	34.2	16	160
147	Fish-clams-canned-solids and liquids	oz	28.4	13	2	1	0	tr	0.1	18	15	40	*	1.2	0.3	*	*	tr	*	0.3	*	*	5.4	23	39
1682	Fish-clams-cooked-moist heat	serv	85	126	22	4	0	2	0.2	57	95	534	16	23.8	2.3	145	19	0.13	0.36	2.9	0.09	16	84.1	78	287
146	Fish-clams-raw-meat only	serv	85	63	11	0	0	1	0.1	29	48	267	8	11.9	1.2	77	11	0.07	0.18	1.5	0.05	14	42	39	144
1396	Fish-cod-Atlantic-cooked-dry heat	piece	180	189	41	0	0	2	0.3	99	141	440	76	0.9	1	25	2	0.16	0.14	4.5	0.51	15	1.89	25	248
1397	Fish-crab cake	item	60	93	12	tr	tr	5	0.9	90	198	195	20	0.7	2.5	49	2	0.05	0.05	1.7	0.1	25	3.56	63	128
148	Fish-crab meat-king-canned-unpacked	cup	135	135	24	1	0	3	0.6	135	675	149	29	1.1	5.8	*	*	0.11	0.11	2.6	*	*	13.5	61	246
1670	Fish-crab-Alaska king-raw	serv	85	71	16	0	0	1	0.1	36	711	173	42	0.5	5.1	6	6	0.04	0.04	0.9	0.13	37	7.65	39	186
1673	Fish-crab-blue-canned	cup	135	134	28	0	0	2	0.3	120	450	505	53	1.1	5.4	3	4	0.11	0.11	1.9	0.2	*	0.62	136	351
1674	Fish-crab-blue-cooked-moist heat	cup	135	138	27	0	0	2	0.3	135	376	437	64	1.2	5.7	3	4	0.14	0.07	4.5	0.24	69	9.86	140	278
1526	Fish-crab-deviled	cup	240	451	27	32	2.3	23	4.8	223	2081	398	64	2.9	5.5	330	14	0.19	0.26	3.6	0.31	88	8.69	113	329
1672	Fish-crab-dungeness-raw	serv	85	73	15	1	0	1	0.1	50	251	301	38	0.3	3.6	23	3	0.04	0.14	2.7	0.13	37	7.65	39	155
1671	Fish-crab-imitation-surimi	serv	85	87	10	9	0	1	0.2	17	715	77	37	0.3	0.3	17	0	0.03	0.02	0.2	0.03	*	1.36	11	240
1527	Fish-crab-imperial	cup	220	323	32	9	0	17	4.2	275	1602	288	57	2	6.4	211	11	0.13	0.26	2.4	0.31	83	10.6	132	365
1399	Fish-crab-steamed-pieces	cup	155	150	30	0	0	2	0.2	151	1662	406	53	1.2	11.8	14	12	0.08	0.09	2.1	0.28	79	17.8	92	434
1675	Fish-crayfish-cooked-moist heat	serv	85	97	20	0	0	1	0.2	151	58	298	26	2.7	1.4	19	0	0.15	0.07	2.5	0.15	*	2.94	84	281
1644	Fish-croaker-breaded-fried	serv	85	188	16	6	0.3	11	3	71	296	289	35	0.7	0.4	19	4	0.16	0.11	3.7	0.22	15	1.79	27	184
1645	Fish-eel-cooked-dry heat	serv	85	201	20	0	0	13	2.6	137	55	297	22	0.5	1.8	966	2	0.16	0.04	3.8	0.07	15	2.45	22	235
1646	Fish-flatfish-cooked-dry heat	serv	85	100	21	0	0	1	0.3	58	89	292	49	0.3	0.5	9	0	0.07	0.1	1.9	0.2	8	2.13	15	246
1735	Fish-gefiltefish-commercial-with broth	piece	42	35	4	3	tr	1	0.2	13	220	38	4	1	0.3	11	tr	0.03	0.03	0.4	0.03	1	0.35	10	31

Code	Food	Measure	g																						
1647	Fish-grouper-cooked-dry heat	serv	85	100	21	0	0	1	0.3	40	45	403	32	1	0.4	43	0	0.07	0.01	0.3	0.3	9	0.59	18	121
150	Fish-haddock-breaded-fried	piece	85	140	17	5	0.3	5	1.4	42	150	296	*	1	*	*	2	0.03	0.06	2.7	*	*	1.1	34	210
1401	Fish-haddock-broiled	serv	85	95	21	0	0	tr	0.1	63	74	339	43	1.2	0.4	16	0	0.03	0.04	3.9	0.29	11	1.18	36	205
1402	Fish-halibut-all types-broiled in butter	piece	125	214	32	0	0	9	*	75	168	656	*	1	*	255	0	0.06	0.09	10.4	*	*	*	20	310
1708	Fish-halibut-cooked-broiled	serv	85	119	23	0	0	2	0.4	35	59	490	91	0.9	0.5	46	*	0.06	0.08	6.1	0.34	12	1.16	51	242
1403	Fish-herring-Atlantic-broiled	serv	85	173	20	0	0	10	2.2	66	98	356	35	1.2	1.1	26	1	0.1	0.25	3.5	0.3	10	11.2	63	258
1649	Fish-herring-Atlantic-raw	serv	85	134	15	0	0	8	1.7	51	76	278	27	0.9	0.8	24	1	0.08	0.2	2.7	0.26	9	11.6	49	201
1404	Fish-herring-canned-solids and liquids	serv	100	208	20	0	0	14	*	98	*	*	*	1.8	*	*	*	0.18	*	*	*	1	2.14	147	297
1405	Fish-herring-pickled-bismarck type	item	50	131	7	5	0	9	1.2	7	435	35	4	0.6	0.3	129	0	0.02	0.07	1.7	0.09	1	2.14	39	45
1407	Fish-lobster newburg	cup	250	485	46	13	0	27	30.1	376	573	428	56	2.3	4.2	530	1	0.18	0.28	1.6	0.17	32	4.11	218	480
1408	Fish-lobster thermidor	serv	157	405	29	15	0	27	18.9	236	360	388	35	1.9	2.6	295	0	0.15	0.51	4.8	0.11	20	2.58	290	451
1676	Fish-lobster-cooked-moist heat	oz	28.4	28	6	tr	0	tr	tr	20	108	100	10	0.1	0.8	7	0	tr	0.02	0.3	0.02	3	0.88	17	53
1406	Fish-lobster-northern-raw	oz	28.4	26	5	tr	0	tr	0.1	27	84	78	8	0.3	0.9	6	0	tr	0.01	0.4	0.01	3	0.26	14	41
1410	Fish-mackerel-Atlantic-canned	cup	190	296	44	0	0	12	3.4	150	720	369	70	3.9	1.9	248	2	0.08	0.4	11.7	0.4	10	13.2	458	572
1409	Fish-mackerel-Atlantic-raw	oz	28.4	58	5	0	0	4	0.9	20	26	89	22	0.5	0.2	14	tr	0.05	0.09	2.6	0.11	tr	2.47	3	62
1650	Fish-mackerel-cooked-dry heat	serv	85	223	20	0	0	15	3.6	64	71	341	83	1.3	0.8	46	tr	0.14	0.35	5.8	0.39	1	16.2	13	236
1651	Fish-mullet-cooked-dry heat	serv	85	128	21	0	0	4	1.2	54	60	389	28	1.2	0.7	36	1	0.09	0.09	5.4	0.42	8	0.21	26	207
1684	Fish-mussel-blue-cooked-moist heat	serv	85	147	20	6	0	4	0.7	48	313	228	32	5.7	2.3	77	12	0.26	0.36	2.6	0.09	64	20.4	28	242
1411	Fish-mussels-Atlantic/Pacific-meat only	oz	28.4	27	4	6	0	1	*	16	81	90	*	1	*	*	12	0.06	0.05	2.4	*	63	18	25	67
1683	Fish-mussels-blue-raw	cup	150	129	18	6	0.1	3	0.6	42	429	479	51	5.9	2.4	72	12	0.24	0.32	2.4	0.1	3	18	39	192
151	Fish-ocean perch-breaded-fried	piece	85	195	16	6	0	11	2.7	32	128	242	*	1.1	*	*	12	0.05	0.1	1.6	*	*	0.85	28	235
1652	Fish-ocean perch-cooked-dry heat	serv	85	103	20	0	0	2	0.3	46	82	298	33	1	0.5	12	1	0.11	0.11	2.1	0.23	9	0.98	117	158
1413	Fish-octopus-raw	serv	85	70	13	2	0	1	0.2	41	196	298	26	4.5	1.4	38	4	0.03	0.03	1.8	0.31	14	17	45	344
1685	Fish-oyster-eastern-canned	cup	248	171	18	10	0	6	1.6	136	278	568	134	16.6	226	223	12	0.37	0.41	3.1	0.24	22	47.5	112	236
1686	Fish-oyster-eastern-cooked-moist heat	serv	85	117	12	7	0	4	1.1	93	190	389	93	11.4	155	145	7	0.25	0.28	2.1	0.08	15	32.5	76	135
1412	Fish-oysters-eastern-cooked-fried	serv	85	167	7	10	0.1	11	2.7	69	355	208	49	5.9	74.1	77	3	0.13	0.17	1.4	0.05	12	13.3	53	344
152	Fish-oysters-eastern-raw-meat only	cup	248	171	18	10	0	6	1.6	136	277	568	135	16.6	226	222	12	0.34	0.41	3.3	0.12	25	47.5	111	138
1687	Fish-oysters-Pacific-raw	serv	85	69	8	4	0	2	0.4	43	90	143	19	4.3	14.1	69	7	0.06	0.2	1.7	0.04	9	13.6	7	218
1653	Fish-perch-cooked-dry heat	serv	85	100	21	0	0	1	0.2	98	67	292	32	1	1.2	9	1	0.07	0.1	1.6	0.12	5	1.87	87	239
1654	Fish-pike-cooked-dry heat	serv	85	96	21	0	0	1	0.1	43	42	281	34	0.6	0.7	20	3	0.06	0.07	2.4	0.12	15	1.96	62	188
1663	Fish-pollock-Atlantic-raw	serv	85	78	17	0	0	1	0.1	60	73	303	57	0.4	0.4	9	0	0.04	0.16	2.8	0.24	3	2.71	51	410
1655	Fish-pollock-cooked-dry heat	serv	85	96	20	0	0	1	0.2	82	99	329	62	0.5	0.5	20	0	0.06	0.07	1.4	0.06	3	3.57	5	290
1656	Fish-pompano-cooked-dry heat	serv	85	179	20	0	0	10	3.8	54	65	541	27	0.6	0.6	31	0	0.58	0.13	3.2	0.2	15	1.02	36	171
1661	Fish-red snapper-cooked-dry heat	serv	85	109	22	0	0	1	0.3	40	48	444	31	0.2	0.4	30	1	0.05	tr	0.3	0.39	5	2.98	34	169
1414	Fish-red snapper-raw	serv	85	85	17	0	0	1	0.2	31	54	355	27	0.2	0.3	26	1	0.04	tr	0.2	0.34	4	2.55	27	169
1415	Fish-rockfish-cooked-dry heat	serv	100	121	24	0	0	2	0.5	44	77	520	34	0.5	0.5	66	1	0.04	0.08	3.9	0.27	10	1.2	12	228
1419	Fish-salmon patty	serv	100	239	16	16	1	12	3.5	64	96	89	34	1.2	0.8	20	4	0.12	0.22	4	0.07	13	3	78	104
1420	Fish-salmon rice loaf	serv	100	122	7	7	0.7	5	2.9	116	753	275	32	1.2	0.9	115	2	0.08	0.28	4.3	0.21	21	2.24	180	262
1417	Fish-salmon-broiled or baked-with butter	serv	100	182	27	0	0	7	1.4	47	116	443	32	1.2	0.7	48	2	0.16	0.06	9.8	0.22	5	2.71	18	418
1657	Fish-salmon-cooked-moist heat	serv	85	157	23	0	0	6	1.2	42	50	454	32	0.8	0.4	15	1	0.16	0.17	7.1	0.39	4	3.06	39	248
153	Fish-salmon-pink-canned-solids & liquids	serv	85	118	17	0	0	5	1.3	47	471	277	29	0.7	0.8	14	0	0.02	0.16	5.6	0.26	13	5.85	181	279
1418	Fish-salmon-smoked	serv	100	117	18	0	0	4	0.9	23	784	175	18	0.9	0.3	26	0	0.02	0.1	4.7	0.28	11	3.26	11	164
154	Fish-sardines-Atlantic-canned in oil	item	12	25	3	0	0	1	0.2	17	61	48	5	0.4	0.2	8	0	0.01	0.03	0.6	0.02	1	1.07	46	59
1421	Fish-sardines-canned in tomato sauce	item	38	68	6	0	0.1	5	1.2	23	157	130	13	0.9	0.5	27	tr	0.02	0.09	1.6	0.05	9	3.42	91	139
1422	Fish-scallops-bay and sea-steamed	oz	28.4	32	7	1	0	tr	*	15	75	135	*	0.9	0.9	*	1	*	*	0.9	*	*	*	33	96
155	Fish-scallops-frozen-breaded-fried	item	15	32	3	2	0.1	2	0.4	9	70	50	9	0.1	0.2	3	tr	0.01	0.02	0.2	0.02	3	0.2	6	35
1688	Fish-scallops-raw	serv	85	75	14	2	0	1	0.1	28	137	274	48	0.8	0.8	13	3	0.01	0.06	1	0.13	14	1.3	20	186
1658	Fish-sea bass-cooked-dry heat	serv	85	105	20	0	0	2	0.6	45	74	279	45	0.3	0.4	54	3	0.11	0.13	1.6	0.39	5	0.26	11	211
156	Fish-shad-baked-butter/margarine & bacon	serv	100	201	23	0	0	11	2.5	69	79	377	*	0.6	0.7	9	*	0.13	0.26	8.6	0.26	5	1.27	24	313
1659	Fish-shark-raw	serv	85	111	18	0	0	4	0.8	43	67	136	42	0.7	0.4	60	0	0.04	0.05	2.5	0.05	3	1.27	29	179
157	Fish-shrimp-canned meat	cup	128	154	30	1	0	3	0.5	222	216	269	53	3.5	1.6	23	3	0.04	0.05	3.5	0.14	2	1.44	75	299

* indicates that no data was available.

Appendix A - Table of Food Composition
(continued)

Item	Food name	Portion	Weight (g)	Food Energy (Kcal)	Protein (gm)	Carbohydrates (gm)	Fiber (gm)	Total Fat (gm)	Saturated Fat (gm)	Cholesterol (mg)	Sodium (mg)	Potassium (mg)	Magnesium (mg)	Iron (mg)	Zinc (mg)	Vitamin A (RE)	Vitamin C (mg)	Thiamin (mg)	Riboflavin (mg)	Niacin (mg)	Vitamin B6 (mg)	Folates (µg)	Vitamin B12 (µg)	Calcium (mg)	Phosphorus (mg)
1677	Fish-shrimp-cooked-moist heat	serv	85	84	18	0	0	1	0.2	166	190	155	29	2.6	1.3	56	2	0.03	0.03	2.2	0.11	3	1.26	33	116
158	Fish-shrimp-french fried	serv	85	206	18	10	0.5	10	1.8	150	292	191	34	1.1	1.2	48	1	0.11	0.12	2.6	0.08	7	1.59	57	185
1423	Fish-smelt-Atlantic-canned	item	20	40	4	0		3						0.3	*									72	74
1660	Fish-smelt-cooked-dry heat	serv	85	105	19	0	0	3	0.5	77	66	316	32	1	1.8	15	0	0.63	0.12	1.5	0.15	4	3.37	66	251
1400	Fish-sole/flounder-baked	serv	127	148	31	0	0	2	0.5	86	133	436	74	0.4	0.8	14	4	0.1	0.15	2.8	0.31	11	3.19	23	368
1690	Fish-squid-cooked-fried	serv	85	149	15	7	0.3	6	1.6	221	260	237	33	0.9	1.5	9	4	0.05	0.39	2.2	0.05	5	1.04	33	213
1689	Fish-squid-raw	serv	85	78	13	3	0	1	0.3	198	37	209	28	0.6	1.3	9	4	0.02	0.35	1.9	0.05	4	1.1	27	188
1424	Fish-sturgeon-steamed	serv	100	135	21	0	0	5	1.2	75	108	364	35	2	0.5	243	0	0.08	0.09	9.8	0.22	17	2.6	40	263
1662	Fish-surimi	serv	85	84	13	6	0	1	0.2	26	95	37	17	0.2	0.3	17	0	0.02	0.02	0.2	0.03	1	1.36	8	240
1425	Fish-swordfish-broiled-butter/margarine	serv	100	174	28	0	0	6	2	4	478	354	33	1.3	1.4	616	3	0.04	0.05	10.9	0.36	3	1.9	7	275
1664	Fish-swordfish-cooked-dry heat	serv	85	132	22	0	0	4	1.2	43	98	314	29	0.9	1.3	35	1	0.04	0.1	10	0.32	2	1.72	5	287
1665	Fish-tilefish-cooked-dry heat	serv	85	125	21	0	0	4	0.7	54	50	435	28	0.3	0.5	18	0	0.12	0.16	3	0.26	15	2.13	22	201
1426	Fish-trout-brook-cooked	serv	100	196	24	tr	0	11	1.5	69	79	602	35	1.1	1.3	96	1	0.12	0.06	2.5	0.44	17	3.25	218	272
1666	Fish-trout-rainbow-cooked-dry heat	serv	85	128	22	0	0	4	0.7	62	29	539	9	2.1	1.2	19	3	0.07	0.19	5.9	0.39	15	2.98	73	273
1667	Fish-tuna-bluefin-cooked-dry heat	serv	85	156	25	0	0	5	1.4	42	43	275	54	1.1	0.7	643	0	0.24	0.26	9	0.45	2	9.25	9	277
159	Fish-tuna-canned in oil-drained solids	serv	85	168	25	0	0	7	1.3	15	301	176	26	1.2	0.8	20	0	0.03	0.1	10.5	0.09	5	1.87	11	264
354	Fish-tuna-dietetic-low sodium-drained	oz	28.4	36	8	tr	0	1	0.1	10	11	74	9	0.3	0.1	7	*	0.01	0.01	3.5	0.11	0	0.4	1	63
355	Fish-tuna-light-canned in water-drained	serv	85	111	25	0	0	tr	0.1	15	303	267	25	2.7	0.4	20	0	0.03	0.1	10.5	0.32	4	1.87	10	158
351	Fish-tuna-white-albacore-canned in water	serv	85	116	23	0	0	2	0.6	35	333	241	29	0.5	0.4	20	0	tr	0.04	4.9	0.37	2	1.87	14	227
1668	Fish-tuna-yellowfin-raw	serv	85	92	20	0	0	1	0.2	38	32	377	43	0.6	0.4	15	1	0.37	0.04	8.3	0.77	*	0.44	14	162
1428	Fish-white perch-fried filet	item	65	108	13	0	0	5	*	*	*	*	*	0.7	*	0	0	0.04	0.05	2.7	*	*	*	9	113
1427	Fish-whitefish-lake-baked-stuffed	serv	100	215	15	6	0.6	14	*	*	195	291	*	0.5	*	601	0	0.11	0.11	2.3	*	*	2.21	*	246
1669	Fish-whiting-cooked-dry heat	serv	85	98	20	0	0	1	0.3	71	113	369	23	0.4	0.5	29	0	0.06	0.05	1.4	0.15	13	2.21	53	242
Frozen dinners																									
1375	Barbecued chicken-Light and Elegant	item	227	300	26	35	3.2	6	3.1	97	900	450	55	1.5	2.9	189	5	0.19	0.15	6.9	0.57	40	0.36	22	896
463	Beef and green peppers-Stouffer dinner	item	220	225	10	18	*	11	*	*	960	420	*	2.3	*	136	0	0.08	0.16	3.9	*	11	0.36	0	*
1331	Beef and spinach pasta shells-Stouffer	item	255	290	19	28	*	11	*	*	1315	485	*	*	*	*	0	*	*	*	*	*	*	0	*
79	Beef burgundy-frozen dinner-Efficienc	item	142	144	17	6	*	5	*	*	411	147	*	0.6	*	449	0	0.04	0.24	4.1	*	*	*	5	*
1371	Beef burgundy-Light and Elegant dinner	item	255	230	23	25	1.6	4	3.5	95	1235	200	55	3.1	8.1	181	1	0.15	0.23	1.7	0.49	25	4.12	14	172
1339	Beef cubes in wine sauce-Hormel entree	oz	28.4	52	4	1	*	4	1.9	15	106	71	4	0.5	1.3	*	tr	0.77	0.05	0.5	0.02	4	0.41	3	23
1454	Beef dinner-Swanson frozen dinner	item	326	320	25	34	3.3	9	9.6	84	1085	616	42	4	4.7	1140	6	0.14	0.27	4.9	0.52	24	2.1	36	283
1372	Beef julienne-Light and Elegant dinner	item	241	260	21	27	*	7	*	*	990	240	*	4.9	*	356	4	0.09	0.1	3.5	*	11	0.52	27	152
1338	Beef short ribs in barbecue sauce-Hormel	oz	28.4	54	5	1	0.8	3	1.7	15	176	92	5	0.7	1.7	11	tr	0.01	0.07	0.7	0.03	11	0.52	3	28
1439	Beef sirloin tips-Le Menu frozen dinner	item	326	400	29	27	*	19	*	*	1100	*	*	*	*	*	*	*	*	*	*	*	*	*	*
1342	Beef stew-Hormel entree	oz	28.4	29	2	2	0.3	1	0.4	9	116	45	3	0.2	0.2	65	tr	0.01	0.03	0.6	0.04	11	0.06	5	29
81	Beef stroganoff-frozen dinner-Efficienc	item	170	192	20	8	2.9	8	*	7	785	316	*	2.9	*	68	2	0.05	0.32	2.9	0.01	6	0.15	23	15
1373	Beef stroganoff-Light and Elegant dinner	item	255	260	24	27	1.3	6	10.6	84	785	230	40	3	4.9	189	2	0.2	0.26	2.2	0.28	19	2.58	45	79
1374	Beef teriyaki-Light and Elegant	item	227	240	18	37	*	3	*	*	625	215	*	5.6	*	24	tr	0.4	0.1	2.5	*	*	0.1	30	152
1341	Cabbage rolls in tomato sauce-Hormel	oz	28.4	23	1	3	*	1	0.3	3	127	87	4	0.3	0.2	*	tr	0.76	0.02	0.3	0.03	3	0.1	6	16
84	Cabbage rolls-frozen dinner-Efficienc	item	227	168	11	17	*	5	*	*	1026	290	*	1.4	*	136	0	0.09	0.16	2.7	*	*	*	49	*
1330	Cheese pasta shells/meat sauce-Stouffer	item	255	320	19	30	1.9	14	8.3	169	1310	465	35	3.4	3.1	209	8	0.24	0.4	4.4	0.26	26	1.34	146	238
1376	Chicken and broccoli-Light and Elegant	item	270	290	19	30	*	11	*	*	805	180	*	1.6	*	75	1	0.11	0.21	1.8	*	*	*	204	240
1347	Chicken and dumplings with gravy-Hormel	oz	28.4	31	3	2	0.3	2	0.4	9	116	45	3	0.2	0.2	65	tr	0.01	0.03	0.6	0.04	11	0.06	5	29
1451	Chicken burgundy-Classic Lite dinner	item	319	240	23	24	2.9	5	*	25	1030	270	*	2.6	*	*	*	*	*	*	*	*	*	*	*
1328	Chicken cacciatore-Stouffer dinner	item	319	310	25	29	2.9	11	8.4	166	1135	300	73	3.9	4.1	176	33	0.24	0.42	18.2	0.95	22	0.57	75	398
360	Chicken chow mein-Lean Cuisine dinner	item	319	250	14	36	*	5	*	25	1040	420	50	2.6	1.1	910	33	0.15	0.19	8	0.46	28	0.19	54	192
1327	Chicken crepes/mushroom sauce-Stouffer	item	234	390	30	19	2.3	22	7.3	76	1610	602	60	2.7	2.6	323	12	0.33	0.39	10.3	0.45	30	0.36	112	295
1456	Chicken dinner-Swanson frozen dinner	item	326	660	26	64	6.2	33	7.4	111	*	*	*	*	*	*	*	*	*	*	*	*	*	*	*
1326	Chicken divan-Stouffer frozen dinner	item	241	335	21	14	1	22	9.2	86	830	415	52	1.7	2	221	20	0.13	0.44	4.6	0.29	41	0.74	269	295
1440	Chicken florentine-Le Menu frozen dinner	item	354	510	28	35	6.7	28	8	121	985	653	66	2.9	2.9	351	13	0.36	0.42	11.2	0.49	33	0.39	122	320
1437	Chicken kiev-Le Menu frozen dinner	item	234	500	21	35	4.4	30	5.3	80	745	432	43	1.9	1.9	232	*	0.24	0.28	7.4	0.33	22	0.26	80	212

The following is a data table of prepared-food nutritional values. Each row lists a food code, a description, a serving unit, and a sequence of numeric values (an asterisk "*" indicates that no data was available).

Code	Food	Unit																					
1441	Chicken parmigiana-Le Menu frozen dinner	item	333	390	26	28	*	19	*	*	900	*	*	7	*	0.2	6.6	*	22	0.53	*	73	*	394
1377	Chicken parmigiana-Light and Elegant	item	227	260	28	23	1.7	6	6.8	172	685	310	55	2.8	2.9	0.33	0.3	7.5	0.45	28	0.39	59	*	226
1329	Chicken pasta shells-Stouffer dinner	item	255	400	26	24	3	22	2.5	165	1060	350	47	3.7	2.2	0.3	0.43	*	7.5	0.35	28	0.39	59	226
387	Chicken-glazed-with rice-Lean Cuisine	item	241	270	26	23	*	8	*	55	810	380	*	1.8	*	*	*	*	*	*	*	*	*	*
1742	Chicken-sweet and sour-Budget Gourmet	serv	284	350	18	53	1.7	7	1.3	40	640	429	45	0.7	1.4	0.12	0.34	3	0.38	13	0.17	60	163	*
1442	Chicken-sweet and sour-Le Menu dinner	item	298	450	20	42	1.8	22	1.3	53	1170	450	47	2	1.5	0.14	0.18	7	0.4	14	0.18	37	171	*
408	Corn souffle frozen side dish	item	113	155	4	19	*	7	*	*	510	190	1	0.4	0.1	0.08	0.16	0.8	0.08	34	*	48	*	*
1325	Cream chipped beef-Stouffer dinner	item	156	235	12	10	0.2	16	4.9	28	900	290	27	1.7	1.7	0.06	0.28	2.2	0.13	9	0.95	127	*	171
410	Creamed spinach-Stouffer side dish	item	128	190	4	9	*	15	*	*	855	585	*	*	*	*	*	*	*	*	*	*	*	*
1470	Egg roll-beef and shrimp-frozen-La Choy	item	12	27	1	4	0.1	1	0.1	2	81	15	2	0.1	0.1	0.01	0.01	0.1	0.01	1	0.02	2	*	5
433	Fettucini alfredo-Stouffer frozen dinner	item	142	270	8	19	*	18	*	100	1195	240	*	1.8	*	0.15	0.43	6	*	*	*	200	*	*
1737	Fettucini-chicken-Budget Gourmet	serv	284	400	23	29	*	21	*	*	740	*	350	*	*	*	*	*	*	*	*	*	*	*
391	Filet of fish divan-Lean Cuisine dinner	item	351	270	31	16	*	10	*	85	780	850	38	*	*	*	*	*	*	*	*	*	*	*
394	Filet of fish florentine-Lean Cuisine	item	255	240	26	13	*	9	*	100	700	540	49	*	*	*	*	*	*	*	*	*	*	*
1471	Fish and chips-Van de Kamps dinner	item	224	500	16	45	4.7	30	6.2	33	551	785	53	2.2	1	0.24	0.14	4.3	0.41	23	0.68	35	271	*
1447	Flounder filet-Le Menu frozen dinner	item	298	350	22	27	*	17	*	53	1125	*	*	4.8	*	0.21	*	7.7	*	*	*	*	348	*
1378	Glazed chicken-Light and Elegant	item	227	230	24	25	*	4	*	*	655	300	38	*	*	0.07	*	*	*	*	18	348	*	*
1324	Ham and swiss cheese crepes-Stouffer	item	213	410	25	23	*	25	*	36	905	345	39	2	2.7	0.21	0.07	7.7	*	*	*	*	*	*
1565	Ham-Banquet frozen dinner	item	284	369	17	48	2.6	12	2	36	1590	125	38	2.5	2.5	0.57	0.23	3.4	0.48	21	0.45	151	*	278
1379	Lasagna florentine-Light and Elegant	item	319	280	34	34	*	5	*	65	975	720	22	3.6	*	0.39	0.38	1.7	*	*	280	*	387	*
1743	Lasagna-3 cheese-Budget Gourmet	serv	284	400	22	38	3.4	17	6.1	80	760	437	49	2.7	1.8	0.38	0.51	4	0.16	24	0.36	500	*	286
1738	Lasagna-sausage-Budget Gourmet	serv	284	284	20	38	3.8	20	9	*	950	591	54	2.7	3.7	0.45	0.43	4	0.28	23	0.91	400	*	348
471	Lasagna-Stouffer frozen dinner	item	298	385	28	36	*	14	*	16	1200	580	*	3.2	*	0.21	0.42	4.2	*	*	*	410	*	*
469	Linguini with clam sauce-Stouffer dinner	item	298	285	17	36	*	8	*	35	1010	115	*	*	*	*	*	*	*	*	*	*	*	*
467	Lobster newburg-Stouffer frozen dinner	item	184	350	15	9	*	29	*	25	700	190	*	*	*	*	*	*	*	*	*	*	*	*
1380	Macaroni and cheese-Light and Elegant	item	255	300	15	9	*	9	*	*	1015	210	*	2	*	0.34	0.43	1.5	*	*	238	*	334	*
1446	Manicotti-cheese-Le Menu frozen dinner	item	241	310	18	29	1.9	13	10	20	840	434	39	3	2.7	0.23	0.46	3.3	0.22	26	1.03	348	*	328
1736	Manicotti-cheese/meat-Budget Gourmet	serv	284	450	20	33	2.4	26	11.1	50	920	484	45	2.7	2.3	0.45	0.51	4	0.23	31	0.72	450	*	376
396	Meatball stew-Lean Cuisine frozen dinner	item	284	240	22	21	*	7	*	65	1250	410	5	*	*	*	*	*	*	*	*	*	*	*
461	Meatballs and noodles-Stouffer dinner	item	312	475	25	33	*	27	*	79	1620	395	*	*	*	*	*	*	*	*	*	*	*	*
1564	Meatloaf-Banquet frozen dinner	item	312	412	21	29	5.4	24	7.5	79	1991	468	64	4.3	3.4	0.16	0.22	4.2	0.36	48	1.21	84	*	243
1453	Mexican dinner-Swanson frozen dinner	item	454	590	29	64	6.7	29	9.5	44	1865	603	75	5.1	3.6	0.35	0.3	3.8	0.3	135	0.83	198	*	340
435	Noodles romanoff-Stouffer frozen dinner	item	113	170	6	16	*	9	*	*	675	95	*	0.8	0.8	0.08	0.16	0.8	0.08	9	*	88	*	*
1333	Ocean fish almondine-Efficienc entree	item	113	236	16	3	*	17	*	35	388	229	0	0.7	*	0.19	0.25	3.1	*	17	*	22	*	93
1334	Ocean fish with lemon sauce-Efficienc	serv	113	262	14	3	0.9	21	1.6	16	370	224	0	0.7	0.5	0.17	0.18	2.8	0.13	18	0.22	15	*	*
398	Oriental beef-Lean Cuisine frozen dinner	item	245	250	18	28	*	7	*	35	1150	270	22	*	*	*	*	*	*	*	*	*	*	*
1739	Pepper steak with rice-Budget Gourmet	serv	284	300	15	39	1.4	9	5.8	25	800	729	49	0.7	6	0.15	0.17	3	0.59	22	3.9	40	*	350
1443	Pepper steak-Le Menu frozen dinner	item	326	360	26	34	*	13	*	9	1045	*	*	0.1	*	0.05	0.02	0.4	*	6	0.06	8	*	23
1431	Pizza-combination-Weight Watchers-frozen	item	205	340	20	38	*	12	*	20	1200	360	*	*	6	*	*	3	*	22	*	40	*	*
1344	Pork loin and gravy-Hormel entree	oz	28.4	40	5	1	*	2	0.9	9	133	82	5	0.2	0.4	0.04	0.04	0.9	0.06	10	0.07	2	*	32
1472	Quiche lorraine-frozen dinner-Mrs Smiths	item	269	720	34	54	0.8	41	34.3	95	1965	610	*	2.7	*	1.01	0.33	6	*	135	0.83	97	*	*
453	Ratatouille-Stouffer frozen side dish	item	142	60	1	9	2.3	3	*	10	1320	505	10	1	*	0.03	0.2	1	*	3	*	*	*	*
1566	Salisbury steak-Banquet frozen dinner	item	312	390	18	24	5.3	25	7.3	86	2059	387	64	3.5	3.6	0.16	0.19	3.6	0.36	48	1.34	90	*	206
402	Salisbury steak-Lean Cuisine	item	269	280	25	11	*	15	*	95	800	650	4	0.1	0.3	0.04	0.06	0.2	0.02	1	0.07	29	*	33
1345	Sausage and gravy-Hormel entree	oz	28.4	31	2	2	tr	2	0.6	2	119	84	4	0.3	0.2	0.05	0.03	0.4	0.02	6	0.06	8	*	23
1343	Scalloped potatoes and ham-Hormel entree	oz	28.4	28	2	3	0.6	1	0.6	4	146	68	4	0.1	0.2	0.05	0.02	3	0.59	22	3.9	40	*	350
1332	Scallops and shrimp mariner-Stouffer	item	291	400	23	40	*	16	*	4	1120	355	4	*	6	*	*	*	*	*	*	*	*	*
400	Scallops/vegetables/rice-Lean Cuisine	item	312	220	17	32	*	3	*	20	1200	360	88	0.2	*	*	*	0.2	0.03	6	0.09	8	*	16
1346	Seafood gumbo-Hormel entree	oz	28.4	10	1	1	*	tr	tr	5	146	82	5	0.2	0.1	0.01	0.02	0.2	0.03	6	0.09	8	*	16
1740	Seafood newburg-Budget Gourmet	serv	284	350	17	43	0.2	12	2	70	660	704	64	0.7	4.7	0.23	0.26	2	0.2	37	4.67	100	*	460
1381	Shrimp creole-Light and Elegant	item	283	200	11	31	2.2	2	2.9	293	1045	200	88	2.5	2.4	0.22	0.03	3.3	0.32	14	1.91	54	*	225

* indicates that no data was available.
©1994 First DataBank—The Hearst Corporation (N-Squared Computing).

Appendix A - Table of Food Composition
(continued)

Item	Food name	Portion	Weight (g)	Food Energy (Kcal)	Protein (gm)	Carbohydrates (gm)	Fiber (gm)	Total Fat (gm)	Saturated Fat (gm)	Cholesterol (mg)	Sodium (mg)	Potassium (mg)	Magnesium (mg)	Iron (mg)	Zinc (mg)	Vitamin A (RE)	Vitamin C (mg)	Thiamin (mg)	Riboflavin (mg)	Niacin (mg)	Vitamin B6 (mg)	Folates (µg)	Vitamin B12 (µg)	Calcium (mg)	Phosphorus (mg)
1741	Sirloin tip/vegetables-Budget Gourmet	serv	284	310	16	21	2.6	18	1.9	40	570	504	35	0.4	4.4	150	2	0.15	0.17	4	0.44	16	1.87	60	195
1449	Sole-light-Van de Kamp's frozen dinner	item	142	293	16	17	1.9	18	0.4	45	412	453	39	0.9	0.6	10	21	0.13	0.13	3.3	0.25	36	1.35	39	200
404	Spaghetti-beef and mushroom-Lean Cuisine	item	326	280	15	38	*	7	*	20	1450	580	*	*	*	*	*	*	*	*	*	*	*	*	252
1383	Spaghetti-Light and Elegant	item	290	290	16	40	*	8	*	8	700	273	*	6	*	157	10	0.25	0.15	3.4	*	9	*	100	*
465	Spinach crepes/cheese sauce-Stouffer	item	269	415	16	30	0.1	25	1.7	8	995	440	6	*	0.4	11	*	*	0.06	*	0.03	27	0.18	15	*
1340	Swedish meatballs in sauce-Hormel entree	serv	28.4	44	3	2	0.4	3	0.7	8	165	87	5	0.5	0.6	76	tr	0.02	0.05	0.5	0.04	*	0.32	5	39
1337	Swiss steak in gravy-Hormel entree	oz	28.4	34	4	1	0.5	2	*	8	110	86	*	0.5	*	54	tr	0.17	0.23	0.9	*	*	*	98	15
459	Tuna noodle casserole-Stouffer dinner	item	163	200	10	18	*	9	*	*	670	210	*	1.2	*	*	*	*	*	3.5	*	*	*	*	*
1450	Turf and surf-Classic Lite frozen dinner	item	283	250	29	15	*	8	*	*	*	*	*	*	*	*	*	*	*	*	*	*	*	*	*
1206	Turkey & gravy-frozen	cup	240	160	14	11	2.7	6	2	43	1328	146	20	2.2	1.7	20	0	0.06	0.31	4.3	0.23	10	0.58	33	194
1744	Turkey a la king/rice-Budget Gourmet	serv	284	390	20	36	2.4	18	4.2	75	740	451	52	1.1	1.9	100	2	0.15	0.4	5	0.56	41	0.3	150	212
1445	Turkey breast-Le Menu frozen dinner	item	319	470	27	36	*	24	*	74	1165	*	*	*	*	*	*	*	*	*	*	*	*	*	*
1455	Turkey dinner-Swanson frozen dinner	item	326	340	20	42	3.6	10	5.7	*	1295	635	56	2.7	2.6	771	13	0.26	0.27	7.9	0.56	42	0.42	84	305
457	Turkey pie-Stouffer frozen dinner	item	284	460	20	35	*	26	*	*	1735	270	*	*	*	*	*	*	*	*	*	*	*	*	*
455	Turkey tetrazzini-Stouffer frozen dinner	item	170	240	12	17	*	14	*	*	620	200	*	0.6	*	41	*	0.12	0.24	2.4	0.12	*	*	72	121
1382	Turkey-sliced-Light and Elegant	item	227	230	20	25	*	5	*	162	1020	280	*	*	*	171	1	0.12	0.14	4.6	0.14	25	1.21	18	401
1335	Veal parmigiana-Efficienc entree	item	213	296	24	17	1.6	14	9	60	973	466	49	1	3.6	123	6	0.3	0.38	6.8	0.43	62	0.85	97	299
1452	Veal steak-Classic Lite frozen dinner	item	312	280	25	27	5.8	8	5.9	39	1738	932	81	2.3	4.2	241	33	0.36	0.43	6.5	0.53	78	0.2	171	274
1438	Vegetable lasagna-Le Menu frozen dinner	item	312	400	15	30	5.1	24	9.4	*	1135	519	82	3.6	1.5	723	62	0.23	0.47	3.3	0.34	*	*	296	*
1444	Yankee pot roast-Le Menu frozen dinner	item	312	360	27	29	*	15	*	*	830	570	*	3.2	*	*	*	*	*	*	*	*	*	*	*
406	Zucchini lasagna-Lean Cuisine	item	312	260	20	28	*	7	*	20	1050	*	*	*	*	*	*	*	*	*	*	*	*	*	*
1448	Zucchini romano-Le Menu frozen dinner	item	234	350	17	27	*	19	*	*	680	*	*	*	*	*	*	*	*	*	*	*	*	*	*
	Fruits																								
881	Apples-can-sweet-heated	cup	204	137	tr	34	5.1	1	0.1	0	7	142	5	0.5	0.1	11	tr	0.02	0.02	0.2	0.09	tr	0	8	11
883	Apples-dried-cooked-unsweetened	cup	255	145	1	39	3.9	tr	tr	0	52	267	10	0.8	0.1	4	3	0.02	0.05	0.3	0.13	0	0	8	23
882	Apples-dried-uncooked	cup	86	209	1	57	8.6	tr	tr	0	75	387	14	1.2	0.2	0	3	0	0.14	0.8	0.11	0	0	12	33
885	Apples-frozen-unsweetened-heated	cup	206	97	1	25	3.9	1	0.1	0	5	156	6	0.4	0.1	4	1	0.03	0.02	0.1	0.07	1	0	9	16
884	Apples-frozen-unsweetened-unheated	cup	173	83	tr	21	3.5	tr	0.1	0	5	134	4	0.1	0.1	6	tr	0.02	0.01	0.1	0.06	1	0	8	13
879	Apples-raw-peeled	item	128	73	tr	19	2.4	tr	0.1	0	0	144	4	0.1	0.1	6	5	0.02	0.02	0.1	0.06	0	0	5	9
880	Apples-raw-peeled-boiled	cup	171	91	tr	23	4.1	1	0.1	0	2	150	5	0.3	0.1	8	tr	0.03	0.02	0.2	0.08	1	0	9	13
224	Apples-raw-sliced-with skin	cup	110	65	tr	17	2.4	tr	0.1	0	2	126	5	0.2	tr	6	6	0.02	0.02	0.1	0.05	3	0	8	8
223	Apples-raw-with skin-2 3/4 inch diameter	item	138	81	tr	21	3	tr	0.1	0	1	159	6	0.3	0.1	7	8	0.02	0.02	0.1	0.07	4	0	10	10
226	Applesauce-canned-sweetened	cup	255	194	tr	51	3.1	tr	0.1	0	8	156	7	0.9	0.1	3	4	0.03	0.07	0.5	0.07	2	0	9	17
227	Applesauce-canned-unsweetened	cup	244	105	tr	28	3.7	tr	tr	0	5	183	7	0.3	0.1	7	3	0.03	0.06	0.5	0.06	1	0	7	17
228	Apricot-raw-without pit	item	35.3	17	tr	4	0.7	tr	tr	0	tr	104	3	0.2	0.1	92	4	0.01	0.01	0.2	0.02	3	0	5	7
229	Apricots-canned-heavy syrup-with skin	cup	258	214	1	55	5.5	tr	tr	0	10	361	18	0.8	0.3	317	8	0.05	0.06	1	0.14	4	0	22	32
888	Apricots-canned-juice pack	cup	248	119	2	31	2.8	tr	tr	0	9	409	24	0.7	0.3	420	12	0.05	0.05	0.9	0.13	4	0	30	50
889	Apricots-canned-light syrup pack	cup	253	159	1	42	1.2	tr	tr	0	10	349	21	1	0.3	334	7	0.04	0.05	0.8	0.14	4	0	28	34
887	Apricots-canned-water pack	cup	243	66	1	16	4.1	tr	tr	0	7	467	17	0.4	0.3	314	8	0.05	0.06	1	0.13	4	0	19	32
231	Apricots-dried-sulfured-cooked-no sugar	cup	250	213	3	55	19.5	tr	tr	0	9	1222	42	4.2	0.7	591	4	0.02	0.08	2.4	0.29	0	0	40	104
230	Apricots-dried-sulfured-uncooked	cup	130	309	5	80	10.1	1	tr	0	13	1791	61	6.1	1	941	3	0.01	0.2	3.9	0.2	13	0	59	152
890	Apricots-frozen-sweetened	cup	242	237	2	61	4.1	tr	tr	0	10	554	22	2.2	0.2	407	22	0.05	0.1	1.9	0.15	4	0	24	46
125	Apricots-halves-with skin-canned-water	serv	28.4	6	tr	2	0.5	tr	tr	0	3	44	3	tr	tr	51	1	0.01	0.01	0.1	0.02	tr	0	5	5
233	Avocado-raw-California	item	173	306	4	12	6.1	30	4.5	0	21	1097	70	2	0.7	106	14	0.19	0.21	3.3	0.48	113	0	19	73
234	Avocado-raw-Florida	item	304	340	5	27	8.3	27	5.3	0	15	1484	103	1.6	1.3	186	24	0.33	0.37	5.8	0.85	162	0	33	119
236	Banana flakes-dehydrated or powdered	tbsp	6.2	22	tr	5	0.5	1	tr	0	tr	92	7	0.1	0.1	2	tr	0.01	0.02	0.2	*	tr	0	1	5
235	Bananas-raw-peeled	item	114	105	1	27	1.8	1	0.2	0	1	451	33	0.4	0.2	9	10	0.05	0.11	0.6	0.66	22	0	7	22
891	Blackberries-canned-heavy syrup pack	cup	256	236	3	59	17.7	tr	0	0	7	254	44	1.7	0.5	56	7	0.07	0.1	0.7	0.09	68	0	54	36
892	Blackberries-frozen-unsweetened	cup	151	97	2	24	7.6	1	tr	0	2	211	33	1.2	0.4	17	5	0.04	0.07	1.8	0.09	51	0	44	45
237	Blackberries-raw	cup	144	75	1	18	8.9	1	0.1	0	0	282	29	0.8	0.4	24	30	0.04	0.06	0.6	0.08	49	0	46	30

893	Blueberries-canned-heavy syrup pack	cup	256	225	2	57	2.8	1	0.1	0	9	102	9	0.8	0.2	16	3	0.09	0.14	0.3	0.09	4	0	14	26
894	Blueberries-frozen-unsweetened	cup	155	79	1	19	4.9	1	tr	0	2	84	8	0.3	0.1	13	4	0.05	0.06	0.8	0.09	10	0	12	17
238	Blueberries-raw	cup	145	81	1	21	3.3	1	0.1	0	9	129	7	0.2	0.2	15	19	0.07	0.07	0.5	0.05	9	0	9	15
895	Boysenberries-canned-heavy syrup pack	cup	256	225	3	57	5.7	tr	*	0	9	230	28	1.1	0.5	10	16	0.07	0.07	0.6	0.1	88	0	46	25
896	Boysenberries-frozen-unsweetened	cup	132	66	1	16	5.2	tr	tr	0	2	183	21	1.1	0.3	9	4	0.07	0.05	1	0.07	84	0	36	36
897	Breadfruit-raw	item	384	396	4	104	46.8	1	0.3	0	8	1882	96	2.1	0.5	15	111	0.42	0.12	3.5	0.36	39	0	65	115
898	Carambola-raw	item	127	42	1	10	1.5	tr	0	0	2	207	12	0.3	0.1	63	27	0.04	0.03	0.5	0.13	11	0	6	20
899	Carissa-raw	item	20	12	tr	3	*	tr	*	0	1	52	3	0.3	*	1	8	0.01	0.01	tr	*	*	0	2	1
900	Cherimoya-raw	item	547	514	7	131	13	2	*	0	*	*	*	2.7	*	6	49	0.55	0.6	7.1	*	*	0	126	219
901	Cherries-sour-canned-water pack	cup	244	88	2	22	0.6	tr	0.1	0	17	239	15	3.3	0.2	184	5	0.04	0.1	0.4	0.11	20	0	27	24
902	Cherries-sour-frozen-unsweetened	cup	155	71	1	17	1.9	1	0.2	0	2	192	14	0.8	0.2	135	3	0.07	0.05	0.2	0.1	7	0	20	25
239	Cherries-sour-red-canned in heavy syrup	cup	256	233	2	60	0.6	tr	0.1	0	18	238	15	3.3	0.2	183	5	0.04	0.1	0.4	0.11	20	0	26	26
904	Cherries-sweet-canned-juice pack	cup	250	135	2	35	0.6	tr	tr	0	8	328	30	1.5	0.3	31	6	0.05	0.06	1	0.08	11	0	35	55
903	Cherries-sweet-canned-water pack	cup	248	114	2	29	0.6	tr	0.1	0	3	325	22	0.9	0.2	40	5	0.06	0.1	1	0.07	10	0	27	38
905	Cherries-sweet-frozen-sweetened	cup	259	231	3	58	8.7	tr	0.1	0	3	515	26	0.9	0.1	49	3	0.07	0.12	0.5	0.09	11	0	31	41
240	Cherries-sweet-raw	item	6.8	5	tr	1	0.1	tr	tr	0	0	15	1	tr	tr	1	tr	tr	tr	tr	tr	tr	0	1	1
1460	Cranapple juice cocktail-Ocean Spray	fl oz	32	5	0	1	0	0	0	0	1	8	1	0.1	tr	*	14	tr	0.01	tr	*	tr	0	1	0
1540	Cranapple juice-canned	cup	253	170	tr	43	0	0	0	0	5	68	5	0.2	0.1	0	81	0.01	0.05	0.2	0.05	1	0	18	8
241	Cranberry juice cocktail-bottled	cup	253	144	0	36	0	tr	0	0	10	46	5	0.4	0.2	0	90	0.02	0.02	0.1	0.05	1	0	8	5
1461	Cranberry juice cocktail-Ocean Spray	fl oz	32	6	tr	5	0	tr	0	0	1	8	1	0.1	tr	0	14	tr	0.01	tr	0.01	tr	0	1	tr
242	Cranberry sauce-canned-sweetened	cup	277	418	1	108	3.2	tr	0.1	0	80	72	8	0.6	0.1	6	11	0.04	0.06	0.3	0.04	*	0	11	17
244	Dates-domestic-natural and dry-chopped	cup	178	490	4	131	15.5	1	0.1	0	5	1161	62	2.1	0.5	9	0	0.16	0.18	3.9	0.34	22	0	57	71
243	Dates-domestic-natural and dry-whole	item	8.3	23	tr	6	0.7	tr	0	0	tr	54	3	0.1	tr	tr	0	0.01	0.01	0.2	0.02	1	0	3	3
906	Elderberries-raw	cup	145	106	1	27	12.3	1	tr	0	9	406	7	2.3	0.2	87	52	0.1	0.09	0.7	0.33	9	0	55	57
909	Figs-canned-heavy syrup pack	cup	259	228	1	59	8.9	tr	0.1	0	3	258	26	0.7	0.3	10	3	0.06	0.1	1.1	0.18	5	0	69	26
908	Figs-canned-water pack	cup	248	131	1	35	5.2	tr	0.1	0	2	255	25	0.7	0.3	10	2	0.06	0.09	1.1	0.17	5	0	69	25
910	Figs-dried-uncooked	cup	199	507	6	130	18.5	2	0.5	0	22	1417	117	4.4	1	26	2	0.14	0.18	1.4	0.45	15	0	287	135
907	Figs-raw	item	50	37	tr	10	3.2	tr	tr	0	1	116	8	0.2	0.1	7	1	0.03	0.03	0.2	0.06	3	0	18	7
245	Fruit cocktail-canned in heavy syrup	cup	255	186	1	48	3.8	tr	tr	0	15	224	14	0.7	0.2	52	5	0.05	0.05	1	0.13	7	0	16	28
912	Fruit cocktail-canned-juice pack	cup	248	114	1	29	1.5	tr	tr	0	10	236	17	0.5	0.2	76	7	0.03	0.04	1	0.13	6	0	20	35
911	Fruit cocktail-canned-water pack	cup	245	78	1	21	1.6	tr	tr	0	10	230	17	0.6	0.2	61	5	0.04	0.03	0.9	0.13	7	0	12	27
127	Fruit cocktail-canned-water-dietetic	oz	28.4	9	tr	2	0.1	tr	0	0	1	26	2	0.1	tr	7	1	0.01	0.06	0.2	0.02	1	0	2	3
1544	Fruit roll up-cherry	item	14.4	50	0	12	*	1	*	0	5	45	*	*	*	*	*	*	*	*	*	*	0	*	*
916	Gooseberries-canned-heavy syrup pack	cup	252	184	2	47	7	1	tr	0	5	194	15	0.8	0.3	35	25	0.05	0.13	0.4	0.03	8	0	40	18
915	Gooseberries-raw	cup	150	66	1	15	4	1	0.1	0	2	297	15	0.5	0.2	44	42	0.06	0.05	0.5	0.12	9	0	38	41
260	Grape drink-canned	cup	253	154	1	38	0	tr	0.1	0	8	334	25	0.6	0.1	2	tr	0.07	0.09	0.7	0.16	7	0	23	28
248	Grapefruit-canned in light syrup	cup	254	152	1	39	1.7	tr	tr	0	4	328	25	1	0.2	0	54	0.1	0.05	0.6	0.05	22	0	36	25
918	Grapefruit-canned-juice pack	cup	249	92	2	23	1.6	tr	tr	0	19	420	26	0.5	0.2	0	84	0.07	0.05	0.6	0.05	22	0	37	30
917	Grapefruit-canned-water pack	cup	244	88	1	22	1.6	tr	tr	0	5	322	24	1	0.2	0	53	0.1	0.05	0.6	0.05	22	0	37	24
246	Grapefruit-pink & red-raw	item	246	74	1	19	3.2	tr	tr	0	0	312	20	0.3	0.2	64	91	0.1	0.05	0.5	0.1	23	0	36	22
247	Grapefruit-white-raw	item	236	78	2	20	2.5	tr	tr	0	0	350	21	0.1	0.2	2	79	0.09	0.05	0.6	0.1	24	0	28	18
256	Grapes-raw-adherent skin (European) type	serv	160	114	1	28	2.6	1	0.3	0	3	296	10	0.4	0.1	12	17	0.15	0.09	0.5	0.18	6	0	17	21
255	Grapes-raw-slip skin (American) type	cup	92	58	1	16	1.5	tr	0.1	0	2	176	5	0.3	tr	9	4	0.09	0.05	0.3	0.1	4	0	13	9
920	Grapes-thompson-canned-heavy syrup pack	cup	256	187	1	50	1.7	tr	0.1	0	14	264	15	2.4	0.1	16	3	0.08	0.06	0.3	0.17	7	0	25	44
919	Grapes-thompson-canned-water pack	cup	245	98	1	25	1.7	tr	0.1	0	15	262	15	2.4	0.1	16	2	0.08	0.06	0.3	0.16	6	0	25	44
921	Guavas-common-raw	item	90	46	1	11	5.4	1	0.2	0	3	256	9	0.3	0.2	71	165	0.05	0.05	1.1	0.13	13	0	18	23
922	Guavas-strawberry-raw	item	6	4	tr	1	0.4	tr	tr	0	2	18	1	tr	tr	1	2	tr	tr	tr	0.01	1	0	1	2
225	Juice apple-canned or bottled	cup	248	116	tr	29	0.5	tr	tr	0	7	296	8	0.9	0.1	tr	2	0.05	0.04	0.2	0.07	tr	0	16	18
886	Juice-apple-frozen-diluted	cup	239	112	tr	28	0.6	tr	tr	0	17	301	12	0.6	0.1	*	1	0.01	0.04	0.1	0.08	1	0	14	17
232	Juice-apricot nectar-canned	cup	251	141	1	36	1.5	tr	tr	0	9	286	13	1	0.2	330	1	0.02	0.04	0.7	*	3	0	17	23
257	Juice-grape-canned & bottled	cup	253	154	1	38	0	tr	0.1	0	8	334	25	0.6	0.1	2	tr	0.07	0.09	0.7	0.16	7	0	23	28

* indicates that no data was available.

©1994 First DataBank—The Hearst Corporation (N-Squared Computing).

Appendix A - Table of Food Composition
(continued)

Item	Food name	Portion	Weight (g)	Food Energy (Kcal)	Protein (gm)	Carbohydrates (gm)	Fiber (gm)	Total Fat (gm)	Saturated Fat (gm)	Cholesterol (mg)	Sodium (mg)	Potassium (mg)	Magnesium (mg)	Iron (mg)	Zinc (mg)	Vitamin A (RE)	Vitamin C (mg)	Thiamin (mg)	Riboflavin (mg)	Niacin (mg)	Vitamin B6 (mg)	Folates (µg)	Vitamin B12 (µg)	Calcium (mg)	Phosphorus (mg)
258	Juice-grape-frozen concentrate	item	216	387	1	96	0.6	1	0.2	0	15	160	32	0.8	0.3	6	179	0.11	0.2	0.9	0.32	10	0	28	32
259	Juice-grape-frozen-diluted	cup	250	128	tr	32	0	tr	0.1	0	5	53	11	0.3	0.1	2	60	0.04	0.07	0.3	0.11	3	0	9	11
251	Juice-grapefruit-canned-sweetened	cup	250	115	1	28	0	tr	tr	0	5	405	25	0.9	0.2	0	67	0.1	0.06	0.8	0.05	26	0	20	28
250	Juice-grapefruit-canned-unsweetened	cup	247	94	1	22	0.4	tr	tr	0	2	378	25	0.5	0.2	2	72	0.1	0.05	0.6	0.05	26	0	17	27
254	Juice-grapefruit-dehydrated-prepared	cup	247	100	1	24	0	0	0	0	2	412	*	0.2	*	2	91	0.1	0.05	0.5	*	*	0	22	40
252	Juice-grapefruit-frozen concentrate	item	207	302	4	72	0	1	0.1	0	6	1002	78	1	0.4	7	248	0.3	0.16	1.6	0.32	26	0	56	101
253	Juice-grapefruit-frozen-diluted	cup	247	101	1	24	0	tr	tr	0	2	336	27	0.3	0.1	2	83	0.1	0.05	0.5	0.11	9	0	20	35
249	Juice-grapefruit-raw	cup	247	96	1	23	0.5	tr	tr	0	2	400	30	0.5	0.1	2	94	0.1	0.05	0.5	0.11	25	0	22	37
263	Juice-lemon-canned & bottled	cup	244	51	1	16	0.7	1	0.1	0	51	249	20	0.3	0.1	4	61	0.1	0.02	0.5	0.11	25	0	27	22
264	Juice-lemon-frozen-single strength	cup	244	54	1	16	0.7	tr	0.1	0	2	217	20	0.3	0.1	3	77	0.14	0.03	0.3	0.15	23	0	20	20
262	Juice-lemon-raw	cup	244	61	1	21	0.7	tr	tr	0	2	303	15	0.1	0.1	5	112	0.07	0.02	0.2	0.12	32	0	17	15
270	Juice-lime-canned & bottled	cup	246	52	1	17	0	1	0.1	0	39	185	17	0.6	0.1	3	16	0.08	0.01	0.4	0.07	19	0	30	25
269	Juice-lime-raw	cup	246	66	1	22	0	tr	tr	0	2	268	15	0.1	0.1	3	72	0.05	0.03	0.2	0.11	20	0	22	17
280	Juice-orange grapefruit-canned	cup	247	106	1	25	0.5	tr	tr	0	7	390	25	1.1	0.2	29	72	0.14	0.07	0.8	0.06	35	0	20	35
281	Juice-orange grapefruit-frozen-diluted	cup	248	110	1	26	0	0	0	0	2	439	24	0.2	0.2	27	102	0.15	0.02	0.7	0.06	*	0	20	32
276	Juice-orange-canned	cup	249	104	1	25	0.3	tr	tr	0	6	436	27	1.1	0.2	44	86	0.15	0.07	0.8	0.22	136	0	21	36
277	Juice-orange-canned-frozen concentrate	item	213	339	5	81	1.7	tr	0.1	0	7	1435	73	0.7	0.4	59	294	0.6	0.14	1.5	0.33	331	0	67	122
279	Juice-orange-dehydrated-prepared	cup	248	115	1	27	0	0	0	0	2	518	24	0.5	*	50	109	0.2	0.07	1	*	*	0	25	40
278	Juice-orange-frozen concentrate-diluted	cup	249	112	2	27	0.5	tr	tr	0	2	474	24	0.2	0.1	19	97	0.22	0.05	0.5	0.11	109	0	22	40
275	Juice-orange-raw	cup	248	111	2	26	2	1	0.1	0	2	496	27	0.5	0.1	50	124	0.22	0.07	1	0.1	136	0	27	42
942	Juice-passion fruit-purple	cup	247	126	2	34	3.4	tr	tr	0	15	687	42	0.6	0.1	177	74	0	0.32	3.6	0.14	19	0	9	31
943	Juice-passion fruit-yellow	cup	247	148	2	36	1.3	tr	tr	0	15	687	42	0.9	0.1	595	45	0	0.25	5.5	0.14	19	0	10	62
299	Juice-pineapple-canned	cup	250	140	1	35	0.3	tr	tr	0	3	335	33	0.7	0.3	1	27	0.14	0.06	0.6	0.24	58	0	43	20
955	Juice-pineapple-frozen-diluted	cup	250	130	1	32	0.3	tr	tr	0	3	340	23	0.8	0.3	3	30	0.18	0.05	0.5	0.19	27	0	28	20
306	Juice-prune-canned & bottled	cup	256	182	2	45	2.6	tr	tr	0	10	707	36	3	0.5	1	11	0.04	0.18	2	0.56	12	1	31	64
317	Juice-tangerine-canned-sweetened	cup	249	125	1	30	0.6	1	tr	0	2	443	20	0.5	0.1	105	55	0.15	0.05	0.2	0.08	12	0	45	35
974	Juice-tangerine-raw	cup	247	106	1	25	0.8	tr	0.1	0	2	440	20	0.5	0.1	104	77	0.15	0.05	0.2	0.1	11	0	44	35
924	Kiwifruit-raw	item	76	46	1	11	2.6	tr	0	0	4	252	23	0.3	0.1	13	75	0.02	0.04	0.4	0.07	29	0	20	30
925	Kumquats-raw	item	19	12	tr	3	1.3	tr	0	0	1	37	2	0.1	tr	6	7	0.02	0.02	0.1	0.01	3	0	8	4
927	Lemon peel-raw	tbsp	6	4	tr	1	0	tr	tr	0	0	10	1	0.1	*	*	8	tr	tr	tr	*	*	0	8	1
265	Lemonade-canned-frozen concentrate	item	219	425	1	112	5.6	tr	tr	0	4	153	*	0.4	*	4	66	0.05	0.06	0.7	*	*	0	9	13
266	Lemonade-frozen concentrate-diluted	cup	248	105	0	28	0.6	0	0	0	4	40	*	0.1	*	1	17	0.01	0.02	0.2	*	12	0	2	3
926	Lemons-raw-unpeeled	item	108	22	1	12	1	0	0	0	3	157	13	0.8	0.1	3	83	0.05	0.04	0.2	0.12	11	0	66	16
261	Lemons-raw-without peel	item	58	17	1	5	0.6	tr	tr	0	1	80	5	0.3	tr	2	31	0.02	0.01	0.1	0.05	6	0	15	9
267	Limeade-canned-frozen concentrate	item	218	410	0	108	2.2	tr	0	0	14	129	*	0.2	*	2	26	0.02	0.02	0.2	*	*	0	11	13
268	Limeade-frozen concentrate-diluted	cup	247	100	0	27	0.5	0	0	0	2	32	*	0	0	0	6	0	0	0	*	*	0	3	3
928	Limes-raw	item	67	20	tr	7	0.4	tr	tr	0	1	68	4	0.4	0.1	1	20	0.02	0.01	0.1	0.03	5	0	22	12
929	Loganberries-frozen	cup	147	81	2	19	7.1	1	tr	0	1	213	31	0.9	0.5	5	23	0.07	0.05	1.2	0.1	38	0	38	38
930	Longans-raw	item	3.2	2	tr	tr	*	tr	tr	0	0	9	tr	tr	tr	*	3	tr	tr	tr	*	*	0	tr	1
931	Loquats-raw	item	9.9	5	tr	1	0.3	tr	tr	0	tr	26	1	tr	tr	15	tr	tr	tr	tr	*	*	0	2	3
932	Lychees-raw	item	9.59	6	tr	2	tr	tr	tr	0	tr	16	1	tr	*	0	7	tr	0.01	0.1	0.01	3	0	tr	3
933	Mangos-raw	item	207	135	1	35	4.8	1	0.1	0	4	322	18	0.3	0.1	806	57	0.12	0.12	1.2	0.28	29	0	21	22
935	Melon balls-frozen	cup	173	57	1	14	2.6	tr	tr	0	54	484	24	0.5	0.3	307	11	0.29	0.04	1.1	0.18	45	0	17	21
271	Melons-cantaloupe-raw-cubed pieces	cup	160	56	1	13	1.3	tr	0	0	14	494	18	0.3	0.3	516	68	0.06	0.03	0.9	0.18	27	0	18	27
934	Melons-casaba-raw	cup	170	44	2	11	2	tr	0	0	20	357	14	0.7	0.3	5	27	0.1	0.03	0.7	0.2	29	0	9	12
272	Melons-honeydew-raw-cubed pieces	cup	170	60	1	16	1.5	tr	tr	0	17	461	12	0.1	*	7	42	0.13	0.03	1	0.1	*	0	10	17
938	Mulberries-raw	cup	140	60	2	14	2.4	1	tr	0	14	271	25	2.6	0.2	4	51	0.04	0.14	0.9	0.07	8	0	55	53
939	Nectarines-raw	item	136	67	1	16	2.2	1	0.1	0	0	288	11	0.2	0.1	100	7	0.02	0.06	1.4	0.03	5	0	7	22
273	Oranges-raw-all common varieties-whole	item	131	62	1	15	3.1	tr	tr	0	0	237	13	0.1	0.1	27	70	0.11	0.05	0.4	0.08	40	0	52	18
274	Oranges-raw-sections without membranes	cup	180	85	2	21	3.6	tr	tr	0	0	326	18	0.2	0.1	37	96	0.16	0.07	0.5	0.11	55	0	72	25
940	Papaya nectar-canned	cup	250	143	tr	36	1.2	tr	0.1	0	13	78	8	0.9	0.4	28	8	0.02	0.01	0.4	0.02	5	0	25	0

#	Food	Measure																							
282	Papayas-raw	cup	140	55	1	14	1.3	tr	0.1	0	4	359	14	0.1	0.1	282	87	0.04	0.05	0.5	0.03	53	0	34	7
941	Passion fruit-purple-raw	item	18	18	tr	4	2.2	tr	tr	0	5	63	5	0.3	tr	13	5	0	0.02	0.3	0.02	3	0	2	12
944	Peach nectar-canned	cup	249	134	1	35	0.4	tr	0.2	0	17	101	11	0.5	0.2	64	13	0.01	0.04	0.7	0.02	3	0	13	16
285	Peaches-canned-heavy syrup pack	cup	256	189	1	51	1.1	tr	0.1	0	15	235	13	0.7	0.1	85	7	0.03	0.06	1.6	0.05	8	0	8	28
286	Peaches-canned-water pack	cup	244	59	1	15	1.1	tr	0.1	0	7	242	12	0.8	0.2	130	7	0.02	0.05	1.3	0.05	8	0	5	24
288	Peaches-dried-cooked-sulfured-no sugar	cup	258	199	3	51	6.7	1	0.1	0	5	826	34	3.4	0.5	51	10	0.01	0.05	3.9	0.1	tr	0	23	98
287	Peaches-dried-uncooked-sulfured	cup	160	382	6	98	14	1	tr	0	11	1594	67	6.5	0.9	346	8	tr	0.34	7	0.11	8	0	45	190
290	Peaches-frozen-sliced-sweetened	cup	250	235	2	60	6	tr	tr	0	16	325	12	0.9	0.1	71	235	0.03	0.09	1.6	0.05	8	0	6	28
49	Peaches-halved-canned in water-dietetic	serv	28.4	7	tr	2	0.4	tr	0	0	1	30	1	0.1	tr	12	1	tr	0.01	0.1	*	*	0	1	3
284	Peaches-raw-sliced	cup	170	73	1	19	2.7	tr	tr	0	0	335	12	0.2	0.2	91	11	0.03	0.07	1.7	0.03	6	0	9	20
283	Peaches-raw-whole	item	87	37	1	10	1.4	tr	tr	0	0	171	6	0.1	0.1	47	6	0.02	0.04	0.9	0.02	3	0	4	10
47	Peaches-sliced-canned in water-dietetic	oz	28.4	7	tr	2	0.4	tr	0	0	1	30	1	0.1	tr	12	1	tr	0.01	0.1	*	*	0	1	3
289	Peaches-spiced-canned-heavy syrup pack	cup	242	182	1	49	1	tr	tr	0	10	206	17	0.7	0.2	77	13	0.03	0.09	1.3	0.05	8	0	15	22
948	Pear nectar-canned	cup	250	150	tr	39	1.6	tr	tr	0	10	33	8	0.7	0.2	tr	3	0.01	0.03	0.3	0.04	3	0	13	8
294	Pears-canned-heavy syrup pack	cup	255	189	1	49	2.4	tr	tr	0	13	166	10	0.6	0.2	0	3	0.03	0.06	0.6	0.04	3	0	13	18
946	Pears-canned-juice pack	cup	248	124	1	32	4.7	tr	tr	0	10	238	17	0.7	0.2	1	4	0.03	0.03	0.5	0.04	3	0	22	30
945	Pears-canned-water pack	cup	244	71	tr	19	4.1	tr	tr	0	5	129	10	0.5	0.2	0	2	0.02	0.02	0.1	0.03	3	0	10	17
947	Pears-dried-uncooked	cup	180	472	3	125	13.8	1	0.1	0	10	959	60	3.8	0.7	1	13	0.01	0.26	2.5	0.13	0	0	60	106
45	Pears-halved-canned in water-dietetic	oz	28.4	9	tr	2	0.4	0	0	0	1	17	1	0.1	0.1	*	1	tr	0.01	0.1	*	*	0	1	2
291	Pears-raw-bartlett-with skin	item	166	98	1	25	4.3	1	tr	0	0	208	10	0.4	0.2	3	7	0.03	0.07	0.2	0.03	12	0	18	18
292	Pears-raw-bosc-with skin	item	141	83	1	21	3.7	1	tr	0	1	176	8	0.4	0.2	3	6	0.03	0.06	0.1	0.03	10	0	16	16
293	Pears-raw-d'anjou-with skin	item	200	118	1	30	5.2	1	0.1	0	1	250	12	0.5	0.2	4	8	0.04	0.08	0.2	0.04	15	0	22	22
950	Persimmons-Japanese-dried	item	34	93	tr	25	0.6	tr	tr	0	1	273	11	0.3	0.1	19	19	0.01	0.01	0.1	0.03	3	0	9	28
949	Persimmons-Japanese-raw	item	168	118	1	31	2.9	tr	0.1	0	3	270	15	0.3	0.2	364	13	0.03	0.03	0.2	0.17	13	0	13	28
951	Persimmons-native-raw	item	25	32	tr	8	0.4	tr	tr	0	1	78	2	0.6	tr	54	17	0.01	0.01	tr	0.03	2	0	7	7
1542	Pineapple grapefruit drink	cup	253	129	1	32	0	tr	0	0	56	139	15	0.8	0.1	0	68	0.05	0.05	0.6	2.02	25	0	15	10
1543	Pineapple orange drink	cup	253	134	1	34	0	0	0	0	8	121	15	0.7	0.2	134	63	0.08	0.05	0.5	0.12	28	0	13	10
296	Pineapple-bits-canned in syrup	cup	252	131	1	34	1.9	tr	tr	0	3	266	40	1	0.3	4	19	0.23	0.06	0.7	0.19	12	0	36	17
952	Pineapple-bits-canned-water pack	cup	246	79	1	20	2	tr	tr	0	4	312	44	1	0.3	4	19	0.23	0.06	0.7	0.18	12	0	37	10
953	Pineapple-canned-juice pack	cup	250	150	1	39	1.9	tr	tr	0	4	304	35	0.7	0.2	10	24	0.24	0.05	0.7	0.19	12	0	34	16
954	Pineapple-frozen-sweetened	cup	245	208	1	54	5.4	tr	0.1	0	5	245	25	1	0.3	7	20	0.25	0.07	0.7	0.18	26	0	22	10
295	Pineapple-raw-diced	cup	155	76	1	19	1.9	1	0.1	0	2	175	22	0.6	0.1	4	24	0.14	0.06	0.7	0.14	16	0	11	11
43	Pineapple-sliced-dietetic-canned/water	oz	28.4	13	tr	4	0.5	0	0	0	1	24	3	0.1	0.1	1	2	0.03	0.01	0.1	*	*	0	3	1
956	Pitanga-raw	item	7	2	tr	1	*	tr	*	0	tr	7	1	tr	*	11	2	tr	tr	tr	*	*	0	3	1
958	Plantains-cooked	cup	154	179	1	48	3.5	tr	0.1	0	8	716	49	0.9	0.2	140	17	0.07	0.08	1.2	0.37	40	0	3	43
957	Plantains-raw	item	179	218	2	57	4.1	1	0.3	0	7	893	66	1.1	0.3	202	33	0.09	0.1	1.2	0.54	39	0	5	61
302	Plums-purple-canned-heavy syrup pack	cup	258	230	1	60	1.1	tr	tr	0	50	234	13	2.2	0.2	67	7	0.04	0.1	0.8	0.07	7	0	24	33
960	Plums-purple-canned-juice pack	cup	252	146	1	38	1	tr	tr	0	3	389	20	0.8	0.3	254	7	0.06	0.15	1.2	0.07	7	0	25	39
959	Plums-purple-canned-water pack	cup	249	102	1	28	1.2	tr	tr	0	2	314	13	0.4	0.2	228	7	0.05	0.1	0.9	0.07	7	0	17	33
300	Plums-raw-Japanese & hybrid	item	66	36	1	9	1.4	tr	tr	0	0	114	5	0.1	0.1	21	6	0.03	0.06	0.3	0.05	1	0	3	7
301	Plums-raw-prune type	item	28.4	20	0	6	0.6	tr	0	0	0	48	2	0.1	tr	8	2	0.01	0.01	0.1	0.02	1	0	5	5
961	Pomegranates-raw	item	154	105	1	26	1.1	1	0.1	0	5	399	5	0.5	0.2	0	9	0.05	0.05	0.5	0.16	9	0	5	12
963	Pricklypears-raw	item	103	42	1	10	5.6	1	tr	0	5	227	88	0.3	0.3	5	14	0.01	0.06	0.5	*	*	0	58	25
962	Prunes-canned-heavy syrup pack	cup	234	246	2	65	8.6	tr	tr	0	7	529	35	1	0.4	187	7	0.08	0.29	2	0.48	tr	0	40	61
297	Prunes-dried-cooked-with sugar	cup	238	295	3	78	7.6	1	tr	0	4	741	45	2.5	0.5	68	6	0.05	0.22	1.6	0.48	tr	0	51	78
305	Prunes-dried-cooked-without sugar	cup	212	227	2	60	7.5	tr	tr	0	6	708	43	2.4	0.5	65	6	0.05	0.21	1.5	0.46	7	0	48	75
304	Prunes-dried-uncooked	cup	161	385	4	101	11	1	0.1	0	6	1200	73	4	0.9	320	5	0.13	0.26	3.2	0.43	6	0	82	127
964	Pummelo-sections-raw	cup	190	72	1	18	1.9	tr	tr	0	2	410	11	0.2	0.2	0	116	0.07	0.05	0.4	0.07	*	0	8	32
965	Quinces-raw	item	92	52	tr	14	1.8	tr	tr	0	4	181	7	0.6	tr	4	14	0.02	0.03	0.2	0.04	3	0	10	16
307	Raisins-seedless	cup	145	435	5	115	7.7	1	0.2	0	17	1089	48	3	0.4	1	5	0.23	0.13	1.2	0.36	5	0	71	141
308	Raisins-seedless-packet	item	14	42	tr	11	0.7	tr	tr	0	2	105	5	0.3	tr	tr	tr	0.02	0.01	0.1	0.04	tr	0	7	14

* indicates that no data was available.

©1994 First DataBank—The Hearst Corporation (N-Squared Computing).

Appendix A – Table of Food Composition (continued)

Item	Food name	Portion	Weight (g)	Food Energy (Kcal)	Protein (gm)	Carbohydrates (gm)	Fiber (gm)	Total Fat (gm)	Saturated Fat (gm)	Cholesterol (mg)	Sodium (mg)	Potassium (mg)	Magnesium (mg)	Iron (mg)	Zinc (mg)	Vitamin A (RE)	Vitamin C (mg)	Thiamin (mg)	Riboflavin (mg)	Niacin (mg)	Vitamin B6 (mg)	Folates (µg)	Vitamin B12 (µg)	Calcium (mg)	Phosphorus (mg)
966	Raspberries-canned-heavy syrup pack	cup	256	234	2	60	6.5	tr	tr	0	9	241	31	1.1	0.4	9	22	0.05	0.08	1.1	0.11	27	0	27	23
310	Raspberries-frozen-sweetened	cup	250	258	2	65	11	tr	tr	0	3	285	33	1.6	0.5	15	41	0.05	0.11	0.6	0.09	65	0	38	43
309	Raspberries-raw	cup	123	60	1	14	5.5	1	tr	0	0	187	22	0.7	0.6	16	31	0.04	0.11	1.1	0.07	32	0	27	15
312	Rhubarb-cooked from frozen-added sugar	cup	240	278	1	75	4.8	tr	0	0	5	230	29	0.5	0.2	17	8	0.04	0.06	0.5	0.05	13	0	348	19
311	Rhubarb-cooked from raw-added sugar	cup	270	380	1	97	5.4	0	0	0	5	548	32	1.6	0.2	22	16	0.05	0.14	0.8	0.05	14	0	211	41
298	Roselle-raw	cup	57	28	1	6	2.3	tr	*	*	3	119	29	0.8	*	16	7	0.01	0.02	0.2	*	*	*	123	21
967	Sapodilla-raw	item	170	140	1	34	9	2	0.2	0	20	328	20	1.4	0.2	10	25	0	0.03	0.3	0.06	24	0	36	20
968	Sapotes-raw	item	225	302	5	76	*	1	*	0	23	774	68	2.3	*	92	45	0.02	0.05	4.1	*	*	*	88	63
923	Sauce-guava-cooked	cup	238	86	1	23	6.8	tr	0.1	0	10	536	17	0.4	0.4	67	348	0.06	0.03	1	*	*	*	17	26
303	Soursop-raw-pulp	cup	225	149	2	38	*	1	*	0	32	626	47	1.4	*	7	46	0.16	0.11	2	0.13	*	0	32	61
969	Strawberries-canned-heavy syrup pack	cup	254	234	1	60	3.1	tr	tr	0	8	218	22	1.2	0.2	7	80	0.05	0.09	0.1	0.12	71	0	33	29
314	Strawberries-frozen-sweetened-sliced	cup	255	245	1	66	19.8	tr	tr	0	8	249	18	1.5	0.1	6	106	0.04	0.13	1	0.08	38	0	28	32
315	Strawberries-frozen-sweetened-whole	cup	255	199	1	54	5.6	tr	tr	0	3	250	15	1.2	0.1	7	101	0.04	0.2	0.7	0.07	10	0	28	31
970	Strawberries-frozen-unsweetened	cup	149	52	1	14	3.9	tr	tr	0	3	221	16	1.1	0.2	7	61	0.03	0.06	0.7	0.04	25	0	24	19
313	Strawberries-raw-whole	cup	149	45	1	11	3.9	tr	tr	0	1	247	15	0.6	0.2	4	85	0.03	0.1	0.3	0.09	26	0	21	28
971	Tamarinds-raw	item	2	5	tr	1	0.1	tr	tr	0	1	13	2	0.1	tr	2	0	0.01	tr	tr	tr	12	0	2	2
972	Tangerines-canned-juice pack	cup	249	92	2	24	1.5	tr	tr	0	13	331	27	0.7	1.3	212	85	0.2	0.07	1.1	0.11	12	0	27	25
973	Tangerines-canned-light syrup pack	cup	252	154	1	41	1.4	tr	tr	0	15	197	20	0.6	0.6	212	50	0.13	0.11	1.1	0.11	12	0	18	25
316	Tangerines-raw-peeled	item	84	37	1	9	1.7	tr	*	0	1	132	10	0.1	0.2	77	26	0.09	0.02	0.1	0.06	17	0	12	8
318	Watermelon-raw	cup	160	51	1	12	0.6	1	*	0	3	186	18	0.3	0.1	59	15	0.13	0.03	0.3	0.23	4	0	13	14
	Grains																								
1774	Barley-dry-uncooked	cup	184	651	23	135	27	4	0.9	0	22	831	244	6.6	5.1	4	0	1.19	0.53	8.5	0.59	35	0	61	485
1775	Barley-pearled-light-cooked	cup	157	193	4	44	8.9	1	0.1	0	5	145	35	2.1	1.3	2	0	0.13	0.1	3.2	0.18	26	0	17	85
321	Barley-pearled-light-uncooked	cup	200	704	20	155	31.2	2	0.5	0	18	560	158	5	4.3	4	0	0.38	0.23	9.2	0.52	46	0	57	442
1465	Bisquick mix-dry	cup	112	480	8	76	3	16	*	*	1400	*	*	1.6	1.2	*	*	*	*	*	*	*	*	*	139
1778	Buckwheat groats-roasted-cooked	cup	198	182	7	40	4	1	0.3	0	8	175	101	1.6	1.2	0	0	0.08	0.08	1.9	0.15	27	0	14	139
1777	Buckwheat groats-roasted-dry	cup	164	567	19	123	12.3	6	1	0	18	525	362	4.1	4	0	0	0.37	0.45	8.4	0.58	69	0	29	523
1776	Buckwheat-raw-whole	cup	170	583	23	122	18.4	6	1.3	0	1	782	393	3.7	4.1	0	0	0.17	0.72	11.9	0.36	51	0	31	590
384	Bulgur-canned-seasoned	cup	135	245	8	44	8.8	4	*	0	621	151		1.9	1	0	0	0.08	0.05	4.1	*	*	*	18	263
1779	Bulgur-cooked	cup	182	152	6	34	6.8	tr	0.1	0	9	124	58	1.8	1	0	0	0.1	0.05	1.8	0.15	33	0	18	73
1497	Bulgur-dry-commercial	cup	140	479	17	106	32	2	0.3	0	23	573	230	3.4	2.7	0	0	0.33	0.16	7.2	0.48	37	0	49	419
1781	Corn bran-crude	cup	76	170	6	65	13	1	0.1	0	5	33	48	2.1	1.2	5	0	0.01	0.08	2.1	0.12	3	0	32	55
1278	Corn chips	oz	28.4	155	2	17	1.7	9	1.5	0	164	43	22	0.4	0.4	11	1	0.05	0.03	0.6	0.05	2	0	37	55
1557	Corn germ-toasted	oz	28.4	130	5	12	2.3	7	*	0	1	*	188	2.2	3	2	1	0.47	0.21	0.6	0.39	26	*	3	444
1783	Corn grits-dry	cup	156	579	14	124	18.6	2	0.3	0	1	213	42	6.1	0.6	1	0	1	0.59	7.7	0.23	7	0	3	114
1780	Corn kernels-whole grain	cup	166	606	16	123	18.5	8	1.1	0	58	476	211	4.5	3.7	78	0	0.64	0.33	6	1.03	32	0	12	349
427	Cornmeal-degermed-enriched-cooked	cup	240	878	20	186	1.9	4	0.5	0	7	389	96	9.9	1.7	98	0	1.72	0.98	12.1	0.62	115	0	12	202
426	Cornmeal-degermed-enriched-dry	cup	138	505	12	107	7.2	2	0.3	0	4	224	55	5.7	1	57	0	0.99	0.56	7	0.35	66	0	7	116
429	Cornmeal-degermed-unenriched-cooked	cup	240	878	20	186	1.9	4	0.5	0	7	389	96	2.6	1.7	98	0	0.34	0.12	5.6	0.62	115	0	12	202
428	Cornmeal-degermed-unenriched-dry	cup	138	505	12	107	7.2	2	0.3	0	4	224	55	1.5	1	57	0	0.19	0.07	1.4	0.35	66	0	7	116
1385	Cornmeal-self rising-degermed	cup	138	490	12	103	7.7	2	0.3	0	1860	235	68	6.5	1.4	57	0	0.94	0.53	6.3	0.54	43	*	483	860
425	Cornmeal-whole grain-bolted	cup	122	407	10	86	13.4	4	0.6	0	1521	311	105	7	2.4	57	0	0.81	0.49	6.5	0.66	70	0	440	981
424	Cornmeal-whole grain-dry	cup	122	442	10	94	18.8	4	0.6	0	43	350	155	4.2	2.2	57	0	0.47	0.25	4.4	0.37	31	0	7	294
1529	Cornstarch	cup	128	488	tr	117	1.2	tr	tr	0	11	4	3	0.6	0.1	0	0	0	0	0	0	0	0	2	16
1785	Couscous-cooked	cup	179	200	7	42	8.3	tr	0.1	0	9	104	14	0.7	0.5	0	0	0.11	0.05	1.8	0.09	27	0	14	39
1784	Couscous-dry	cup	184	692	24	142	28.4	1	0.2	0	18	305	81	2	1.5	0	0	0.3	0.14	6.4	0.2	37	0	44	313
1475	Croutons-herb seasoned	cup	30	100	4	20	1.4	1	0	0	372	39	11	1.5	0.3	0	0	0.13	0.2	1.7	0.1	0	0	29	42
1786	Farina-enriched-dry	cup	176	649	19	137	10.2	1	0.1	0	5	165	23	6.5	0.9	*	*	1.01	0.63	7.1	0.01	42	0	25	202
1773	Flour-arrowroot	cup	128	457	tr	113	5.1	tr	tr	0	2	14	4	0.4	0.1	0	0	tr	tr	0	0.01	9	0	51	7
1466	Flour-barley	cup	112	401	11	86	20.2	2	0.3	0	3	179	157	4.8	2.8	0	0	0.62	0.13	4.8	0.36	54	0	46	417
383	Flour-buckwheat-whole groat	cup	120	402	15	85	16.9	4	0.8	0	3	692	301	4.9	3.8	0	0	0.5	0.23	7.4	0.7	64	0	49	404

Code	Food	Unit	1	2	3	4	5	6	7	8	9	10	11	12	13	14	15	16	17	18	19	20	21	22	23	24
1630	Flour-carob	cup	103	185	5	92	10.9	1	0.1	0	36	852	56	3	0.9	2	2	tr	0.06	0.48	2	0.38	30	0	359	81
1467	Flour-corn-masa-sifted	cup	114	416	11	87	6.5	4	0.6	0	6	340	125	8.2	2	55	0	0	1.63	0.86	11.2	0.42	28	0	161	255
1782	Flour-corn-whole grain	cup	117	422	8	90	18	5	0.6	0	6	369	109	2.8	2	55	0	0	0.29	0.09	2.2	0.43	30	0	8	318
1029	Flour-potato	cup	179	628	14	143	6.4	1	0.4	0	61	2843	158	30.8	2.9	0	34	0	0.75	0.25	6.1	0.01	91	0	59	319
1798	Flour-rice-brown	cup	158	574	11	121	5.5	4	0.9	0	12	456	177	3.1	3.9	0	0	0	0.7	0.13	10	1.16	25	0	18	533
1468	Flour-rice-white	cup	158	578	9	127	3	2	0.6	0	1	120	55	0.6	1.3	0	0	0	0.22	0.03	4.1	0.69	6	0	16	155
1800	Flour-rye-dark	cup	128	415	18	88	4	3	0.4	0	2	934	318	8.3	7.2	0	0	0	0.4	0.32	5.5	0.57	77	0	72	809
1801	Flour-rye-light	cup	102	374	9	82	3.7	2	0.1	0	2	238	72	1.8	1.8	0	0	0	0.34	0.09	0.8	0.24	23	0	21	198
1481	Flour-sesame-lowfat	cup	100	333	50	36	6	2	0.2	0	39	397	338	14.2	10	6	0	0	2.52	0.27	12.5	0.14	29	0	149	757
1495	Flour-soybean-lowfat	cup	88	313	38	32	7	6	*	0	1	1636	*	8	*	7	0	0	0.73	0.32	2.3	*	*	0	231	558
1804	Flour-triticale-whole grain	cup	130	439	17	95	7.1	2	0.4	0	3	606	199	3.4	3.5	0	0	0	0.49	0.17	3.7	0.52	96	0	46	417
502	Flour-wheat-enriched-sifted	cup	115	419	12	88	3.1	1	0.2	0	2	123	25	5.3	0.8	0	0	0	0.9	0.57	6.8	0.05	30	0	17	124
503	Flour-wheat-enriched-unsifted	cup	125	455	13	95	3.4	1	0.2	0	2	134	27	5.8	0.9	0	0	0	0.98	0.62	7.4	0.06	33	0	18	135
504	Flour-wheat-white-cake/pastry-enriched	cup	109	395	9	85	2.6	1	0.1	0	2	115	18	8	0.7	0	0	0	0.97	0.47	7.4	0.04	21	0	16	93
1813	Flour-wheat-white-for bread	cup	137	495	16	99	4.5	2	0.3	0	2	136	34	6	1.2	0	0	0	1.11	0.7	10.4	0.05	40	0	21	133
505	Flour-wheat-white-self rising-enriched	cup	125	443	12	93	3.4	1	0.2	0	1588	155	24	5.8	0.8	0	0	0	0.84	0.52	7.3	0.06	53	0	423	744
1814	Flour-wheat-white-tortilla mix	cup	111	450	11	75	3.4	12	4.6	0	751	111	23	7.8	0.7	7	0	0	0.82	0.55	6.5	0.04	26	0	228	233
506	Flour-wheat-whole grain-stirred	cup	120	407	16	87	15.1	2	0.4	0	6	486	166	4.7	3.5	0	0	0	0.54	0.26	7.6	0.41	52	0	40	415
1787	Hominy-canned	cup	160	115	2	23	4.6	1	0.2	0	336	14	26	1.7	1.7	0	0	0	tr	0.01	0.1	0.01	1	0	15	56
438	Macaroni-cooked-firm stage-hot	cup	130	183	6	37	2.1	1	0.1	0	1	41	23	1.8	0.7	0	0	0	0.27	0.13	2.2	0.05	1	0	1	71
439	Macaroni-cooked-tender stage-cold	cup	105	148	5	30	1.7	1	0.1	0	1	33	19	1.5	0.6	*	0	0	0.22	0.1	1.8	0.04	8	0	8	57
440	Macaroni-cooked-tender stage-hot	cup	140	197	7	40	2.2	1	0.1	0	1	44	25	2	0.7	0	0	0	0.29	0.14	2.3	0.05	10	0	10	76
1822	Macaroni-vegetable-cooked	cup	134	172	6	36	2.7	tr	tr	0	8	42	26	0.7	0.6	7	0	0	0.15	0.08	1.4	0.03	8	0	15	67
1390	Macaroni-whole wheat-cooked	cup	140	174	7	37	2.8	1	0.1	0	4	61	42	1.5	1.1	0	0	0	0.15	0.06	1	0.11	7	0	21	124
1769	Matzos-American crackers-Manischewitz	serv	28.4	115	3	22	0.8	2	0.1	0	1	52	12	1	0.5	0	0	0	0.16	0.09	1.1	0.03	10	0	6	40
1768	Matzos-daily thin tea-Manischewitz	piece	25.5	103	3	22	0.7	tr	*	0	*	34	*	1	*	0	*	*	*	*	*	*	*	0.37	*	*
1770	Matzos-matzo meal-Manischewitz	cup	135	514	13	109	3.9	1	8.1	0	3	149	13	4.1	0.7	87	tr	0	0.1	0.29	0.9	0.08	24	0	37	101
1789	Millet-cooked	cup	240	286	8	57	11.4	2	0.4	0	5	148	105	1.5	2.2	0	0	0	0.25	0.2	3.2	0.26	46	0	7	240
1788	Millet-raw	cup	200	756	22	146	29.2	8	1.5	0	10	390	227	6	3.4	7	0	0	0.84	0.58	9.4	0.77	170	0	17	569
1387	Noodles-cellophane/long rice-dry	cup	140	491	tr	121	*	14	tr	0	14	14	4	2.1	0.3	0	0	0	0.21	0.07	0.3	0.07	3	0	35	45
449	Noodles-chow mein-enriched	cup	45	237	4	26	1.8	14	2	0	197	54	23	2.1	0.6	0	4	0	0.26	0.19	2.7	0.05	10	0	9	72
1389	Noodles-egg-cooked	cup	160	213	8	40	3	2	0.5	53	11	45	30	2.5	1	0	10	0	0.3	0.13	2.4	0.06	11	0.14	19	110
448	Noodles-egg-enriched-cooked	cup	160	200	7	37	3.5	2	*	50	3	70	43	1.4	*	7	11	0	0.22	0.13	1.9	0.14	19	0	16	94
1388	Noodles-egg-spinach-cooked	cup	160	211	8	39	0.4	3	0.6	52	20	59	38	1.7	1	0	34	0	0.39	0.2	2.4	0.18	34	0.22	30	91
1548	Noodles-ramen-oriental	cup	227	207	6	31	2	9	0.4	36	829	69	17	1.8	0.6	221	tr	0	0.16	0.1	1.4	0.07	8	0.01	18	70
1550	Noodles-soba-buckwheat-dry	oz	28.4	95	4	21	0.5	tr	tr	0	225	72	27	0.8	0.5	0	0	0	0.14	0.04	0.9	0.07	17	0	10	72
1549	Noodles-somen-wheat-dry	oz	28.4	101	3	21	0.5	tr	tr	0	523	47	8	0.4	0.1	0	0	0	0.03	0.01	0.2	0.01	4	0	7	23
1791	Oat bran-raw	cup	94	231	16	62	12.5	7	1.3	0	4	532	221	5.1	2.9	0	0	0	1.1	0.21	0.9	0.16	49	0	55	690
1790	Oats-whole grain-uncooked	cup	156	607	26	104	20.8	11	1.9	0	3	669	276	7.4	6.2	0	0	0	1.19	0.22	1.5	0.19	87	0	84	816
1817	Pasta-corn-cooked	cup	140	176	4	39	1.8	1	0.1	0	1	43	50	0.3	0.9	8	0	0	0.07	0.03	0.8	0.08	9	0	2	106
1818	Pasta-fresh-plain-cooked	oz	28.4	38	1	7	0.3	tr	tr	2	2	7	5	0.3	0.2	2	0	0	0.06	0.04	0.3	0.01	2	0.04	2	18
1819	Pasta-fresh-spinach-cooked	oz	28.4	37	1	7	0.3	tr	0.1	2	2	11	7	0.2	0.2	4	0	0	0.05	0.04	0.3	0.03	5	0.04	5	16
1820	Pasta-homemade-with egg-cooked	oz	28.4	37	2	7	0.3	1	0.1	24	2	6	4	0.3	0.1	12	0	0	0.05	0.05	0.4	0.01	6	0.03	3	15
1821	Pasta-homemade-without egg-cooked	oz	28.4	35	1	7	0.3	tr	tr	0	21	5	4	0.3	0.1	21	0	0	0.05	0.04	0.4	0.01	5	0	2	11
477	Popcorn-popped-oil & salt	cup	9	40	1	5	0.4	2	*	0	174	*	16	0.2	0.4	174	*	0	*	0.01	0.2	*	*	*	1	19
476	Popcorn-popped-plain	cup	35	25	2	5	0.4	0	0	0	0	*	*	0.2	0.5	*	0	0	*	*	0.1	0.01	*	0	1	17
478	Popcorn-popped-sugar coated	cup	35	135	2	30	1.4	1	0.5	0	0	*	*	0.5	*	0	0	0	*	0.02	0.4	*	*	0	2	47
479	Pretzel-dutch-twisted	item	16	60	2	12	*	1	*	0	258	21	4	0.2	0.2	0	0	0	0.05	0.04	0.7	tr	3	0	4	21
481	Pretzel-thin-stick	item	0.3	1	tr	tr	*	tr	0	0	5	tr	tr	tr	tr	0	0	0	tr	tr	tr	0	tr	0	tr	tr
480	Pretzel-thin-twisted	item	6	24	1	5	*	tr	*	0	97	6	1	0.1	0.1	0	0	0	0.02	0.02	0.3	tr	1	0	2	5
1794	Quinoa-whole or ground	cup	170	636	22	117	8.8	10	1	0	36	1258	357	15.7	5.6	0	0	0	0.34	0.67	5	0.38	83	0	102	697

* indicates that no data was available.
©1994 First DataBank—The Hearst Corporation (N-Squared Computing).

Appendix A - Table of Food Composition
(continued)

Item	Food name	Portion	Weight (g)	Food Energy (Kcal)	Protein (gm)	Carbohydrates (gm)	Fiber (gm)	Total Fat (gm)	Saturated Fat (gm)	Cholesterol (mg)	Sodium (mg)	Potassium (mg)	Magnesium (mg)	Iron (mg)	Zinc (mg)	Vitamin A (RE)	Vitamin C (mg)	Thiamin (mg)	Riboflavin (mg)	Niacin (mg)	Vitamin B6 (mg)	Folates (µg)	Vitamin B12 (µg)	Calcium (mg)	Phosphorus (mg)
1571	Rice bran	oz	28.4	80	5	16	6.1	tr	1.2	0	5	593	408	4.6	1.7	0	0	0.78	0.08	9.7	1.16	18	0	16	119
1797	Rice bran-crude	cup	83	262	11	41	8.2	17	3.5	0	4	1232	648	15.4	5	0	0	2.29	0.24	28.2	3.38	52	0	47	1392
1547	Rice cake-low sodium	item	9.31	35	1	8	0.2	tr	1.2	0	tr	26	3	0.2	0.1	0	tr	tr	tr	0.1	0.01	1	0	7	10
1546	Rice cake-regular	item	9.31	35	1	8	0.2	tr	1.2	0	11	27	3	0.2	0.1	0	tr	tr	tr	0.1	0.01	1	0	7	10
129	Rice-brown-long grain-cooked	cup	195	216	5	45	3.3	2	0.4	0	9	83	83	0.8	1.2	0	0	0.19	0.05	3	0.28	8	0	20	161
131	Rice-brown-long grain-raw	cup	185	685	15	143	10.7	5	1.1	0	13	413	265	2.7	3.7	0	0	0.74	0.17	9.4	0.94	36	0	43	616
1348	Rice-brown-Uncle Ben's	cup	146	220	5	46	2.5	2	0.5	0	2	172	*	0.9	*	0	0	0.18	0.04	4.2	*	*	*	16	222
1508	Rice-spanish-home recipe	cup	245	213	4	41	1.8	4	8.3	0	774	566	50	1.5	2.9	162	37	0.1	0.07	1.7	0.33	11	2.12	34	96
482	Rice-white-instant-hot	cup	165	162	3	35	1.3	tr	0.1	0	5	7	8	1	0.4	0	0	0.12	0.08	1.5	0.02	6	0	13	23
484	Rice-white-long grain-cooked	cup	205	264	6	57	2.1	1	0.2	0	4	80	26	2.3	0.9	0	0	0.33	0.03	3	0.19	7	0	23	95
483	Rice-white-long grain-raw	cup	185	675	13	148	1.9	1	0.3	0	9	213	46	8	2	0	0	1.07	0.09	7.8	0.3	16	0	52	213
486	Rice-white-parboiled-cooked	cup	175	199	4	43	0.9	tr	0.1	0	6	66	20	2	0.5	0	0	0.44	0.03	2.5	0.03	6	0	33	73
485	Rice-white-parboiled-dry	cup	185	686	13	151	3.3	1	0.3	0	9	222	57	6.6	1.8	0	0	1.1	0.13	6.7	0.65	31	0	112	252
1795	Rice-white-short grain-cooked	cup	205	267	5	59	2.7	tr	0.1	0	*	54	17	3	0.8	0	0	0.34	0.03	3.1	0.12	3	0	2	67
1796	Rice-white-with pasta-cooked	cup	202	246	5	43	2	6	1.1	1	1147	85	24	1.9	0.6	0	tr	0.25	0.16	3.6	0.2	15	0.12	16	75
1816	Rice-wild-cooked	cup	164	166	7	35	2.6	1	0.1	0	6	166	52	1	2.2	*	0	0.09	0.14	2.1	0.22	43	0	5	134
1799	Rye-whole-dry	cup	169	566	25	118	8.9	4	0.5	0	10	446	204	4.5	6.3	0	0	0.53	0.42	7.2	0.5	101	0	56	632
1802	Semolina	cup	167	601	21	122	*	2	0.3	0	2	311	79	7.3	1.8	0	0	1.35	0.95	10	0.17	120	0	28	227
1362	Shake 'n Bake-package-General Foods	oz	28.4	116	2	18	*	4	*	*	984	57	*	0.7	*	62	tr	0.16	0.18	2.2	*	*	*	14	44
1803	Sorghum-whole-dry	cup	192	651	22	143	28.6	6	0.9	0	12	672	*	8.5	*	0	0	0.46	0.27	5.6	0.08	16	0	54	551
493	Spaghetti-cooked-firm stage-al dente-hot	cup	130	190	7	39	2.1	1	*	0	1	103	25	1.4	0.7	0	0	0.23	0.13	1.8	0.09	17	0	14	85
494	Spaghetti-cooked-tender stage-hot	cup	140	155	5	32	2.2	1	0.2	0	*	85	24	1.3	0.7	0	0	0.2	0.11	1.5	0.06	3	0	11	70
1360	Stuffing mix-chicken-General Foods	oz	28.4	107	4	21	0.1	6	*	15	488	77	6	1.1	0.4	5	tr	0.15	0.09	1.3	*	*	0.05	29	37
1530	Stuffing mix-dry form	cup	30	111	4	22	*	1	*	*	399	52	*	1	*	0	0	0.07	0.08	1	*	3	*	37	57
1531	Stuffing mix-prepared	cup	140	501	9	50	*	31	*	0	1254	126	11	2.2	*	91	0	0.13	0.17	2.1	0.04	3	*	92	136
1279	Taco shells	item	11	50	1	7	0.9	2	0.3	0	20	27	21	0.3	0.1	5	0	0.03	0.02	0.2	*	*	*	16	25
1469	Tortilla chips-Doritos	oz	28.4	139	2	19	1.9	7	1.4	0	180	51	21	0.5	0.2	5	0	0.03	0.03	tr	0.1	4	0	30	59
1280	Tortilla-corn	item	30	67	2	13	1.6	1	0.1	0	53	52	20	0.6	0.4	5	0	0.05	0.03	0.4	0.09	6	0	42	55
1492	Tortilla-flour	item	30	95	3	17	0.8	2	0.6	0	113	30	7	1.1	0.2	tr	0	0.01	0.08	1	0.01	4	0	46	25
1811	Wheat bran-crude	cup	60	130	9	39	7.7	3	0.4	0	2	710	366	6.3	4.4	0	0	0.31	0.35	8.2	0.78	48	0	44	608
1812	Wheat germ-crude	cup	115	414	27	60	11.9	11	1.9	0	14	1026	275	7.2	14.1	0	0	2.17	0.57	7.8	1.5	324	0	44	968
1810	Wheat-durum	cup	192	651	26	137	10.3	5	0.9	0	3	827	277	6.8	8	0	0	0.8	0.23	12.9	0.8	83	0	65	975
1805	Wheat-hard red-spring	cup	192	632	30	131	9.8	4	0.6	0	4	653	238	6.9	5.3	0	0	0.97	0.21	11	0.65	83	0	48	637
1806	Wheat-hard red-winter	cup	192	628	24	137	10.3	3	0.5	0	4	697	243	6.1	5.1	0	0	0.74	0.22	10.5	0.58	72	0	56	552
1808	Wheat-hard white	cup	192	657	22	146	6.6	3	0.5	0	4	829	179	8.8	6.4	0	0	0.74	0.21	8.4	0.71	72	0	61	682
1807	Wheat-soft red-winter	cup	192	556	17	125	9.4	3	0.5	0	4	667	212	5.4	4.4	0	0	0.66	0.16	8.1	0.46	68	0	46	828
1809	Wheat-soft white	cup	168	571	18	127	5.7	3	0.6	0	3	730	151	9	5.8	0	0	0.69	0.18	8	0.63	68	0	57	675
1815	Wheat-sprouted	cup	108	214	8	46	3.4	1	0.2	0	18	182	89	2.3	1.8	*	3	0.24	0.17	3.3	0.29	41	0	30	216
Vitamins																									
1613	Vitamin-Centrum-advanced formula	item	1.3	*	*	*	*	*	*	0	*	8	100	27	22.5	5000	90	2.25	2.6	20	3	400	9	162	125
1616	Vitamin-Flintstone-complete childrens	item	1.2	*	*	*	*	*	*	*	*	20	20	18	15	5000	60	1.5	1.7	20	2	400	6	100	100
1614	Vitamin-Geritol complete	item	1.2	*	*	*	*	*	*	*	*	8	100	50	15	5000	60	1.5	1.7	20	2	400	6	162	125
1622	Vitamin-Nature Made-multi	item	1.3	*	*	*	*	*	*	0	0	*	65	12	1.5	1000	200	10	10	100	5	*	5	20	*
1619	Vitamin-One a Day a Day-maximum formula	item	1.3	*	*	*	*	*	*	0	*	38	100	18	15	5000	60	1.5	1.7	20	2	400	6	130	100
1615	Vitamin-One a Day a Day-Stressgard	item	1.3	*	*	*	*	*	*	*	*	*	*	18	15	5000	600	15	10	100	5	400	12	*	*
1621	Vitamin-Safeway-daily plus iron	item	1.2	*	*	*	*	*	*	*	*	*	*	18	*	5000	60	1.5	1.7	20	2	400	6	*	*
1620	Vitamin-Safeway-one tab daily	item	1.2	*	*	*	*	*	*	0	0	*	*	*	*	5000	60	1.5	1.7	20	2	400	6	*	*
1618	Vitamin-Shaklee-Vita Lea	item	1.2	*	*	*	*	*	*	0	*	*	50	4.5	3.8	1250	23	0.53	0.6	5	0.5	100	2.25	150	113
1617	Vitamin-Stresstabs 600	item	1.2	*	*	*	*	*	*	*	*	*	*	*	*	*	600	15	15	100	5	400	12	*	*

No.	Meats																										
1297	Bacon bits	tbsp	6	2	2	0.6	2	0.2	0	0	165	9	6	0.3	0.1	tr	0	0	0.03	0.02	0.1	0.01	8	0.07	8	18
161	Bacon-pork-broiled/pan-fried/roasted	slice	6.3	27	2	0	3	1.1	5	5	101	31	6	0.1	0.2	2	0	0	0.04	0.02	0.5	0.02	tr	0.11	1	21
1234	Barbecue loaf-pork and beef	slice	23	40	4	1	2	0.7	9	9	307	76	4	0.3	0.6	4	2	0	0.08	0.06	0.5	0.06	2	0.39	13	30
162	Beef cuts-lean and fat-simmered/roasted	slice	85	297	21	0	23	9.5	78	78	50	244	18	2.2	4.7	0	0	0.07	0.18	2.9	0.26	6	2.03	8	164
163	Beef cuts-lean only-simmered/roasted	slice	85	347	19	0	30	12.3	78	78	55	186	14	1.9	4.5	0	0	0.05	0.15	2.4	0.2	5	1.91	8	147
176	Beef-dried-cured-chipped	serv	71	117	21	1	3	1.1	65	65	2464	315	23	3.2	3.7	*	0	0.05	0.23	2.7	*	*	1.31	4	124
181	Beef-heart-cooked-simmered	slice	85	149	25	tr	5	1.4	164	164	54	198	21	6.4	2.7	0	1	0.12	1.31	3.5	0.18	8	12.2	5	213
188	Beef-liver-fried in margarine	slice	85	184	23	7	7	2.4	410	410	90	309	20	5.3	4.6	9216	19	0.18	3.52	12.3	1.22	187	95	9	392
1577	Beef-pot roast-chuck-arm cut-cooked	slice	100	231	33	0	10	3.8	101	101	66	289	24	3.8	8.7	0	0	0.08	0.29	3.7	0.33	11	3.4	9	268
1578	Beef-pot roast-chuck-blade cut-cooked	slice	100	270	31	0	15	6.2	106	106	71	263	23	3.7	10.3	0	0	0.08	0.29	2.7	0.29	6	2.47	13	235
1579	Beef-rib steak-cooked	slice	100	221	28	0	11	4.8	80	80	69	394	27	2.6	7	0	0	0.11	0.22	4.8	0.4	8	3.32	13	208
1573	Beef-steak-chicken fried	item	100	389	18	12	30	6.6	97	97	815	126	30	2.3	4.9	8	0	0.11	0.14	2.7	0.5	11	3.27	11	110
1580	Beef-tenderloin steak-broiled	item	100	204	28	0	9	3.6	84	84	63	419	30	3.6	5.6	0	4	0.13	0.3	3.9	0.38	8	0.44	7	238
1235	Beerwurst-beer salami-beef	slice	6	20	1	tr	2	0.8	4	4	62	10	1	0.1	0.1	0	1	tr	0.01	0.2	0.01	tr	0.12	1	6
1219	Beerwurst-beer salami-pork	slice	6	14	1	0	1	0.4	4	4	74	15	1	tr	0.1	0	2	0.03	0.02	0.2	0.02	tr	0.05	tr	6
1236	Bockwurst-raw-link	item	65	200	9	0	18	6.6	38	38	718	176	12	0.4	1	4	0	0.27	0.11	2.7	0.15	4	0.53	10	95
198	Bologna-cured pork-4 by 1/8 inch slice	slice	23	57	4	tr	5	1.6	14	14	272	65	3	0.2	0.5	0	8	0.12	0.04	0.9	0.06	1	0.21	3	32
1212	Bratwurst-pork-cooked-link	item	85	256	12	2	22	7.9	51	51	473	180	12	1.1	2	0	1	0.43	0.16	2.7	0.18	2	0.81	38	126
199	Braunschweiger-liver sausage-cured pork	slice	18	65	2	1	6	2	28	28	206	36	2	1.7	0.5	759	2	0.05	0.28	1.5	0.06	8	3.62	2	30
1572	Brisket-lean-cooked	slice	100	241	29	0	13	4.6	93	93	72	287	23	2.8	6.9	0	0	0.07	0.22	3.8	0.3	8	2.55	6	239
1220	Canadian bacon-pork-grilled	slice	23.3	43	6	tr	2	0.7	14	14	360	91	5	0.2	0.4	0	5	0.19	0.05	1.6	0.11	1	0.18	3	69
1237	Cheesefurter-pork and beef	item	43	141	6	1	13	4.5	29	29	465	89	5	0.5	1	16	8	0.11	0.07	1.3	0.05	1	0.74	25	76
1214	Chitterlings-pork-simmered	oz	28.4	86	3	0	8	2.9	41	41	11	2	3	1.1	1.4	0	0	0	0.02	tr	tr	1	0.29	8	13
1238	Chorizo-pork and beef-link	item	60	273	15	1	23	8.6	53	53	741	239	11	1	2.1	0	0	0.38	0.18	3.1	0.32	5	1.2	5	90
175	Corned beef hash-canned	cup	220	400	19	24	25	11.9	50	50	1188	440	*	4.4	*	*	*	0.02	0.2	4.6	*	*	*	29	147
1239	Corned beef loaf-jellied	slice	28.4	44	7	0	2	0.7	13	13	270	29	3	0.6	1.2	0	2	0	0.03	0.5	0.03	2	0.36	3	21
174	Corned beef-canned	serv	85	213	23	1	13	5.3	73	73	855	116	12	1.8	3	0	tr	0.02	0.2	2.9	0.11	3	1.38	17	94
202	Frankfurter (hot dog)-no bun-beef & pork	item	57	183	6	1	17	6.1	29	29	639	95	6	0.7	1.1	0	15	0.11	0.07	1.5	0.08	2	0.74	6	49
1554	Frog legs-fried-flour coated	item	24	70	4	2	5	0.7	32	32	119	65	6	0.3	0.3	1	1	0.03	0.06	0.3	0.03	6	0.11	5	39
1222	Ham and cheese loaf/roll	slice	28.4	74	5	tr	6	2.1	16	16	381	84	5	0.3	0.6	7	7	0.17	0.05	1	0.07	1	0.23	17	72
1223	Ham and cheese spread	tbsp	15	37	2	tr	3	1.3	9	9	179	24	3	0.1	0.3	14	1	0.05	0.03	0.3	0.02	tr	0.11	33	74
1226	Ham salad spread	tbsp	15	32	2	2	2	0.8	6	6	137	23	2	0.1	0.2	0	8	0.07	0.02	0.3	0.02	1	0.11	1	18
190	Ham-boiled-regular-11% fat-luncheon meat	slice	28.4	52	5	1	3	1	16	16	373	94	5	0.3	0.6	0	8	0.24	0.07	1.5	0.1	1	0.24	2	70
191	Ham-boiled-chopped-luncheon meat	slice	21	50	3	tr	4	1.3	10	10	287	60	3	0.2	0.4	0	6	0.11	0.04	0.7	0.07	1	0.15	1	29
1225	Ham-canned-extra lean-4% fat	cup	140	190	30	1	7	2.2	42	42	1589	487	29	1.3	3.1	0	39	1.45	0.35	6.9	0.63	7	0.99	8	293
801	Ham-canned-roasted-13% fat	cup	140	316	29	1	21	7.1	87	87	1317	500	24	1.9	3.5	0	20	1.15	0.36	7.4	0.42	7	1.48	11	340
201	Ham-deviled-canned-luncheon meat	tbsp	13	45	2	0	4	1.5	10	10	160	*	2	0.3	0.2	0	*	0.02	0.01	0.2	0.04	*	0.09	1	12
1224	Ham-extra lean-5% fat-roasted	cup	140	203	29	2	8	2.5	74	74	1684	402	20	2.1	4	0	29	1.06	0.28	5.6	0.56	5	0.91	11	275
1227	Ham-lean only-roasted	cup	140	220	35	0	8	2.6	77	77	1858	442	31	1.3	3.6	0	tr	0.95	0.36	7	0.66	6	0.98	10	318
806	Ham-minced-pork	slice	21	55	3	tr	4	1.5	15	15	261	65	3	0.2	0.4	6	6	0.15	0.04	0.9	0.06	tr	0.2	2	33
189	Ham-roasted-regular-11% fat-boneless	cup	140	249	32	0	13	4.4	83	83	2100	573	30	1.9	3.5	0	32	1.02	0.46	8.6	0.43	4	0.98	12	393
164	Hamburger patty-broiled-extra lean beef	item	85	218	22	0	14	5.5	71	71	60	266	18	2	4.6	0	6	0.05	0.23	4.2	0.23	8	1.84	6	137
165	Hamburger patty-broiled-medium-lean beef	serv	85	231	21	0	16	6.2	74	74	65	256	18	1.8	4.6	9	0	0.04	0.18	4.4	0.22	8	2	9	134
1704	Hamburger-ground-regular-baked	serv	85	244	20	0	18	7	74	74	51	188	13	2.1	4.2	0	0	0.03	0.14	4	0.2	7	1.99	8	117
1705	Hamburger-ground-regular-fried	serv	85	260	20	0	19	7.5	75	75	71	255	17	2.1	4.3	0	0	0.03	0.17	5	0.2	8	2.3	10	145
1228	Headcheese-pork	slice	28.4	60	5	tr	4	1.4	23	23	357	9	3	0.3	0.4	*	6	0.01	0.05	0.3	0.05	1	0.3	5	17
1213	Italian sausage-pork-link	item	67	216	13	1	17	6.1	52	52	618	204	12	1	1.6	0	0	0.42	0.16	2.8	0.22	3	0.87	16	114
1240	Kielbasa-pork and beef	slice	26	81	3	1	7	2.6	17	17	280	71	4	0.4	0.5	0	5	0.06	0.06	0.7	0.05	1	0.42	11	39
1241	Knockwurst-pork and beef-link	item	68	209	8	1	19	6.9	39	39	687	136	8	0.6	1.1	0	18	0.23	0.1	1.9	0.11	1	0.8	7	67
182	Lamb chop-rib-broiled-lean and fat	serv	85	307	19	0	25	10.8	84	84	64	230	20	1.6	3.4	0	0	0.08	0.19	6	0.09	12	2.16	16	151
183	Lamb chop-rib-broiled-lean only	serv	57	134	16	0	7	2.7	52	52	49	178	17	1.3	3	0	0	0.06	0.14	3.7	0.09	12	1.5	9	121

* indicates that no data was available.
©1994 First DataBank—The Hearst Corporation (N-Squared Computing).

Appendix A - Table of Food Composition (continued)

Item	Food name	Portion	Weight (g)	Food Energy (Kcal)	Protein (gm)	Carbohydrates (gm)	Fiber (gm)	Total Fat (gm)	Saturated Fat (gm)	Cholesterol (mg)	Sodium (mg)	Potassium (mg)	Magnesium (mg)	Iron (mg)	Zinc (mg)	Vitamin A (RE)	Vitamin C (mg)	Thiamin (mg)	Riboflavin (mg)	Niacin (mg)	Vitamin B6 (mg)	Folates (µg)	Vitamin B12 (µg)	Calcium (mg)	Phosphorus (mg)
184	Lamb-leg-roasted-lean and fat	slice	85	219	22	0	0	14	5.9	79	56	266	20	1.7	3.7	*	*	0.09	0.23	5.6	0.13	17	2.2	9	162
185	Lamb-leg-roasted-lean only	slice	71	136	20	0	0	6	2	63	48	240	19	1.5	3.5	*	*	0.08	0.21	4.5	0.12	16	1.87	6	146
186	Lamb-shoulder-roasted-lean and fat	slice	85	235	19	0	0	17	7.2	78	56	214	19	1.7	4.4	*	*	0.08	0.2	5.2	0.11	18	2.24	17	156
187	Lamb-shoulder-roasted-lean only	slice	64	131	16	0	0	7	2.6	56	44	170	16	1.4	3.9	*	*	0.06	0.17	3.7	0.1	16	1.73	12	128
1229	Liver cheese-pork	slice	38	116	6	1	0	10	3.4	66	466	86	5	4.1	1.4	1996	1	0.08	0.85	4.5	0.18	40	9.33	3	79
1230	Liverwurst-liver sausage-pork	slice	18	59	3	tr	0	5	1.9	28	215	36	2	1.2	0.5	760	2	0.05	0.19	1.5	0.03	5	2.42	5	41
1242	Mortadella-pork and beef	slice	15	47	2	tr	0	4	1.4	8	187	25	2	0.2	0.3	0	4	0.02	0.02	0.4	0.02	tr	0.22	3	15
1231	Olive loaf-pork	slice	28.4	67	3	3	0	5	1.7	11	421	84	5	0.2	0.4	6	3	0.08	0.07	0.5	0.07	1	0.36	31	36
1243	Pepperoni-pork and beef	slice	5.5	27	1	tr	0	2	0.9	4	112	19	1	0.1	0.1	0	tr	0.02	0.01	0.3	0.01	tr	0.14	1	7
1232	Pimento/pickle loaf-pork	slice	28.4	74	3	2	*	6	2.2	11	394	97	5	0.3	0.4	2	4	0.08	0.07	0.6	0.05	1	0.34	27	40
1233	Polish sausage-pork	item	227	740	32	4	0	65	23.4	159	1989	538	32	3.3	4.4	0	2	1.14	0.34	7.8	0.43	5	2.22	27	309
192	Pork chop-loin-broiled-lean and fat	item	82	284	19	0	0	22	8.1	77	54	287	20	0.7	2	2	tr	0.69	0.29	4.3	0.31	4	0.81	5	193
193	Pork chop-loin-broiled-lean only	item	66	169	18	0	0	10	3.5	63	49	276	19	0.6	1.9	2	tr	0.64	0.28	3.9	0.3	4	0.71	5	184
194	Pork-center loin-roasted-lean and fat	item	88	268	22	0	0	19	6.9	80	56	284	17	0.9	1.8	2	tr	0.73	0.21	4.4	0.35	1	0.53	5	173
195	Pork-center loin-roasted-lean only	item	72	173	21	0	0	9	3.3	66	50	261	15	0.8	1.6	2	tr	0.65	0.19	3.9	0.32	1	0.43	4	158
1221	Pork-feet-pickled	oz	28.4	58	4	tr	0	5	1.6	26	262	67	1	0.2	0.4	0	0	tr	0.01	0.1	0.11	1	0.18	9	10
1215	Pork-feet-simmered	oz	28.4	55	5	0	0	4	1.2	28	9	42	1	0.1	0.3	0	0	tr	0.02	0.1	0.03	tr	0.05	13	14
1216	Pork-kidneys-braised	cup	140	211	36	0	0	7	2.1	673	111	200	25	7.4	5.8	109	15	0.55	2.22	8.1	0.65	57	10.9	18	337
1217	Pork-liver-braised	oz	28.4	47	7	1	0	1	0.4	101	14	43	4	5.1	1.9	1531	7	0.07	0.62	2.4	0.16	46	5.3	3	68
197	Pork-shoulder-roasted-lean only	cup	140	342	36	0	0	21	7.2	136	106	493	28	2.1	5.9	3	tr	0.82	0.51	6	0.56	7	1.23	11	323
1321	Pork-spareribs-braised	oz	28.4	113	8	0	0	9	3.3	34	26	91	7	0.5	1.3	1	0	0.12	0.11	1.6	0.1	1	0.31	13	74
196	Pork-tenderloin-roasted-lean only	oz	28.4	47	8	0	0	1	0.5	26	19	153	7	0.4	0.9	1	tr	0.27	0.11	1.3	0.12	2	0.16	3	82
1218	Pork-tongue-braised	serv	85	230	21	0	0	16	5.5	124	93	201	17	4.2	3.9	0	1	0.27	0.43	4.5	0.2	3	2.03	16	148
203	Potted meat-canned-beef/chicken/turkey	tbsp	13	30	2	0	*	2	0.8	15	156	*	*	*	0.4	3	*	0	0.03	0.2	*	*	*	*	*
1507	Rabbit-stewed-boneless-skinless	serv	85	175	26	0	*	7	2.1	73	32	255	17	2	2	0	0	0.05	0.15	6.1	0.29	8	5.53	17	192
169	Roast beef-bottom round-cooked-lean only	slice	78	173	25	0	0	7	2.7	75	40	240	20	2.7	4.3	0	0	0.06	0.2	3.2	0.28	9	1.93	4	212
168	Roast beef-bottom round-cooked-lean and fat	slice	85	222	25	0	0	13	4.8	81	43	248	20	2.8	4.4	0	0	0.06	0.21	3.3	0.29	9	2.04	5	217
166	Roast beef-rib-broiled-lean and fat	slice	85	308	18	0	0	26	10.8	73	52	257	17	1.8	4.3	0	0	0.07	0.15	2.7	0.25	5	2.37	10	140
167	Roast beef-rib-broiled-lean only	slice	51	122	14	0	0	7	3	41	38	192	13	1.3	3.5	0	0	0.04	0.11	2.1	0.15	4	1.49	5	109
206	Salami-cooked-beef-4 by 1/8 inch slice	slice	23	60	3	1	0	5	2.1	15	270	52	3	0.5	0.5	0	4	0.02	0.04	0.7	0.05	tr	1.11	2	26
205	Salami-dry or hard-pork-slice	slice	10	41	2	tr	0	3	1.2	8	226	38	2	0.1	0.4	0	0	0.09	0.03	0.6	0.06	tr	0.28	1	23
204	Sausage-link-cooked-pork	item	13	48	3	tr	0	4	1.4	11	168	47	2	0.2	0.3	0	0	0.1	0.03	0.6	0.04	tr	0.22	4	24
200	Sausage-patty-cooked-fresh pork	item	27	100	5	tr	0	8	2.9	22	349	97	5	0.3	0.7	0	1	0.2	0.07	1.2	0.09	1	0.47	9	50
207	Sausage-vienna-canned-beef and pork	item	16	45	2	tr	0	4	1.5	8	152	16	1	0.1	0.3	0	0	0.01	0.02	0.3	0.02	1	0.16	2	8
170	Steak-sirloin-broiled-lean and fat	item	85	238	23	0	0	15	6.4	77	54	306	24	2.6	4.9	15	0	0.1	0.22	3.3	0.34	8	2.26	9	185
171	Steak-sirloin-broiled-lean only	slice	56	116	17	0	0	5	2	50	37	226	18	1.9	3.7	3	0	0.07	0.17	2.4	0.25	6	1.6	6	137
172	Steak-top round-broiled-lean and fat	slice	85	179	26	0	0	7	2.8	72	51	365	26	2.4	4.6	0	0	0.1	0.22	5	0.46	10	2.08	5	203
173	Steak-top round-broiled-lean only	slice	68	130	22	0	0	4	1.5	57	42	301	21	2	3.8	0	0	0.08	0.18	4.1	0.38	8	1.69	4	167
1509	Sweetbreads-calf-braised	serv	85	143	28	0	*	3	*	*	*	*	*	*	*	*	*	0.05	0.14	2.5	0.14	tr	*	*	264
1244	Thuringer/cervelat-pork	slice	23	77	4	tr	0	7	2.8	17	286	62	26	0.6	0.6	0	5	0.04	0.08	1	0.06	13	1.27	3	26
208	Veal-leg-top round-pan fried	serv	85	179	27	0	0	7	2.7	89	64	362	22	0.8	2.8	0	tr	0.06	0.3	1	0.41	14	1.23	5	237
209	Veal-rib-separable lean only-braised	serv	85	185	29	0	0	7	2.2	123	84	270	23	1.2	5.1	0	0	0.05	0.26	6.7	0.29	15	1.3	20	186
1384	Veal-shoulder-arm-lean only-roasted	serv	85	139	22	0	0	5	2	93	77	302	23	1	3.7	*	*	0.06	0.28	7	0.25	*	1.33	23	192
1556	Venison-dried-salted	serv	100	142	31	0	0	1	*	82	*	*	*	1.9	*	*	*	0.09	0.34	10	*	0	*	60	298
1555	Venison-roasted	slice	100	146	30	0	0	2	2.1	82	70	336	29	3.5	4.5	0	0	0.37	0.28	7.4	0.26	7	6.22	20	264
Miscellaneous																									
683	Baking powder-low sodium	tsp	4.3	7	tr	2	*	0	0	0	tr	471	0	0	*	*	*	*	0	0	*	*	*	207	314
680	Baking powder-no calcium sulfate	tsp	3	4	tr	1	*	0	0	0	329	5	0	0	*	*	*	*	0	0	*	*	*	58	87
682	Baking powder-straight phosphate	tsp	3.8	5	tr	1	*	0	0	0	312	6	0	0	*	*	*	*	0	0	*	*	*	239	359
681	Baking powder-with calcium sulfate	tsp	2.9	3	tr	1	*	0	0	0	290	4	0	0	*	*	*	*	0	0	*	*	*	183	45
1434	Baking soda	tsp	3	0	0	0	0	0	0	0	821	0	0	0	0	0	0	0	0	0	0	0	0	tr	0
1524	Chewing gum-candy coated	item	1.7	5	0	2	0	tr	0	0	tr	0	0	0	0	0	0	0	0	0	0	0	0	tr	0

Code	Food	Meas.	g	Cal	Prot	Carb	Fib	Fat	Sat	Na	K															Ca	
1489	Chewing gum-Wrigleys	item	3	10	0	2	0	0	0	0	0	0	0	0	0	0	0	0	0	0	0	0	0	0	3	0
698	Gelatin dessert-prepared	cup	240	140	4	34	0	0	0	0	0	0	3	0	tr	0	tr	0	0	0	0	0	0	0	5	46
1459	Gelatin-d zerta-low calorie-prepared	cup	240	16	4	0	0	0	0	0	0	3	180	0.1	tr	0	0	0	0	0	0	0	0	0	6	0
697	Gelatin-dry-envelope	item	7	25	6	0	0	0	0	0	0	2	*	*	*	4	*	*	*	*	tr	0	tr	0	0	*	*
1458	Gelatin-Jello-sugar free-prepared	item	4	16	tr	0	0.1	0	0	0	0	1	120	tr	*	0	*	*	*	*	*	0	*	0	0	2	1
700	Olives-green-pickled-canned	item	4	4	tr	tr	0.1	0.1	*	81	2	tr	*	0	0	tr	tr	0	tr	tr	0	0	0	0	2	1
701	Olives-Mission-ripe-canned	item	3	5	tr	tr	0.1	0.2	tr	19	1	1	tr	tr	1	tr	0	0	0	tr	tr	0	0	0	3	tr
33	Pickle relish-hamburger-Heinz	oz	28.4	30	0	7	*	0	0.2	325	*	*	*	*	*	*	*	*	*	*	*	0	*	*	*	6	4
31	Pickle relish-hot dog-Heinz	oz	28.4	35	0	8	*	0	0.2	200	*	*	*	*	*	*	*	*	*	*	*	0	*	*	*	6	4
705	Pickle relish-sweet-chopped	tbsp	15	20	0	5	0.3	0	0.1	124	30	1	tr	2	1	tr	tr	tr	tr	tr	0	1	0	0	tr	3	2
702	Pickle-dill-cucumber-medium sized	item	65	5	0	1	0.8	0	0.7	928	130	8	0.7	7	4	0.2	0.01	0.01	0.01	0.01	1	1	0	0	1	17	14
703	Pickle-fresh pack-cucumber-sliced	item	7.5	5	0	2	0.1	0	0.2	50	15	tr	0.2	1	1	tr	tr	tr	tr	tr	tr	tr	0	0	tr	3	2
704	Pickle-sweet/gherkin-small-whole	item	15	20	0	5	0.2	0	0.2	128	30	tr	0.2	1	1	tr	tr	tr	tr	tr	tr	tr	0	0	tr	2	2
706	Popsicle	item	95	70	0	18	0	0	0	tr	4	0	0	0	0	0	tr	*	*	0	*	0	0	*	0	0	*
1725	Vanilla-pure	tsp	4.7	14	0	1	0	0	*	2	6	0	*	0	0	0	0	0	0	0	*	0	0	0	0	1	1
726	Vinegar-cider	tbsp	15	2	0	1	0	0	0.1	tr	15	3	0.1	0	0	tr	0	0	0	0	0	0	0	0	0	14	22
1496	Vinegar-distilled	cup	240	29	0	12	0	0	1.4	2	36	0	1.4	0	0	0	0	0	0	0	0	0	0	0	0	3	90
728	Yeast-baker's-dry-active-package	serv	7	20	3	3	2.2	0	1.1	1	140	4	1.1	0	0	0.16	0.38	0.16	2.6	0.14	0	286	0	0	0.16	3	90
729	Yeast-brewer's-dry	tbsp	8	25	3	3	2.5	0	1.4	9	152	18	0.6	0	0	0.6	1.25	0.34	3	0.2	0	313	0	0	1.25	17	140

Nuts & seeds

Code	Food	Meas.	g	Cal	Prot	Carb	Fib	Fat	Sat	Na	K														Ca	
1071	Almond butter-plain	tbsp	16	101	2	3	1.8	9	0.9	2	121	48	0.6	0.5	0	tr	1	0.1	0.02	0.01	0.5	0.1	0	10	0	0	43	84
521	Nut-filbert/hazel-dried-chopped	cup	115	727	15	18	5.3	72	5.3	8	512	328	3.8	2.8	8	1	4	0.13	0.7	0.58	1.3	0.13	0	83	0	0	216	359
531	Nut-walnut-persian/english	cup	120	770	17	22	6.7	74	6.7	15	602	203	2.9	3.3	15	4	3	0.18	0.67	0.46	1.3	0.18	0	79	0	0	113	380
507	Nuts-almonds-unblanched-shelled-chopped	cup	130	766	26	27	12.1	68	6.4	14	952	385	4.8	3.8	0	1	4	1.01	0.15	0.27	4.4	0.15	0	76	0	0	346	676
508	Nuts-almonds-unblanched-shelled-slivered	cup	115	677	23	24	10.7	60	5.7	13	842	340	4.2	3.4	0	1	3.9	0.9	0.13	0.24	3.9	0.13	0	68	0	0	306	598
1072	Nuts-beechnuts-dried	oz	28.4	164	2	10	2.6	14	1.6	11	289	0	0.7	0.1	4	tr	0.2	0.11	0.09	0.19	0.2	0.11	0	32	0	0	tr	0
517	Nuts-brazil-dried-shelled	cup	140	918	20	18	10.8	93	22.6	3	840	315	4.8	6.4	1	1	2.3	1.4	0.35	0.17	2.3	0.35	0	6	0	0	246	840
1073	Nuts-butternuts-dried	oz	28.4	174	7	3	2.4	16	0.4	19	119	67	1.1	0.9	3	3	0.3	0.11	0.04	0.27	0.3	0.16	0	19	0	0	15	127
1074	Nuts-cashews-dry roasted	cup	137	786	21	45	10	64	12.5	22	774	356	8.2	7.7	0	7	1.9	0.27	0.27	0.35	1.9	0.35	0	95	0	0	62	671
518	Nuts-cashews-oil roasted	cup	130	749	21	37	7.8	63	12.4	22	689	332	5.3	6.2	0	1	2.3	0.55	0.23	0.23	2.3	0.23	0	88	0	0	53	554
1090	Nuts-hickory-dried	oz	28.4	187	4	5	2.4	18	2	tr	124	49	0.6	1.2	4	1	0.3	0.25	0.04	0.06	0.3	0.04	1	11	0	0	17	95
1091	Nuts-macadamia-dried	cup	134	941	11	18	12.4	99	14.8	7	493	155	3.2	2.3	0	18	2.9	0.47	0.15	0.26	2.9	0.15	0	21	0	0	94	182
1092	Nuts-macadamia-oil roasted	cup	134	962	10	17	9.3	103	15.4	9	441	157	2.4	1.5	1	17	2.7	0.29	0.15	0.27	2.7	0.27	0	60	0	0	96	268
1093	Nuts-mixed-dry roasted	cup	137	814	24	35	11.6	71	9.5	16	817	308	5.2	5.1	2	35	6.4	0.27	0.27	0.41	6.4	0.27	1	69	0	0	96	596
1094	Nuts-mixed-oil roasted	cup	142	876	24	30	12.8	80	12.4	16	825	333	7.2	4.6	3	30	7.2	0.71	0.32	0.34	7.2	0.34	1	118	0	0	153	659
523	Nuts-peanuts-oil roasted	cup	144	837	38	27	12.8	71	9.9	8	982	266	2.6	9.6	0	27	20.6	0.36	0.16	0.37	20.6	0.16	0	181	0	0	127	744
1585	Nuts-peanuts-oil roasted-salted	cup	144	837	38	27	12.8	71	9.9	624	982	266	2.6	9.6	0	27	20.6	0.36	0.16	0.37	20.6	0.16	0	181	0	0	127	744
1095	Nuts-peanuts-spanish-dried	cup	146	828	38	24	11.7	72	10	26	1029	245	6.7	4.8	0	37	17.6	0.93	0.2	0.51	17.6	0.2	0	350	0	0	134	549
526	Nuts-pecans-dried-halves	cup	108	720	8	20	7	73	5.9	1	423	138	2.3	5.9	14	2	2.3	0.92	0.14	0.2	1	0.14	2	42	0	0	39	314
1096	Nuts-pecans-oil roasted	cup	110	754	8	18	8.5	78	6.3	1	395	142	2.3	6.1	*	9	6.1	0.34	0.11	0.21	1	0.11	1	43	0	0	37	324
1097	Nuts-pistachio-dried	cup	128	739	26	32	13.8	62	7.8	7	1399	28	8.7	1.7	30	9	1.7	1.05	0.22	0.32	1.4	0.22	0	74	0	0	173	644
1098	Nuts-pistachio-dry roasted	cup	128	776	19	35	13.8	68	8.6	8	1242	166	4.1	1.7	31	9	1.8	0.54	0.32	0.33	1.8	0.32	0	76	0	0	90	609
1099	Nuts-soybean kernels-roasted	cup	108	489	40	33	9.2	26	3.4	4	1588	187	4.8	3.9	22	2	3.9	0.11	0.16	0.32	1.9	0.11	0	244	0	0	149	392
529	Nuts-walnut-black-dried-chopped	cup	125	759	30	15	8.1	71	4.5	2	655	252	3.8	4.3	37	4	0.9	0.27	0.14	0.69	0.9	0.14	0	82	0	0	72	580
530	Nuts-walnuts-finely ground	cup	80	486	20	10	5.2	45	2.9	2	419	161	2.5	2.7	24	3	0.6	0.18	0.09	0.44	0.6	0.09	0	52	0	0	46	371
1706	Peanut butter-chunk style	tbsp	16.1	95	4	3	1.1	8	1.5	78	121	26	0.3	0.4	0	24	2.2	0.02	0.02	0.07	2.2	0.07	0	15	0	0	7	51
1462	Peanut butter-low sodium-Peter Pan	tbsp	16	95	5	3	1.7	9	1.4	5	110	28	0.3	0.5	0	0	2.2	0.02	0.02	0.06	2.2	0.06	0	13	0	0	5	60
1707	Peanut butter-old fashioned	tbsp	16	95	4	3	1.1	8	1.5	75	110	30	0.3	0.5	0	0	2.3	0.01	0.02	0.06	2.3	0.06	0	13	0	0	5	60
524	Peanut butter-smooth type	tbsp	16	94	4	3	1	8	1.5	77	115	25	0.3	0.3	*	0	2.1	0.02	0.02	0.06	2.1	0.06	0	13	0	0	5	52
1100	Seeds-breadfruit-roasted	oz	28.4	59	2	11	0.2	1	0.2	8	307	18	0.3	0.3	8	2	2.1	0.12	0.07	0.12	2.1	0.12	0	17	0	0	24	50

* indicates that no data was available.
©1994 First DataBank—The Hearst Corporation (N-Squared Computing).

Appendix A - Table of Food Composition (continued)

Item	Food name	Portion	Weight (g)	Food Energy (Kcal)	Protein (gm)	Carbohydrates (gm)	Fiber (gm)	Total Fat (gm)	Saturated Fat (gm)	Cholesterol (mg)	Sodium (mg)	Potassium (mg)	Magnesium (mg)	Iron (mg)	Zinc (mg)	Vitamin A (RE)	Vitamin C (mg)	Thiamin (mg)	Riboflavin (mg)	Niacin (mg)	Vitamin B6 (mg)	Folates (µg)	Vitamin B12 (µg)	Calcium (mg)	Phosphorus (mg)
527	Seeds-pumpkin/squash-dried	cup	138	747	34	25	14.8	63	12	0	24	1114	738	20.7	10.3	53	3	0.29	0.44	2.4	0.12	79	0	59	1620
1101	Seeds-pumpkin/squash-roasted	cup	64	285	14	34	29.4	12	2.4	0	12	588	168	2.1	6.6	4	tr	0.02	0.03	0.2	0.02	6	0	35	59
1102	Seeds-sesame-dried-whole	cup	144	825	26	34	21.6	72	10	0	16	674	505	21	11.2	1	0	1.14	0.36	6.5	1.14	139	0	1404	906
1103	Seeds-sesame-roasted-whole	oz	28.4	161	5	7	5.3	14	1.9	0	3	135	101	4.2	2	tr	0	0.23	0.07	1.3	0.23	28	0	281	181
528	Seeds-sunflower-dried	cup	144	821	33	27	9.8	71	7.5	0	4	992	509	9.8	7.3	7	2	3.29	0.36	6.5	1.81	327	0	168	1015
1104	Seeds-sunflower-oil roasted	cup	135	830	29	20	9.2	78	8.1	0	4	652	171	9.1	7	7	2	0.43	0.38	5.6	1.07	316	0	76	1538
Poultry																									
1184	Chick-breast-no skin-roasted	item	172	284	53	0	0	6	1.7	146	126	440	50	1.8	1.7	11	0	0.12	0.2	23.6	1.02	6	0.58	26	392
1189	Chick-thigh-no skin-roasted	item	52	109	14	0	0	6	1.6	49	46	124	12	0.7	1.3	10	tr	0.04	0.12	3.4	0.18	4	0.16	6	95
1201	Chicken frankfurter	item	45	116	6	3	0	9	2.5	45	617	38	5	0.9	0.5	17	0	0.03	0.05	1.4	0.14	2	0.11	43	48
1203	Chicken roll-light	slice	28.4	45	6	1	0	2	0.6	14	166	65	5	0.3	0.2	7	0	0.02	0.04	1.5	0.06	1	0.04	12	45
1204	Chicken spread-canned	tbsp	13	25	2	1	0	2	1.7	7	50	14	2	0.3	0.2	3	0	tr	0.02	0.4	0.02	tr	0.02	16	12
1179	Chicken-back-fried-flour coated	item	144	477	40	9	0.2	30	8.1	128	130	325	33	2.3	3.6	53	0	0.15	0.34	10.5	0.44	12	0.4	35	239
1180	Chicken-back-stewed	item	122	316	27	0	0	22	6.1	96	78	178	20	1.5	2.4	113	0	0.05	0.18	5.3	0.18	6	0.22	22	146
1183	Chicken-breast-no skin-fried	item	172	322	58	1	0	8	2.2	156	136	474	54	2	1.9	12	0	0.14	0.22	25.4	1.1	8	0.62	28	424
1181	Chicken-breast-roasted	item	196	386	58	0	0	15	4.3	166	138	480	54	2.1	2	55	0	0.13	0.23	24.9	1.08	6	0.64	28	420
1182	Chicken-breast-stewed	item	220	404	60	0	0	16	4.6	166	136	390	48	2.1	2.1	54	0	0.09	0.25	17.2	0.64	6	0.46	28	344
212	Chicken-breast-with skin-fried in batter	item	280	728	70	25	*	37	9.9	238	770	564	68	3.5	2.7	57	0	0.32	0.41	29.5	1.2	16	0.82	56	516
210	Chicken-breast-with skin-fried in flour	item	196	436	62	3	0.1	17	4.8	176	150	506	58	2.3	2.1	29	0	0.16	0.26	26.9	1.14	8	0.68	32	456
213	Chicken-canned-boneless-with broth	item	142	234	31	0	0	11	3.1	78	714	196	17	2.3	2	100	3	0.02	0.18	9	0.5	6	0.42	20	350
1193	Chicken-capon-roasted	item	1274	2914	369	0	0	148	41.6	1098	626	3252	308	18.9	22.1	260	0	0.89	2.17	114	5.5	70	4.14	182	3140
211	Chicken-drumstick-with skin-fried/flour	item	49	120	13	1	0	7	1.8	44	44	112	11	1.2	1.4	12	0	0.04	0.11	3	0.17	4	0.16	6	86
1174	Chicken-giblets-fried-flour coated	cup	145	402	47	6	*	20	5.5	647	164	478	37	15	9.1	5195	13	0.14	2.21	15.9	0.88	550	19.3	26	414
1175	Chicken-giblets-simmered	cup	145	228	38	1	0	7	2.2	570	85	229	30	9.3	6.6	3234	12	0.13	1.38	6	0.49	545	14.7	18	331
1176	Chicken-gizzard-simmered	cup	145	222	39	2	0	5	1.5	281	97	259	29	6	6.4	82	2	0.04	0.35	5.8	0.17	77	2.81	14	225
1177	Chicken-heart-simmered	cup	145	268	38	tr	0	12	3.3	350	70	192	29	13.1	10.6	12	3	0.1	1.07	4.1	0.47	116	10.6	27	289
1186	Chicken-leg-no skin-roasted	item	95	182	26	0	0	8	2.2	89	87	230	23	1.2	2.7	18	0	0.07	0.22	6	0.35	8	0.31	12	174
1187	Chicken-leg-no skin-stewed	item	101	187	27	0	0	8	2.2	90	78	192	21	1.4	2.8	18	0	0.06	0.22	4.9	0.22	8	0.23	11	151
1185	Chicken-leg-roasted	item	114	265	30	0	0	15	4.2	105	99	256	26	1.5	3	46	0	0.08	0.24	7.1	0.37	8	0.35	14	199
1202	Chicken-liver pate-canned	tbsp	13	26	2	1	0	2	0.5	51	50	12	2	1.2	0.3	28	1	0.01	0.18	1	0.03	42	1.05	1	23
1178	Chicken-liver-simmered	cup	140	219	34	1	0	8	2.6	883	71	196	29	11.9	6.1	6886	22	0.21	2.45	6.2	0.82	107	27.1	20	437
1188	Chicken-thigh-fried-flour coated	item	62	162	17	2	tr	9	2.5	60	55	147	15	0.9	1.6	18	0	0.06	0.15	4.3	0.21	5	0.19	8	116
1772	Chicken-thin sliced-smoked-Land o Frost	serv	28.4	60	5	1	0	4	1	21	182	49	5	0.4	0.5	0	0	0.02	0.03	1.6	0.07	2	0.06	0	39
1190	Chicken-wing-fried-flour coated	item	32	103	8	1	0	7	1.9	26	25	57	6	0.4	0.6	12	0	0.02	0.04	2.1	0.13	1	0.09	5	48
1191	Chicken-wing-roasted	item	34	99	9	0	0	7	1.9	29	28	62	7	0.4	0.6	16	0	0.01	0.04	2.3	0.14	1	0.1	5	51
1192	Chicken-wing-stewed	item	40	100	9	0	0	7	1.9	28	27	56	6	0.5	0.7	16	0	0.02	0.04	1.9	0.09	1	0.07	5	48
1194	Duck-flesh & skin-roasted	item	764	2574	145	0	0	217	73.9	640	454	1560	124	20.6	14.2	483	0	1.33	2.06	36.9	1.4	50	2.26	86	1190
1195	Duck-no skin-roasted	item	442	890	104	0	0	50	18.4	396	286	1114	88	11.9	11.5	103	0	1.15	2.08	22.5	1.1	44	1.76	52	898
1196	Goose-flesh & skin-roasted	item	1548	4721	389	0	0	339	106	1416	1084	5092	341	43.8	40.6	325	0	1.19	5	64.5	5.73	31	6.35	201	4180
1205	Goose-liver pate-smoked-canned	tbsp	13	60	1	2	0	6	*	20	91	18	2	0.7	0.1	130	tr	0.01	0.04	0.3	0.01	8	1.22	8	26
1197	Goose-no skin-roasted	item	1182	2813	342	0	0	150	53.9	1138	898	4586	296	33.9	499	142	0	1.09	4.61	48.2	5.5	142	5.56	165	3652
1207	Turkey ham-cured thigh meat	slice	28.4	37	5	tr	0	1	0.5	16	283	92	5	0.4	0.8	0	0	0.02	0.07	1	0.07	1	0.57	3	54
1208	Turkey loaf-breast	serv	28.4	31	6	0	0	tr	0.1	12	406	79	6	0.1	0.3	0	0	0.01	0.03	2.4	0.1	1	0.57	2	65
1209	Turkey pastrami	slice	28.4	40	5	tr	0	2	0.6	15	297	74	4	0.5	0.6	0	0	0.02	0.07	1	0.08	1	0.07	3	57
1210	Turkey roll-light	oz	28.4	42	5	tr	0	2	0.6	12	139	71	5	0.4	0.4	0	0	0.03	0.06	2	0.09	1	0.07	11	52
1211	Turkey roll-light and dark	oz	28.4	42	5	1	0	2	0.6	16	166	77	5	0.4	0.6	0	0	0.03	0.08	1.4	0.08	1	0.07	11	48
222	Turkey-breast-no skin-roasted	item	612	826	184	0	0	5	1.4	510	318	1784	178	9.4	10.6	0	0	0.26	0.8	45.9	3.42	38	2.36	76	1370
219	Turkey-dark meat-no skin-roasted	cup	140	262	40	0	0	10	3.4	119	110	406	34	3.3	6.3	0	0	0.09	0.35	5.1	0.5	13	0.52	45	286
1198	Turkey-giblets-simmered	cup	145	242	39	3	0	7	2.2	606	86	290	25	9.7	5.3	2629	3	0.07	1.31	6.5	0.47	501	34.8	19	296
1199	Turkey-gizzard-simmered	cup	145	236	43	1	0	6	1.6	336	79	306	27	7.9	6	81	2	0.05	0.47	4.5	0.17	75	2.76	22	186
220	Turkey-light meat-no skin-roasted	cup	140	219	42	0	0	5	1.4	97	89	426	39	1.9	2.9	0	0	0.09	0.18	9.6	0.75	8	0.52	27	307
221	Turkey-light/dark meat-no skin-roasted	cup	140	238	41	0	0	7	2.3	107	99	418	37	2.5	4.3	0	0	0.09	0.26	7.6	0.64	10	0.52	35	298

ID	Food	Measure	Wt (g)																						
1200	Turkey-liver-simmered	cup	140	237	34	5	0	8	2.6	876	89	272	21	10.9	4.3	5288	3	0.07	1.99	8.3	0.73	66.5	932	15	381
1771	Turkey-thin sliced-smoked-Land o Frost	serv	28.4	50	5	1	0	3	0.8	23	283	80	7	0.4	0.8	0	0	0	0.03	1.2	0.12	0.1	2	40	58

Sauces & dips

ID	Food	Measure	Wt (g)																						
35	Catsup-tomato-Heinz lite	tbsp	15	8	tr	*	*	2	0	*	110	54	*	0.1	*	21	2	0.01	0.01	0.2	*	*	*	7	8
37	Catsup-tomato-low sodium-Heinz	tbsp	15	8	tr	*	*	2	0	*	90	54	*	0.1	*	21	2	0.01	0.01	0.2	*	*	*	7	8
337	Dip-bacon and horseradish-Kraft	tbsp	15	30	1	2	*	3	*	3	100	*	*	*	*	*	*	*	*	*	*	*	*	*	*
331	Dip-buttermilk-Kraft	tbsp	15	40	1	4	*	1	*	4	135	*	*	*	*	*	*	*	*	*	*	*	*	*	*
339	Dip-clam-Kraft	tbsp	15	30	1	2	*	2	*	2	115	*	*	*	*	*	*	*	*	*	*	*	*	*	*
333	Dip-french onion-Kraft	tbsp	15	30	1	2	*	2	*	2	120	*	*	*	*	*	*	*	*	*	*	*	*	*	*
342	Dip-garlic-Kraft	tbsp	15	30	1	2	*	2	*	2	80	*	*	*	*	*	*	*	*	*	*	*	*	*	*
335	Dip-green onion-Kraft	tbsp	15	25	1	2	*	2	*	2	85	*	*	*	*	*	*	*	*	*	*	*	*	*	*
328	Dip-guacamole-Kraft	tbsp	15	25	1	2	*	2	*	2	108	*	*	*	*	*	*	*	*	*	*	*	*	*	*
1574	Dip-jalapeno bean-Fritos	oz	28.4	33	2	1	1.9	5	0.2	1	163	77	9	0.1	*	4	0	0.02	0.03	1.1	0.03	0	20	7	23
326	Dip-jalapeno pepper-Kraft	tbsp	15	25	1	2	*	1	*	2	80	*	*	*	*	*	*	*	*	*	*	*	*	*	*
776	Gravy-beef-canned	cup	233	123	9	5	0.1	11	2.7	7	1305	189	14	1.6	2.3	0	0	0.08	0.08	1.5	0.02	0.23	5	14	70
779	Gravy-brown-from dry-prepared with water	cup	258	75	2	2	tr	13	0.8	3	1076	57	10	0.2	0.3	0	0	0.04	0.09	0.8	0	0	10	66	44
777	Gravy-chicken-canned	cup	238	188	5	14	2.1	13	3.4	5	1373	260	5	1.1	1.9	264	5	0.04	0.1	1.1	0.02	0.24	5	48	69
778	Gravy-mushroom-canned	cup	238	119	3	6	1	13	1	5	1357	252	3	1.6	1.7	0	29	0.08	0.15	1.6	0.05	0	29	17	36
781	Gravy-pork-from dry-prepared with water	cup	258	77	6	5	*	13	0.7	3	1235	57	10	0.3	0.3	0	3	0.05	0.06	0.8	0.03	0.16	5	31	44
780	Gravy-turkey-canned	cup	238	121	6	5	1.5	12	1.5	5	1373	259	5	1.7	1.9	0	5	0.05	0.19	3.1	0.02	0	5	10	69
1464	Horseradish-prepared	tbsp	15	6	tr	*	0.3	1	0	0	165	44	3	0.1	0.1	0	tr	tr	0.02	tr	0.01	0.01	11	9	5
1505	Mustard-brown-prepared	cup	250	228	15	13	2.1	13	7.7	0	3268	325	46	4.5	0.8	0	11	0.07	*	0.4	0.09	0.09	11	310	335
1536	Mustard-low sodium-Featherweight	tsp	5	4	tr	tr	0	tr	0	0	1	7	2	0.1	*	*	tr	*	*	tr	*	*	*	4	4
699	Mustard-yellow-prepared	tsp	5	5	tr	tr	0.1	tr	0	0	65	7	2	0.1	*	*	tr	*	*	*	*	*	*	4	4
684	Sauce-barbecue-ready to serve	cup	250	188	5	5	2.3	32	0.7	0	2032	435	45	2.3	0.5	218	10	0.08	0.05	2.3	0.19	0	10	48	50
767	Sauce-bearnaise-from dry mix-milk/butter	cup	255	701	8	68	0.1	18	41.8	189	1265	298	26	0.3	0.8	757	10	0.08	0.26	0.3	0.08	0.51	10	230	186
768	Sauce-cheese-from dry mix-milk/butter	cup	279	307	16	17	0.1	23	9.3	53	1566	554	47	0.3	1	117	13	0.15	0.56	0.3	0.14	1.12	13	570	437
27	Sauce-chili-bottled	tbsp	15	16	tr	*	*	4	0	0	201	56	*	0.1	*	21	*	0.01	0.01	0.2	*	*	*	3	8
1537	Sauce-chili-low sodium	tbsp	14.2	8	0	*	*	2	0	0	10	10	*	*	*	*	*	*	*	*	*	*	*	3	*
769	Sauce-curry-from dry mix-made with milk	cup	272	269	11	15	0.9	26	6	35	1276	495	46	1.1	1.1	41	16	0.11	0.54	0.5	0.11	1.09	16	484	280
770	Sauce-hollandaise-dry mix-made with milk	cup	255	703	8	68	0.1	18	41.9	189	1134	309	26	0.2	0.8	696	10	0.08	0.33	0.2	0.08	0.51	10	240	194
1056	Sauce-marinara-canned	cup	250	170	4	8	*	26	1.2	0	1573	1060	60	2	0.7	240	34	0.11	0.15	4	0.62	0	34	45	88
771	Sauce-mushroom-dry mix-made with milk	cup	267	227	11	10	0.5	24	5.4	34	1535	494	37	0.5	1.3	94	40	0.19	0.8	4.8	0.19	0.8	40	302	166
348	Sauce-picante-canned	fl oz	16	9	tr	1	*	2	0	0	218	77	*	0.3	*	23	16	0.02	0.01	0.2	*	*	16	4	8
347	Sauce-salsa with green chilies-canned	fl oz	16	10	tr	1	*	2	0	0	111	87	*	0.3	*	39	16	0.02	0.01	0.3	*	*	16	4	9
1268	Sauce-sour cream-from mix-with milk	cup	314	509	19	30	2.1	45	16.1	91	1007	733	44	0.6	1.4	144	16	0.13	0.7	0.6	0.13	0.94	16	546	*
775	Sauce-soy	tbsp	18	10	2	tr	0	2	tr	0	1029	32	6	0.4	0.1	0	0	0.01	0.02	0.6	0.03	0	3	20	20
1637	Sauce-soy-tamari	tbsp	18	11	2	tr	0	1	tr	0	1005	38	7	0.4	0.1	0	0	0.01	0.03	0.7	0.04	0	3	4	23
1064	Sauce-spaghetti-tomato based-canned	cup	249	271	5	12	*	40	1.7	0	1235	956	60	1.6	0.5	306	54	0.14	0.15	3.8	0.88	0	54	70	90
29	Sauce-steak-Heinz 57	tbsp	15	15	tr	tr	*	3	*	0	265	*	*	0.3	*	*	*	*	0.01	0.2	*	*	*	*	*
772	Sauce-stroganoff-from mix-prepared	cup	296	272	12	11	1.2	34	6.8	39	1829	672	39	1.3	1.1	127	9	0.86	0.77	0.8	0.12	0.59	9	521	302
773	Sauce-sweet/sour-from mix-prepared	cup	313	294	1	tr	1.9	73	tr	0	779	66	9	1.6	0.1	66	2	0.03	0.1	0.9	0.31	0	2	41	188
1478	Sauce-tabasco	tsp	5	0	tr	0	*	tr	*	0	22	3	1	tr	tr	3	1	0	0.01	0	0.01	*	1	tr	*
346	Sauce-taco-canned	fl oz	16	11	tr	1	*	2	*	0	128	88	*	0.3	*	4	6	0.02	0.01	0.3	*	*	54	6	10
141	Sauce-tartar-regular	tbsp	14	75	0	8	*	1	1.5	9	98	11	*	0.1	*	3	0	0	0	0	*	*	8	3	4
1436	Sauce-teriyaki-bottled-ready to serve	tbsp	18	15	1	tr	tr	3	tr	0	690	41	11	0.3	tr	0	4	0.01	0.01	0.2	0.02	0	4	5	28
774	Sauce-teriyaki-from mix-prepared-water	cup	283	130	4	1	0.1	28	0.1	0	4791	216	85	2.8	0.1	0	28	0.03	0.09	1.3	0.14	0	28	113	215
1533	Sauce-tomato-canned-low sodium-s&w	cup	226	90	4	tr	3.4	18	0.1	0	65	838	43	1.7	0.6	221	20	0.16	0.14	2.6	0.36	0	20	32	72
1059	Sauce-tomato-canned-salt added	cup	245	74	3	tr	3.7	18	0.1	0	1482	908	32	1.9	0.6	240	32	0.16	0.14	2.8	0.38	0	23	34	78
1060	Sauce-tomato-spanish-canned	cup	244	81	4	1	3.7	18	0.1	0	1152	900	21	1.9	0.8	242	21	0.18	0.15	3.2	0.43	0	33	42	117
1061	Sauce-tomato-with herbs/cheese-canned	cup	244	144	5	5	3.7	25	1.5	*	1325	869	46	2.1	0.9	240	25	0.19	0.3	3	0.05	0	20	90	132

Item	Food name	Portion	Weight (g)	Food Energy (Kcal)	Protein (gm)	Carbohydrates (gm)	Fiber (gm)	Total Fat (gm)	Saturated Fat (gm)	Cholesterol (mg)	Sodium (mg)	Potassium (mg)	Magnesium (mg)	Iron (mg)	Zinc (mg)	Vitamin A (RE)	Vitamin C (mg)	Thiamin (mg)	Riboflavin (mg)	Niacin (mg)	Vitamin B6 (mg)	Folates (µg)	Vitamin B12 (µg)	Calcium (mg)	Phosphorus (mg)
1062	Sauce-tomato-with mushrooms-canned	cup	245	86	4	21	3.7	tr	tr	0	1107	931	47	2.2	0.5	233	30	0.18	0.27	3.1	0.33	23	0	32	78
1063	Sauce-tomato-with onions-canned	cup	245	103	4	24	3.7	tr	0.1	0	1350	1012	47	2.3	0.6	208	31	0.18	0.33	3	0.65	55	0	42	96
1435	Sauce-white-dehydrated-prepared-milk	cup	264	240	10	21	0.1	14	6.4	34	797	443	264	0.3	0.5	92	3	0.08	0.45	0.5	0.07	16	1.06	425	256
727	Sauce-white-medium-with enriched flour	cup	250	405	10	22	0.4	31	19.3	33	796	348	38	0.5	tr	115	2	0.12	0.43	0.7	0.06	12	0.7	288	233
1477	Sauce-worcestershire	tbsp	15	12	tr	3	*	0	0	0	147	120	2	0.9	tr	5	27	0	0.03	0.2	0	1	0	15	9
673	Tomato catsup	tbsp	15	15	0	4	0.2	0	0	0	156	54	4	0.1	tr	21	3	0.01	0.01	0.2	0.02	1	0	3	8

Soups

Item	Food name	Portion	Weight (g)	Food Energy (Kcal)	Protein (gm)	Carbohydrates (gm)	Fiber (gm)	Total Fat (gm)	Saturated Fat (gm)	Cholesterol (mg)	Sodium (mg)	Potassium (mg)	Magnesium (mg)	Iron (mg)	Zinc (mg)	Vitamin A (RE)	Vitamin C (mg)	Thiamin (mg)	Riboflavin (mg)	Niacin (mg)	Vitamin B6 (mg)	Folates (µg)	Vitamin B12 (µg)	Calcium (mg)	Phosphorus (mg)
710	Soup-bean with bacon-canned-with water	cup	253	173	8	23	3.2	6	1.5	3	952	403	44	2.1	1	89	2	0.09	0.03	0.6	0.04	32	0.05	81	132
711	Soup-beef broth-canned-ready to eat	cup	240	17	3	tr	0	1	0.3	0	782	130	5	0.4	0	0	2	0.01	0.05	1.9	0.02	5	0.17	14	31
721	Soup-beef broth-dehydrated-cubed	item	3.6	6	1	1	0	tr	0.1	tr	864	15	2	0.1	tr	1	0	0.01	0.01	0.5	0.01	1	0.04	2	8
712	Soup-beef noodle-prepared-water	cup	244	84	5	9	1.5	3	1.2	5	952	99	6	1.1	0.6	63	2	0.07	0.06	1.1	0.04	4	0.2	15	46
1246	Soup-beef-chunky-canned-ready to serve	cup	240	170	12	20	*	5	2.6	14	866	336	5	2.3	2.6	261	7	0.06	0.15	2.7	0.13	13	0.61	31	120
1245	Soup-black bean-canned-prepared-water	cup	247	116	6	20	*	2	0.4	0	1198	273	42	2.2	1.4	49	0	0.08	0.05	0.5	0.09	25	0.02	45	107
759	Soup-cheese-canned-prepared with milk	cup	251	230	9	16	2	15	9.1	48	1020	340	20	0.8	0.7	147	1	0.06	0.33	0.5	0.08	10	0.44	288	250
1247	Soup-chicken and dumplings-canned-milk	cup	241	96	6	6	0.7	6	1.3	34	860	116	5	0.6	0.4	52	0	0.02	0.07	1.8	0.04	2	0.16	15	60
760	Soup-chicken broth-canned-prepared-water	cup	244	39	5	1	0	1	0.4	1	776	210	2	0.5	0.2	0	0	0.01	0.07	3.4	0.02	5	0.24	9	73
761	Soup-chicken noodle-canned-with water	cup	241	75	4	9	1.5	2	0.7	7	1106	55	5	0.8	0.4	72	tr	0.05	0.06	1.4	0.03	2	0.15	17	36
1591	Soup-chicken noodle-low sodium	cup	240	91	5	10	1.4	2	0.7	7	36	106	5	1.2	0.4	109	tr	0.17	0.14	2.6	0.03	2	0.14	17	36
723	Soup-chicken noodle-prepared from dry	cup	252	53	3	7	0.2	1	0.3	3	1283	30	8	0.5	0.2	6	tr	0.07	0.06	0.9	0.01	2	0.25	33	33
1248	Soup-chicken-chunky-canned-ready to eat	cup	251	178	13	17	0.8	7	2	30	887	176	8	1.7	1	130	1	0.09	0.17	4.4	0.05	5	0.25	24	113
1592	Soup-chicken-chunky-low sodium	cup	251	173	13	15	*	5	*	*	78	264	*	1.8	*	94	2	0.13	0.25	4.8	*	*	*	28	*
1249	Soup-chicken/rice-canned-ready to serve	cup	240	127	12	13	1.4	3	1	12	888	108	10	1.9	1.4	586	4	0.02	0.1	4.1	0.05	4	0.31	35	72
1250	Soup-chili-beef-canned-prepared-water	cup	250	170	7	22	*	7	3.4	13	1035	525	30	2.1	1.4	151	4	0.06	0.08	1.1	0.16	18	0.32	43	148
713	Soup-clam chowder-Manhattan style-water	cup	244	78	2	12	2.1	2	0.4	2	578	188	12	1.6	1	96	4	0.03	0.04	0.8	0.1	10	4.05	27	42
762	Soup-clam chowder-New England-with milk	cup	248	163	9	17	1.5	7	3	22	992	300	23	1.5	0.8	40	4	0.07	0.24	1	0.13	10	10.3	187	157
1251	Soup-clam chowder-New England-with water	cup	244	95	5	12	1.5	3	0.4	5	915	146	7	1.5	0.8	1	2	0.02	0.04	1	0.08	4	8	44	54
1252	Soup-consomme-canned-prepared with water	cup	241	29	3	2	*	0	0	0	636	154	0	0.5	0.4	0	1	0.02	0.03	0.7	0.02	3	0	10	31
1593	Soup-corn-canned-low sodium-Campbells	serv	305	191	3	31	*	5	*	*	33	164	*	0.8	*	93	6	0.1	0.15	1.9	*	*	*	28	*
1253	Soup-crab-canned-ready to serve	cup	244	76	5	10	*	2	0.4	10	1234	326	88	1.2	1.5	50	4	0.2	0.07	1.3	0.12	15	0.2	66	88
757	Soup-cream of asparagus-canned-with milk	cup	248	161	6	16	0.8	8	3.3	22	1041	359	20	0.9	0.9	83	3	0.1	0.28	0.9	0.06	30	0.5	175	153
758	Soup-cream of celery-canned-with milk	cup	248	164	6	15	0.8	10	3.9	32	1009	310	22	0.7	0.2	68	1	0.07	0.25	0.4	0.06	9	0.5	186	151
707	Soup-cream of chicken-canned-with milk	cup	248	191	7	15	0.5	12	4.6	27	1046	273	18	0.7	0.7	94	1	0.07	0.26	0.9	0.07	8	0.55	180	152
714	Soup-cream of chicken-canned-with water	cup	244	117	3	9	0.5	7	2.1	10	986	88	2	0.6	0.6	56	tr	0.03	0.06	0.8	0.02	2	0.1	34	37
708	Soup-cream of mushroom-canned-with milk	cup	248	203	6	15	0.5	14	5.1	20	1076	270	20	0.6	0.6	38	2	0.08	0.28	0.7	0.06	10	0.5	178	156
715	Soup-cream of mushroom-canned-with water	cup	244	129	2	9	0.9	9	2.4	2	1031	101	5	0.5	0.6	0	1	0.05	0.09	0.7	0.02	5	0.05	46	50
765	Soup-cream of potato-canned-with milk	cup	248	148	6	17	0.5	6	3.8	22	1060	323	17	0.5	0.7	67	1	0.08	0.24	0.6	0.09	9	0.5	166	160
766	Soup-cream of shrimp-canned-with milk	cup	248	164	7	14	0.2	9	5.8	35	1036	248	22	0.6	0.8	54	1	0.06	0.23	0.5	0.45	10	1.04	164	337
1254	Soup-escarole-canned-ready to serve	cup	248	27	2	2	*	2	0.5	2	3864	265	5	0.7	2.2	217	4	0.07	0.05	2.3	0.22	35	0.5	32	79
763	Soup-gazpacho-canned-ready to serve	cup	244	57	9	1	*	2	0.3	0	1183	224	7	1	0.2	20	3	0.05	0.02	0.9	0.15	10	0	24	37
1255	Soup-lentil with ham-canned-ready to eat	cup	248	139	9	20	*	3	1.1	7	1319	357	22	2.7	0.7	36	4	0.17	0.11	1.4	0.22	50	0.3	42	184
716	Soup-minestrone-canned-prepared-water	cup	241	82	4	11	1.9	3	0.6	2	911	313	7	0.9	0.7	234	1	0.05	0.04	0.9	0.1	16	0	34	55
1256	Soup-onion-canned-prepared with water	cup	241	58	4	8	*	2	0.3	0	1053	68	2	0.7	0.6	0	tr	0.03	0.02	0.6	0.05	15	0	27	12
722	Soup-onion-dehydrated-packet	serv	39	115	5	21	2.2	2	0.5	2	3493	260	25	0.6	0.2	1	1	0.11	0.24	2	0.04	6	0	55	126
724	Soup-onion-dehydrated-prepared-water	cup	246	27	1	5	0.4	1	0.1	0	849	64	5	0.1	0.1	0	tr	0.03	0.06	0.5	0	1	0	12	30
764	Soup-oyster stew-canned-prepared-milk	cup	245	134	6	10	*	8	5.1	32	1040	235	21	1	10.3	45	4	0.07	0.23	0.3	0.06	10	2.63	167	162
1257	Soup-oyster stew-canned-prepared-water	cup	241	58	2	4	*	4	2.5	15	981	48	5	1	10.3	7	3	0.02	0.04	0.2	0.01	2	2.19	22	48
1258	Soup-pea green-canned-prepared with milk	cup	254	239	13	32	2.8	7	4	18	1048	377	55	2	1.8	58	3	0.16	0.27	1.3	0.1	8	0.44	173	238
1259	Soup-pea green-canned-prepared/water	cup	250	165	9	27	2.8	3	1.4	0	988	190	39	2	1.7	20	2	0.11	0.07	1.2	0.05	15	0	28	124
1269	Soup-pea green-low sodium-canned-water	cup	250	165	9	27	0.8	3	1.4	0	33	190	39	2	1.7	20	2	0.11	0.07	1.2	0.05	2	0	28	124
717	Soup-pea-split-canned-prepared-water	cup	253	189	10	28	2.8	4	1.8	8	1008	399	48	2.3	1.3	44	1	0.15	0.08	1.5	0.07	3	0	22	213
1260	Soup-pepperpot-canned-prepared/water	cup	241	103	6	9	*	5	2.1	10	970	152	5	0.9	1.2	87	1	0.05	0.05	1.2	0.06	10	0.17	23	42
1262	Soup-tomato beef & noodle-canned/water	cup	244	139	4	21	1.5	4	1.6	5	917	221	8	1.1	0.8	53	2	0.08	0.09	1.9	0.09	7	0.19	17	56

1263	Soup-tomato bisque-canned-prepared/milk	cup	251	198	6	29	*	7	3.1	22	1108	604	25	0.9	0.6	110	7	0.11	0.27	1.3	0.14	21	0.44	186	174
1432	Soup-tomato bisque-low sodium-with water	cup	247	123	2	24	*	3	0.5	4	30	417	9	0.8	0.6	72	6	0.07	0.07	1.2	0.09	15	0	40	60
1264	Soup-tomato rice-canned-prepared/water	cup	247	119	2	22	1.7	3	0.5	2	815	330	5	0.8	0.5	76	15	0.06	0.05	1.1	0.08	14	0	22	33
725	Soup-tomato vegetable-prepared from dry	cup	253	56	2	10	1.1	1	0.4	0	1146	103	20	0.6	0.2	20	6	0.06	0.05	0.8	0.05	10	0	8	29
709	Soup-tomato-canned-prepared with milk	cup	248	161	6	22	0.8	6	2.9	17	932	449	22	1.8	0.3	108	68	0.13	0.25	1.5	0.16	21	0.44	159	149
718	Soup-tomato-canned-prepared with water	cup	244	85	2	17	0.9	2	0.4	0	871	263	8	1.8	0.2	69	66	0.09	0.05	1.4	0.11	15	0	12	34
1266	Soup-turkey noodle-canned-prepared/water	cup	244	68	4	9	0.7	2	0.6	5	815	75	5	0.9	0.6	29	tr	0.07	0.06	1.4	0.04	2	0.15	12	48
1433	Soup-turkey noodle-low sodium-with water	cup	244	68	4	9	*	2	0.6	5	42	75	5	0.9	0.6	29	tr	0.07	0.06	1.4	0.04	2	0.15	12	48
1267	Soup-turkey vegetable-canned-water	cup	241	72	3	9	1	3	0.9	2	905	175	4	0.8	0.6	244	0	0.03	0.04	1	0.05	5	0.17	17	40
1265	Soup-turkey-chunky-canned-ready to serve	cup	236	135	10	14	2.5	4	1.2	9	923	361	24	1.9	2.1	716	6	0.04	0.11	3.6	0.31	11	2.12	50	104
1590	Soup-vegetable beef-canned-low sodium	serv	305	165	12	18	1.2	4	1.1	6	57	455	8	1.4	1.9	553	11	0.24	0.33	4.2	0.1	13	0.39	49	50
719	Soup-vegetable beef-canned-with water	cup	245	78	6	10	1	2	0.9	5	960	174	5	1.1	1.6	189	2	0.04	0.05	1	0.08	11	0.31	17	42
1510	Soup-vegetable-canned-low sodium	cup	240	98	2	14	3.1	0	0	0	38	185	7	1	0.5	371	3	0.05	0.05	1.2	0.06	11	0	19	35
720	Soup-vegetarian-canned-prepared-water	cup	241	72	2	12	1.2	2	0.3	0	823	209	7	1.1	0.5	300	1	0.05	0.05	0.9	0.06	11	0	21	35
1261	Soup-vichyssoise-canned-prepared/milk	cup	248	148	6	17	*	6	3.8	22	1060	323	17	0.5	0.7	67	1	0.08	0.24	0.6	0.09	9	0.5	166	160
	Sugars & sweets																								
1583	Apple butter	tbsp	20	37	tr	9	0.2	tr	tr	0	0	50	2	0.1	tr	0	tr	tr	tr	tr	0.01	tr	0	3	4
1608	Candy-Almond Joy	oz	28.4	151	2	19	0.3	8	1.7	1	22	114	13	0.3	0.4	3	tr	0.02	0.1	0.2	0.02	4	0.18	60	68
1607	Candy-Bit o Honey	oz	28.4	121	1	21	*	4	1.7	*	*	*	*	0.3	*	*	*	0	0.13	1.4	*	*	*	13	*
537	Candy-caramels-plain/chocolate	oz	28.4	115	1	22	0.8	3	1.6	0	74	54	1	0.4	0.2	0	0	0.01	0.05	0.1	0.01	2	0.04	42	35
540	Candy-chocolate coated peanuts	oz	28.4	160	5	11	*	12	4	0	16	143	*	0.4	*	0	0	0.1	0.05	2.1	*	*	*	33	84
539	Candy-chocolate-semisweet	cup	170	860	7	97	8.8	61	36.2	0	3	553	192	4.4	2.6	9	0	0.02	0.14	0.9	0.07	5	0	51	255
541	Candy-fondant-uncoated	oz	28.4	105	0	25	0	1	0.1	0	60	1	tr	0.3	0	0	0	0	0	0	0	0	0	4	2
542	Candy-fudge-chocolate-plain	oz	28.4	115	1	21	0.4	3	1.3	0	54	42	13	0.3	0.1	0	0	0.01	0.03	0.1	0.01	1	0.06	22	24
543	Candy-gum drops	oz	28.4	100	0	25	0	0	0	0	10	1	tr	0.1	tr	0	0	0	0	0	0	0	0	2	0
544	Candy-hard	oz	28.4	110	0	28	0	0	0	0	9	1	*	0.5	*	0	0	0	0	0	*	*	*	6	2
1609	Candy-jelly beans	item	2.8	7	0	3	0	0	0	0	tr	0	*	tr	*	0	0	0	*	*	*	*	*	tr	tr
1606	Candy-Kit Kat bar	item	43	210	3	25	0.6	11	5.6	3	38	129	19	0.6	0.4	9	0	0.03	0.11	0.1	0.02	3	0.07	65	78
1602	Candy-Life Savers	item	2	8	0	2	0	tr	0	0	1	0	*	tr	*	0	0	0	0	0	*	*	*	tr	tr
1612	Candy-lollipop	item	28.4	108	0	28	0	0	0	0	*	*	*	0	*	0	0	0	0	0	*	*	*	0	0
1603	Candy-M & M-plain-package	item	45	220	3	31	*	10	*	*	*	*	*	*	*	*	*	*	*	*	*	*	*	*	*
1534	Candy-milk chocolate bar-no sugar	item	10.1	60	1	5	*	4	*	*	10	*	*	*	*	*	*	*	*	*	*	*	*	*	*
1499	Candy-milk chocolate with almonds	oz	28.4	151	3	15	1.3	10	4.1	5	23	125	27	0.5	0.4	21	0	0.02	0.12	0.2	0.01	4	0.15	65	77
1498	Candy-milk chocolate with peanuts	oz	28.4	154	4	13	*	11	5.2	*	19	138	*	0.4	*	15	0	0.07	0.07	1.4	*	*	*	49	83
538	Candy-milk chocolate-plain	oz	28.4	145	2	16	*	9	5.5	0	28	109	16	0.3	*	24	0	0.02	0.1	0.1	*	2	*	65	65
1605	Candy-Milky Way bar	item	60	260	3	43	0.1	9	5.1	4	114	157	20	0.4	0.4	4	tr	0.02	0.14	0.3	0.02	4	0.22	79	79
1610	Candy-peanut brittle	oz	28.4	123	2	20	0.5	4	1.9	0	9	43	11	0.6	0.3	2	0	0.02	0.01	1.3	0.02	14	0	11	35
1611	Candy-peanut butter cup	piece	17	92	2	9	0.8	5	2.8	3	55	68	15	0.2	0.2	1	0	0.05	0.03	0.8	0.03	17	0.04	15	41
1604	Candy-Snickers bar	item	57	270	6	33	1.4	13	4.7	9	145	189	37	0.5	0.6	3	0	0.03	0.1	1.7	0.06	29	0.17	66	102
696	Chocolate-bitter-for baking	oz	28.4	145	3	8	4.3	15	8.9	0	1	235	82	1.9	0.3	6	0	0.01	0.07	0.4	0.01	3	0	22	109
1088	Coconut cream-raw	cup	240	792	9	16	1.6	83	73.8	0	10	781	41	5.5	2.3	0	7	0.07	0	2.1	0.07	34	0	26	293
1089	Coconut milk-raw	cup	240	552	6	13	1.1	57	50.7	0	37	630	89	3.9	1.6	0	7	0.06	0	1.8	0.08	39	0	39	240
548	Honey-strained/extracted	tbsp	21	65	0	17	0.1	0	0	0	1	11	1	0.1	tr	0	0	0	0.01	0.1	tr	0	0	1	1
534	Icing-cake-chocolate-prepared from mix	cup	275	1035	9	185	*	38	23.4	0	882	536	*	3.3	*	174	1	0.06	0.28	0.6	*	*	*	165	305
535	Icing-cake-fudge-prepared from mix/water	cup	245	830	7	183	*	16	5.1	0	568	238	*	2.7	*	0	0	0.05	0.2	0.7	*	*	*	96	218
532	Icing-cake-white-boiled	cup	94	295	1	75	0	0	0	0	134	17	*	0	*	0	0	0	0.03	0	*	*	*	2	2
536	Icing-cake-white-uncooked	cup	319	1200	2	260	0	21	12.7	0	156	57	*	0	*	258	0	0	0.06	0	*	*	*	48	38
533	Icing-cake-white/coconut-boiled	cup	166	605	3	124	*	13	11	0	195	277	*	0.8	*	0	0	0.02	0.07	0.3	*	*	*	10	50
562	Jam/preserves-strawberry-low calorie	tsp	6	8	0	2	0.1	0	0	0	6	5	tr	tr	tr	tr	1	tr	tr	tr	tr	1	0	1	tr
549	Jams/preserves-regular	tbsp	20	55	0	14	0.2	0	0	0	2	18	1	0.2	tr	0	0	0	0.01	0	tr	2	0	4	2
550	Jams/preserves-regular-packet size	item	14	40	0	10	0.1	0	0	0	1	12	1	0.1	tr	0	0	0	0	0	tr	1	0	3	1
551	Jellies-regular	tbsp	18	50	0	13	0	0	0	0	3	14	1	0.3	tr	0	1	0	0.01	0	tr	tr	0	4	1

* indicates that no data was available.

Appendix A - Table of Food Composition
(continued)

Item	Food name	Portion	Weight (g)	Food Energy (Kcal)	Protein (gm)	Carbohydrates (gm)	Fiber (gm)	Total Fat (gm)	Saturated Fat (gm)	Cholesterol (mg)	Sodium (mg)	Potassium (mg)	Magnesium (mg)	Iron (mg)	Zinc (mg)	Vitamin A (RE)	Vitamin C (mg)	Thiamin (mg)	Riboflavin (mg)	Niacin (mg)	Vitamin B6 (mg)	Folates (µg)	Vitamin B12 (µg)	Calcium (mg)	Phosphorus (mg)
552	Jellies-regular-packet size	item	14	40	0	11	0	0	0	0	2	11	1	0.2	tr	0	0	0	0	0	tr	tr	0	3	1
545	Marshmallows	oz	28.4	90	1	23	0	0	0	0	11	2	1	0.5	tr	0	0	0	0	0	0	0	0	5	2
556	Molasses-cane-blackstrap	tbsp	20	45	0	11	0	0	0	0	18	585	9	3.2	0.1	0	0	0.02	0.04	0.4	0.04	0	0	137	17
555	Molasses-cane-light	tbsp	20	50	0	13	0	0	0	0	3	183	9	0.9	0.1	0	0	0.01	0.01	0.4	0.04	0	0	33	9
519	Nuts-coconut-dried-flaked-canned	cup	77	341	3	32	4.4	24	21.6	0	15	249	38	1.4	1.2	0	0	0.02	0.02	0.2	0.18	5	0	11	79
1087	Nuts-coconut-dried-shredded	cup	93	466	3	44	3.9	33	29.3	0	244	313	47	1.8	1.7	0	1	0.03	0.02	0.4	0.25	8	0	14	99
520	Nuts-coconut-raw-shredded	cup	80	283	3	12	7.2	27	23.8	0	16	285	26	1.9	0.9	0	3	0.05	0.02	0.4	0.04	21	0	12	90
557	Sorghum	tbsp	21	55	0	14	0	0	0	0	2	37	tr	2.6	tr	0	0	0.03	0.02	0	0	0	0	35	5
559	Sugar-brown-pressed down	cup	220	820	0	212	0	0	0	0	66	757	44	7.5	0.6	0	0	0.02	0.07	0.4	0.09	0	0	187	42
1582	Sugar-Equal-packet size	item	1	4	0	1	0	0	0	0	4	0	*	0	0	0	0	0	0	0	0	0	0	0	0
1581	Sugar-Sweet & Low-packet size	item	1	4	0	1	0	0	0	0	4	3	*	0	0	0	0	0	0	0	0	0	0	0	0
561	Sugar-white-granulated	tbsp	12	45	0	12	0	0	0	0	tr	0	0	tr	tr	0	0	0	0	0	0	0	0	0	0
563	Sugar-white-powdered-sifted	cup	100	385	0	100	0	0	0	0	1	3	*	0.1	0	0	0	0	0	0	0	0	0	0	0
554	Syrup-chocolate flavored-fudge-thick	fl oz	38	125	2	20	*	5	3.1	0	27	107	21	0.5	0.3	18	0	0.02	0.08	0.2	*	*	*	48	60
553	Syrup-chocolate flavored-thin	fl oz	38	83	1	22	0.1	tr	0.2	0	20	106	21	0.6	0.3	0	0	0.01	0.03	0.2	tr	2	0	6	35
558	Syrup-corn-table blends-light and dark	tbsp	21	60	0	15	0	0	0	0	15	1	tr	0.8	tr	0	0	0	0	0	0	0	0	9	3
560	Syrup-pancake-Karo	tbsp	20.5	60	0	15	0	0	0	0	35	1	tr	0.8	tr	0	0	0	0	0	0	0	0	9	3
1457	Syrup-pancake-light-Aunt Jemima	fl oz	39	60	0	15	0	0	0	0	18	7	1	0.1	tr	0	0	tr	0.01	0	tr	0	0	1	4
Vegetables																									
975	Alfalfa seeds-sprouted-raw	cup	33	10	1	1	0.7	tr	tr	0	2	26	9	0.3	0.3	5	3	0.03	0.04	0.2	0.01	12	0	11	23
977	Amaranth-boiled-drained	cup	132	28	3	5	2.5	tr	0.1	0	28	846	73	3	1.2	366	54	0.03	0.18	0.7	0.23	75	0	276	95
976	Amaranth-raw	cup	28	7	1	1	2.7	tr	tr	0	5	171	15	0.7	0.3	82	12	0.01	0.04	0.2	0.05	24	0	60	14
978	Artichokes-boiled-drained	item	120	60	4	13	4	tr	0.1	0	114	425	72	1.6	0.6	22	12	0.08	0.08	1.2	0.13	61	0	54	103
1514	Asparagus-canned-dietary pack-low sodium	cup	244	34	4	5	3.9	1	0.1	0	849	373	22	1.4	1.2	115	40	0.13	0.22	2.1	0.24	208	0	34	93
568	Asparagus-canned-spears-drained solids	cup	242	46	5	6	3.5	2	0.4	0	944	416	24	4.4	1	128	45	0.15	0.24	2.3	0.27	231	0	39	104
567	Asparagus-frozen-boiled-drained-spears	cup	180	50	5	9	2.2	1	0.2	0	7	392	23	1.2	1	147	44	0.12	0.19	1.9	0.04	242	0	41	99
565	Asparagus-frozen-boiled-drained-tips	cup	180	50	5	9	2.2	1	0.2	0	7	392	23	1.2	1	148	44	0.12	0.19	1.9	0.04	242	0	41	99
566	Asparagus-raw-boiled-drained-spears	cup	180	45	5	8	2.2	1	0.1	0	7	558	34	1.2	0.9	149	49	0.18	0.22	1.9	0.25	177	0	43	110
564	Asparagus-raw-boiled-drained-tips	cup	180	45	5	8	1.2	1	0.1	0	7	558	34	1.2	0.9	149	49	0.18	0.22	1.9	0.25	177	0	43	110
979	Balsam pear-leafy tips-boiled-drained	cup	58	20	2	4	2.5	tr	tr	0	8	349	55	0.6	0.2	149	32	0.09	0.16	0.6	0.44	51	0	24	45
980	Balsam pear-pods-boiled-drained	cup	124	24	1	5	2.2	tr	tr	0	7	396	20	0.5	1	14	41	0.06	0.07	0.3	0.05	63	0	11	45
982	Bamboo shoots-boiled-drained	cup	120	14	2	2	2.5	tr	0.1	0	5	640	4	0.3	0.6	0	1	0.02	0.06	0.4	0.12	3	0	14	24
983	Bamboo shoots-canned-drained	cup	131	25	2	4	3.4	1	0.1	0	9	105	5	0.4	0.9	1	1	0.03	0.03	0.2	0.18	4	0	11	33
981	Bamboo shoots-raw	cup	151	41	4	8	3.9	tr	0.1	0	6	805	5	0.8	1.7	3	6	0.23	0.11	0.9	0.36	11	0	20	89
1623	Beans-adzuki-boiled	cup	230	294	17	57	14.3	tr	0	0	18	1224	120	4.6	4.1	*	1	0.27	0.15	1.7	0.22	279	0	63	385
1624	Beans-adzuki-canned-sweetened	cup	296	702	11	163	13.7	tr	0	0	646	353	91	3.3	3.6	3	0	0.3	0.17	1.9	0.25	316	0	66	220
1626	Beans-baked beans-canned	cup	254	236	12	52	19.6	1	0.3	0	1008	752	81	0.7	3.6	3	8	0.39	0.15	1.1	0.34	61	0	127	264
1625	Beans-baked beans-home recipe	cup	253	382	14	54	19.5	13	4.9	13	1068	907	110	5	1.8	tr	3	0.34	0.12	1	0.23	122	0.03	155	275
1627	Beans-black-cooked-boiled	cup	172	227	15	41	7.2	1	0.2	0	1	611	121	3.6	1.9	1	0	0.42	0.1	0.9	0.12	256	0	47	241
1628	Beans-french-cooked-boiled	cup	177	228	13	43	14.9	1	0.1	0	11	655	99	1.9	1.1	1	2	0.23	0.11	1	0.19	132	0	111	181
123	Beans-garbanzo-canned-reconstituted	serv	28.4	28	1	5	1.4	1	0.1	0	113	55	9	0.7	0.3	tr	*	tr	0.01	0.1	*	*	0	11	30
1501	Beans-garbanzo-dry-raw	cup	200	720	41	122	*	10	*	0	52	1594	*	13.8	*	1	*	0.62	0.3	4	0.3	*	0	300	662
509	Beans-great northern-dry-cooked-drained	cup	180	210	14	38	9.7	1	tr	0	12	749	86	4.9	1.8	*	0	0.25	0.13	1.3	1.01	63	0	90	266
1511	Beans-green-canned-dietary-low sodium	cup	136	26	2	6	1.8	tr	tr	0	3	148	18	1.2	0.4	31	6	0.02	0.08	0.3	*	43	0	32	26
573	Beans-green-frozen-boiled-french style	cup	135	35	2	8	2.2	tr	tr	0	18	151	28	1.1	0.8	72	11	0.07	0.1	0.6	0.08	11	0	61	32
1535	Beans-kidney-canned-dietary-low sodium	cup	255	230	15	42	12.5	1	0	0	10	673	10	4.6	1.9	3	8	0.13	0.1	1.5	1.12	36	0	74	278
570	Beans-lima-baby-frozen-boiled-drained	cup	180	189	12	35	13	1	0.1	0	52	740	101	3.5	1	43	10	0.13	0.1	1.4	0.21	28	0	50	202
1513	Beans-lima-canned-dietary-low sodium	cup	248	186	11	34	10.4	1	0.2	0	10	668	84	3.9	1.6	43	22	0.07	0.11	1.3	0.15	40	0	70	176
984	Beans-lima-canned-solids & liquids	cup	248	186	11	34	10.4	1	0.2	0	618	668	84	3.9	1.6	43	22	0.07	0.11	1.3	0.15	40	0	70	176
569	Beans-lima-frozen-boiled-drained	cup	170	170	10	32	8.3	1	0.1	0	90	694	58	2.3	0.7	32	22	0.12	0.1	1.8	0.21	111	0	38	153
515	Beans-lima-raw-boiled-drained	cup	170	209	12	40	12.2	1	0.1	0	29	969	126	4.2	1.3	63	17	0.24	0.16	1.8	0.33	45	0	54	221
579	Beans-mung-sprouted-boiled	cup	125	26	3	5	2.7	tr	tr	0	13	126	18	0.8	0.6	1	14	0.06	0.13	1	0.07	37	0	15	35

Code	Food	Unit																							
578	Beans-mung-sprouted-raw	cup	104	31	3	6	1.6	tr	tr	0	6	155	22	0.9	0.4	2	14	0.09	0.13	0.8	0.09	63	0	14	56
510	Beans-navy pea-dry-cooked-drained	cup	190	225	15	40	9.3	1	0.2	0	13	790	97	5.1	1.8	0	0	0.27	0.13	1.3	1.06	67	0	95	281
985	Beans-navy-sprouted-boiled	oz	28.4	22	2	4	1.4	tr	tr	0	4	90	32	0.6	0.3	tr	5	0.11	0.07	0.4	0.06	30	0	5	29
986	Beans-pinto-frozen-boiled	oz	28.4	46	3	9	1.4	tr	tr	0	24	183	15	0.8	0.2	0	tr	0.08	0.03	0.2	0.06	10	0	15	28
514	Beans-red kidney-canned-solids & liquids	cup	255	230	15	42	12.5	1	1.2	0	833	673	10	4.6	1.9	1	8	0.13	0.1	1.5	1.12	36	0	74	278
1632	Beans-refried	cup	253	271	16	47	11.6	3	1	0	1073	994	99	4.5	3.5	0	15	0.14	0.14	1.2	0.25	211	0	116	213
1558	Beans-refried-canned-sausage-Old El Paso	cup	200	388	14	26	6	26	6.9	16	624	600	88	4.2	1.8	0	6	0.31	0.14	0.6	0.31	254	0	88	258
987	Beans-shellie-canned	cup	245	74	4	15	12	tr	0.1	0	818	267	37	2.4	0.7	56	8	0.12	0.13	0.5	0.12	44	0	71	74
1629	Beans-small white-boiled	cup	179	254	16	46	7.9	1	0.3	0	4	828	122	5.1	2	0	0	0.23	0.11	0.5	0.23	245	0	131	302
574	Beans-snap-green-canned-drained-cuts	cup	135	27	2	6	1.8	tr	tr	0	339	147	18	1.2	0.4	47	7	0.02	0.08	0.3	0.05	43	0	35	34
41	Beans-snap-green-canned-dietetic-low sodium	oz	28.4	4	tr	1	0.4	tr	0	0	18	24	3	0.2	0.1	10	11	0.01	0.01	0.1	*	*	0	7	6
572	Beans-snap-green-frozen-boiled-cuts	cup	135	35	2	8	2.2	tr	0.1	0	4	151	28	1.1	0.8	72	11	0.07	0.1	0.6	0.08	11	0	61	32
571	Beans-snap-green-raw-boiled	cup	125	44	2	10	2.3	tr	0.1	0	4	374	31	1.6	0.5	84	12	0.09	0.12	0.8	0.07	42	0	58	49
577	Beans-snap-yellow/wax-canned	cup	136	27	2	6	1.8	tr	tr	0	341	148	18	1.2	0.4	48	7	0.02	0.08	0.3	0.05	43	0	35	26
576	Beans-snap-yellow/wax-frozen-boiled	cup	135	35	2	8	2.2	tr	tr	0	18	151	28	1.1	0.8	72	11	0.07	0.1	0.6	0.08	11	0	61	32
575	Beans-snap-yellow/wax-raw-boiled	cup	125	44	2	10	2.3	tr	0.1	0	4	374	31	1.6	0.5	84	12	0.09	0.12	0.8	0.07	42	0	58	48
584	Beet greens-boiled-drained	cup	145	39	4	8	4.4	tr	tr	0	349	1318	99	2.8	0.7	740	36	0.17	0.42	0.7	0.19	21	0	165	60
1512	Beets-canned-dietary pack-low sodium	cup	246	71	2	17	2.7	tr	tr	0	113	349	39	1.7	0.6	2	9	0.03	0.09	0.5	0.14	71	0	34	39
581	Beets-sliced-boiled-drained	cup	170	53	2	11	3.4	tr	tr	0	83	530	63	1.1	0.4	2	2	0.05	0.02	0.3	0.05	90	0	19	53
583	Beets-sliced-canned-drained	cup	170	53	2	12	2.9	tr	tr	0	466	252	29	3.1	0.4	2	7	0.02	0.07	0.3	0.1	51	0	26	29
580	Beets-whole-boiled-drained	item	50	16	1	3	1.1	tr	tr	0	25	156	19	0.3	0.1	1	3	0.02	0.01	0.1	0.02	27	0	6	12
582	Beets-whole-canned	cup	246	71	2	17	2.7	tr	tr	0	647	349	39	1.7	0.6	91	10	0.03	0.09	0.4	0.14	71	0	34	39
590	Broccoli-frozen-boiled-drained	cup	185	52	6	10	7.3	tr	tr	0	44	333	37	1.1	0.6	350	74	0.1	0.15	0.8	0.24	104	0	94	102
587	Broccoli-raw	cup	88	25	3	5	2.5	tr	tr	0	24	286	22	0.8	0.4	136	82	0.06	0.11	0.6	0.14	63	0	42	58
588	Broccoli-raw-boiled-drained	cup	155	43	5	8	4	1	0.1	0	40	453	37	1.3	0.6	215	116	0.09	0.18	0.9	0.22	78	0	71	92
592	Brussels sprouts-frozen-boiled	cup	155	65	6	13	4.5	1	0.1	0	36	504	37	1.2	0.6	92	71	0.16	0.18	0.8	0.45	157	0	37	84
591	Brussels sprouts-raw-boiled	cup	156	61	4	14	6.7	1	0.2	0	33	495	31	1.9	0.5	112	97	0.17	0.12	0.9	0.28	94	0	56	87
988	Burdock root-boiled-drained	item	166	146	3	35	*	tr	*	0	7	597	65	1.3	0.6	4	4	0.07	0.1	0.5	0.46	32	0	82	154
598	Cabbage-celery-raw	cup	76	12	1	2	0.8	tr	tr	0	7	181	10	0.2	0.2	21	21	0.03	0.04	0.3	0.18	60	0	59	22
595	Cabbage-common-boiled-drained	cup	145	31	1	7	4	tr	tr	0	28	297	22	0.6	0.2	35	35	0.08	0.08	0.3	0.09	29	0	48	36
594	Cabbage-common-raw-shredded	cup	90	22	1	5	1.8	tr	tr	0	16	221	14	0.5	0.2	11	43	0.05	0.03	0.3	0.09	51	0	42	21
593	Cabbage-common-raw-sliced	cup	70	17	1	4	1.5	tr	tr	0	13	172	11	0.4	0.1	9	33	0.04	0.02	0.2	0.07	40	0	33	16
596	Cabbage-red-raw-shredded	cup	70	19	1	4	1.4	tr	tr	0	8	144	11	0.3	0.1	3	40	0.04	0.02	0.2	0.15	15	0	36	29
597	Cabbage-savoy-raw-shredded	cup	70	19	1	4	1.5	tr	tr	0	20	161	20	0.3	0.2	70	22	0.05	0.02	0.2	0.13	56	0	25	29
599	Cabbage-white mustard-boiled	cup	170	20	3	3	2.7	tr	tr	0	58	631	19	1.8	0.3	437	44	0.05	0.11	0.7	0.28	69	0	158	49
589	Cabbage-white mustard-raw	cup	70	9	2	2	0.7	tr	tr	0	46	176	13	0.6	0.1	210	69	0.03	0.05	0.4	0.14	46	0	74	26
989	Carrot juice-canned	cup	246	98	1	23	5.9	tr	0.1	0	71	718	34	1.1	0.4	6335	21	0.23	0.14	1	0.53	9	0	59	103
601	Carrot-raw-scraped-shredded	cup	110	47	2	11	3.5	tr	tr	0	39	355	17	0.6	0.2	3094	10	0.11	0.06	1	0.16	15	0	30	48
600	Carrot-raw-scraped-whole	item	72	31	2	7	2.3	tr	tr	0	25	233	11	0.4	0.1	2025	7	0.07	0.04	0.7	0.11	10	0	19	32
602	Carrots-boiled-drained-sliced	cup	156	70	1	16	5.8	tr	0.1	0	103	354	20	1	0.5	3830	4	0.05	0.09	0.8	0.38	22	0	48	47
1515	Carrots-canned-dietary pack-low sodium	cup	246	57	2	12	2.7	tr	tr	0	96	426	22	1.5	0.7	3239	7	0.05	0.07	1	0.28	20	0	62	49
603	Carrots-canned-sliced-drained	cup	146	34	1	8	2.2	tr	tr	0	352	261	12	0.9	0.4	2010	4	0.03	0.04	0.9	0.16	13	0	37	35
633	Carrots-frozen-boiled-drained	cup	146	53	3	12	5.4	tr	tr	0	86	231	15	0.7	0.4	2584	4	0.04	0.05	0.7	0.19	16	0	41	38
606	Cauliflower-frozen-boiled	cup	180	34	2	7	3.2	tr	0.1	0	32	250	16	0.7	0.2	4	56	0.07	0.1	0.7	0.16	74	0	31	43
605	Cauliflower-raw-boiled-drained	cup	124	30	2	6	2.7	tr	tr	0	8	400	14	0.5	0.3	2	69	0.08	0.06	0.6	0.25	63	0	34	44
604	Cauliflower-raw-chopped	cup	100	24	2	5	2.4	tr	tr	0	15	355	14	0.6	0.2	2	72	0.06	0.06	0.6	0.23	66	0	29	46
608	Celery-pascal-raw-diced	cup	120	19	1	4	1.9	tr	tr	0	104	344	13	0.4	0.2	16	8	0.05	0.05	0.4	0.1	34	0	48	30
607	Celery-pascal-raw-stalk	item	40	6	tr	1	0.6	tr	tr	0	35	115	4	0.2	0.1	5	3	0.02	0.02	0.1	0.04	11	0	16	10
991	Chard-swiss-boiled-drained	cup	175	35	3	7	3.7	tr	0	0	313	961	150	4	0.6	549	32	0.06	0.15	0.6	0.15	15	0	102	58
990	Chard-swiss-raw	cup	36	7	1	1	0.6	tr	0	0	64	198	31	0.8	0.1	113	6	0.01	0.03	0.1	0.03	3	0	21	12
992	Chicory greens-raw-chopped	cup	180	41	3	8	4.3	1	0.1	0	81	756	54	1.6	0.8	720	43	0.11	0.18	0.9	0.19	197	0	180	85

* indicates that no data was available.

Appendix A - Table of Food Composition (continued)

Item	Food name	Portion	Weight (g)	Food Energy (Kcal)	Protein (gm)	Carbohydrates (gm)	Fiber (gm)	Total Fat (gm)	Saturated Fat (gm)	Cholesterol (mg)	Sodium (mg)	Potassium (mg)	Magnesium (mg)	Iron (mg)	Zinc (mg)	Vitamin A (RE)	Vitamin C (mg)	Thiamin (mg)	Riboflavin (mg)	Niacin (mg)	Vitamin B6 (mg)	Folates (µg)	Vitamin B12 (µg)	Calcium (mg)	Phosphorus (mg)
993	Chicory roots-raw	item	60	44	1	11	1.4	tr	tr	0	30	174	13	0.5	0.2	3	3	0.02	0.02	0.2	0.15	14	0	25	37
995	Chives-freeze dried	tbsp	0.2	1	tr	tr	tr	tr	tr	0	tr	6	1	tr	tr	14	1	tr	tr	tr	tr	tr	0	2	1
994	Chives-raw-chopped	tbsp	3	1	tr	tr	0.1	tr	tr	0	tr	8	2	tr	tr	19	2	tr	0.01	0.01	0.01	tr	0	2	2
610	Collards-frozen-boiled-drained	cup	170	61	5	12	5.2	1	*	0	85	427	51	1.9	0.5	1017	45	0.08	0.2	1.1	0.19	129	0	357	46
609	Collards-raw-boiled-drained	cup	128	35	2	8	2.1	1	tr	0	21	168	9	0.2	0.1	349	16	0.03	0.07	0.4	0.07	8	0	29	10
1503	Corn fritter	item	35	132	3	14	0.6	8	2	25	167	47	8	0.6	0.2	14	1	0.06	0.07	0.6	0.02	11	0.06	22	54
1516	Corn-creamed-canned-dietary-low sodium	cup	256	184	4	46	3.1	1	0.2	0	8	343	44	1	1.4	26	12	0.06	0.14	2.5	0.16	115	0	8	131
612	Corn-ear-frozen-boiled-drained	item	126	117	4	28	2.7	1	0.1	0	5	316	37	0.8	0.8	27	6	0.22	0.09	1.9	0.28	38	0	4	95
613	Corn-frozen-boiled-drained-kernels	cup	165	134	5	34	3.5	tr	tr	0	8	228	30	0.5	0.6	41	4	0.11	0.12	2.1	0.16	33	0	4	78
611	Corn-kernels from one ear-boiled-drained	item	77	83	3	19	2.9	1	0.2	0	13	192	25	0.5	0.6	17	5	0.17	0.06	1.2	0.05	36	0	2	79
616	Corn-sweet-canned-drained	cup	165	134	4	31	2.3	2	0.3	0	533	322	33	1.4	0.6	26	14	0.05	0.13	2	0.08	80	0	8	107
1502	Corn-sweet-canned-low sodium	cup	256	156	5	38	2.1	1	0.2	0	8	392	41	0.9	0.9	31	17	0.07	0.16	2.4	0.1	98	0	10	131
615	Corn-sweet-canned-vacuum packed	cup	210	166	5	41	9.5	1	0.2	0	572	390	48	0.9	1	51	17	0.09	0.15	2.5	0.12	104	0	10	134
614	Corn-sweet-cream style-canned	cup	256	184	4	46	3.1	1	0.2	0	730	343	44	1	1.4	26	12	0.06	0.14	2.5	0.16	115	0	8	131
997	Corn-with red and green peppers-canned	cup	227	170	5	41	5.1	1	0.2	0	788	347	57	1.8	0.8	52	20	0.05	0.18	2.2	0.22	77	0	11	141
999	Cress-garden-raw	cup	50	16	1	3	0.6	tr	tr	0	8	304	19	0.7	0.2	465	35	0.04	0.13	0.5	0.12	40	0	40	38
618	Cucumber-raw-sliced	cup	104	14	1	3	1	tr	tr	0	2	155	11	0.3	0.2	15	5	0.03	0.02	0.3	0.05	15	0	15	18
617	Cucumber-raw-whole	item	301	39	2	9	3	tr	0.1	0	6	448	33	0.8	0.7	1229	14	0.09	0.06	0.9	0.16	42	0	42	51
619	Dandelion greens-boiled	cup	105	35	2	7	4.1	1	0.1	0	46	244	25	1.9	0.3	1229	19	0.14	0.18	0.5	0.17	13	0	147	44
1000	Eggplant-boiled-drained	cup	96	27	1	6	2.7	tr	tr	0	3	238	13	0.3	0.2	6	1	0.07	0.02	0.6	0.08	14	0	6	21
620	Endive-raw-chopped	cup	50	9	1	2	1.2	tr	tr	0	11	157	8	0.4	0.4	103	3	0.04	0.04	0.2	0.01	71	0	26	14
1727	Frijoles-beans with cheese	cup	167	226	11	29	*	8	4.1	36	882	605	85	2.2	1.7	46	2	0.14	0.33	1.5	0.19	111	0.68	188	175
1001	Garlic-raw-clove	clove	3	4	tr	1	0.1	tr	tr	0	1	12	1	0.1	tr	0	tr	0.01	tr	tr	0.04	tr	0	5	5
1002	Ginger root-raw-sliced	cup	96	66	2	15	0.7	1	0.2	0	13	398	41	0.5	0.3	0	5	0.02	0.03	0.7	0.15	11	0	17	26
1003	Gourd-white flowered-boiled	cup	146	22	1	5	1.6	tr	tr	0	3	248	16	0.4	1	0	12	0.04	0.03	0.6	0.06	6	0	35	19
1636	Hummus	cup	246	421	12	50	0	21	3.1	0	600	428	71	3.9	2.7	5	19	0.23	0.13	1	0.98	146	0	123	275
1004	Jerusalem artichokes-raw	cup	150	114	3	26	0	tr	0	0	6	644	26	5.1	2	0	6	0.3	0.09	2	0.12	20	0	21	117
622	Kale-frozen-boiled-drained	cup	130	39	4	7	3.8	1	0.1	0	20	417	23	1.2	0.2	826	33	0.06	0.15	0.9	0.11	19	0	179	36
621	Kale-raw-boiled-drained	cup	130	42	2	7	4.3	1	0.1	0	30	296	23	1.2	0.3	962	53	0.07	0.09	0.7	0.18	17	0	94	36
1006	Kohlrabi-boiled-drained	cup	165	48	3	11	3.3	tr	tr	0	35	561	31	0.7	0.5	7	89	0.07	0.03	0.6	0.25	20	0	41	74
1005	Kohlrabi-raw	cup	140	38	2	9	2.5	tr	tr	0	28	490	27	0.6	tr	6	87	0.07	0.03	0.6	0.21	23	0	34	64
1008	Leeks-boiled-drained	item	124	38	1	9	4	tr	tr	0	12	108	17	1.4	0.2	6	5	0.03	0.03	0.2	0.14	30	0	37	21
1007	Leeks-raw	item	124	76	2	18	2.5	tr	0.1	0	25	223	35	2.6	0.1	12	15	0.06	0.04	0.5	0.29	80	0	73	43
1009	Lentils-sprouted-raw	cup	77	82	7	17	6.2	tr	tr	0	8	248	29	2.5	1.2	4	13	0.18	0.1	0.9	0.15	77	0	19	133
522	Lentils-whole-cooked	cup	198	231	18	40	9.8	1	0.1	0	4	731	71	6.6	2.5	2	3	0.34	0.15	2.1	0.35	358	0	37	356
623	Lettuce-butterhead-head	item	163	21	2	4	1.6	tr	tr	0	8	419	21	0.5	0.3	158	13	0.1	0.1	0.5	0.08	119	0	52	38
624	Lettuce-butterhead-leaves	leaf	15	2	tr	tr	0.2	tr	tr	0	1	39	2	tr	0.1	15	1	0.01	0.01	tr	0.01	11	0	5	3
627	Lettuce-iceberg-raw-chopped	cup	55	7	1	1	0.6	tr	tr	0	5	87	5	0.3	0.1	18	2	0.03	0.02	0.1	0.02	31	0	11	11
625	Lettuce-iceberg-raw-head	item	539	70	5	11	5.4	1	0.1	0	49	852	49	2.7	1.2	178	21	0.25	0.16	1	0.22	302	0	102	108
626	Lettuce-iceberg-raw-leaves	piece	20	3	tr	tr	0.2	tr	tr	0	2	32	2	0.1	tr	7	1	0.01	0.01	tr	0.01	11	0	4	4
628	Lettuce-looseleaf-raw	cup	55	10	1	2	0.8	tr	tr	0	5	145	6	0.8	0.2	105	10	0.03	0.04	0.2	0.03	27	0	37	14
1488	Lettuce-romaine-raw-shredded	oz	28.4	9	1	1	1	tr	0.1	0	4	162	3	0.6	0.1	146	13	0.06	0.06	0.3	0.03	76	0	20	25
1011	Lotus root-boiled-drained	item	115	19	tr	17	0.9	tr	tr	0	13	103	6	0.3	0.1	0	8	0.04	tr	0.1	0.06	2	0	7	22
1010	Lotus root-raw	cup	115	64	3	20	3.5	tr	tr	0	46	639	27	1.3	0.4	0	51	0.18	0.25	0.5	0.21	15	0	52	115
1575	Miso-fermented soybeans	cup	275	567	33	77	9.9	17	2.4	0	1003	451	116	7.5	9.1	25	0	0.27	0.69	2.4	0.59	91	0	182	421
1013	Mushrooms-boiled-drained	item	12	3	tr	tr	0.3	tr	tr	0	tr	43	1	0.2	0.1	15	1	0.01	0.04	0.5	0.01	2	0	1	10
1014	Mushrooms-canned-drained	item	12	3	tr	1	0.2	tr	tr	0	51	16	2	0.1	0.2	18	2	0.01	tr	0.2	0.01	1	0	1	8
629	Mushrooms-raw-chopped	cup	70	18	2	3	0.9	tr	tr	0	3	259	7	0.9	0.5	0	2	0.07	0.31	2.9	0.07	15	0	4	73
630	Mustard greens-boiled-drained	cup	140	21	3	3	2.7	tr	tr	0	22	283	21	1	0.2	424	35	0.06	0.09	0.6	0	103	0	103	58
1576	Natto-fermented soybeans	cup	280	468	47	32	9.7	21	4.5	0	20	697	322	10.4	8.5	0	0	0.07	0.5	1.1	0.36	22	0	103	182
1076	Nuts-chestnuts-chinese-dried	oz	28.4	103	2	23	2.2	1	0.1	0	2	206	39	0.7	0.4	9	17	0.07	0.08	0.4	0.19	31	0	8	44

Code	Food	Measure	Wt (g)	Cal	Prot	Carb	Fiber	Fat	Chol	Sod	Cal	Iron	A	C	Thia	Ribo	Niac	B6	Fol	B12?	Potas	Magn
1075	Nuts-chestnuts-chinese-raw	oz	28.4	64	1	14	2.2	tr	0	1	24	0.2	6	10	0.05	0.05	0.2	0.12	19	0	5	27
1086	Nuts-chestnuts-roasted	oz	28.4	68	1	15	2.2	tr	0	1	26	0.3	tr	11	0.04	0.03	0.4	0.12	21	0	5	29
631	Okra-raw-boiled-drained	cup	160	51	3	12	2	0.1	0	8	91	0.9	92	26	0.21	0.09	1.4	0.3	73	0	101	90
1015	Onion rings-frozen-prepared-heated	item	10	41	1	4	0.4	0.9	3	38	2	0.2	2	tr	0.03	0.01	0.4	0.01	1	0	3	8
634	Onions-mature-boiled-drained	cup	210	92	3	21	1.7	0.1	0	6	23	0.5	0	11	0.03	0.05	0.3	0.27	32	0	46	74
632	Onions-mature-raw-chopped	cup	160	61	2	14	2.6	tr	0	5	16	0.4	0	10	0.07	0.03	0.2	0.19	30	0	32	53
635	Onions-young green	item	5	1	tr	tr	0.1	tr	0	tr	1	0.1	25	2	tr	0.01	tr	tr	1	0	3	2
636	Parsley-raw-chopped	tbsp	4	1	tr	tr	0.2	tr	0	tr	2	0.2	21	4	tr	tr	0.1	tr	7	0	5	2
637	Parsnips-sliced-boiled-drained	cup	156	126	2	31	7.6	0.1	0	16	46	0.9	0	20	0.13	0.08	1.1	0.15	91	0	58	108
516	Peas-blackeye/cowpeas-boiled-drained	cup	165	179	13	30	15.8	1	0	6	83	2.4	105	3	0.11	0.18	1.8	0.08	173	0	46	197
586	Peas-blackeye/cowpeas-frozen-boiled	cup	170	224	14	40	9.8	1	0	9	85	3.6	13	5	0.44	0.11	1.2	0.16	240	0	40	208
585	Peas-blackeye/cowpeas-raw-boiled	cup	165	160	5	34	11	1	0	7	86	1.9	130	4	0.17	0.24	2.3	0.11	210	0	211	84
639	Peas-edible podded-raw	cup	145	61	4	11	3.8	tr	0	6	35	3	20	87	0.22	0.12	0.9	0.23	61	0	62	77
1517	Peas-green-canned-dietary-low sodium	cup	170	117	8	21	5.8	0.1	0	3	29	1.6	131	16	0.21	0.13	1.2	0.11	75	0	34	114
638	Peas-green-canned-drained	cup	170	117	8	21	5.8	0.1	0	372	29	1.6	131	16	0.21	0.13	1.2	0.11	75	0	34	114
640	Peas-green-frozen-boiled-drained	cup	160	125	8	23	6.1	0.1	0	139	46	2.5	107	16	0.45	0.16	2.4	0.18	94	0	38	144
525	Peas-split-dry-cooked	cup	200	230	16	42	10.5	0.1	0	8	72	3.4	8	1	0.3	0.18	1.8	0.1	129	0	22	178
39	Peas-sweet-canned in water-dietetic	oz	28.4	12	1	2	0.6	0	0	1	5	0.2	16	3	0.02	0.02	0.2	*	*	0	6	17
1486	Peppers-hot chili-canned	cup	136	34	1	8	2.1	tr	0	1595	19	0.7	83	92	0.03	0.07	1.1	0.21	14	0	10	24
1487	Peppers-hot chili-raw	cup	150	60	3	14	3.6	0.1	0	10	38	1.8	116	364	0.14	0.14	1.4	0.42	35	0	26	68
641	Peppers-hot-red-dried	tsp	2	5	0	1	0.7	tr	0	20	3	0.3	130	0	0	0.02	0.2	tr	tr	0	5	4
1020	Peppers-jalapeno-canned-chopped	item	136	33	1	1	2	0.1	0	1990	16	3.8	231	18	0.04	0.07	0.7	0.28	18	0	35	23
643	Peppers-sweet-boiled-drained	item	73	20	1	5	0.7	tr	0	1	7	0.3	43	54	0.02	0.02	0.3	0.17	11	0	7	13
642	Peppers-sweet-raw	item	74	20	1	5	1.2	tr	0	1	7	0.3	47	66	0.05	0.02	0.4	0.18	16	0	7	14
1506	Pimientos-4 ounce can or jar	item	113	31	1	7	2.6	0.1	0	35	6	1.7	260	107	0.02	0.07	0.5	0.19	14	0	8	19
1021	Poi-taro root product	cup	240	269	1	65	4.8	0.1	0	28	58	2.1	5	10	0.31	0.1	2.6	0.66	51	0	37	94
653	Potato chips-salt added	item	2	11	tr	1	tr	0.2	0	1	tr	tr	0	1	0	0	0.1	0.01	1	0	1	3
1030	Potato pancakes-home recipe	item	76	495	5	26	1.4	3.4	93	388	24	1.2	9	tr	0.1	0.1	1.6	0.29	22	0.22	21	78
1031	Potato puffs-frozen-heated	item	7	16	tr	2	0.2	0.4	1	52	1	0.1	tr	1	0.01	0.01	0.2	0.02	1	0	2	3
1022	Potato skin-baked	item	58	115	2	27	3	tr	0	12	25	4.1	0	8	0.07	0.06	1.8	0.36	13	0	20	59
1023	Potato-au gratin-home recipe	cup	245	323	12	28	4.4	19	56	1061	49	1.6	93	24	0.16	0.28	2.4	0.43	20	0.49	292	277
1024	Potato-au gratin-prepared from mix	oz	28.4	26	1	4	0.5	1	*	125	4	0.1	9	1	0.01	0.02	0.3	0.01	2	0	24	27
1078	Potato-baked-flesh & skin-whole	item	202	220	5	51	4.9	tr	0	16	55	2.8	0	26	0.22	0.07	3.3	0.7	22	0	20	115
644	Potato-baked-peeled after baking	item	156	145	3	34	3.7	tr	0	8	39	0.6	0	20	0.16	0.03	2.2	0.47	14	0	8	78
645	Potato-boiled-peeled after boiling	item	136	118	3	27	2	tr	0	5	30	0.4	0	18	0.14	0.03	2	0.41	14	0	7	60
646	Potato-boiled-peeled before boiling	item	135	116	2	27	1.5	tr	0	7	26	0.4	0	10	0.13	0.03	1.8	0.36	12	0	10	54
1077	Potato-canned-drained	item	35	21	tr	5	0.9	tr	0	91	5	0.4	0	2	0.02	0.01	0.3	0.07	2	0	2	10
648	Potato-french fried-prepared from frozen	item	5	11	tr	2	0.2	0.2	0	1	1	0.1	0	1	0.01	tr	0.1	0.01	1	0	tr	4
647	Potato-french fried-prepared from raw	item	5	14	tr	2	0.2	0.2	0	11	1	0.1	0	1	0.01	tr	0.2	0.01	tr	0	1	6
1025	Potato-hash brown-prepared from raw	cup	156	239	4	12	3.1	8.5	0	37	31	1.3	0	9	0.12	0.03	3.1	0.43	12	0	13	66
649	Potato-hashed brown-prepared from frozen	cup	156	340	5	44	1.5	7	0	54	26	2.3	0	10	0.17	0.03	3.8	0.2	39	0	24	112
1734	Potato-hush puppies	serv	78	256	5	35	1.9	2.7	135	965	16	1.4	9	0	0	0.02	2	0.1	21	0.18	69	190
652	Potato-mashed-from dehydrated-with milk	cup	210	166	4	28	1.2	1.4	4	491	34	1.3	19	6	0.06	0.11	1.7	0.42	15	0.11	65	92
650	Potato-mashed-from raw-with milk	cup	210	162	4	37	1.2	0.7	0	636	39	0.6	4	14	0.19	0.08	2.4	0.49	17	0.11	55	100
651	Potato-mashed-home recipe-milk/butter	cup	210	223	4	35	3.2	2.2	4	620	38	0.5	42	13	0.18	0.08	2.3	0.47	17	0	55	97
1026	Potato-o'brien-home recipe	cup	194	157	5	30	*	1.6	7	421	35	0.9	93	32	0.11	0.11	2	0.41	16	0.16	70	97
1027	Potato-scalloped-home recipe	cup	245	211	7	26	4.4	5.5	29	821	47	1.4	47	26	0.17	0.23	2.6	0.44	21	0	140	154
1028	Potato-scalloped-prepared from mix	oz	28.4	26	1	4	0.5	0.7	*	97	4	0.1	6	1	0.01	0.02	0.3	0.01	tr	0	10	16
1032	Pumpkin pie mix-canned	cup	270	281	3	71	*	0.2	0	562	43	2.9	2241	9	0.04	0.32	1	0.43	95	0	100	122
1595	Pumpkin-boiled-drained-mashed	cup	245	49	2	12	6.7	0.1	0	3	22	1.4	265	12	0.08	0.19	0.6	0.11	21	0	37	74
655	Pumpkin-canned	cup	245	83	3	20	5	0.4	0	12	56	3.4	5404	10	0.06	0.13	0.9	0.14	30	0	64	86

* indicates that no data was available.
©1994 First DataBank—The Hearst Corporation (N-Squared Computing).

Appendix A - Table of Food Composition
(continued)

Item	Food name	Portion	Weight (g)	Food Energy (Kcal)	Protein (gm)	Carbohydrates (gm)	Fiber (gm)	Total Fat (gm)	Saturated Fat (gm)	Cholesterol (mg)	Sodium (mg)	Potassium (mg)	Magnesium (mg)	Iron (mg)	Zinc (mg)	Vitamin A (RE)	Vitamin C (mg)	Thiamin (mg)	Riboflavin (mg)	Niacin (mg)	Vitamin B6 (mg)	Folates (µg)	Vitamin B12 (µg)	Calcium (mg)	Phosphorus (mg)
1528	Pumpkin-raw-cubed	cup	116	30	1	8	2	tr	0.1	0	1	1	14	0.9	0.4	186	10	0.06	0.13	0.7	0.06	16	0	24	51
1482	Radish-daikon-sliced-boiled-drained	cup	147	25	1	5	2.9	tr	0.1	0	19	419	13	0.2	0.2	0	22	0	0.03	0.2	0.06	26	0	25	35
656	Radishes-raw	item	4.5	1	tr	tr	0.1	tr	tr	0	1	10	1	tr	tr	0	1	tr	tr	tr	tr	1	0	1	1
1033	Rutabagas-boiled-drained	cup	170	58	2	13	2.5	tr	tr	0	31	488	36	0.8	0.5	0	37	0.12	0.06	1.1	0.15	26	0	71	83
657	Sauerkraut-canned	cup	236	45	2	10	6.1	tr	0.1	0	1560	401	31	3.5	0.4	5	35	0.05	0.06	0.3	0.31	56	0	71	47
1034	Seaweed-agar-dried	serv	28.4	87	2	23	0.9	tr	tr	0	29	320	219	6.1	1.7	0	0	tr	0.06	0.1	0.09	165	0	178	15
1035	Seaweed-irishmoss-raw	oz	28.4	14	5	3	1	tr	tr	0	19	18	41	2.5	0.6	3	3	tr	0.13	0.2	0.02	52	0	20	45
1036	Seaweed-kelp (kombu)-raw	oz	28.4	12	tr	3	1.2	tr	0.1	0	66	25	34	0.8	0.3	3	1	0.01	0.04	0.1	tr	51	0	48	12
1037	Seaweed-laver (nori)-raw	oz	28.4	10	2	1	1	tr	tr	0	14	101	1	0.5	0.3	148	11	0.03	0.13	0.4	0.05	42	0	20	17
1038	Seaweed-spirulina-dried	oz	28.4	82	16	7	1.4	2	0.8	0	298	387	55	8.1	0.6	16	3	0.68	1.04	3.6	0.1	27	0	34	34
1039	Seaweed-wakame-raw	oz	28.4	13	1	3	1.2	tr	tr	0	248	14	30	0.6	0.1	10	1	0.02	0.07	0.5	0.02	56	0	43	23
1041	Shallots-freeze dried	tbsp	0.9	7	tr	2	0.1	tr	tr	0	1	15	2	0.1	tr	51	1	0.01	tr	tr	0.04	1	0	2	3
1040	Shallots-raw	tbsp	10	7	tr	2	*	tr	tr	0	4	33	2	0.1	tr	125	0	0.01	0.04	tr	*	3	0	4	6
1493	Soybeans-dry-cooked	cup	180	234	20	19	*	10	*	0	4	972	*	4.9	*	5	0	0.38	0.16	1.1	0.11	*	0	131	322
1042	Soybeans-green-boiled-drained	cup	180	254	22	20	*	12	1.3	0	25	970	108	4.5	1.6	29	31	0.47	0.28	2.3	0.19	201	0	261	284
1043	Soybeans-sprouted-steamed	cup	94	76	8	6	1	5	0.5	0	25	334	56	1.2	1	0	32	0.19	0.05	1	0.21	75	0	56	127
1521	Spinach-canned-dietary pack-low sodium	cup	234	45	5	7	5.1	1	0.1	0	746	538	131	3.7	1	1505	32	0.04	0.25	0.6	0.19	136	0	194	75
662	Spinach-canned-drained	cup	214	50	6	7	6.8	1	0.2	0	57	740	162	4.9	1	1878	31	0.03	0.3	0.8	0.3	209	0	271	94
1520	Spinach-canned-solids and liquids	cup	234	45	5	7	5.1	1	0.1	0	746	538	131	3.7	1	1505	32	0.04	0.25	0.6	0.28	136	0	194	75
660	Spinach-frozen-boiled-chopped	cup	205	57	6	11	4.5	1	0.1	0	176	611	141	3.1	1.4	1596	25	0.12	0.34	0.9	0.44	220	0	299	98
661	Spinach-leaf-frozen-boiled-drained	cup	190	53	6	10	4	tr	0.1	0	164	566	131	2.9	1.3	1479	23	0.11	0.32	0.8	0.11	204	0	277	91
659	Spinach-raw-boiled-drained	cup	180	41	5	7	4	tr	tr	0	126	839	157	6.4	1.4	1474	16	0.17	0.43	0.9	0.4	262	0	245	101
658	Spinach-raw-chopped	cup	56	12	2	2	1.5	tr	tr	0	44	312	44	1.5	0.3	376	22	0.04	0.11	0.4	0.25	108	0	55	27
1485	Squash-acorn-baked	cup	205	115	2	30	4.3	tr	0.1	0	9	896	87	1.9	0.4	88	31	0.34	0.03	1.8	0.24	38	0	90	93
1484	Squash-butternut-baked	cup	205	82	2	22	3.5	tr	tr	0	8	582	60	1.2	0.3	1435	31	0.15	0.04	2	0.12	39	0	84	55
1483	Squash-hubbard-boiled-mashed	cup	236	71	3	15	4.2	1	0.2	0	12	505	32	0.7	0.2	946	15	0.1	0.07	0.8	0.15	23	0	24	33
663	Squash-summer-boiled-sliced	cup	180	36	2	8	2.5	1	0.1	0	2	346	44	0.6	0.7	52	10	0.08	0.07	0.9	0.35	36	0	48	69
664	Squash-winter-bake-mashed	cup	205	80	3	18	5.7	1	0.3	0	2	896	16	0.7	0.5	730	20	0.17	0.05	1.4	0.14	57	0	29	41
1047	Squash-zucchini-frozen-boiled	cup	223	38	3	8	3.2	tr	0.1	0	4	433	29	1.1	0.4	96	5	0.09	0.09	0.9	0.12	17	0	38	56
1048	Squash-zucchini-italia-canned	cup	227	66	2	16	7	tr	0.1	0	850	622	31	1.5	0.6	123	5	0.1	0.09	1.2	0.22	69	0	39	66
1046	Squash-zucchini-raw-boiled	cup	180	29	1	7	2.3	tr	tr	0	5	455	40	0.6	0.3	43	8	0.07	0.07	0.8	0.14	30	0	23	72
1045	Squash-zucchini-raw-sliced	cup	130	18	2	4	2	tr	tr	0	4	322	29	0.5	0.3	44	12	0.09	0.04	0.5	0.12	29	0	20	42
1049	Succotash-boiled-drained	cup	192	221	10	47	14	tr	0.3	0	33	787	102	2.9	1.2	56	16	0.32	0.18	2.6	0.22	63	0	33	225
665	Sweet potato-baked-peeled	item	114	117	2	28	3.4	tr	0.1	0	11	397	23	0.5	0.3	2487	28	0.08	0.15	0.7	0.28	26	0	32	63
666	Sweet potato-boiled-mashed	cup	328	344	5	80	9.8	1	0.2	0	42	602	32	1.8	0.9	5594	56	0.17	0.46	2.1	0.8	36	0	70	88
667	Sweet potato-candied	piece	105	144	1	29	1.1	3	1.4	0	73	198	12	1.2	0.2	440	7	0.02	0.04	0.4	0.04	12	0	27	27
668	Sweet potato-canned-mashed	cup	255	258	5	59	4.6	1	0.1	0	191	536	61	3.4	0.5	3857	13	0.07	0.23	2.4	0.17	27	0	76	133
669	Sweet potato-canned-vacuum pack	cup	200	182	3	42	4.8	tr	0.1	0	106	624	44	1.8	0.4	1596	53	0.07	0.11	1.5	0.38	33	0	44	98
1051	Taro root-cooked-sliced	cup	132	187	1	46	6	tr	tr	0	20	638	40	1	0.4	0	7	0.14	0.04	0.7	0.44	25	0	24	100
1050	Taro root-raw-sliced	cup	104	111	2	28	*	tr	tr	0	11	615	34	0.6	0.2	0	5	0.1	0.03	0.6	0.29	23	0	45	87
1634	Tempeh-soybean product	cup	166	330	32	28	*	13	1.8	0	10	609	116	3.8	3	114	0	0.22	0.18	7.7	0.5	86	1.66	154	342
1639	Tofu-fried	piece	13	35	2	1	0.2	3	0.4	0	2	19	8	0.6	0.3	0	0	0.02	0.01	tr	0.03	3	0	48	37
1640	Tofu-okara	cup	122	94	4	15	5	2	0.2	0	11	259	32	1.6	0.7	0	0	0.02	0.02	0.1	0.01	32	0	98	73
1638	Tofu-raw-firm	cup	252	365	40	11	3	22	3.2	0	35	597	237	26.4	4	43	1	0.4	0.26	1	0.14	74	0	517	479
1494	Tofu-soybean curd	piece	120	86	9	3	1.4	5	2.6	0	8	50	115	2.3	1	0	0	0.07	0.04	0.1	0.06	21	0.03	154	151
674	Tomato juice-canned	cup	244	42	2	10	2.9	tr	tr	0	881	537	27	1.4	0.3	137	45	0.11	0.08	1.6	0.27	49	0	22	46
75	Tomato juice-low sodium	cup	244	42	2	10	2.8	tr	tr	0	24	537	27	1.4	0.3	137	45	0.11	0.08	1.6	0.27	49	0	22	46
1057	Tomato paste-canned-low sodium	cup	262	220	10	49	11.3	2	0.3	0	172	2442	134	7.8	2.1	647	111	0.41	0.5	8.4	1	59	0	92	207
1522	Tomato paste-canned-salt added	cup	262	220	10	49	11.3	2	0.3	0	2070	2442	134	7.8	2.1	647	111	0.41	0.5	8.4	1	59	0	92	207
675	Tomato powder	oz	28.4	86	4	21	0.7	tr	tr	0	38	547	51	1.3	0.5	490	33	0.26	0.22	2.6	0.13	34	0	47	84
1058	Tomato puree-canned-low sodium	cup	250	103	4	25	5.8	tr	tr	0	50	1050	60	2.3	0.6	340	88	0.18	0.14	4.3	0.38	28	0	38	100

Code	Food	Measure																							
1523	Tomato puree-canned-salt added	cup	250	103	4	25	5.8	tr	tr	0	998	1050	60	2.3	0.6	340	88	0.18	0.14	4.3	0.38	28	0	38	100
1518	Tomato-canned-dietary pack-low sodium	cup	240	48	2	10	1.7	1	0.1	0	31	530	29	1.5	0.4	144	36	0.11	0.07	1.8	0.22	19	0	62	46
1053	Tomato-cooked-stewed-home recipe	cup	101	80	2	13	1	3	0.5	0	460	249	15	1.1	0.2	68	18	0.11	0.08	1.1	0.09	11	0	26	38
1054	Tomato-red-canned-stewed	cup	255	66	2	17	2	tr	0.1	0	648	609	31	1.9	0.4	140	34	0.12	0.09	1.8	0.04	14	0	84	51
671	Tomato-red-canned-whole	cup	240	48	2	10	1.9	1	0.1	0	391	530	29	1.5	0.4	144	36	0.11	0.07	1.8	0.22	19	0	62	46
1055	Tomato-red-canned-with green chilies	cup	241	36	2	9	0.9	tr	tr	0	966	258	27	0.6	0.3	94	15	0.08	0.05	1.5	0.25	22	0	48	34
1052	Tomato-red-raw-boiled	cup	240	65	3	14	2.1	1	0.1	0	26	670	34	1.3	0.3	178	55	0.17	0.14	1.8	0.23	31	0	14	74
670	Tomato-red-ripe-raw	item	123	26	1	6	1.6	tr	0.1	0	11	273	14	0.6	0.1	76	24	0.07	0.06	0.8	0.1	19	0	6	30
1386	Tomatoes-green-raw	item	123	30	1	6	0.6	tr	tr	0	16	251	12	0.6	0.1	79	29	0.07	0.05	0.6	0.1	11	0	16	34
678	Turnip greens-frozen-boiled	cup	164	49	5	8	5.1	1	0.2	0	25	367	43	3.2	0.7	1309	36	0.09	0.12	0.8	0.11	65	0	249	56
677	Turnip greens-raw-boiled	cup	144	29	2	6	4.5	tr	0.1	0	42	292	32	1.2	0.2	792	40	0.07	0.1	0.6	0.26	171	0	197	42
676	Turnips-boiled-drained-diced	cup	156	28	1	8	3.1	tr	tr	0	78	211	13	0.3	0.3	0	18	0.04	0.04	0.5	0.11	14	0	34	30
1065	Vegetable juice-canned	cup	242	46	2	11	2.7	tr	tr	0	883	467	27	1	0.5	283	67	0.1	0.07	1.8	0.34	51	0	27	41
118	Vegetable juice-Snap e Tom-tomato	cup	243	46	2	9	1.9	0	0	0	1298	688	27	1.9	0.5	103	10	0.1	0.07	2.4	0.34	51	0	37	41
15	Vegetable juice-V-8 cocktail-low sodium	cup	243	51	0	10	2.7	0	0	0	58	571	*	1.5	*	437	53	0.05	0.07	1.9	*	*	0	39	*
1323	Vegetable juice-V-8-regular	cup	243	49	0	10	2.4	0	0	0	819	513	27	1.5	0.5	342	49	0.05	0.05	1.7	0.34	51	0	29	41
1068	Waterchestnuts-chinese-canned	cup	140	70	1	17	*	tr	tr	0	12	164	6	1.2	0.5	1	2	0.02	0.03	0.5	0.22	8	0	6	28
1067	Waterchestnuts-chinese-raw	cup	124	131	2	30	*	tr	tr	0	17	724	27	0.1	0.6	0	5	0.17	0.25	1.2	0.41	20	0	14	78
1069	Watercress-raw	cup	34	4	1	tr	0.4	tr	tr	0	14	112	8	0.1	tr	160	15	0.03	0.04	0.1	0.04	3	0	40	20
1012	Yam-mountain-Hawaii-steamed	cup	145	119	3	29	5.6	tr	tr	0	18	717	15	0.6	0.5	0	17	0.13	0.02	0.2	0.3	18	0	11	57
1070	Yams-boiled or baked-drained	cup	136	158	2	38	3.3	tr	tr	0	11	911	25	0.7	0.3	0	17	0.13	0.04	0.8	0.31	22	0	19	66

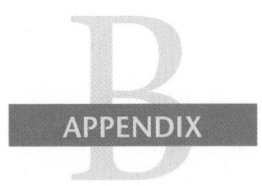

Nutrition Information–Reliable Resources

Turn to a Further Reading section of any chapter in this book. Notice that information on nutrition comes from a wide range of journals and books. This Appendix groups the major sources of nutrition information to assist you in further reading in your university or college library. It also provides addresses of newsletters, professional organizations, government and international agencies, and local sources of nutrition information.

The following are sources of reliable information on nutrition and on food and the environment as they relate to nutrition.

Scientific and Medical Journals

Journals with one or more articles on nutrition in each issue

American Journal of Clinical Nutrition
Annual Review of Nutrition
Appetite
British Food Journal
British Journal of Nutrition
Ecology of Food and Nutrition
FDA Consumer
Human Nutrition: Applied Nutrition
Human Nutrition: Clinical Nutrition
Journal of the American Dietetic Association
Journal of the Canadian Dietetic Association

Journal of Nutrition
Journal of Nutrition Education
Journal of Nutrition for the Elderly
Journal of Nutritional Biochemistry
Nutrition
Nutrition Research Reviews
Nutrition Reviews
Nutrition Today
Proceedings of the Nutrition Society
World Review of Nutrition and Dietetics

Journals with periodic coverage of nutrition issues

American Journal of Epidemiology
American Journal of Medicine
American Journal of Nursing
American Journal of Physiology
American Journal of Psychiatry
American Journal of Public Health
American Scientist
Annals of Internal Medicine
Annual Review of Medicine
Archives of Disease in Childhood
British Medical Journal
Cancer
Cancer Research
Circulation
Diabetes
Food Chemical Toxicology
Food Technology
Gastroenterology
Geriatrics

Gut
Journal of the American Geriatric Society
Journal of the American Medical Association
Journal of Applied Physiology
Journal of the National Cancer Institute
Journal of Pediatrics
Lancet
Mayo Clinic Proceedings
Medicine and Science in Sports and Exercise
Nature
New England Journal of Medicine
New Scientist
Pediatrics
Physician and Sportsmedicine
Postgraduate Medicine
Proceedings of the Society for Experimental Biology and Medicine
Science
Scientific American

Newsletters

The following newsletters cover nutrition issues on a regular basis (* = free, ** = inexpensive).

CNI Nutrition Week
Community Nutrition Institute
2001 S. St. NW
Washington, DC 20009

** *Dairy Council Digest*
National Dairy Council
6300 River Rd.
Rosemont, IL 60018

Dietetic Currents
Ross Laboratories
Director of Professional Services
625 Cleveland Ave.
Columbus, OH 43216

Environmental Nutrition
2112 Broadway
New York, NY 10023

FDA Consumer
Superintendent of Documents
Government Printing Office
Washington, DC 20402

Food and Nutrition News
National Livestock and Meat Board
444 Michigan Ave.
Chicago, IL 60610

Harvard Medical School Health Letter
Department of Continuing Education
25 Shattuck St.
Boston, MA 02115

Healthline
830 Menlo Ave. #100
Menlo Park, CA 94025

National Council Against Health Fraud Newsletter
NCAHF
P.O. Box 1276
Loma Linda, CA 92354

Nutrition & the M.D.
P.O. Box 2160
Van Nuys, CA 91404

Nutrition Forum
George Stickley Co.
210 Washington Square
Philadelphia, PA 19106

Sports Science Exchange
Gatorade Sports Science Institute
P.O. Box 049005
Chicago, IL 60604-9005

Tufts University Diet & Nutrition Letter
P.O. Box 57857
Boulder, CO 80322-7857

Professional and Lay Organizations Dealing with Nutrition Issues

American Academy of Pediatrics
P.O. Box 1034
Evanston, IL 60204

American Cancer Society
1599 Clifton Rd.
Atlanta, GA 30329

American Council on Science and
Health
1995 Broadway
New York, NY 10023

American Dental Association
211 East Chicago Ave.
Chicago, IL 60611

American Diabetes Association
Diabetes Information Service Center
1660 Duke St.
Alexandria, VA 22314

American Dietetic Association
216 W. Jackson Blvd.
Suite 800
Chicago, IL 60606-6995

American Geriatric Society
770 Lexington Ave., Suite 400
New York, NY 10021

American Heart Association
7320 Greenville Ave.
Dallas, TX 75231

American Institute of Nutrition
9650 Rockville Pike
Bethesda, MD 20014

American Medical Association
Nutrition Information Section
535 N. Dearborn St.
Chicago, IL 60610

American Public Health Association
1015 Fifteenth St. N.W.
Washington, DC 20005

Canadian Diabetes Association
123 Edward St., Suite 601
Toronto, Ontario M5G 1E2, Canada

Canadian Dietetic Association
480 University Avenue
Toronto, Ontario M5G 1V2, Canada

Canadian Society for Nutritional
Science
Department of Foods and Nutrition
University of Manitoba
Winnipeg, Manitoba, R3T 2N2
Canada

Food and Nutrition Board
Institute of Medicine
National Academy of Sciences
2101 Constitution Ave. NW
Washington, DC 20418

Institute of Food Technologists
221 N. LaSalle St.
Chicago, IL 60601

National Council on Aging
1828 L St., NW
Washington, DC 20036

National Institute of Nutrition
1335 Carling Ave., Suite 210
Ottawa, Ontario, K1Z 0L2 Canada

Nutrition Foundation, Inc.
1126 Sixteenth St. NW, Suite 111
Washington, DC 20036

Nutrition Today Society
428 Preston St.
Baltimore, MD 21202

Society for Nutrition Education
1736 Franklin St.
Oakland, CA 94612

Government and International Agencies Dealing with Nutrition

United States

Agricultural Research Service
USDA
3700 East West Highway
Hyattsville, MD 20782

Consumer Information Center
Department 609K
Pueblo, CO 81009

Department of Agriculture (USDA)
Extension Services
3 South Building, Room 6007
Washington, DC 20250

Food and Drug Administration (FDA)
5600 Fishers Lane
Rockville, MD 20852

Food and Nutrition Information
National Agricultural Library
10301 Baltimore Blvd.
Beltsville, MD 20705

Health Nutrition Information Service
Federal Center Building
Hyattsville, MD 20782

Office of Cancer Communications
National Cancer Institute
Bldg. 31, Room 10A29
9000 Rockville Pike
Bethesda, MD 20892

Canada

Department of Community Health
1075 Ste-Foy Road, Seventh Floor
Quebec, Quebec G1S 2M1

Health and Welfare Canada
Canadian Government Publishing
Center
Minister of Supply and Services
Ottawa, Ontario K1A 0S9

Nutrition Services
P.O. Box 6000
Fredericton, New Brunswick E3B 5H1

Nutrition Services
P.O. Box 488
Halifax, Nova Scotia B3J 2R8

Public Health Resource Service
15 Overlea Blvd., Fifth Floor
Toronto, Ontario M4H 1A9

United Nations

Food and Agricultural Organization
(FAO)
North American Regional Office
1325 C St., SW
Washington, DC 20025
or
Viale delle Terme di Caracalla
00100 Rome, Italy

World Health Organization (WHO)
1211 Geneva 27, Switzerland

Local Resources

Cooperative extension agents. Contact county extension offices.
Dietitians. Contact your local or state dietetics association for information.
Nutrition faculty. Contact departments of nutrition, foods and nutrition, food science, or home economics
for a list of faculty expertise.
Dietitians associated with local hospitals, utilities, food processing companies, and city, county, and state
agencies.

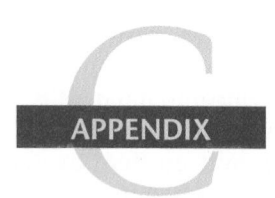

APPENDIX

Nutrition/Environment Interface– Additional Readings

Some of the suggested readings listed on this page can be purchased in your local bookstore, some as paperbacks. Your university or college library should have these books, or they can obtain them by inter-library loan.

General

The following books give useful information on issues such as the effects of environmental contamination on nutrition status, environmental factors in food production, new uses for crops that do not harm the environment, global warming and food production, and the effect of food packaging on the environment. All of these issues impact, either directly or indirectly, the availability and utilization of nutrients.

Publications of Governments and International Organizations

National Academy of Sciences. *One Earth, One Future–Our Changing Global Environment.* National Academy Press, Washington, DC, 1990.

U.S. Department of Agriculture. *Agriculture and the Environment, The 1991 Yearbook of Agriculture.* Superintendent of Documents, U.S. Government Printing Office, Washington, DC, 1991.

U.S. Department of Agriculture. *New Crops, New Uses, New Markets, The 1992 Yearbook of Agriculture.* Superintendent of Documents, U.S. Government Printing Office, Washington, DC, 1992.

British Medical Association. *The BMA Guide to Pesticides, Chemicals, and Health.* Edward Arnold, London, 1992.

World Health Organization. *Our Planet, Our Health.* Report of the WHO Commission on Health and Environment, World Health Organization, Geneva, Switzerland, 1992.

World Health Organization. *Safe Use of Pesticides.* Fourteenth Report of the WHO Expert Committee on Vector Biology and Control. World Health Organization, Geneva, Switzerland, 1991.

World Health Organization. *WHO Commission on Health and Environment, Report of the Panel on Food and Agriculture.* World Health Organization, Geneva, Switzerland, 1992.

Books

Carson, P., and Moulden, J. *Green is Gold. Business Talking to Business About the Environmental Revolution.* Harper Business, Toronto, 1991.

Gaull, G. E., and Goldberg, R. A., eds. *New Technologies and the Future of Food and Nutrition.* John Wiley & Sons, Inc., New York, 1991.

Gordon, A., and Suzuki, D. *It's a Matter of Survival.* Harper Collins, London, 1991.

Kennedy, P. *Preparing for the Twenty-First Century.* Vintage Books, New York, 1993.

Rathje, W., and Murphy, C. *Rubbish. The Archaeology of Garbage.* Harper Perennial, New York, 1992.

Rodricks, J. V. *Calculated Risks. The Toxicity and Human Health Risks of Chemicals in Our Environment.* Cambridge University Press, Cambridge, England, 1994.

Stilwell, E. J., and others. *Packaging for the Environment.* Amacom, New York, 1991.

Environmental Issues

Some of the following books take a critical look at whether there is an environmental problem; others claim not enough attention is given to environmental issues; others question whether food production will be adversely affected by deterioration in environmental quality; and some are critical of current agricultural practices and their impact on the environment. This sampling of books demonstrates the many environmental issues influencing food production and nutrient availability. It demonstrates also the wisdom in reading widely on this subject because of the many differing opinions and solutions to the problems.

References

Bailey, R. *Ecoscam. The False Prophets of Ecological Apocalypse*. St. Martin's Press, New York, 1993.

Ray, D. L. *Environmental Overkill*. Harper Perennial, New York, 1993.

Durning, A. T. *How Much is Enough?* W.W. Norton & Company, New York, 1992.

Ray, D. L. *Trashing the Planet*. Harper Perennial, New York, 1990.

Lacey, R. *Unfit for Human Consumption*. Grafton, London, 1992.

Caldicott, H. *If You Love This Planet*. W.W. Norton & Company, New York, 1992.

Brown, L. R. ed. *The World-Watch Reader on Global Environmental Issues*. W.W. Norton & Company, New York, 1991.

Fox, M. W. *Agricide*. Schocken Books, New York, 1986.

Meadows, D. H., Meadows, D. L., and Randers, J. *Beyond the Limits*. Chelsea Green Publishing Company, Post Mills, Vermont, 1992.

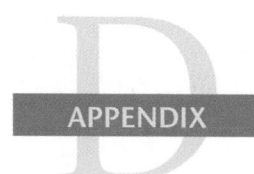

Exchange Lists for Meal Planning

The reason for dividing food into six different groups is that foods vary in their carbohydrate, protein, fat, and calorie content. Each exchange list contains foods that are alike–each choice contains about the same amount of carbohydrate, protein, fat, and calories.

The following chart shows the amount of these nutrients in one serving from each exchange list.

Exchange List	Carbohydrate (grams)	Protein (grams)	Fat (grams)	Calories
Starch/bread	15	3	trace	80
Meat				
Lean	...	7	3	55
Medium-fat	...	7	5	75
High-fat	...	7	8	100
Vegetable	5	2	...	25
Fruit	15	...	...	60
Milk				
Skim	12	8	trace	90
Lowfat	12	8	5	120
Whole	12	8	8	150
Fat	...	...	5	45

As you read the exchange lists, you will notice that one choice often is a larger amount of food than another choice from the same list. Because foods are so different, each food is measured or weighed so the amount of carbohydrate, protein, fat, and calories is the same in each choice.

You will notice symbols on some foods in the exchange groups. Foods that are high in fiber (3 grams or more per exchange) have a green ■ symbol. High-fiber foods are good for you. It is important to eat more of these foods.

Foods that are high in sodium (400 milligrams or more of sodium per exchange) have a red ● symbol; foods that have 400 mg or more of sodium if two or more exchanges are eaten have a blue ◆ symbol. It's a good idea to limit your intake of high-salt foods, especially if you have high blood pressure.

If you have a favorite food that is not included in any of these groups, ask your dietitian about it. That food can probably be worked into your meal plan, at least now and then.

Starch/Bread List

Each item in this list contains approximately 15 grams of carbohydrate, 3 grams of protein, a trace of fat, and 80 calories. Whole grain products average about 2 grams of fiber per exchange. Some foods are higher in fiber. Those foods that contain 3 or more grams of fiber per exchange are identified with the fiber symbol ■.

You can choose your starch exchanges from any of the items on this list. If you want to eat a starch food that is not on this list, the general rule is that:
- 1/2 cup of cereal, grain, or pasta is one exchange
- 1 ounce of a bread product is one exchange

Your dietitian can help you be more exact.

Cereals/Grains/Pasta

■ Bran cereals, concentrated (such as Bran Buds®, All Bran®)	1/3 cup
■ Bran cereals, flaked	1/2 cup
Bulgur (cooked)	1/2 cup
Cooked cereals	1/2 cup
Cornmeal (dry)	2 1/2 Tbsp.
Grape-Nuts®	3 Tbsp.
Grits (cooked)	1/2 cup
Other ready-to-eat unsweetened cereals	3/4 cup
Pasta (cooked)	1/2 cup
Puffed cereal	1 1/2 cup
Rice, white or brown (cooked)	1/3 cup
Shredded wheat	1/2 cup
■ Wheat germ	3 Tbsp.

Dried Beans/Peas/Lentils

■ Beans and peas (cooked) (such as kidney, white, split, blackeye)	1/3 cup
■ Lentils (cooked)	1/3 cup
■ Baked beans	1/4 cup

Starchy Vegetables

■ Corn	1/2 cup
■ Corn on cob, 6 in. long	1
■ Lima beans	1/2 cup
■ Peas, green (canned or frozen)	1/2 cup
■ Plantain	1/2 cup
Potato, baked	1 small (3 oz.)
Potato, mashed	1/2 cup
■ Squash, winter (acorn, butternut)	1 cup
Yam, sweet potato, plain	1/3 cup

Bread

Bagel	1/2 (1 oz.)
Bread sticks, crisp, 4 in. long x 1/2 in.	2 (2/3 oz.)
Croutons, lowfat	1 cup
English muffin	1/2
Frankfurter or hamburger bun	1/2 (1 oz.)
Pita, 6 in. across	1/2
Plain roll, small	1 (1 oz.)
Raisin, unfrosted	1 slice (1 oz.)
Rye, pumpernickel	1 slice (1 oz.)
Tortilla, 6 in. across	1
White (including French, Italian)	1 slice (1 oz.)
Whole wheat	1 slice (1 oz.)

Crackers/Snacks

Animal crackers	8
Graham crackers, 2 1/2 in. square	3
Matzoh	3/4 oz.
Melba toast	5 slices
Oyster crackers	24
Popcorn (popped, no fat added)	3 cups
Pretzels	3/4 oz.
■ Rye crisp, 2 in. x 3 1/2 in.	4
Saltine-type crackers	6
■ Whole-wheat crackers, no fat added (crisp breads, such as Finn®, Kavli®, Wasa®)	2–4 slices (3/4 oz.)

Starch Foods Prepared with Fat

(Count as 1 starch/bread exchange, plus 1 fat exchange.)

Biscuit, 2 1/2 in. across	1
Chow mein noodles	1/2 cup
Corn bread, 2 in. cube	1 (2 oz.)
Cracker, round butter type	6
French fried potatoes, 2 in. to 3 1/2 in. long	10 (1 1/2 oz.)
Muffin, plain, small	1
Pancake, 4 in. across	2
Stuffing, bread (prepared)	1/4 cup
Taco shell, 6 in. across	2
Waffle, 4 1/2 in. square	1
■ Whole-wheat crackers, fat added (such as Triscuit®)	4–6 (1 oz.)

■ 3 grams or more of fiber per exchange

Meat List

Each serving of meat and substitutes on this list contains about 7 grams of protein. The amount of fat and number of calories varies, depending on what kind of meat or substitute you choose. The list is divided into three parts based on the amount of fat and calories: lean meat, medium-fat meat, and high-fat meat. One ounce (one meat exchange) of each of these includes:

	Carbohydrate (grams)	Protein (grams)	Fat (grams)	Calories
Lean	0	7	3	55
Medium-fat	0	7	5	75
High-fat	0	7	8	100

Lean Meat and Substitutes

(One exchange is equal to any one of the following items.)

Beef	USDA Select or Choice grades of lean beef, such as round, sirloin, and flank steak; tenderloin; and chipped beef ●	1 oz.
Pork	Lean pork, such as fresh ham; canned, cured or boiled ham ●; Canadian bacon ●, tenderloin.	1 oz.
Veal	All cuts are lean except for veal cutlets (ground or cubed). Examples of lean veal are chops and roasts.	1 oz.
Poultry	Chicken, turkey, Cornish hen (without skin)	1 oz.
Fish	All fresh and frozen fish	1 oz.
	Crab, lobster, scallops, shrimp, clams (fresh or canned in water)	2 oz.
	Oysters	6 medium
	Tuna ◆ (canned in water)	1/4 cup
	Herring ◆ (uncreamed or smoked)	1 oz.
	Sardines (canned)	2 medium
Wild game	Venison, rabbit, squirrel	1 oz.
	Pheasant, duck, goose (without skin)	1 oz.
Cheese	Any cottage cheese ◆	1/4 cup
	Grated parmesan	2 Tbsp.
	Diet cheeses ● (with less than 55 calories per ounce)	1 oz.
Other	95% fat-free luncheon meat ●	1 1/2 oz.
	Egg whites	3 whites
	Egg substitutes with less than 55 calories per 1/2 cup	1/2 cup

Medium-Fat Meat and Substitutes

(One exchange is equal to any one of the following items.)

Beef	Most beef products fall into this category. Examples are: all ground beef, roast (rib, chuck, rump), steak (cubed, Porterhouse, T-bone), and meatloaf.	1 oz.
Pork	Most pork products fall into this category. Examples are: chops, loin roast, Boston butt, cutlets.	1 oz.
Lamb	Most lamb products fall into this category. Examples are: chops, leg, and roast.	1 oz.
Veal	Cutlet (ground or cubed, unbreaded)	1 oz.

Poultry	Chicken (with skin), domestic duck or goose (well drained of fat), ground turkey	1 oz.
Fish	Tuna ◆ (canned in oil and drained)	1/4 cup
	Salmon ◆ (canned)	1/4 cup
Cheese	Skim or part-skim milk cheeses, such as:	
	Ricotta	1/4 cup
	Mozzarella	1 oz.
	Diet cheeses ● (with 56–80 calories per ounce)	1 oz.
Other	86% fat-free luncheon meat ◆	1 oz.
	Egg (high in cholesterol, limit to 3 per week)	1
	Egg substitutes with 56–80 calories per 1/4 cup	1/4 cup
	Tofu (2 1/2 in. × 2 3/4 in. × 1 in.)	4 oz.
	Liver, heart, kidney, sweetbreads (high in cholesterol)	1 oz.

High-Fat Meat and Substitutes

Remember, these items are high in saturated fat, cholesterol, and calories, and should be used only three (3) times per week.

(One exchange is equal to any one of the following items.)

Beef	Most USDA Prime cuts of beef, such as ribs, corned beef ◆	1 oz.
Pork	Spareribs, ground pork, pork sausage ● (patty or link)	1 oz.
Lamb	Patties (ground lamb)	1 oz.
Fish	Any fried fish product	1 oz.
Cheese	All regular cheeses, such as American ●, Blue ●, Cheddar ◆, Monterey Jack ◆, Swiss	1 oz.
Other	Luncheon meat ●, such as bologna, salami, pimento loaf	1 oz.
	Sausage ●, such as Polish, Italian smoked	1 oz.
	Knockwurst ●	1 oz.
	Bratwurst ◆	1 oz.
	Frankfurter ● (turkey or chicken)	1 frank (10/lb.)
	Peanut butter (contains unsaturated fat)	1 Tbsp.

Count as one high-fat meat plus one fat exchange:

	Frankfurter ● (beef, pork, or combination)	1 frank (10/lb.)

● 400 mg or more of sodium per exchange

◆ 400 mg or more of sodium if two or more exchanges are eaten

Vegetable List

Each vegetable serving on this list contains about 5 grams of carbohydrate, 2 grams of protein, and 25 calories. Vegetables contain 2–3 grams of dietary fiber. Vegetables which contain 400 mg or more of sodium per exchange are identified with a ● symbol.

Unless otherwise noted, the serving size for vegetables (one vegetable exchange) is:
- 1/2 cup of cooked vegetables or vegetable juice
- 1 cup of raw vegetables

Artichoke (1/2 medium)	Mushrooms, cooked
Asparagus	Okra
Beans (green, wax, Italian)	Onions
Bean sprouts	Pea pods
Beets	Peppers (green)
Broccoli	Rutabaga
Brussels sprouts	Sauerkraut ●
Cabbage, cooked	Spinach, cooked
Carrots	Summer squash (crookneck)
Cauliflower	Tomato (one large)
Eggplant	Tomato/vegetable juice ●
Greens (collard, mustard, turnip)	Turnips
Kohlrabi	Water chestnuts
Leeks	Zucchini, cooked

Starchy vegetables such as corn, peas, and potatoes are found on the Starch/Bread List.

For free vegetables, see Free Food List

Fruit List

Each item on this list contains about 15 grams of carbohydrate and 60 calories. Fresh, frozen, and dried fruits have about 2 grams of fiber per exchange. Fruits that have 3 or more grams of fiber per exchange have a ■ symbol. Fruit juices contain very little dietary fiber.

The carbohydrate and calorie content for a fruit exchange are based on the usual serving of the most commonly eaten fruits. Use fresh fruits or fruits frozen or canned without sugar added. Whole fruit is more filling than fruit juice and may be a better choice for those who are trying to lose weight. Unless otherwise noted, the serving size for one fruit exchange is:
- 1/2 cup of fresh fruit or fruit juice
- 1/4 cup of dried fruit

Fresh, Frozen, and Unsweetened Canned Fruit

Apple (raw, 2 in. across)	1 apple
Applesauce (unsweetened)	1/2 cup
Apricots (medium, raw)	4 apricots
Apricots (canned)	1/2 cup, or 4 halves
Banana (9 in. long)	1/2 banana
■ Blackberries (raw)	3/4 cup
■ Blueberries (raw)	3/4 cup
Cantaloupe (5 in. across) (cubes)	1/3 melon 1 cup
Cherries (large, raw)	12 cherries
Cherries (canned)	1/2 cup
Figs (raw, 2 in. across)	2 figs
Fruit cocktail (canned)	1/2 cup
Grapefruit (medium)	1/2 grapefruit
Grapefruit (segments)	3/4 cup
Grapes (small)	15 grapes
Honeydew melon (medium) (cubes)	1/8 melon 1 cup
Kiwi (large)	1 kiwi
Mandarin oranges	3/4 cup
Mango (small)	1/2 mango
■ Nectarine (2 1/2 in. across)	1 nectarine
Orange (2 1/2 in. across)	1 orange
Papaya	1 cup
Peach (2 3/4 in. across)	1 peach, or 3/4 cup
Peaches (canned)	1/2 cup or 2 halves
Pear	1/2 large, or 1 small
Pears (canned)	1/2 cup, or 2 halves
Persimmon (medium, native)	2 persimmons
Pineapple (raw)	3/4 cup
Pineapple (canned)	1/3 cup
Plum (raw, 2 in. across)	2 plums
■ Pomegranate	1/2 pomegranate
■ Raspberries (raw)	1 cup
■ Strawberries (raw, whole)	1 1/4 cup
■ Tangerine (2 1/2 in. across)	2 tangerines
Watermelon (cubes)	1 1/4 cup

Dried Fruit

■ Apples	4 rings
■ Apricots	7 halves
Dates	2 1/2 medium
■ Figs	1 1/2
■ Prunes	3 medium
Raisins	2 Tbsp.

Fruit Juice

Apple juice/cider	1/2 cup
Cranberry juice cocktail	1/3 cup
Grapefruit juice	1/2 cup
Grape juice	1/3 cup
Orange juice	1/2 cup
Pineapple juice	1/2 cup
Prune juice	1/3 cup

■ 3 or more grams of fiber per exchange

Milk List

Each serving of milk or milk products on this list contains about 12 grams of carbohydrate and 8 grams of protein. The amount of fat in milk is measured in percent (%) of butterfat. The calories vary, depending on what kind of milk you choose. The list is divided into three parts based on the amount of fat and calories: skim/very lowfat milk, lowfat milk, and whole milk. One serving (one milk exchange) of each of these includes:

	Carbohydrate (grams)	Protein (grams)	Fat (grams)	Calories
Skim/very lowfat	12	8	trace	90
Lowfat	12	8	5	120
Whole	12	8	8	150

Skim and Very Lowfat Milk

Skim milk	1 cup
1/2% milk	1 cup
1% milk	1 cup
Lowfat buttermilk	1 cup
Evaporated skim milk	1/2 cup
Dry nonfat milk	1/3 cup
Plain nonfat yogurt	8 oz.

Lowfat Milk

2% milk	1 cup fluid
Plain lowfat yogurt (with added nonfat milk solids)	8 oz.

Whole Milk

Whole milk	1 cup
Evaporated whole milk	1/2 cup
Whole plain yogurt	8 oz.

Fat List

Each serving on the fat list contains about 5 grams of fat and 45 calories.

The foods on the fat list contain mostly fat, although some items may also contain a small amount of protein. All fats are high in calories and should be carefully measured. Everyone should modify fat intake by eating unsaturated fats instead of saturated fats. The sodium content of these foods varies widely. Check the label for sodium information.

Unsaturated Fats

Avocado	1/8 medium
Margarine	1 tsp.
◆ Margarine, diet	1 Tbsp.
Mayonnaise	1 tsp.
◆ Mayonnaise, reduced-calorie	1 Tbsp.
Nuts and seeds:	
Almonds, dry roasted	6 whole
Cashews, dry roasted	1 Tbsp.
Pecans	2 whole
Peanuts	20 small or 10 large
Walnuts	2 whole
Other nuts	1 Tbsp.
Seeds, pine nuts, sunflower (without shells)	1 Tbsp.
Pumpkin seeds	2 tsp.
Oil (corn, cottonseed, safflower, soybean, sunflower, olive, peanut)	1 tsp.
◆ Olives	10 small or 5 large
Salad dressing, mayonnaise-type	2 tsp.
Salad dressing, mayonnaise-type, reduced-calorie	1 Tbsp.
◆ Salad dressing (oil varieties)	1 Tbsp.
● Salad dressing, reduced-calorie	2 Tbsp.

(Two tablespoons of low-calorie salad dressing is a free food.)

Saturated Fats

Butter	1 tsp.
◆ Bacon	1 slice
Chitterlings	1/2 ounce
Coconut, shredded	2 Tbsp.
Coffee whitener, liquid	2 Tbsp.
Coffee whitener, powder	4 tsp.
Cream (light, coffee, table)	2 Tbsp.
Cream, sour	2 Tbsp.
Cream (heavy, whipping)	1 Tbsp.
Cream cheese	1 Tbsp.
◆ Salt pork	1/4 ounce

● 400 mg or more of sodium per exchange

◆ 400 mg or more of sodium if two or more exchanges are eaten

Combination Foods

Much of the food we eat is mixed together in various combinations. These combination foods do not fit into only one exchange list. It can be quite hard to tell what is in a certain casserole dish or baked food item. This is a list of average values for some typical combination foods. This list will help you fit these foods into your meal plan. Ask your dietitian for information about any other foods you'd like to eat. The *American Diabetes Association/American Dietetic Association Family Cookbooks* and the *American Diabetes Association Holiday Cookbook* have many recipes and further information about many foods, including combination foods. Check your library or local bookstore.

Food	Amount	Exchanges
Casseroles, homemade	1 cup (8 oz.)	2 starch, 2 medium-fat meat, 1 fat
Cheese pizza ●, thin crust	1/4 of 15 oz. or 1/4 of 10 in.	2 starch, 1 medium-fat meat, 1 fat
Chili with beans ■, ● (commercial)	1 cup (8 oz.)	2 starch, 2 medium-fat meat, 2 fat
Chow mein ● (without noodles or rice)	2 cups (16 oz.)	1 starch, 2 vegetable, 2 lean meat
Macaroni and cheese ●	1 cup (8 oz.)	2 starch, 1 medium-fat meat, 2 fat
Soup:		
Bean ■, ●	1 cup (8 oz.)	1 starch, 1 vegetable, 1 lean meat
Chunky, all varieties ●	10 3/4 oz. can	1 starch, 1 vegetable, 1 medium-fat meat
Cream ● (made with water)	1 cup (8 oz.)	1 starch, 1 fat
Vegetable ● or broth-type ●	1 cup (8 oz.)	1 starch
Spaghetti and meatballs ● (canned)	1 cup (8 oz.)	2 starch, 1 medium-fat meat, 1 fat
Sugar-free pudding (made with skim milk)	1/2 cup	1 starch
If beans are used as a meat substitute:		
Dried beans ■, peas ■, lentils ■	1 cup (cooked)	2 starch, 1 lean meat

■ 3 grams or more of fiber per exchange

● 400 mg or more of sodium per exchange

Free Foods

A free food is any food or drink that contains less than 20 calories per serving. You can eat as much as you want of those items that have no serving size specified. You may eat two or three servings per day of those items that have a specific serving size. Be sure to spread them out through the day.

Drinks:

Bouillon ● or broth without fat

Bouillon, low-sodium

Carbonated drinks, sugar-free

Carbonated water

Club soda

Cocoa powder, unsweetened (1 Tbsp.)

Coffee/tea

Drink mixes, sugar-free

Tonic water, sugar-free

Nonstick Pan Spray

Fruit:

Cranberries, unsweetened (1/2 cup)

Rhubarb, unsweetened (1/2 cup)

Vegetables:

(raw, 1 cup)

Cabbage

Celery

Chinese cabbage ■

Cucumber

Green onion

Hot peppers

Mushrooms

Radishes

Zucchini ■

Salad Greens:

Endive

Escarole

Lettuce

Romaine

Spinach

Sweet Substitutes:

Candy, hard, sugar-free

Gelatin, sugar-free

Gum, sugar-free

Jam/jelly, sugar-free (less than 20 cal./2 tsp.)

Pancake syrup, sugar-free (1–2 Tbsp.)

Sugar substitutes (saccharin, aspartame)

Whipped topping (2 Tbsp.)

Condiments:

Catsup (1 Tbsp.)

Horseradish

Mustard

Pickles ●, dill, unsweetened

Salad dressing, low-calorie (2 Tbsp.)

Taco sauce (3 Tbsp.)

Vinegar

Seasonings can be very helpful in making food taste better. Be careful of how much sodium you use. Read the label, and choose those seasonings that do not contain sodium or salt.

Basil (fresh)
Celery seeds
Chili powder
Chives
Cinnamon
Curry
Dill

Flavoring extracts (vanilla, almond, walnut, peppermint, butter, lemon, etc.)
Garlic
Garlic powder
Herbs
Hot pepper sauce
Lemon

Lemon juice
Lemon pepper
Lime
Lime juice
Mint
Onion powder
Oregano
Paprika
Pepper

Pimento
Spices
Soy sauce ●
Soy sauce ● low-sodium ("lite")
Wine, used in cooking (1/4 cup)
Worcestershire sauce

● 400 mg or more of sodium per exchange

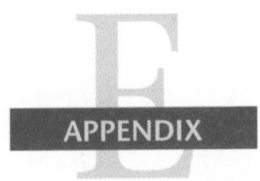

APPENDIX

Summary of Examples of Recommended Nutrients for Canadians Based on Energy, Expressed as Daily Rates

Age	Sex	Energy (kcal)	Thiamin (mg)	Riboflavin (mg)	Niacin (NE)[a]	n-3 PUFA[b] (g)	n-6 PUFA (g)
Months							
0–4	Both	600	0.3	0.3	4	0.5	3
5–12	Both	900	0.4	0.5	7	0.5	3
Years							
1	Both	1,100	0.5	0.6	8	0.6	4
2–3	Both	1,300	0.6	0.7	9	0.7	4
4–6	Both	1,800	0.7	0.9	13	1.0	6
7–9	M	2,200	0.9	1.1	16	1.2	7
	F	1,900	0.8	1.0	14	1.0	6
10–12	M	2,500	1.0	1.3	18	1.4	8
	F	2,200	0.9	1.1	16	1.1	7
13–15	M	2,800	1.1	1.4	20	1.4	9
	F	2,200	0.9	1.1	16	1.2	7
16–18	M	3,200	1.3	1.6	23	1.8	11
	F	2,100	0.8	1.1	15	1.2	7
19–24	M	3,000	1.2	1.5	22	1.6	10
	F	2,100	0.8	1.1	15	1.2	7
25–49	M	2,700	1.1	1.4	19	1.5	9
	F	2,000	0.8	1.0	14	1.1	7
50–74	M	2,300	0.9	1.3	16	1.3	8
	F	1,800	0.8[c]	1.0[c]	14[c]	1.1[c]	7[c]
75+	M	2,000	0.8	1.0	14	1.0	7
	F[d]	1,700	0.8[c]	1.0[c]	14[c]	1.1[c]	7[c]
Pregnancy (additional)							
1st Trimester		100	0.1	0.1	0.1	0.05	0.3
2nd Trimester		300	0.1	0.3	0.2	0.16	0.9
3rd Trimester		300	0.1	0.3	0.2	0.16	0.9
Lactation (additional)		450	0.2	0.4	0.3	0.25	1.5

[a] Niacin Equivalents
[b] PUFA, polyunsaturated fatty acids.
[c] Level below which intake should not fall
[d] Assumes moderate physical activity

Source: Health Canada. Excerpts from RNI Table 1990, *Recommended Nutrients for Canadians*.
Reproduced with permission of the Minister of Supply and Services Canada, 1994.

Summary of Examples of Recommended Nutrients for Canadians Based on Energy, Expressed as Daily Rates (continued)

Age	Sex	Weight (kg)	Protein (g)	Vit. A (RE)[a]	Vit. D (µg)	Vit. E (mg)	Vit. C (mg)	Folate (µg)	Vit. B12 (µg)	Calcium (mg)	Phos-phorus (mg)	Mag-nesium (mg)	Iron (mg)	Iodine (µg)	Zinc (mg)
Months															
0–4	Both	6.0	12[b]	400	10	3	20	50	0.3	250[c]	150	20	10.3[d]	30	2[d]
5–12	Both	9.0	12	400	10	3	20	50	0.3	400	200	32	7	40	3
Years															
1	Both	11	19	400	10	3	20	65	0.3	500	300	40	6	55	4
2–3	Both	14	22	400	5	4	20	80	0.4	550	350	50	6	65	4
4–6	Both	18	26	500	2.5	5	25	90	0.5	600	400	65	8	85	5
7–9	M	25	30	700	2.5	7	25	125	0.8	700	500	100	8	110	7
	F	25	30	700	2.5	6	25	125	0.8	700	500	100	8	95	7
10–12	M	34	38	800	5	8	25	170	1.0	900	700	130	8	125	9
	F	36	40	800	5	7	25	180	1.0	1,100	800	135	8	110	9
13–15	M	50	50	900	5	9	30	150	1.5	1,100	900	185	10	160	12
	F	48	42	800	5	7	30	145	1.5	1,000	850	180	13	160	9
16–18	M	62	55	1,000	5	10	40[e]	185	1.9	900	1,000	230	10	160	12
	F	53	43	800	2.5	7	30[e]	160	1.9	700	850	200	12	160	9
19–24	M	71	58	1,000	2.5	10	40[e]	210	2.0	800	1,000	240	9	160	12
	F	58	43	800	2.5	7	30[e]	175	2.0	700	850	200	13	160	9
25–49	M	74	61	1,000	2.5	9	40[e]	220	2.0	800	1,000	250	9	160	9
	F	59	44	800	2.5	6	30[e]	175	2.0	700	850	200	13	160	9
50–74	M	73	60	1,000	5	7	40[e]	220	2.0	800	1,000	250	9	160	12
	F	63	47	800	5	6	30[e]	190	2.0	800	850	210	8	160	9
75+	M	69	57	1,000	5	6	40[e]	205	2.0	800	1,000	230	9	160	12
	F	64	47	800	5	5	30[e]	190	2.0	800	850	210	8	160	9
Pregnancy (additional)															
1st Trimester			5	100	2.5	2	0	300	1.0	500	200	15	0	25	6
2nd Trimester			20	100	2.5	2	10	300	1.0	500	200	45	5	25	6
3rd Trimester			24	100	2.5	2	10	300	1.0	500	200	45	10	25	6
Lactation (additional)			20	400	2.5	3	25	100	0.5	500	200	65	0	50	6

[a] Retinol Equivalents
[b] Protein is assumed to be from breast milk and must be adjusted for infant formula.
[c] Infant formula with high phosphorous should contain 375 mg calcium.
[d] Breast milk is assumed to be the source of the mineral.
[e] Smokers should increase vitamin C by 50%.

Source: Health Canada. Excerpts from RNI Table 1990, *Recommended Nutrients for Canadians*.
Reproduced with permission of the Minister of Supply and Services Canada, 1994.

Canada's Food Guide to Healthy Eating (1992)

For people four years and over

Different People Need Different Amounts of Food

The amount of food you need every day from the four food groups and other food depends on your age, body size, activity level, whether you are male or female and if you are pregnant or breast feeding. That's why the Food Guide gives a lower and higher number of servings for each food group. For example, young children can choose the lower number of servings, while male teenagers can go to the higher number. Most other people can choose servings somewhere in between.

Food Group	Servings per Day	Examples of One Serving	Examples of Two Servings
Grain products	5–12	1 slice bread 30 g cold cereal 175 ml (3/4 cup) hot cereal	1 bagel, pita, or bun 20 ml (1 cup) pasta or rice
Vegetables and fruit	5–10	1 medium size vegetable or fruit 125 ml (1/2 cup) fresh, frozen, or canned vegetables or fruit 250 ml (1 cup) salad 125 ml (1/2 cup) juice	
Milk products	Children, 4–9: 2–3 Youth, 10–16: 3–4 Adults: 2–4 Pregnant & Breast feeding Women: 3–4	250 ml (1 cup) milk 50 g (3" × 1" × 1") cheese 50 g (2 slices) cheese 175 g (3/4 cup) yogourt	
Meat and alternatives	2–3	50–100 g meat, poultry, or fish 50–100 g (1/3–2/3 can) fish 1–2 eggs 125–250 ml beans 100 g (1/3 cup) tofu 30 ml (2 tbsp) peanut butter	

Other Foods

Taste and enjoyment can also come from other foods and beverages that are not part of the four food groups. Some of these foods are higher in fat or calories, so use these foods in moderation.

Enjoy eating well, being active and feeling good about yourself. That's VITALITY®

Adapted from *Canada's Food Guide to Healthy Eating*, Health Canada, 1992.
Reproduced with permission of the Minister of Supply and Services Canada, 1994.

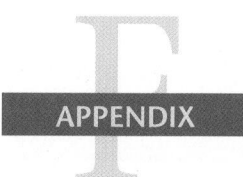

WHO/FAO Recommended Nutrient Reference Values for Food Labelling Purposes

World Health Organization (WHO) and Food and Agriculture Organization of the United Nations (FAO) are United Nations agencies that make recommendations for worldwide use on issues in nutrition, food, agriculture, health, disease, environment, and related topics.

WHO/FAO recognize that standards for nutrient intake have varied terminology in different countries. For example, Recommended Dietary Allowances (RDAs) in the United States may have a different title in other countries. Also, recommended intakes for specific nutrients vary among countries. A common reference standard, the Nutrient Reference Values (NRVs), was proposed by WHO/FAO to avoid this international confusion. NRVs provide consumers, and the scientific community, a uniform standard for easy comparison of the nutrient content of foods. This is important because of increased exportation of food from one country to another.

WHO/FAO recognize that individual requirements for the intake of specific nutrients are a function of a person's age, gender, body weight, and physiological status. However, they also recognize that, for the most part, the same foods are eaten by all members of the population above three years of age. For this reason, a single NRV is established for individual nutrients. These NRVs do *not* represent the specific requirements of individuals in the population.

Nutrient	Unit	Nutrient Reference Value
Protein	g	50
Vitamin A	µg	800
Vitamin D	µg	5[a]
Vitamin C	mg	60
Thiamin	mg	1.4
Riboflavin	mg	1.6
Niacin	mg	18[a]
Vitamin B-6	mg	2
Folic acid	µg	200
Vitamin B-12	µg	1
Calcium	mg	800
Magnesium	mg	300
Iron	mg	14
Zinc	mg	15
Iodine	µg	150[a]
Copper	Value to be established	
Selenium	Value to be established	

[a] Nutrient Reference Values for vitamin D, niacin, and iodine may not be applicable for countries where national nutrition policies or local conditions provide sufficient allowance to ensure that individual requirements are satisfied.

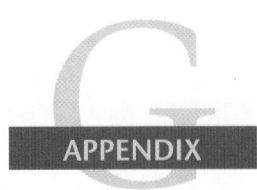

Activities in Diet Easy for Windows™ Software

Activities	Kilocalories Burned Per Kilogram Per Hour	Activities	Kilocalories Burned Per Kilogram Per Hour
Aerobics, heavy	8	Jazzercize, heavy	8
Aerobics, light	3	Jazzercize, light	3
Aerobics, medium	5	Jazzercize, medium	5
Archery	3.5	Jog (9 min/mile)	11
Backpacking	9	Jog (10 min/mile)	10
Badminton, doubles	4	Jog (12 min/mile)	8.5
Badminton, singles	5.1	Jog (13 min/mile)	7
Basketball, nonvigorous	9.5	Jog (14 min/mile)	6
Basketball, vigorous	11	Jog (15 min/mile)	5
Bicycling (6 mph)	3.5	Jog (17 min/mile)	4
Bicycling (10 mph)	5.5	Lawn mowing (hand)	6.5
Bicycling (11 mph)	6.5	Lawn mowing (power)	3.6
Bicycling (12 mph)	7.5	Music playing	2.5
Bicycling (13 mph)	8.5	Racquetball, social	8.5
Billiards	2	Racquetball, vigorous	10
Bowling	3.9	Roller skating	5.1
Boxing, competition	3.3	Rowboating (2.5 mph)	4.4
Boxing, sparring	8.3	Rowing (11 mph)	13
Calisthenics, heavy	8	Run (5 min/ mile)	18
Calisthenics, light	4	Run (6 min/mile)	15.5
Canoeing (2.5 mph)	3.3	Run (7 min/mile)	13.5
Canoeing (5 mph)	7.5	Run (8 min/mile)	12
Carpentry	5	Sailing	3.5
Climbing, mountain	10	Shuffleboard/skeet	3
Disco dancing	6	Skiing (cross-country)	10
Ditch digging, hand	5.8	Skiing, downhill	8
Fencing	7.5	Square dancing	6
Fishing (bank/boat)	3.5	Swimming, compete	15
Fishing (in waders)	5.5	Swimming, fast	9.4
Football, touch	7.5	Swimming, slow	7.7
Gardening	3.2	Table tennis	5.2
Golf (carry clubs)	5	Tennis, doubles	5
Golf (pull cart)	3.6	Tennis, singles	6.5
Golf (ride in cart)	2.5	Tennis, vigorous	8.5
Handball, vigorous	10	Volleyball	5.1
Hiking (across country)	5.5	Walking (20 min/mile)	3.5
Hiking, mountain	7.5	Walking (26 min/mile)	3
Horseback, trotting	5.1	Water skiing	7
Housework	4	Weightlifting, heavy	9
Hunting (carry load)	6	Weightlifting, light	4
Ice hockey, vigorous	10	Wood chopping, sawing	6.5
Ice skating (10 mph)	5.8		

Credits for Art and Text

Contents

Fig. C-1. Michigan State University–Agricultural Experiment Station (MSU-AES).

Fig. C-2. U.S. Department of Agriculture–Agricultural Research Service (USDA-ARS).

Fig. C-3. MSU-AES.

Fig. C-4. Food and Agriculture Organization of the United Nations (FAO).

Figs. C-5 and C-6. USDA-ARS.

Fig. C-7. Kurt Stepnitz. MSU-AES.

Fig. C-8. FAO.

Fig. C-9. ©Peter Beck/Frozen Images.

Preface

Fig. P-1. U.S. Department of Agriculture–Agricultural Research Service (USDA-ARS).

Fig. P-2. Food and Agriculture Organization of the United Nations (FAO).

Fig. P-3. Calorie Control Council (left) and National Institutes of Health (right).

Fig. P-4. Archer Daniels Midland Co.

Fig. P-5. USDA-ARS.

Fig. P-6. FAO.

Fig. P-7. USDA.

Page xiii. Poem printed by permission of David Kritchevsky.

Chapter 1

Fig. 1-1 and Table 1-1. U.S. Department of Agriculture (USDA).

Fig. 1-2. Adapted from data provided by the United Nations Population Fund and the Population Reference Bureau.

Page 4, quotation. Francis Crick, *Life Itself–Its Origins and Nature.* Simon and Schuster, New York, 1981.

Fig. 1-3. USDA.

Fig. 1-4. Watson Food Company, Inc.

Table 1-2. Adapted from G. Campbell-Platt, *Food Science and Technology Today* 2(2):95, 1988.

Fig. 1-5. USDA–Agricultural Research Service (ARS).

Fig. 1-6. The Pillsbury Co.

Table 1-3. Adapted from *Wall Street Journal*, December 26, 1991.

Table 1-4. V. Hegarty, *Decisions in Nutrition*. Times Mirror/Mosby College Publishing, St. Louis, MO, 1988.

Figs. 1-7 and 1-8. USDA-ARS.

Table 1-5. Adapted from R. J. Scheuplein, *Global Food Progress 1991*, D. A. Avery, ed., p. 155. Hudson Institute, Indianapolis, IN, 1991.

Fig. 1-9. ©Teri McDermott, 1994.

Fig. 1-10. ©A. & H.-F. Michler, Science Photo Library/Photo Researchers.

Figs. 1-11 and 1-12. USDA-ARS.

Fig. 1-13. Photo courtesy of *Prepared Foods*.

Fig. 1-14. Groth, E., III, *Food Technology* 45(5):248, 1991.

Fig. 1-15. Photo courtesy of *Prepared Foods*.

Chapter 2

Fig. 2-1. Office of War Information, Washington, DC., U.S. Government Printing Office, 1943.

Page 27, quotation. Faculty of Environmental Studies, York University, North York, Ontario, Canada.

Fig. 2-2. U.S. Department of Agriculture (USDA).

Table 2-1. World Health Organization (WHO).

Fig. 2-3. Food and Agriculture Organization of the United Nations (FAO).

Figs. 2-4 and 2-5. FAO.

Fig. 2-6 and Table 2-2. Based on material in *The BMA Guide to Pesticides, Chemicals and Health*. Edward Arnold, London, 1992.

Page 35, quotation. From WHO report *Chemical Contaminants in Food: Global Situation and Trends*.

Fig. 2-7. G. E. Dunaif and E. P. Krysinski, *Food Technology* 46(3):72, 1992.

Fig. 2-8. The Food Network, University of Guelph.

Fig. 2-9. Cartoon by G. M. Gadd, University of Dundee, Scotland. From *Trends in Food Science and Technology*, March 1992 (Vol. 3), p. 57. ©Elsevier Science Publishers Ltd., Barking, Essex, U.K.

Tables 2-3 and 2-4. S. Harlander and R. G. Garner, *1986 Yearbook of Agriculture, Research for Tomorrow*. USDA, 1986.

Fig. 2-10 and 2-11. Monsanto Co.

Fig. 2-12. USDA-ARS.

Fig. 2-13. FAO.

Fig. 2-14. *Dairy Foods*.

Fig. 2-15. Nordion International Inc.

Table 2-5. U.S. Food and Drug Administration (FDA).

Fig. 2-16. Pfizer, Inc.

Fig. 2-17. S. C. Delaney/U.S. Environmental Pollution Agency (EPA).

Fig. 2-18. USDA Soil Conservation Service.

Fig. 2-19. W. D. Gibson, *Chemical Marketing Reporter*, June 15, 1992, p. 26. Schnell Publishing Co., Inc.

Table 2-6. FDA.

Pages 52–53, list. ©The American Dietetic Association. Reprinted by permission from *Journal of The American Dietetic Association*, Vol. 90, 1990.

Fig. 2-20. *Food Technology* 45(2):30, 1991.

Table 2-7. FDA.

Chapter 3

Fig. 3-1. Courtesy of the Commonwealth of Pennsylvania.

Fig. 3-2. ©Dan Ford Connolly-MERCURY.

Table 3-1. D. P. Richardson, *Bibliotheca Nutrio et Dieta* 45:143, 1990. By permission of S. Karger AG, Basel, Switzerland.

Figs 3-3A and 3-3B. Adapted from L. H. Rappoport and others, *Ecology of Food and Nutrition* 28:171, 1992.

Figs. 3-4 and 3-5. Provesta Corporation.

Fig. 3-6. ©Greg Edwards Photography, St. Paul, MN.

Pages 64–65, quotation. J. Postgate, *Microbes and Man*, 3rd ed. Cambridge University Press, 1992. Reprinted with permission of Cambridge University Press.

Figs. 3-7A and 7B. Medallion Laboratories.

Figs. 3-8 and 3-9. Adapted from M. M. Cody and M. Keith, *Food Safety for Professionals: A Reference and Study Guide*. The American Dietetic Association, Chicago, 1991.

Tables 3-2 and 3-3. Centers for Disease Control.

Fig. 3-10. U.S. Department of Agriculture–Agricultural Research Service (USDA-ARS).

Fig. 3-11. USDA–Federal Grain Inspection Service.

Fig. 3-12. ©Teri McDermott, 1994.

Fig. 3-13. *Nature*, cover for December 3, 1992. ©Macmillan Magazines, Ltd., London.

Fig. 3-15. Photo from USDA-ARS. Drawings adapted from V. Hegarty, *Decisions in Nutrition*. Times Mirror/Mosby College Publishing, St. Louis, MO, 1988.

Fig. 3-16. Adapted from V. Hegarty, *Decisions in Nutrition*. Times Mirror/Mosby College Publishing, St. Louis, MO, 1988.

Fig. 3-17. Food and Agriculture Organization of the United Nations.

Chapter 4

Fig. 4-1. Food and Agriculture Organization of the United Nations (FAO).

Fig. 4-2. Gulf States Paper Corporation.

Fig. 4-3. *Maclean's Magazine;* Hunter Mclean Ltd.; October 22, 1990.

Fig. 4-4. World Health Organization (WHO) and FAO.

Fig. 4-5. Data from WHO.

Table 4-1. FAO.

Figs. 4-6 and 4-7. U.S. Department of Agriculture (USDA).

Tables 4-2, 4-4, 4-5, 4-6, 4-7, and 4-8. USDA.

Fig. 4-8. National Livestock and Meat Board.

Tables 4-9, 4-10, and 4-11. USDA.

Table 4-12. Adapted from the American Diabetes Association and The American Dietetic Association, *Exchange Lists for Meal Planning*, 1989.

Figs. 4-9, 4-10, 4-11, and 4-12, 4-13, and 4-14. International Diabetes Center, Minneapolis, MN.

Page 98, quotation. From J. V. G. A. Durnin and others, *Nature* 242:418, 1973.

Fig. 4-15. Adapted from V. Hegarty, *Decisions in Nutrition*. Times Mirror/Mosby College Publishing, St. Louis, MO, 1988.

Figs. 4-16 and 4-17. U.S. Food and Drug Administration (FDA).

Table 4-13 and margin information on p. 104. FDA.

Fig. 4-18. ©*Cereal Foods World*.

Fig. 4-19. *Native American Foods*. Courtesy of NATIONAL DAIRY COUNCIL.

Fig. 4-21. Courtesy of Archer Daniels Midland Co.

Fig. 4-22. USDA–Agricultural Research Service (ARS).

Fig. 4-23. Courtesy of Rodale Institute.

Table 4-14. Adapted from S. J. Crockett and D. L. Stuber, *Ecology of Food and Nutrition* 27:51, 1992.

Fig. 4-24. A. B. Caragay, *Food Technology* 46(4):65, 1992.

Fig. 4-25. Canadian Dietetic Association.

Chapter 5

Figs. 5-1A and B. Dr. Norbert Hirschhorn.

Figs. 5-2A and B. Dr. Ann P. Streissguth, University of Washington School of Medicine.

Fig. 5-3. Michigan State University–Agricultural Experiment Station (MSU-AES).

Fig. 5-4. Food and Agriculture Organization of the United Nations (FAO).

Fig. 5-5. Photograph: ©Science Source/Photo Researchers.

Fig. 5-6. S. C. Delaney/U.S. Environmental Pollution Agency (EPA).

Fig. 5-8. FAO.

Fig. 5-9. U.S. Department of Agriculture–Agricultural Research Service (USDA-ARS).

Fig. 5-10. FAO.

Fig. 5-11. S. C. Delaney/U.S. EPA.

Fig. 5-12. California Prune Board.

Table 5-1. Adapted from H.-D. Belitz and W. Grosch, *Food Chemistry*. Springer Verlag, Berlin, 1987.

Fig. 5-13. U.S. Food and Drug Administration (FDA).

Fig. 5-15. Adapted from B. F. Grant and others, *Seminars in Liver Diseases* 8(1):12, 1988.

Fig. 5-16. Reprinted by permission of *The New England Journal of Medicine* from C. S. Lieber, *New England Journal of Medicine* 319:1639, Figure 2. ©1988, Massachusetts Medical Society.

Figs. 5-17 and 5-18. USDA-ARS.

Chapter 6

Fig. 6-1. Photo courtesy of The NutraSweet Company.

Fig. 6-2. Used with permission of Ross Products Division, Abbott Laboratories, Columbus, OH 43216, ©1990, Ross Products Division, Abbott Laboratories.

Fig. 6-4. *Food Technology*, Feb. 1991.

Fig. 6-7. The Procter & Gamble Company.

Fig. 6-8, right. Unilever.

Fig. 6-9. Medallion Laboratories.

Fig. 6-11. Archer Daniels Midland Co.

Table 6-2 and Fig. 6-12. U.S. Department of Agriculture (USDA).

Fig. 6-14. ©Teri McDermott, 1994.

Fig. 6-15. Figure courtesy of Kellogg Company.

Fig. 6-16. ©*Cereal Foods World*.

Fig. 10-18. USDA.

Fig. 10-19. ©1991, Newsweek, Inc. All rights reserved. Reprinted by permission.

Fig. 10-20. *The All-American Guide to Calcium-Rich Foods.* Courtesy of NATIONAL DAIRY COUNCIL.

Chapter 11

Fig. 11-1. Dairy Council of Wisconsin.

Fig. 11-2. U.S. Department of Agriculture (USDA).

Fig. 11-3. Adapted from E. T. Poehlman, ©*Journal of Nutrition* 122:2057, 1992. American Institute of Nutrition.

Fig. 11-4. S. B. Heymsfield and others, ©*Journal of Nutrition* 123:432, 1993. American Institute of Nutrition.

Table 11-3. Food and Agriculture Organization of the United Nations (FAO).

Table 11-4. Adapted from *Recommended Dietary Allowances*, 10th ed., National Academy Press, Washington, DC, 1989.

Fig. 11-5. University of Minnesota, Minnesota Extension Service.

Table 11-5. Adapted from P. M. Kris-Etherton, *Nutrition Today* 21:6, 1986.

Figs. 11-6 and 11-7. USDA-Agricultural Research Service.

Table 11-6. Adapted from W. D. McArdle and others, *Exercise Physiology*, 2nd ed. Lea & Febiger, Philadelphia, 1986.

Chapter 12

Fig. 12-1. ©Linda Winchester/Superstock.

Page 298, quotation. From S. B, Eaton and others, *The Paleolithic Prescription: A Program of Diet and Exercise and a Design for Living.* Harper and Row, New York, 1989.

Fig. 12-2. ©Teri McDermott, 1994.

Table 12-1. Adapted from M. C. Linder, *Nutritional Biochemistry and Metabolism*, 2nd ed. Elsevier, New York, 1991.

Fig. 12-3. U.S. Department of Agriculture–Agricultural Research Service (USDA-ARS).

Table 12-2. Gatorade Sports Science Institute.

Table 12-3. Adapted from C. D. Jensen and others, *Journal of The American Dietetic Association* 92:986, 1992.

Fig. 12-4. Kurt Stepnitz. Michigan State University–Agricultural Experiment Station (MSU-AES).

Fig. 12-5. National Institutes of Health.

Fig. 12-7. ©Blair Seitz/Photo Researchers.

Fig. 12-8 and Table 12-4. Gatorade Sports Science Institute.

Fig. 12-9. ©NIBSC/Science Photo Library/Photo Researchers.

Page 310, list of sports nutrition tips. ©The American Dietetic Association. Reprinted by permission from *Journal of The American Dietetic Association*, 92:419, 1992.

Table 12-5. Adapted from J. A. McSherry, American Family Physician 29:141, 1984.

Fig. 12-10. USDA-ARS.

Table 12-6. Adapted from R. M. Philen and others, *Journal of the American Medical Association* 268:1008, 1992. ©American Medical Association.

Fig. 12-11. University of Minnesota, Minnesota Extension Service.

Table 12-7. Gatorade Sports Science Institute.

Chapter 13

Fig. 13-1. ©1993 by Consumers Union of U.S., Inc., Yonkers, NY 10703-1057. Reprinted by permission from *Consumer Reports*, June 1993.

Fig. 13-2. World Health Organization (WHO).

Page 318, data on obesity in different countries. Adapted from G. Bray, *Annals of the New York Academy of Science* 249:14, 1987.

Fig. 13-3. Kurt Stepnitz. Michigan State University–Agricultural Experiment Station (MSU-AES).

Table 13-1. National Institutes of Health (NIH).

Table 13-2. NIH.

Table 13-3. Adapted from P. J. Brown and M. Konner, *Annals of the New York Academy of Science* 499:29, 1987.

Fig. 13-4. C. Oberg. Michigan State University.

Fig. 13-6. Adapted from J. Garrow, *British Medical Journal* 303:704, 1991.

Table 13-5. Adapted from Anne Meyer, *Prepared Foods* 159(10):57, 1990. Data from Marketdata Enterprises.

Fig. 13-7. Based on data of Thomas A. Wadden.

Table 13-7. Michigan Department of Public Health.

Figs. 13-8 and 13-9. WHO.

Fig. 13-10. U.S. Department of Agriculture–Agricultural Research Service.

Fig. 13-11. Food and Agriculture Organization of the United Nations (FAO).

Fig. 13-13. *Penn State Agriculture*, p. 14, winter, 1992. James McClure, Penn State.

Page 339, tips for parents. The American Anorexia/Bulimia Association.

Table 13-8. *Lifesteps: Weight Management: A Summary of Current Theory and Practice.* Courtesy of NATIONAL DAIRY COUNCIL. Based on: 1) D. W. Swanson and F. A. Dinello. Severe obesity as a habituation syndrome. In: *Overweight and Obesity: Causes, Fallacies, and Treatment.* B. O. Hafen, ed., p. 94. Brigham Young University Press, Provo, UT, 1975. 2) M. Simonson and J. R. Heilman. *The Complete University Medical Diet.* Rawson and Associates, New York, 1983. 3) D. Craddock, *Obesity and Its Management.* Churchill Livingstone, New York, 1978. 4) J. Wise and S. K. Wise, *The Overeaters: Eating Styles and Personality.* Human Sciences Press, New York, 1979. 5) H. Bruch, Thin fat people. In: *Overweight and Obesity: Causes, Fallacies, and Treatment.* B. Q. Hafen, ed., p. 108. Brigham Young University Press, Provo, UT, 1975. 6) L. Salzman, Obesity–Understanding the Compulsion. In: *Overweight and Obesity: Causes, Fallacies, and Treatment.* B. Q. Hafen, ed., p. 89. Brigham Young University Press, Provo, UT, 1975. 7) I. Rodin, Responsiveness of the obese to external stimuli. In: *Obesity in Perspective*, Vol. 2, part 2. G. A. Bray, ed., p. 61. Department of Health, Education, and Welfare, Washington, DC, 1973.

Chapter 14

Fig. 14-1. National Institutes of Health/©1992 Custom Medical Stock Photo.

Fig. 14-2. National Center for Health Statistics, Centers for Disease Control.

Fig. 14-3. World Health Organization (WHO).

Table 14-1. Adapted from D. J. Raiten, *Nutrition in Clinical Practice* 6:1S, 1991.

Table 14-2 and Fig. 14-4. Courtesy Mead Johnson Nutritional Group.

Fig. 14-5. Adapted from K. C. H. Fearon, *Proceedings of the Nutrition Society* 51:251, 1992.

Fig. 14-6. American Institute for Cancer Research.

Table 14-3. National Institutes of Health (NIH).

Fig. 14-7 and list on pp. 351–352. Used by permission, ©1985 American Cancer Society, *Taking Control.*

Fig. 14-8. Lilly Research Laboratories, A Division of Eli Lilly and Company.

Fig. 14-9. Anonymous, *Journal of Nutritional Biochemistry* 2:37, 1991.

Table 14-4. Adapted from T. M. S. Wolever and D. J. A. Jenkins, in: *Diet, Nutrition, and Health*, K. K. Carroll, ed., p. 103. McGill-Queen's University Press, Montreal, 1990. By permission of The Royal Society of Canada.

Fig. 14-10. British Diabetic Association.

Page 356, Target Nutritional Goals. From *Diabetes Care* 10:126, 1987. Position statement of the American Diabetes Association.

Fig. 14-11. Calorie Control Council.

Tables 14-5 and 14-6. Reprinted from *Low-calorie Foods Handbook*, A. M. Altschul, ed., pp. 93 and 94, 1993. Courtesy of Marcel Dekker, Inc., New York.

Fig. 14-12. Rhône-Poulenc Food Ingredients.

Chapter 15

Fig. 15-1. Michigan State University–Agricultural Experiment Station (MSU-AES).

Fig. 15-2. Food and Agriculture Organization of the United Nations (FAO).

Fig. 15-3. Adapted from *Recommended Dietary Allowances*, 10th ed., National Academy Press, Washington, DC, 1989.

Fig. 15-4. National Livestock and Meat Board.

Fig. 15-5. World Health Organization (WHO).

Table 15-1. Reprinted with permission from: *Nutrition During Pregnancy and Lactation: An Implementation Guide.* ©1992 by the National Academy of Sciences. Courtesy of the National Academy Press, Washington, DC.

Table 15-2. Reprinted with permission from *Nutrition During Lactation.* ©1991 by the National Academy of Sciences. Courtesy of the National Academy Press, Washington, DC.

Fig. 15-6. U.S. Department of Agriculture (USDA).

Figs. 15-7, 15-8, 15-9 and 15-10. WHO.

Fig. 15-11. USDA.

Table 15-3. M. Sigman-Grant, *Nutrition Today*, 27(4):13-17, 1992.

Fig. 15-12. WHO.

Table 15-4. USDA.

Table 15-5. K. Stanek and others. ©The American Dietetic Association. Reprinted by permission from *Journal of the American Dietetic Association* 90:1583, 1990.

Fig. 15-13. FAO.

Page 385, list. "Position of the American Dietetic Association: Child Nutrition Services." ©The American Dietetic Association. Reprinted by permission from *Journal of the American Dietetic Association* 93(3):334, 1993.

Fig, 15-14. Minnesota Department of Health, WIC program.

Fig. 15-5. Washington Apple Commission.

Chapter 16

Fig. 16-1. *Food Business* magazine, Putman Publishing Co., Chicago, IL. Photograph by Barry Rustin Photography/ Glenview, IL.

Table 16-1. Department of Health and Human Services, Public Health Services, Office of Disease Prevention and Health Promotion, Centers for Disease Control, and National Institute on Drug Abuse.

Fig. 16-2. *Fast Food: Today's Guide to Healthy Choices.* Courtesy of NATIONAL DAIRY COUNCIL.

Fig. 16-3. Nabisco Foods Group. Data compiled by Scholastic, Inc.

Fig. 16-4. Photograph courtesy of Polaroid Corporation.

Fig. 16-5. U.S. Department of the Interior, National Park Service, Edison National Historic Site.

Fig. 16-6. University of Minnesota, Minnesota Extension Service.

Pages 399–400, list. ©The American Dietetic Association. Reprinted by permission.

Table 16-2. Adapted from A. A. Hertzler and R. Frary, *Journal of The American Dietetic Association* 92:867, 1992.

Figure 16-7. McDonald's Corporation.

Page 403, quotation. Reprinted with permission of Charles Scribner's Sons, an imprint of Macmillan Publishing Company, from *The Fragile Species* by Lewis Thomas. ©1992 by Lewis Thomas.

Table 16-3. From J. Dwyer and others, *Nutrition Today* 26(5):21-24, 1991.

Table 16-4. V. Hegarty, *Decisions in Nutrition.* Times Mirror/Mosby College Publishing, St. Louis, MO, 1988.

Page 408, list. From M. Matsutani, *Nutrition Reviews* 50(12):472, 1992.

Table 16-5. Adapted from J. E. Kerstetter and others, *Journal of The American Dietetic Association* 92:1109, 1992.

Fig. 16-8. American Institute of Baking.

Table 16-6. B. M. Popkin and others, *American Journal of Clinical Nutrition* 55:823, 1992. ©American Society for Clinical Nutrition.

Chapter 17

Fig. 17-1. Courtesy Mead Johnson Nutritional Group.

Fig. 17-2. G. Pelto, *Journal of Nutrition Education* 13:S2, 1981.

Table 17-1. Adapted from M. A. Drake, *Public Health Reports* 107:312, 1992.

Fig. 17-3. Food and Agriculture Organization of the United Nations (FAO).

Fig. 17-4. Michigan State University–Agricultural Experiment Station (MSU-AES).

Table 17-2. "Low-Fat Fast Foods." ©1993 by Consumers Union of U.S., Inc., Yonkers, NY 10703-1057. Adapted with permission from *Consumer Reports*, September 1993. Although this material originally appeared in *Consumer Reports*, the selective adaptation and resulting conclusions presented are those of the author and are not sanctioned or endorsed in any way by Consumers Union, the publisher of *Consumer Reports*.

Fig. 17-5. FAO.

Fig. 17-6. U.S. Department of Agriculture–Agricultural Research Service.

Figs. 17-7, 17-8 and Tables 17-3, 17-4. FAO.

Fig. 17-9. *Food Engineering*, Chilton Company.

Fig. 17-10. Stacie Bird, Penn State University.

Table 17-5. E. Pestano-Binghay and others, *Journal of Nutrition Education* 25:144, 1993.

Fig. 17-11. University of Minnesota, Minnesota Extension Service.

Appendix A. ©1994. First DataBank—The Hearst Corporation (N-Squared Computing).

Appendix D. Reprinted by permission. Copyright ©1989 by American Diabetes Association Inc., and The American Dietetic Association.

Appendix E. Pages A60–A61. Health Canada. Excerpts from RNI Table 1990, *Recommended Nutrients for Canadians*. Reproduced with permission of the Minister of Supply and Services Canada, 1994. Page A62. Adapted from *Canada's Food Guide to Healthy Eating*, Health Canada, 1992. Reproduced with permission of the Minister of Supply and Services Canada, 1994.

Appendix F. From *Recommended Nutrient Reference Values for Food Labelling Purposes*, Report of a Joint FAO/WHO Expert Consultation on Recommended Allowances of Nutrients for Food Labelling Purposes, 1988.

Appendix G. ©1994. First DataBank—The Hearst Corporation (N-Squared Computing).

Page facing back cover. Adapted from National Research Council, National Academy of Sciences, *Recommended Dietary Allowances*, 10th edition, National Academy of Sciences, Washington, DC, 1989.

Inside back cover. Adapted from National Research Council, National Academy of Sciences, *Recommended Dietary Allowances*, 10th edition, National Academy of Sciences, Washington, DC, 1989.

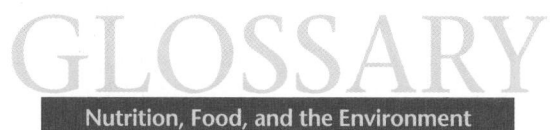

Glossary

Acidulation: Increasing the acid content of a food.

Acne: A skin disorder consisting of pimples and inflammation.

Acquired immunodeficiency syndrome (AIDS): A disease of the human immune system caused by infection with the human immunodeficiency virus (HIV), usually resulting in death.

Acute exposure to a toxin: A high dose of a toxin, resulting in poisoning.

Adenosine triphosphate (ATP): The main energy reserve for enzyme activity, muscular contraction, pumping chemicals against a concentration gradient, and other work required of cells. Energy is released when one phosphate unit is removed from ATP, thus forming **adenosine diphosphate (ADP)**.

Adipose tissue: Tissue in which fat is stored.

Adrenal gland: Gland that influences the metabolism of carbohydrates, body water, muscle, bone, the nervous system, the GI tract, and the cardiovascular system. Located near the kidney. Produces epinephrine (adrenaline).

Aerobic: Requiring oxygen.

Aflatoxin: Toxic substances produced by a mold; a strong carcinogen.

Alcoholism: A primary, chronic disease evidenced by continuous or periodic excessive consumption of alcoholic beverages with genetic, psychosocial, and environmental factors influencing its development and manifestations.

Algae: A class of mainly aquatic plants that includes seaweeds. Derivatives of algae hold water and are used by the food industry as thickeners, stabilizers, and gelling agents.

Algins: Substances found in many seaweeds; form viscous solutions; hold large amounts of water and are useful as thickeners and stabilizers in foods such as ice cream and synthetic cream.

Alkaloids: Specific nitrogen-containing compounds of plant origin, such as found in potatoes and tomatoes. Alkaloids used in medicine include morphine and quinine.

Allergen: Any substance that causes allergy. Common allergens include foods, inhalants (dust, pollen, smoke), some drugs, infectious agents (bacteria, viruses, fungi), contactants (chemicals, animals, plants), and physical agents (heat, cold, light).

Allergy: An abnormal tissue reaction to a specific foreign substance (allergen) that, in similar amounts, produces no effect in nonsensitive persons.

Alzheimer's disease: An irreversible degenerative disease of the central nervous system characterized by loss of memory, mainly in 40–60 year olds.

Amino acid: An organic acid containing both an amino (-NH$_2$) and an acidic (-COOH) group. The approximately 20 different amino acids can be linked in varying combinations to form proteins in humans, animals, plants, and microorganisms.

Amniotic fluid: The liquid that protects the developing fetus.

Anaerobic: ("without oxygen") Not requiring oxygen.

Anemia: A lower than normal level of red blood cells or of hemoglobin in the blood.

Anorexia: Loss of appetite.

Anorexia nervosa: An eating disorder usually associated with puberty. Involves a psychological loss of appetite and self-starvation. May be produced by a distorted body image and by social pressures, especially those associated with body weight.

Antacid: An agent that neutralizes acidity in the GI tract.

Antibiotics: Substances produced by living organisms that inhibit the growth of other organisms. Penicillin is a good example of an antibiotic.

Antioxidants: Substances that prevent oxygen from combining with other substances to cause damage to cells, or cause fat in foods to become rancid.

Appetite: A pleasant sensation based on previous experiences causing a person to seek food for taste and enjoyment.

Aquaculture: Fish farming.

Arthritis: Inflammation of a joint, usually accompanied by pain and frequently by changes in bone structure.

Balanced diet: A diet providing the recommended intake of all nutrients and containing a wide variety of foods.

Basal metabolic rate (BMR): Energy needed to maintain vital body processes for a given period of time; measured in kilocalories.

Basal metabolism: Metabolic processes needed to sustain life.

Beriberi: Deficiency of thiamin, producing edema, cardiovascular changes, muscle weakness, nerve degeneration, and loss of appetite.

BHT (butylated hydroxytoluene) and BHA (butylated hydroxyanisole): Compounds used in foods to prevent fats from becoming rancid.

Bioavailability: Degree to which a substance is able to be digested and utilized by the body in the amount or form in which it is present; usually refers to nutrients in foods.

Bioconcentration: Increasing concentrations of a chemical (toxin, pesticide, pollutant) in organisms further up the food chain. The food chain goes from simple forms of life and small species to larger animals, fish, birds, and ultimately to people.

Biotechnology: Application of the techniques of science and engineering to organisms, cells, and parts of cells to produce products and services, including food (bio = life).

Blood coagulation: Formation of a blood clot; stops bleeding; vitamin K is needed for coagulation.

Body composition: Relative proportions of fat, bone, and lean tissue (muscle, kidneys, liver, brain, and other soft tissues) in the body.

Body mass index (BMI): A measure for ideal weight and for obesity used by some nutritionists. Determined as body weight (in kilograms) divided by height (in meters) squared.

Bomb calorimeter: Instrument that measures energy (caloric content) present in a substance by burning it in oxygen and measuring the heat released.

Botulism: Paralytic disease caused by ingesting a toxin produced by the bacteria *Clostridium botulinum*. Foods most affected are improperly home-canned foods, sausages, and bacon.

Bovine somatotropin (BST): A natural hormone produced by cattle that can be produced also by biotechnology. It is injected into cattle, resulting in higher milk yields.

Bran: Outer layers of cereal grain; largely removed in milling to make white flour or white rice; contains fiber, vitamins, and iron.

Brown adipose tissue (BAT): Fat tissue with brown color given by a high concentration of mitochondria, which are energy-producing subcellular structures; found in high concentrations in hibernating animals such as bears and in newborn humans.

Buffers: Substances that resist change in acidity or alkalinity.

Bulimia: An eating disorder involving consumption of large quantities of food at one time (bingeing), followed by purging from the body by vomiting, use of laxatives, or other means.

Calcitonin: A hormone from the thyroid gland that decreases high blood calcium levels by depositing the extra calcium in bones.

Calorie: The term "calorie" is the popular usage for the term "kilocalorie" (kcalorie, kcal) or "Calorie," which is a measure of energy. One kilocalorie equals the amount of heat required to raise the temperature of 1 kilogram of water by 1°C. This book uses "calorie" to represent "kilocalorie."

Caramel: Brown material formed by heating carbohydrates in the presence of acid or alkali.

Carbohydrate loading: Consumption of carbohydrates (600 grams per day or 70% of total energy intake as carbohydrate, whichever is larger) for 6–7 days before certain athletic events to increase glycogen stores; also known as glycogen loading or glycogen supercompensation.

Carcinogens: Substances that cause cancer.

Carotenoids: One of a group of pigments (such as carotene) ranging in color from light yellow to purple; widely distributed in plants.

Catabolism: The breakdown of complex chemicals into their simpler units in living organisms. For example, glycogen is catabolized into its basic unit, glucose.

Cataracts: Dimming or fuzzing of the lens in the eye, thereby decreasing vision.

Cell: Unit of structure of all animals and plants; the physical basis of all life processes.

Cell membrane: A thin, soft layer of tissue surrounding a cell or lining a tube or cavity.

Cellulose: A straight-chain polysaccharide found only in plants; it forms supporting structures for plants.

Chemical senses: The senses of taste and smell, which work by the effect of chemicals in food and drink on the nervous system.

Chemotherapy: In the treatment of disease, the application of chemicals that have a specific and toxic effect on the disease-causing agent.

Chlorophyll: Green coloring matter found in all plants; involved in the manufacture of foods for the plant.

Chronic diseases: Disease having a slow onset and lasting a long time—e.g., coronary heart disease, cancer, hypertension.

Chronic exposure to a toxin: Long-term low or intermittent doses of a toxin, resulting in poisoning.

Coenzymes: Substances needed to assist certain enzymes.

Collagen: An insoluble protein that gives rigidity to cells and tissues; found in skin, bone, ligaments, and cartilage.

Colostrum: The milk secreted within the first two or three days of lactation; so-called "first milk."

Complementing or mutual supplementation effect: An outcome in which foods that individually are low in one or more of the essential amino acids (EEAs) collectively provide adequate amounts of all EEAs.

Complex carbohydrates: Polysaccharides, such as starch.

Coronary heart disease (CHD): The most common type of heart disease, caused by narrowing of the arteries that feed the heart.

Creatine: A nitrogen-containing compound; an essential part of the energy release system of muscle. Present in meat and some soups.

Creatine phosphate: A high-energy compound used to reform ATP from ADP; also known as phosphocreatine.

Cretinism: Severe mental and physical retardation of infants caused by iodine deficiency during pregnancy.

Cross-linking: Formation of bonds between amino acids in adjacent peptide chains.

Daily Value (DV): Figures on food labels showing how a food fits into the overall daily diet.

Deforestation: The permanent clearing of forest land and its conversion to nonforest uses.

Dementia: Irreversible mental degeneration, including loss of memory.

Denatured protein: A protein in which the molecular structure has been modified so that its properties and biological activity are destroyed or diminished.

Dental caries: Tooth decay.

Desertification: A process by which the biological productivity of land is reduced, thus causing the spread of desertlike conditions.

Developed countries: Countries with established industries, agriculture, and services. Includes North America, Australia, New Zealand, Japan, and most of Europe.

Developing countries: Countries in which industries, agriculture, and services are in the developmental stage. Includes most of the countries in Asia, Africa, and Central and South America.

Diet: The usual pattern of food and drink intake by a person or animal.

Dietary fiber: Collective term for the structural parts of plants that are not digested by humans.

Dietary thermogenesis: Energy needed to digest, absorb, transport, and store nutrients in food; also known as specific dynamic action of food, or thermic effect of food.

Dipeptide: Two amino acids joined by a peptide bond.

Disaccharide: Two monosaccharides linked together; includes sucrose, lactose, and maltose.

Diuretics: Substances that increase the excretion of urine.

DNA (deoxyribonucleic acid): A nucleic acid that contains hereditary information in humans, animals, plants, and microbes. Directs protein synthesis.

Eating disorder: Unusual pattern of food intake. Anorexia nervosa is self-induced denial of food, and bulimia is binge eating followed by vomiting.

Edema: Excessive accumulation of fluid in tissues.

Electrolytes: Compounds that ionize in water, which can then conduct electricity.

Emaciated: Excessively thin.

Emulsion: Mixture of two immiscible compounds such as oil and water, where one is dispersed in the other in the form of fine droplets. They stay mixed because of the presence of an **emulsifying agent.** These include gums, egg yolk, albumin and casein (both proteins), and lecithin. Emulsifying agents are used in margarine, ice cream, and salad dressing.

Endorphins: Chemicals produced by the brain to stimulate appetite and to control pain.

Energy: The capacity of the body, a tissue, or a cell to do work. Measured in kilocalories ("calories" in popular terminology).

Enteral feeding: Feeding a liquid diet down a tube through the nose into the GI tract, or directly into the stomach or intestine ("within the intestine").

Environment: The conditions under which any person lives. More broadly, the earth's ecosystem.

Enzyme: A protein that speeds up biochemical reactions in humans, animals, plants, and microorganisms without otherwise becoming part of the reaction.

Eosinophilia-myalgia syndrome (EMS): A blood disorder caused by suspected contamination of supplements of L-tryptophan. Caused muscle pain, fatigue, weakness, headache, fever, and death in a number of people.

Epidemiology: The study of disease patterns, including diet-related disease, in different populations.

Epilepsy: A condition characterized by disturbed brain function, usually with convulsions.

Epithelial cells: Layer of cells forming the epidermis, which is the external layer of skin, and the mucous membranes.

Ergogenic aids: Products supposed to increase physical performance.

Essential amino acids: Amino acids that must be provided by the diet because they cannot be synthesized in the body at a rate sufficient to meet the body's requirement for growth and maintenance.

Essential fatty acids (EFAs): Fatty acids that are not synthesized in the body and must be provided in the diet to maintain health. These are linoleic acid, alpha-linolenic acid, and docosahexaenoic acid.

Esters: Compounds produced from the combination of organic acids and alcohols. For example, acetic acid combined with ethyl alcohol gives ethyl ester. Fats are esters because of the combination of fatty acids with glycerol, which is a type of alcohol.

Estrogen: A female sex hormone responsible for development of secondary sexual characteristics; used to prevent osteoporosis.

Exchange lists: Lists of interchangeable foods with similar caloric contents. Used in diet planning and weight-loss programs.

Extracellular fluid: The fluid outside cells.

Facultative thermogenesis: Energy expended in response to changes in ambient temperature, food intake, emotional stress, and other factors.

Feces: Also called stools. Body waste including undigested food, bacteria, and dead cells from the GI tract.

Fermentation: Chemical and sensory changes in foods in the presence or absence of oxygen, usually with the assistance of microbes.

Fetal alcohol syndrome (FAS): Lifelong disabilities and malformations, especially to the face, caused by alcohol use by the mother during pregnancy. FAS is the leading known cause of mental retardation in the United States.

Fiber: Collective term for indigestible or partially digestible structural parts of plants.

Flatulence: Gas production in the GI tract. Undigested sugars serve as substrates for intestinal bacteria, which produce methane, carbon dioxide, and hydrogen.

Food: Substances taken into the body that maintain life and growth by supplying energy and building and replacing tissues.

Food additives: All material deliberately added to food to assist in its manufacture and preservation and to improve palatability and appearance.

Food allergy or food hypersensitivity: Abnormal or exaggerated response of the immune system due to eating certain foods.

Food composition: The amount of nutrients, chemicals, and ingredients in a food.

Food Guide Pyramid: A research-based food guidance system, developed by the USDA, in which foods necessary in large amounts are at the base of the pyramid and foods to be eaten sparingly are at the top.

Food intolerance: A reaction to a food or food additive that does not involve the immune system.

Food poisoning: An imprecise term for an illness caused by ingestion of foods containing poisonous substances.

Food spoilage: Any change in food causing undesirable appearances, flavors, and textures in foods.

Fortified foods: Foods with added nutrients, usually vitamins and minerals.

Gallbladder: Pear-shaped sac near the liver holding bile from the liver until it is discharged into the GI tract.

Gastric mucus: "Gastric" means relating to the stomach. Mucus is a viscous fluid.

Gastrointestinal (GI) tract: The entire digestive tract from the mouth to the anus.

Genitourinary: Pertaining to the genitals and urinary organs.

Geophagy or pica: Cravings for substances not fit for food, especially clay. Pregnant women are known to consume clay, starch, ashes, and plaster. Common throughout the world, especially in lower socioeconomic groups.

Germ: The sprouting part of a cereal grain. In wheat, it is rich in thiamin, riboflavin, and vitamin B-6 and contains most of the fat in the grain; is separated along with the bran during milling to make white flour.

Ghee: Clarified butter fat made by heating and separating the water; made from milk of cow, buffalo, goat, or sheep; does not become rancid as rapidly as butter; popular in India.

Glycemic index: A scale identifying the rate and extent to which various foods influence blood glucose concentration.

Glycerol: An organic alcohol that, when combined with fatty acids, forms a fat.

Glycogen: Storage form of carbohydrates in humans and animals; a branched polysaccharide with many glucose units linked together.

Glycolipid: Fatty acids combined with a carbohydrate; found mainly in the myelin sheath around nerve fibers.

Glycolysis: The anaerobic series of reactions by which glucose is broken down to pyruvic acid, a three-carbon unit that is an intermediate chemical in the liberation of energy from glucose. For microbes, called "fermentation."

Goiter: An enlargement of the thyroid gland in the neck usually caused by dietary iodine deficiency.

Goitrogens: Substances that interfere with the normal functioning of the thyroid gland; found especially in cabbages, peanuts, and soybeans.

Golgi complex: A structure situated near the nucleus in most cells. It concentrates and packages newly formed cell material.

Gout: Metabolic disease resulting in arthritis and inflammation of the joints, usually in the knees and feet.

GRAS (Generally Recognized As Safe): Term applied to a group of historically common food additives judged by the FDA to be safe in food use.

Gums: Substances that can disperse in water to become viscous; used to stabilize emulsions such as salad dressings and processed cheese and as a thickener in foods. Gums used by the food industry may be extracted from certain seeds, sap of some plants, or seaweeds, or the gums may be synthetic.

Hazard: Danger to health and life; involves risk. Measured by the frequency of contact multiplied by the amount of exposure.

Hazard analysis and critical control points (HACCP): A method of monitoring food safety by anticipation and prevention of problems. (Other monitoring methods use inspection of finished products.)

Heartburn: A burning sensation caused by acid liquid from the stomach being forced into the esophagus.

Hedonic: Describing the extent of liking or disliking for a food.

Hemicellulose: Complex carbohydrates found together with cellulose and lignin in plant cell walls. Most gums and mucilages belong to this group of compounds.

Hemoglobin: The oxygen-carrying, iron-containing protein in red blood cells. (*Hemo* = blood, *globin* = globular protein)

Hemolytic anemia: Anemia resulting from the breaking of red blood cells. Hemoglobin is liberated from the red blood cell and cannot perform its oxygen-carrying function.

Hemorrhage: Abnormal bleeding.

Hepatitis: Inflammation of the liver caused by a virus.

Hereditary hemochromatosis: A genetic defect causing excess deposits of iron in the body, especially in the liver. Consequences include liver damage, heart failure, and diabetes; usually develops in middle age.

High fructose corn syrup (HFCS): Glucose syrups containing more than 40% fructose.

High-density lipoprotein (HDL): A lipoprotein with a high protein content; considered the "good" type of cholesterol.

Hominy: Corn kernels that have been soaked in a caustic solution, such as lye, to remove the hulls. Grits are ground hominy.

Hops: Dried flowers of a perennial plant containing bitter resins and essential oils used in brewing.

Human milk banks: Expressed human milk saved for future use; found in many countries, including the United Kingdom.

Humectants: Substances that absorb moisture. They can be used to maintain the water content of foods such as bakery goods.

Hunger: A physiological response to lack of food. Hunger pains coincide with powerful contractions of stomach muscles.

Hydration: The addition or absorption of water.

Hydrogenation: Treatment of liquid oils with hydrogen to saturate some double bonds in the fatty acid chains, which increases the melting point and hardens the fat. Cottonseed, corn, and sunflower are among the oils commonly hydrogenated for use in margarine and cooking fats.

Hydrolysis: (Literally, "breaking with water.") A process that occurs when the OH^- and H^+ ions that make up a water molecule (H_2O) split a substance into two parts. For example, table sugar (sucrose, $C_{12}H_{22}O_{11}$) is hydrolyzed by the addition of H_2O into $C_6H_{12}O_6$ (glucose) and $C_6H_{12}O_6$ (fructose).

Hydrophilic: Literally means "water loving." Refers to something that chemically attracts water.

Hydrophobic: Literally means "water hating." Refers to something that chemically repels water.

Hydroxyapatite: The hard substance between cells in bones and teeth consisting of calcium, phosphorus, hydrogen, and oxygen.

Hypertension: High blood pressure.

Hyperthyroidism: Overactivity of the thyroid gland.

Hypoglycemia: An abnormally low level of blood glucose (hypo = under, glyc = sweet, emia = blood).

Hypothalamus: Part of the brain that influences body-water balance, carbohydrate and fat metabolism, and the regulation of body temperature.

Hypothyroidism: Deficiency of thyroid secretions, including the iodine-containing thyroid hormones, resulting in lower basal metabolism.

Immune system: A system in the body that protects against certain infectious diseases.

In vitro: "Vitro" is Latin for "glass"; therefore, the term means literally "in the test-tube." In contrast, *in vivo* means "in life" or "in the living body of a plant or animal."

Insoluble fiber: Sometimes called roughage; includes cellulose, lignin, and some hemicellulose.

Insulin-dependent diabetes: A disorder characterized by inadequate production of insulin, causing alterations in carbohydrate metabolism and resulting in the loss of glucose in the urine.

Intracellular fluid: The fluid within cells.

Intrinsic factor: A substance synthesized in the GI tract that assists in the absorption of vitamin B-12.

Ion: An atom or group of atoms with an electrical charge. Ions are created when a salt such as NaCl is put into solution, where it is ionized into sodium (Na^+) and chlorine (Cl^-) ions.

Irradiation: Ultraviolet, ionizing, and microwave irradiation are used to preserve food. Ionizing irradiation from radioactive isotopes destroys microorganisms and insects and inhibits sprouting in plants. It *cannot* make the food radioactive.

Irritable bowel syndrome: A group of symptoms including diarrhea, heartburn, flatulence, loss of appetite, nausea, vomiting, and/or abdominal distention after meals. Causes are unknown, but emotional stress may be a factor.

Keratinization: Hardening of cells until they are rough and dry.

Kidney dialysis: Mechanical purification of blood to remove liquids and chemicals that the kidneys would normally remove if they were not diseased.

Kinesiology: The study of muscles and muscular movement.

Kosher foods: Foods specially selected and prepared to meet traditional Jewish ritual and dietary laws.

Krebs cycle: A series of biochemical reactions in the liberation of energy from the energy nutrients; also known as the citric acid cycle or the tricarboxylic acid cycle.

Kwashiorkor: A form of malnutrition in infants caused by severe deficiency of protein associated with inadequate intake of energy. Symptoms include poor growth, edema, wasting of muscles, and mental apathy.

Lactase: Intestinal enzyme that digests lactose by splitting it into glucose and galactose.

Lactic acid: An organic acid formed at the mid-point in the breakdown of glucose to energy, carbon dioxide, and water. It causes fatigue when it builds up in muscles during exercise.

Laetrile: Sometimes called vitamin B-17; it is not a vitamin but was sold in the 1970s as a possible cancer treatment. Contains the poison cyanide.

Lecithin: A phospholipid consisting of glycerol, fatty acids, phosphoric acid, and choline; common in many foods such as soybeans, peanuts, and corn.

Leukocytes: White blood cells; act as scavengers in the body and thereby help to combat infection.

Lignin: A noncarbohydrate associated with carbohydrates in cell walls of plants.

Limiting amino acid: The essential amino acid in a protein that is in the smallest amount relative to dietary needs. Lysine is the limiting amino acid in cereal proteins, and the sulfur amino acid methionine is the limiting amino acid in most animal and vegetable proteins.

Lipid oxidation: The process that makes fat rancid, producing off-odors and off-tastes in foods.

Lipophilic: (literally, "lipid-loving") Having the ability to combine with lipids.

Lipoprotein: A protein combined with lipids such as cholesterol, phospholipids, and triglycerides; water-soluble for transportation in the blood.

Lipoprotein (a): A genetic variant of low-density lipoprotein (LDL).

Liposuction: Surgical removal of fat deposits; not considered a safe way to lose weight.

Low-density lipoprotein (LDL): A lipoprotein with a high cholesterol content; considered the "bad" type of cholesterol.

Lysosomes: Tiny particles within cells; contain enzymes to break down proteins and certain carbohydrates within cells.

Macrominerals: Minerals recommended in amounts greater than 100 milligrams per day. They are calcium, phosphorus, sodium, potassium, chloride, magnesium, and sulfur.

Malaria: An infectious disease that affects red blood cells; has negative effects on the digestive and nervous systems; transmitted by mosquitoes, especially in equatorial parts of the world.

Malnutrition: Poor nutritional status produced by nutrient intake either below or above the beneficial range of intake.

Malt: Grain that has been moistened, sprouted, and then dried under controlled conditions, containing a mixture of starch breakdown products, mainly maltose (malt sugar). Prepared from barley or wheat.

Marasmus: Starvation symptoms of no body fat and muscle wasting, due to little or no intake of dietary protein and energy.

Medicaid: A U.S. government program covering medical expenses of low-income individuals.

Megaloblastic anemia: Anemia in which red blood cells are large, underdeveloped, and have reduced oxygen-carrying capacity.

Megavitamin supplements: Vitamin intake greater than 10 times the RDA, taken in pill, powder, or liquid form.

Menarche: The onset of menstruation.

Metabolic disorders: Unfavorable alterations in energy changes and in the chemical changes that are associated with growth, maturity, and aging.

Methane: A colorless and odorless gas produced by the fermentation of waste matter in the GI tract.

Microbes (bacteria, germs): Tiny one-celled forms of life, producing fermentation, spoilage, decay, and disease.

Microminerals: Also called trace elements. Minerals recommended in amounts less than 20 milligrams per day. They include iron, zinc, iodine, selenium, fluoride, and copper.

Microsomes: Microscopic particles from the endoplasmic reticulum (a connecting network within cells).

Millet: A cereal with high fiber content grown in parts of Africa, South America, and in India. Used as a gruel or made into a flour and cooked as flat cakes. Usually considered not as attractive in taste as rice or wheat.

Miso: A food paste originally made in Japan by fermenting moldy rice with soybeans and salt.

Mitochondria: Tiny rods within a cell; "power houses" of cells because they produce energy. They are involved in protein synthesis and lipid metabolism.

Modified atmosphere packaging: Changing the atmosphere within a package by extracting air and/or using various gases (such as nitrogen) to extend the shelf life of a food.

Molasses: Residue left after sugar refining.

Monosaccharides: A group name for the simplest carbohydrates, including glucose, fructose, and galactose. Glucose is the most important monosaccharide. (Mono = one, saccharide = sugar)

Monosodium glutamate: A flavor enhancer often added to meats, soups, and sauces such as soy sauce. Increases sodium intake.

Morbidity: The state of being diseased.

Mucilages: Viscous products of some plants.

Mutation: Changes in DNA structure so that the normal genetic message is usually not transmitted.

Myelin sheath: The covering around nerves; consists of fatty acids, cholesterol, phospholipids, and glycolipids.

Neophobia: Dread of or aversion to novelty.

Neural tube defect: A defect in the tube formed where the brain and spinal chord develop, causing brain and motor injury.

Neurological disturbances: Dysfunction of the nervous system.

Neurons: Nerve cells; involved in the transmission of nerve impulses.

Neurotransmitters: Chemicals (30–40 different ones) produced in and released from nerves that influence the transmission of the nerve impulse.

Nitrites: Salts added to foods such as bacon to prevent botulism. Nitrosamines, which are carcinogens, are formed when nitrites combine with amines in the stomach and also during cooking.

Nitrogen balance: The difference between the intake of nitrogen as dietary protein and the excretion of nitrogen as urea and other waste nitrogen compounds. May be positive, negative, or in equilibrium.

Nitrogen-fixing bacteria: A special type of bacteria; forms nodules in roots of legumes (beans, peas, and lentils) that "fix" or convert nitrogen from the air. This nitrogen is available to the plant for conversion into amino acids.

Non-insulin-dependent diabetes: A disorder in which adequate amounts of insulin are produced by the pancreas but the insulin is not used normally.

Nonvitamins: Chemicals not meeting all criteria to be called vitamins but marketed as vitamins.

Nucleus: The essential part of a cell; involved in growth, metabolism, reproduction, and transmission of characteristics of a cell.

Nutrient: A nourishing substance or ingredient.

Nutritional status: The extent to which the body's need for nutrients is being met.

Obesity: Body weight of 20% or more in excess of ideal body weight. This condition has several negative health effects.

Opsin: A protein in the eye involved in vision.

Oral rehydration therapy (ORT): Feeding a mixture of sugar, salt, and clean water to dehydrated children, especially those with severe diarrhea.

Organic foods: No single definition. Description of foods as "organic" implies the use of organic rather than synthetic or artificial fertilizers and no use of pesticides. "Organically processed" foods implies that they have received no treatment with antibiotics, hormones, synthetic additives, preservatives, colorants, or waxes.

Osmotic pressure: Pressure that develops when two solutions of different concentrations (such as the blood and the extracellular fluid) are separated by a semipermeable membrane (such as the wall of the blood vessel).

Osteomalacia: Softening of bones, making them brittle; caused by a deficiency or loss of body calcium; increased by vitamin D deficiency.

Osteoporosis: Softening of bone during aging; develops mainly in women after menopause.

Over-the-counter drugs: Medications not requiring a prescription; for example, aspirin, antacids, and cold relief medications.

Oxidation: Gain in oxygen, or loss of hydrogen from a chemical compound. An important oxidation process is the use of oxygen from the air to convert carbohydrates, lipids, and proteins in the body into energy, carbon dioxide, and water.

Ozone layer: A layer in the upper atmosphere consisting of ozone, a highly reactive gas. Protects life on earth by filtering out harmful ultraviolet radiation from the sun.

Pancreas: A gland behind the stomach and connected to the upper portion of the small intestine. Produces pancreatic juice (important in digestion) and hormones–insulin and glucagon.

Parasitic diseases: Diseases caused by parasites, organisms that live within, upon, or at the expense of the host. An example with nutritional implications is the loss of blood (and therefore iron) to hookworms in the GI tract.

Parathyroid hormone: A hormone secreted by the parathyroid gland located close to the thyroid gland in the neck; moves calcium from bone to blood when blood levels of calcium are low.

Parenteral feeding: Feeding nutrients into veins ("outside the intestines"). Also referred to as total parenteral nutrition (TPN) or hyperalimentation.

Pasteurization: The killing of food-spoiling bacteria by mild heat treatment. It prolongs shelf life of foods, but usually for a limited period only. Sterilization, which requires higher temperatures, kills all bacteria and spores.

Pathogen: A microorganism or substance capable of producing a disease.

Pectins: A soluble fiber that provides firmness in plants by cementing the cell walls together; used as a setting agent in jellies and jams, an emulsifier in ice cream, and an antistaling agent in cakes. Fruits rich in pectin include plums, apples, and oranges.

Pellagra: Deficiency of niacin resulting in the three D's—diarrhea, dermatitis, and dementia (and in several cases, death).

Pepsin: An enzyme secreted in the stomach to digest dietary proteins.

Peptide: Two or more amino acids joined together. It may be part of a protein.

Peptide bond: The chemical link between amino acids in a peptide or protein; forms the backbone of protein molecules.

Periodontal disease: Degeneration of bone and gum tissue around teeth.

Peristalsis: Coordinated muscle contractions that move food along the GI tract.

Pesticides: Any substances intended to control or destroy unwanted animals and plants during production, storage, transportation, distribution, and processing of food, agricultural commodities, or animal feeds.

pH: Abbreviation for potential hydrogen. A measure of the concentration of hydrogen ions (H^+) in a substance, which in turn measures its acidity or alkalinity.

Phenolic compounds: Compounds combined with phenol, which is a relative of benzene.

Phenylketonuria (PKU): Genetic defect in which the essential amino acid phenylalanine is incompletely metabolized, causing brain damage and mental retardation. May be prevented by strict limitation of dietary phenylalanine.

Phospholipid: A lipid substance containing phosphorus and fatty acids; lecithin is a good example.

Photosynthesis: Manufacture of glucose from water, carbon dioxide (from the air), and energy (from the sun).

Phytic acid: An organic acid in cereals, especially bran, dried legumes, and some nuts.

Pituitary gland: A small gland located at the base of the brain. Secretes hormones that regulate growth, reproduction, and many metabolic activities. Often referred to as the "master gland."

Placenta: The organ linking the uterus to the fetus. Nutrients are transferred to the fetus through it.

Plasmid: A small circular form of DNA that carries certain genes and can reproduce independently in a host cell.

Polychlorinated biphenyls (PCBs): A group of at least 50 widely used compounds containing chlorine. Can accumulate in food chains and may cause a variety of harmful effects including damage to the reproductive cycle of animals and plants.

Polymers: Compounds formed by the combination of two or more molecules of the same substance, in this case many molecules of modified glucose.

Polysaccharide: Many glucose units joined together; starch and glycogen are the best known.

Precursor: A substance from which another substance is formed.

Premenstrual syndrome (PMS): Physical and emotional symptoms experienced before and during menstruation by some women; includes water retention.

Preservatives: Materials that protect food from deterioration caused by microorganisms, enzymes, and oxidation.

Prostaglandins: "Local hormones" made in all tissues in the body. Involved in contraction of the uterus during labor, in the control of inflammation, and in blood pressure maintenance.

Psyllium: (Pronounced "sillium.") A grain similar to oats, corn, and wheat, grown mainly in India; its husk is a soluble form of fiber.

Recombinant DNA (rDNA): DNA altered to produce a slightly different protein from that produced by the unaltered form.

Recommended Dietary Allowance (RDA): The daily intake of energy and selected nutrients recommended for the U.S. population.

Rennet: An extract of calf stomach containing the enzyme rennin, which clots milk; used in cheese-making.

Requirement: Minimal amount of a nutrient needed to maintain health and to avoid nutrient deficiency.

Retinol binding protein (RBP): A protein synthesized in the liver to transport vitamin A to cells, including those in the eye.

Rhodopsin (visual purple): A protein pigment involved in vision; occurs in the outer parts of the rods in the retina of the eye; important in night vision.

Ribosomes: Tiny structures in cells that synthesize proteins.

Rickets: Deficiency of vitamin D; causes softening of bones due to low calcium content.

Rods: Long slender bodies in the eye that respond to faint light.

Salty peptide: A group of specific amino acids forming a peptide that gives a salty flavor.

Satiety: The condition of being full to satisfaction.

Scurvy: Deficiency disease of vitamin C; causes soft, spongy, bleeding gums.

Sensory analysis: Measurement of the taste, odor, appearance, texture, and sound of food and drink.

Serotonin: An important neurotransmitter in the brain; made from the amino acid tryptophan.

Shelf life: The period during which foods can be stored without spoiling.

Sibling: One of two or more children of the same parents.

Sickle cell anemia: A hereditary form of **anemia** with abnormally shaped red blood cells caused by an amino acid alteration in hemoglobin. Decreases the capacity to deliver oxygen to cells and to remove carbon dioxide.

Soluble fiber: Consists of pectins, gums, mucilages, and some hemicelluloses; constitutes about one-third of the total fiber in typical diets.

Solutes: Substances dissolved in a liquid.

Somatotropin: A growth hormone.

Sorghum: Cereal grown in semiarid regions of Africa, India, and China. Used for animal feed in the United States and Australia.

Special Supplemental Food Program for Women, Infants, and Children (WIC): A government-funded program in the United States that provides food, as well as nutritional and medical support, for low-income women during pregnancy and the first few years of the child's life.

Spina bifida: Birth defects in the spine resulting in a tumor and deformity.

Spirulina **("blue-green manna"):** A type of algae supposed to contain vitamin B-12 and to depress appetite. There is no evidence for these claims.

Starter culture: A culture of bacteria used to start bacterial growth in milk for cheese production, or in butter to develop the flavor, or in any fermentation.

Starvation: The condition of being without food for a long period of time.

Sterol: One of the group of lipids that includes vitamin D, cholesterol, and male and female sex hormones.

Sugar alcohols: Better known to us on food labels as mannitol, xylitol, and sorbitol, which are absorbed more slowly than most other sugars.

Sulfites: Chemicals widely used as preservatives in fruit juices and syrups, on fruits, and in sausage, beer, and wine. They give an unpleasant taste to food. Are driven off by boiling or cooking.

Superoxide dismutase: An enzyme preventing oxidative damage in body tissues.

Systolic and diastolic blood pressure: The pressure existing in the large arteries at the height of the pulse wave. High blood pressure exists when persistent systolic and diastolic blood pressures are above 140 and 100 millimeters of mercury, respectively. Blood pressure reports give systolic pressure as the top number and diastolic pressure as the bottom number.

T cell: (T lymphocyte) A type of white blood cell that fights infections within the body.

Tannins: Specific chemicals present in teas and unripe fruits; used to clarify beers and wines. Also called tannic acid.

Teratogen: Anything that causes the development of a severely deformed fetus.

Thyroid gland: Gland in the neck that secretes thyroid hormones, which are involved in energy metabolism.

Thyroid hormone: Iodine-containing hormone secreted by the thyroid gland, located in the neck.

Thyroxin: One of the iodine-containing hormones produced by the thyroid gland.

Tissue: A group or collection of similar cells that act together to perform a particular function; e.g., muscles and nerves are each classified as tissues.

Tocopherols: Chemical name for some forms of vitamin E.

Tortillas: Large, flat pancake made from ground corn or wheat.

Toxicants: Chemicals that harm people, animals, or plants.

Toxicity: The extent, quality, or degree of being poisonous.

Trans and *cis* **fatty acids:** Fatty acids with the same molecular and structural formulas but existing in different geometric forms. The *cis* form is the natural form and can be metabolized by the body. *Trans* forms are suspected of being involved in coronary heart disease.

Unconventional medicine: Medical practice not taught widely at U.S. medical schools or generally available at U.S. hospitals.

Urea: Waste nitrogen excreted in the urine. Formed by the liver and excreted by the kidneys.

Uterus: The organ that contains and nourishes the embryo and fetus from time of conception until time of birth.

Vascular system: The heart, blood vessels, lymphatic system, and their parts considered collectively.

Vegans: People who consume no foods of animal origin, as contrasted with vegetarians, who often consume dairy products and eggs.

Viscosity: The property of a liquid that makes it resistant to flow. (For instance, syrup is more **viscous** than water and therefore flows more slowly.)

Water activity of food: The amount of water available in a food, measured as the ratio between the vapor pressure of water in food and that of pure water at the same temperature.

Water of metabolism: Water produced in the body when carbohydrates, lipids, proteins, and alcohol are broken down for energy.

Xerophthalmia: Deficiency of vitamin A that causes drying of the membranes in the eye, resulting in blindness.

Yeasts: Organisms used in brewing, wine-making, and baking. Rich in B-complex vitamins. Grouped with the fungi, although they are unicellular.

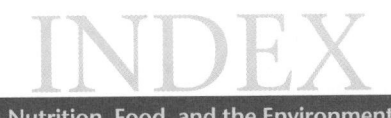

Index

Italic page numbers indicate illustrations.

Estimated Safe and Adequate Daily Dietary Intakes of Selected Vitamins and Minerals[a]

| Category | Age (years) | Vitamins | | Trace Elements[b] | | | | |
		Biotin (µg)	Pantothenic Acid (mg)	Copper (mg)	Manganese (mg)	Fluoride (mg)	Chromium (µg)	Molybdenum (µg)
Infants	0–0.5	10	2	0.4–0.6	0.3–0.6	0.1–0.5	10–40	15–30
	0.5–1	15	3	0.6–0.7	0.6–1.0	0.2–1.0	20–60	20–40
Children and adolescents	1–3	20	3	0.7–1.0	1.0–1.5	0.5–1.5	20–80	25–50
	4–6	25	3–4	1.0–1.5	1.5–2.0	1.0–2.5	30–120	30–75
	7–10	30	4–5	1.0–2.0	2.0–3.0	1.5–2.5	50–200	50–150
	11+	30–100	4–7	1.5–2.5	2.0–5.0	1.5–2.5	50–200	75–250
Adults		30–100	4–7	1.5–3.0	2.0–5.0	1.5–4.0	50–200	75–250

[a] Because there is less information on which to base allowances, these figures are not given in the main table of RDA and are provided here in the form of ranges of recommended intakes.

[b] Because the toxic levels for many trace elements may be only several times usual intakes, the upper levels for the trace elements given in this table should not be habitually exceeded.

Estimated Sodium, Chloride, and Potassium Minimum Requirements of Healthy Persons[a]

Age	Weight (kg)[a]	Sodium (mg)[a,b]	Chloride (mg)[a,b]	Potassium (mg)[c]
Months				
0–5	4.5	120	180	500
6–11	8.9	200	300	700
Years				
1	11.0	225	350	1,000
2–5	16.0	300	500	1,400
6–9	25.0	400	600	1,600
10–18	50.0	500	750	2,000
>18[d]	70.0	500	750	2,000

[a] No allowance has been included for large, prolonged losses from the skin through sweat.

[b] There is no evidence that higher intakes confer any health benefit.

[c] Desirable intakes of potassium may considerably exceed these values (~3,500 mg for adults).

[d] No allowance included for growth. Values for those below 18 years assume a growth rate at the 50th percentile reported by the National Center for Health Statistics and averaged for males and females.